2015

The Year Book of
PEDIATRICS®

Editor

Michael D. Cabana, MD, MPH

*Professor of Pediatrics, Epidemiology & Biostatistics and Chief, UCSF Division
of General Pediatrics, University of California, San Francisco; Core Faculty,
Philip R. Lee Institute for Health Policy Studies, San Francisco, California*

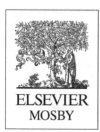

ELSEVIER
MOSBY

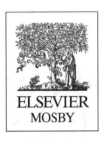

ELSEVIER
MOSBY

Vice President, Global Medical Reference: Mary E. Gatsch
Acquisitions Editor: Kerry Holland
Developmental Editor: Susan Showalter
Production Supervisor, Electronic Year Books: Donna M. Skelton
Electronic Article Manager: Mike Sheets
Illustrations and Permissions Coordinator: Dawn Vohsen

2015 EDITION

Printed in the United States of America
Composition by TNQ Books and Journals Pvt Ltd, India
Printing/binding by Sheridan Books, Inc.

Editorial Office:
Elsevier
Suite 1800
1600 John F. Kennedy Blvd.
Philadelphia, PA 19103-2899

International Standard Serial Number: 0084-3954
International Standard Book Number: 978-0-323-35551-3

Contributing Editors

Mandy A. Allison, MEd, MD, MSPH
Assistant Professor of Pediatrics, University of Colorado, Boulder, Colorado and Children's Hospital Colorado, Aurora, Colorado

Roger W. Apple, PhD
Licensed Psychologist, Apple & Associates LLC, Kalamazoo, Michigan

Smita Awasthi, MD
Departments of Dermatology and Pediatrics, University of California, Davis, Davis, California

Anna I. Bakardjiev, MD
Associate Professor of Pediatrics, UCSF Benioff Children's Hospital and University of California, San Francisco, San Francisco, California

Sophie J. Balk, MD
Attending Pediatrician, Children's Hospital at Montefiore; Professor of Clinical Pediatrics, Albert Einstein College of Medicine, New York, New York

Naomi S. Bardach, MD, MAS
Division of General Pediatrics, Department of Pediatrics, Philip R. Lee Institute for Health Policy Studies, University of California San Francisco, San Francisco, California

Elizabeth S. Barnert, MD, MPH, MS
Department of Pediatrics, University of California, Los Angeles, Los Angeles, California

Laurence S. Baskin, MD
Frank Hinman, Jr., MD, Distinguished Professorship in Pediatric Urology; Chief Pediatric Urology, UCSF Benioff Children's Hospital; KURe Director, University of California, San Francisco, San Francisco, California

Arpi Bekmezian, MD
Associate Clinical Professor, Department of Pediatrics, UCSF Benioff Children's Hospital, University of California, San Francisco, San Francisco, California

Eric G. Benotsch, PhD
Department of Psychology, Virginia Commonwealth University, Richmond, Virginia

Loren Berman, MD, MHS
Nemours-duPont Hospital for Children, Thomas Jefferson University School of Medicine, Philadelphia, Pennsylvania

Vinod K. Bhutani, MD, FAAP
Professor of Pediatrics, Stanford Children's Health, Lucile Packard Children's Hospital Stanford, Stanford University School of Medicine, Stanford, California

Alona Bin-Nun, MD
Senior Neonatologist, Department of Neonatology, Shaare Zedek Medical Center, Jerusalem, Israel

Seth Bokser, MD, MPH
Associate Professor of Pediatrics and Informatics, University of California, San Francisco, San Francisco California

Sonia Lomeli Bonifacio MD
Director, Neuro-Intensive Care Nursery and Assistant Professor of Pediatrics, UCSF Benioff Children's Hospital, University of California, San Francisco, San Francisco, California

Faith Boninger, PhD
University of Colorado Boulder, Boulder, Colorado

William Bor, MBBS, DPM, FRANZCP
Director of Research, Kids in Mind; Mater Research, Mater Hospital, Brisbane Australia

Susan L. Bratton, MD, MPH
Professor of Pediatrics, Division Pediatric Critical Care Medicine, University of Utah, Salt Lake City, Utah

Nelson Branco, MD, FAAP
Tamalpais Pediatrics, Greenbrae, California; Member, AAP Committee on Native American Child Health; Assistant Clinical Professor, Pediatrics, University of California, San Francisco, San Francisco, California

Timothy E. Bunchman, MD
Professor & Director Pediatric Nephrology & Transplantation, Children's Hospital of Richmond, Virginia Commonwealth University School of Medicine, Richmond, Virginia

Merlin G. Butler, MD, PhD
Director, Division of Research; Director, KUMC Genetics Clinic, and Professor of Psychiatry, Behavioral Sciences and Pediatrics, University of Kansas Medical Center, Lawrence, Kansas

Arlene M. Butz, ScD, CRNP
Professor of Pediatrics, Johns Hopkins University Schools of Medicine and Nursing, Baltimore, Maryland

Michael D. Cabana, MD, MPH
Professor of Pediatrics, Epidemiology & Biostatistics and Chief, UCSF Division of General Pediatrics, University of California, San Francisco; Core Faculty, Philip R. Lee Institute for Health Policy Studies, San Francisco, California

John Carlin, BSc, AM, PhD
Murdoch Children's Research Institute; Department of Paediatrics, Melbourne School of Population & Global Health, University of Melbourne, Melbourne, Australia

Aaron B. Caughey, MD, PhD
Professor and Chair, Department of Obstetrics and Gynecology, Oregon Health & Science University, Portland, Oregon

Linda H. Chaudron, MD, MS
School of Medicine and Dentistry, University of Rochester, Rochester, New York

Mike K. Chen, MD
Farley Endowed Chair, Professor and Vice Chairman, Department of Surgery and Director, Division of Pediatric Surgery, Children's Hospital of

Alabama, University of Alabama at Birmingham School of Medicine, Birmingham, Alabama

Cindy W. Christian, MD
Chair, Child Abuse and Neglect Prevention, Children's Hospital of Philadelphia; Professor, Pediatrics, Perelman School of Medicine, University of Pennsylvania, Philadelphia, Pennsylvania

Paul J. Chung, MD, MS
Departments of Pediatrics and Health Policy & Management, Children's Discovery & Innovation Institute, Mattel Children's Hospital UCLA, University of California, Los Angeles; RAND Health, RAND Corporation, Santa Monica, California

Eve R. Colson, MD, MHPE
Professor of Pediatrics, Yale School of Medicine, New Haven, Connecticut

Dalton Conley, MPA, PhD (Sociology), PhD (Biology)
University Professor and Professor of Sociology, Medicine and Public Policy, New York University, New York, New York

Kelly M. Cordoro, MD
Associate Professor of Dermatology and Pediatrics, University of California, San Francisco, San Francisco, California

Patricia B. Crawford DrPH, RD
Adjunct Professor, Director, Dr. Robert C. and Veronica Atkins Center for Weight and Health, and Cooperative Extension Specialist, Nutritional Sciences and Toxicology, University of California, Berkeley School of Public Health, Berkeley, California

Michael Crocetti, MD, MPH
Assistant Professor of Pediatrics, Johns Hopkins Children's Center and Chief of Pediatrics, Johns Hopkins Community Physicians, Johns Hopkins University, Balimore, Maryland

Stephen R. Dager, MD
Professor of Radiology and Bioengineering (Adjunct) and Associate Director, UW Center on Human Development and Disabilities, University of Washington School of Medicine, Seattle, Washington

Donna M. D'Alessandro, MD
Department of Pediatrics, University of Iowa, Iowa City, Iowa

Lisa Ross DeCamp, MD, MSPH
Assistant Professor, Department of Pediatrics, Center for Child and Community Health Research, Johns Hopkins University, Baltimore, Maryland

Girish Deshpande, FRACP, MSc
Department of Neonatal Paediatrics, Nepean Hospital Sydney; Sydney Medical School Nepean, University of Sydney, Sydney, Australia

Linda A. DiMeglio, MD, MPH
Department of Pediatrics, Section of Pediatric Endocrinology and Diabetology, Indiana University School of Medicine, Indianapolis, Indiana

Rebecca R. Dixon, MD
Division of Pediatric Critical Care, University of Utah, Salt Lake City, Utah

Peter R. Donald, FCP (SA), FRCP (Edin), MD
Paediatrics and Child Health Faculty of Health Sciences, Stellenbosch University, Tygerberg, South Africa

George J. Dover, MD
Professor and Director of Pediatrics, Johns Hopkins University School of Medicine, Baltimore, Maryland

Lyn Downe, FRACP
Department of Neonatal Paediatrics, Nepean Hospital Sydney; Sydney Medical School Nepean, University of Sydney, Sydney, Australia

R. Adams Dudley, MD, MBA
Professor of Medicine and Health Policy, Director, UCSF Center for Healthcare Value, and Associate Director, Research, Philip R. Lee Institute for Health Policy Studies, University of California, San Francisco, San Francisco, California

Lauren McCarl Dutra, ScD
Center for Tobacco Control Research and Education, University of California, San Francisco, San Francisco, California

Kathryn M. Edwards, MD
Sarah H. Sell and Cornelius Vanderbilt Chair in Pediatrics, Vanderbilt Vaccine Research Program, Vanderbilt University, Nashville, Tennessee

Lawrence F. Eichenfield, MD
Professor of Pediatrics and Medicine (Dermatology) and Chief, Pediatric and Adolescent Dermatology, Rady Children's Hospital, University of California, San Diego, San Diego, California

Rochelle M. Eime, PhD
Associate Professor and VicHealth Research Practice Fellow, Federation University Australia Victoria University, Victoria Australia

Scott A. Elisofon, MD
Department of Gastroenterology, Hepatology and Nutrition, Boston Children's Hospital; Instructor in Pediatrics, Harvard Medical School, Boston, Massachusetts

Conrad L. Epting, MD
Assistant Professor of Pediatrics and Pathology, Northwestern University, Evanston, Illinois; Pediatric Critical Care Medicine, Ann & Robert H. Lurie Children's Hospital of Chicago, Chicago, Illinois

Avroy A. Fanaroff, MD, FRCPCH
Eliza Henry Barnes Professor of Neonatology, Rainbow Babies & Children's Hospital; Emeritus Professor of Pediatrics, Case Western Reserve University School of Medicine, Cleveland, Ohio

Donna M. Ferriero, MD, MS
W.H. and Marie Wattis Distinguished Professor, Chair, Department of Pediatrics, and Physician-in-Chief, UCSF Benioff Children's Hospital, University of California, San Francisco, San Francisco, California

Chris Feudtner, MD, PhD, MPH
Division of General Pediatrics and Department of Medical Ethics, Children's Hospital of Philadelphia, Philadelphia, Pennsylvania

Philip R. Fischer, MD
Professor of Pediatrics, Mayo Clinic, Rochester, Minnesota

Marisa M. Fisher, MD
Pediatric Endocrinology Fellow, Riley Hospital for Children, Indiana University, Indianapolis, Indiana

Valerie Flaherman, MD, MPH
Assistant Professor of Pediatrics and Epidemiology and Biostatistics, University of California, San Francisco, San Francisco, California

Marc D. Foca, MD
Associate Professor of Pediatrics, Columbia University Medical Center; Division of Infectious Diseases, Department of Pediatrics, Children's Hospital of New York Presbyterian, New York, New York

Robert D. Foss, PhD
Director, Center for the Study of Young Drivers, Highway Safety Research Center, University of North Carolina at Chapel Hill, Chapel Hill, North Carolina

John G. Frohna, MD, MPH
Professor of Pediatrics and Medicine, University of Wisconsin School of Medicine and Public Health, Madison, Wisconsin

Adam Frymoyer, MD, FAAP
General Pediatrics & Neonatal and Developmental Medicine, Stanford University, Stanford, California

Susan Fuchs, MD, FAAP, FACEP
Professor of Pediatrics, Feinberg School of Medicine, Northwestern University; Division of Emergency Medicine, Ann & Robert H Lurie Children's Hospital of Chicago, Chicago, Illinois

Elena Fuentes-Afflick, MD, MPH
University of California, San Francisco, San Francisco, California

Heather J. Fullerton, MD, MAS
Professor of Neurology and Pediatrics, UCSF Benioff Children's Hospital, University of California, San Francisco, San Francisco, California

Estelle B. Gauda, MD
Professor of Pediatrics, Johns Hopkins University School of Medicine, Baltimore, Maryland

Jeffrey S. Gerber, MD, PhD
Assistant Professor of Pediatrics, University of Pennsylvania School of Medicine; Division of Infectious Diseases, Children's Hospital of Philadelphia, Philadelphia, Pennsylvania

Mark A. Gilger, MD
Pediatrician-in-Chief, Children's Hospital of San Antonio, San Antonio; Professor and Vice Chair, Department of Pediatrics, Baylor College of Medicine, Houston, Texas

Stanton A. Glantz, PhD
Distinguished Professor of Medicine, American Legacy Foundation; Director, Center for Tobacco Control Research and Education, University of California, San Francisco, San Francisco, California

Christine A. Gleason, MD
W. Alan Hodson Endowed Chair in Pediatrics, Professor of Pediatrics, and Chief, Division of Neonatology, University of Washington and Seattle Children's Hospital, Seattle, Washington

Michael H. Goodstein, MD, FAAP
Attending Neonatologist and Clinical Associate Professor of Pediatrics, Penn State University; Director, York County Cribs for Kids Program, York Hospital Office of Newborn Medicine, York Pennsylvania

Catherine M. Gordon, MD, MSc
Director, Division of Adolescent Medicine, Hasbro Children's Hospital; Professor and Vice Chair for Clinical Research, Department of Pediatrics, Alpert Medical School, Brown University, Providence, Rhode Island

Donald E. Greydanus, MD, Dr HC (ATHENS)
Professor & Founding Chair, Department of Pediatric & Adolescent Medicine, Homer Stryker M.D. School of Medicine, Western Michigan University, Kalamazoo, Michigan

Stefano Guandalini, MD
Professor and Chief, Section of Pediatric Gastroenterology, University of Chicago; Founder and Medical Director, Celiac Disease Center, Chicago, IL

Neera Gupta, MD, MAS
Pediatric Gastroenterology and Nutrition, New York-Presbyterian Phyllis and David Komansky Center for Children's Health; Weill Cornell Medical Center, New York, New York

J. Austin Hamm, MD
Department of Genetics, University of Alabama at Birmingham, Birmingham, Alabama

Cathy Hammerman, MD, FAAP
Director Newborn Nurseries, Shaare Zedek Medical Center; Professor of Pediatrics, Hebrew University Faculty of Medicine, Jerusalem, Israel

William W. Hay, Jr., MD
Professor of Pediatrics, University of Colorado School of Medicine and Children's Hospital Colorado, Aurora, Colorado

Robert L. Hendren, DO
Professor, Vice Chair, and Director, Child and Adolescent Psychiatry, University of California, San Francisco, San Francisco, California

Adam L. Hersh, MD, PhD
Pediatric Infectious Diseases, University of Utah, Salt Lake City, Utah

Harriet Hiscock, MBBS, FRACP, MD
Centre for Community Child Health at The Royal Children's Hospital; Murdoch Childrens Research Institute, Melbourne, Australia

Paul L. Hofman, MD

Professor of Paediatric Endocrinology, Liggins Institute, University of Auckland, Auckland, New Zealand

Tannie Q. Huang, MD

Assistant Professor, Pediatric Hematology, University of California, San Francisco, San Francisco, California

James N. Huang, MD

Department of Pediatrics, University of California, San Francisco and UCSF Benioff Children's Hospital, San Francisco, California

Michelle F. Huffaker, MD

Brigham and Women's Hospital; Boston Children's Hospital, Harvard Medical School, Boston, Massachusetts

Loris Y. Hwang, MD

Assistant Professor of Pediatrics, University of California, San Francisco; Division of Adolescent and Young Adult Medicine, Department of Pediatrics, UCSF Benioff Children's Hospital, San Francisco, California

Renee R. Jenkins, MD, FAAP

Professor Emerita, Howard University College of Medicine; Principal Investigator, DC-Baltimore Research Center on Child Health Disparities, Washington, DC

Hilary Jericho, MD, MSCI

University of Chicago, Comer Children's Hospital, Chicago, Illinois

Amie E. Jones, MD

Department of Pediatric and Adolescent Medicine, Mayo Clinic, Rochester Minnesota

Bengt Källén, MD, PhD

Professor Emeritus, Tornblad Institute, Lund University, Sweden

Mitul Kapadia, MD, MSc

Assistant Clinical Professor of Physical Medicine & Rehabilitation and Pediatrics and Medical Director, Pediatric Rehabilitation Medicine, UCSF Benioff Children's Hospital, University of California, San Francisco, San Francisco, California

Debra K. Katzman, MD, FRCPC

Professor of Pediatrics, Department of Pediatrics and University of Toronto; Senior Associate Scientist, Research Institute, Hospital for Sick Children, Toronto, Canada

Geoffrey S. Kelly, MD

Pediatrics House Staff, Johns Hopkins Children's Center, Baltimore, Maryland

Lawrence C. Kleinman, MD, MPH

Professor of Pediatrics and Population Health Science and Policy, Vice Chair for Research & Education, Department of Population Health Science and Policy, and Director, Collaboration for Advancing Pediatric Quality Measures, Icahn School of Medicine at Mount Sinai, New York, New York

Scott D. Krugman, MD, MS
Chairman, Department of Pediatrics, MedStar Franklin Square Medical Center, Baltimore, Maryland

Anda K. Kuo, MD
Associate Professor, Department of Pediatrics and Director, Pediatric Leadership for the Underserved, University of California, San Francisco, San Francisco, California

Cynthia R. LaBella, MD
Medical Director, Institute for Sports Medicine, Ann & Robert H. Lurie Children's Hospital of Chicago; Associate Professor of Pediatrics, Northwestern University's Feinberg School of Medicine, Chicago, Illinois

Susan Landers, MD, FAAP, FABM
Pediatrix Medical Group, Seton Family of Hospitals, Austin, Texas

Josephine S. Lau, MD, MPH
Assistant Professor of Pediatrics, Division of Adolescent & Young Adult Medicine, UCSF Benioff Children's Hospital, University of California, San Francisco, San Francisco, California

Daniel Le Grange, PhD
Professor of Psychiatry and Pediatrics, UCSF School of Medicine, University of California, San Francisco, San Francisco, California

Harvey L. Leo, MD
Associate Research Scientist, Center for Managing Chronic Disease, University of Michigan School of Public Health, Ann Arbor, Michigan

Jessica R. Levi, MD
Assistant Professor, Department of Otolaryngology Head and Neck Surgery and Assistant Professor, Department of Pediatrics, Boston University/Boston Medical Center, Boston Massachusetts

Paul H. Lipkin, MD
Kennedy Krieger Institute and Johns Hopkins University School of Medicine, Baltimore, Maryland

Tobias Loddenkemper, MD
Associate Professor of Neurology, Harvard Medical School; Director of Clinical Research, Division of Epilepsy and Clinical Neurophysiology, Boston Children's Hospital, Boston, Massachusetts

Debra S. Lotstein, MD, MPH
Medical Director, Palliative Care Program, Children's Hospital of Los Angeles; Associate Clinical Professor of Pediatrics and Anesthesia, USC Keck School of Medicine, Los Angeles, California

Stephanie Lovinsky-Desir, MD
Assistant Professor of Pediatric Pulmonology, Columbia University Medical Center, New York, New York

Jaspreet Loyal, MD, MS
Department of Pediatrics, Yale School of Medicine, New Haven, Connecticut

Robert H. Lustig, MD, MSL

Professor of Pediatrics, Division of Endocrinology and Member, Institute for Health Policy Studies, University of California, San Francisco; Adjunct Faculty, UC Hastings College of the Law, San Francisco, California

Sheryl Magzamen, PhD, MPH

Assistant Professor, Department of Environmental and Radiological Health Sciences, Colorado State University, Boulder, Colorado

M. Jeffrey Maisels, MB, BCh, DSc

Chair Emeritus and Professor and Director, Academic Affairs, Department of Pediatrics, Oakland University William Beaumont School of Medicine, Beaumont Children's Hospital, Royal Oak, Michigan

Renée Marquardt, MD

Department of Psychiatry, University of California, San Francisco, San Francisco, California

Suzanna M. Martinez, PhD, MS

Division of General Pediatrics, University of California, San Francisco, San Francisco, California

Nobutake Matsuo, MD

Emeritus Professor of Pediatrics, Keio University Medical School, Tokyo, Japan

Dan Merenstein, MD

Associate Professor and Director of Research Programs, Department of Family Medicine, Georgetown University Medical Center, Washington, DC

Marlene R. Miller, MD, MSc

Professor, Pediatrics and Health Policy & Management and Vice Chair, Quality and Patient Safety, Johns Hopkins Children's Center; Chief Quality Officer, Pediatrics, Johns Hopkins Medicine, Baltimore, Maryland

Rachel L. Miller, MD, FAAAAI

Professor of Medicine (Pediatrics) and Environmental Health Sciences, Columbia University Medical Center, New York, New York

Alex Molnar, PhD

University of Colorado Boulder, Boulder, Colorado

Rachel Y. Moon, MD

Children's National Medical Center, George Washington University School of Medicine and Health Sciences, Washington, DC

Anna-Barbara Moscicki, MD

Professor of Pediatrics, University of California, San Francisco, San Francisco, California

Kirstin A. M. Nackers, MD

Assistant Professor of Pediatrics, University of Wisconsin School of Medicine and Public Health and American Family Children's Hospital, Madison, Wisconsin

Thomas B. Newman, MD, MPH

Professor of Epidemiology & Biostatistics and Pediatrics, University of California, San Francisco, San Francisco, California

Kimberly G. Noble, MD, PhD
Assistant Professor of Pediatrics, Columbia University, New York, New York

Richard L. Oken, MD, FAAP
Clinical Professor of Pediatrics, University of California, San Francisco, San Francisco, California

Maria Oliva-Hemker, MD
Chief, Division of Pediatric Gastroenterology and Nutrition, Stermer Family Professor of Pediatric Inflammatory Bowel Disease, and Professor of Pediatrics, Johns Hopkins University School of Medicine, Baltimore, Maryland

Natasha T. O'Malley, FRCS (Tr & Orth)
Assistant Professor of Orthopaedics, Golisano Children's Hospital, University of Rochester Medical Center, Rochester, New York

Douglas J. Opel, MD, MPH
University of Washington School of Medicine, Seattle, Washington

Jane A. Oski, MD, MPH
Tuba City Regional Health Care Corporation; and Member, AAP Committee on Native American Child Health, Tuba City, Arizona

Anisha Patel, MD, MSPH, MSHS
Assistant Professor, Division of General Pediatrics, University of California, San Francisco, San Francisco, California

Minal R. Patel, PhD, MPH
Department of Health Behavior & Health Education, University of Michigan, Ann Arbor, Michigan

Sanjay Patole, MD, DCH, FRACP, MSc, DrPH
Centre for Neonatal Research and Education and Head, Department of Neonatal Paediatrics, King Edward Memorial Hospital for Women, Perth, Western Australia

Ian M. Paul, MD, MSc
Professor of Pediatrics & Public Health Sciences, Penn State College of Medicine, Hershey, Pennsylvania

Wanda Phipatanakul, MD, MS
Associate Professor of Pediatrics, Harvard Medical School; Director, Asthma Clinical Research Center, Boston Children's Hospital, Boston, Massachusetts

Frank S. Pidcock, MD
Vice President of Rehabilitation, Kennedy Krieger Institute; Associate Professor of Physical Medicine & Rehabilitation and Pediatrics, Johns Hopkins University School of Medicine, Baltimore, Maryland

Jared L. Pomeroy MD, MPH
Jefferson University Headache Center, Philadelphia, Pennsylvania

Valerie G. Press, MD, MPH
Assistant Professor, University of Chicago, Chicago, Illinois

Jenny S. Radesky, MD
Division of Developmental and Behavioral Pediatrics, Department of Pediatrics, Boston University Medical Center, Boston, Massachusetts

William J. Ravekes, MD
Division of Pediatric Cardiology, Johns Hopkins University School of Medicine, Baltimore, Maryland

Michael X. Repka, MD, MBA
David L Guyton, MD and Feduniak Professor of Ophthalmology and Professor of Pediatrics, Johns Hopkins University School of Medicine, Baltimore, Maryland

Kenneth B. Roberts, MD
Professor Emeritus of Pediatrics, University of North Carolina School of Medicine, Chapel Hill, NC; Cone Health System, Greensboro, NC

Nathaniel H. Robin, MD
Professor, Department of Genetics, Pediatrics, and Otolaryngology, University of Alabama at Birmingham, Birmingham, Alabama

Paul J. Rozance, MD
Associate Professor of Pediatrics, Neonatal Medicine, Perinatal Research Center, University of Colorado School of Medicine, Boulder, Colorado

Mark L. Rubinstein, MD
Associate Professor, Division of Adolescent & Young Adult Medicine, UCSF Benioff Children's Hospital, University of California, San Francisco, San Francisco, California

Jerry L. Rushton, MD, MPH
Associate Professor of Pediatrics, Indiana University, Indianapolis, Indiana

Robert T. Russell, MD, MPH
Assistant Professor of Pediatric Surgery, Children's of Alabama, University of Alabama at Birmingham, Birmingham, Alabama

George W. Rutherford, MD, AM
Salvatore Pablo Lucia Professor of Epidemiology, Preventive Medicine, Pediatrics and History Vice Chair, Department of Epidemiology and Biostatistics, and Head, Division of Infectious Disease Epidemiology, University of California, San Francisco, San Francisco, California

Iván Sánchez Fernández, MD
Epilepsy Fellow, Division of Epilepsy and Clinical Neurophysiology, Department of Neurology, Boston Children's Hospital, Boston, Massachusetts

James O. Sanders, MD
Professor of Orthopedics and Pediatrics, University of Rochester and the Golisano Children's Hospital at Strong, Rochester, New York

Pascal Scemama de Gialluly, MD, MBA
Assistant in Anesthesiology, Interim Director of Pediatric Pain, Massachusetts General Hospital; Instructor, Harvard Medical School, Boston, Massachusetts

H. Simon Schaaf, MBChB, DCM, MMed (Paed), FCPaed (SA), MD (Paed)

Desmond Tutu TB Centre, Department of Paediatrics and Child Health, Faculty of Medicine and Health Sciences, Stellenbosch University, Cape Town, South Africa

Alan R. Schroeder, MD

Chief, Pediatric Inpatient Services, Santa Clara Valley Medical Center, San Jose, California; Assistant Clinical Professor, Affiliate Department of Pediatrics, Stanford University School of Medicine, Stanford, California

Kathleen B. Schwarz, MD

Department of Pediatrics, Division of Pediatric Gastroenterology and Nutrition, Johns Hopkins University School of Medicine, Baltimore, Maryland

Malcolm R. Sears, MBChB, FRACP, FRCPC, FAAAAI

Professor of Medicine and AstraZeneca Chair in Respiratory Epidemiology, Firestone Institute for Respiratory Health, McMaster University, Ontario Canada

Dennis W.W. Shaw, MD

Professor of Radiology, University of Washington; Radiologist, Seattle Children's Hospital, Seattle, Washington

Eyal Shemesh, MD

Associate Professor of Pediatrics and Psychiatry and Chief, Division of Behavioral and Developmental Pediatrics, Department of Pediatrics and Kravis Children's Hospital, Icahn School of Medicine at Mount Sinai, New York, New York

Budd N. Shenkin, MD, MAPA

Affiliated Faculty, Philip R Lee Institute of Health Policy Studies, University of California, San Francisco, San Francisco, California

Emilia Shin, MD

Pediatric Gastroenterology and Nutrition, Johns Hopkins University, Baltimore, Maryland

Timothy R. Shope, MD, MPH

Associate Professor of Pediatrics, General Academic Pediatrics, Children's Hospital of Pittsburgh, Pittsburgh, Pennsylvania

Scott H. Sicherer, MD

Elliot and Roslyn Jaffe Professor of Pediatrics, Allergy and Immunology and Chief, Division of Pediatric Allergy and Immunology, Jaffe Food Allergy Institute, Icahn School of Medicine at Mount Sinai, New York, New York

Stephen D. Silberstein, MD

Professor, Department of Neurology and Director, Headache Center, Jefferson Medical College, Thomas Jefferson University Hospital, Philadelphia, Pennsylvania

Edward M. Sills, MD

Director, Pediatric Rheumatology, Johns Hopkins University School of Medicine and Johns Hopkins Hospital, Baltimore, Maryland

Marion R. Sills, MD, MPH

Associate Professor of Pediatrics and Emergency Medicine, University of Colorado School of Medicine; Physician, Emergency Department, Children's Hospital Colorado; Principal Investigator, Children's Outcomes Research Program, Boulder, Colorado

Julie Ann Sosa, MD, MA, FACS

Professor of Surgery and Medicine and Chief, Section of Endocrine Surgery, Duke University School of Medicine, Durham, North Carolina

Arvind I. Srinath, MD

Division of Pediatric Gastroenterology, Hepatology, & Nutrition, Children's Hospital of Pittsburgh, Pittsburgh, Pennsylvania

Martin T. Stein, MD

Professor Emeritus of Pediatrics, Division of General Academic Pediatrics, Child Development and Community Health, University of California, San Diego, Rady Children's Hospital, San Diego, California

Martina Steurer, MD, MAS

Assistant Professor, Department of Pediatrics, University of California, San Francisco, San Francisco, California

Gina S. Sucato, MD, MPH

Associate Professor, Pediatrics and Adolescent Medicine, University of Pittsburgh School of Medicine, Pittsburgh, Pennsylvania

Hania Szajewska

Department of Paediatrics, Medical University of Warsaw, Warsaw, Poland

John I. Takayama, MD, MPH

Professor of Clinical Pediatrics, University of California, San Francisco, UCSF Benioff Children's Hospital, San Francisco, California

Howard Taras, MD

Department of Pediatrics, University of California, San Diego, San Diego, California

Joseph Telfair, DrPH, MSW, MPH

Professor and Dual Chair, Department of Community Health and Department of Environmental Health Sciences and Karl E. Peace Distinguished Chair of Public Health, Jiann-Ping Hsu College of Public Health, Georgia Southern University, Statesboro, Georgia

Lisa Swartz Topor, MD, MMSc

Division of Pediatric Endocrinology, Hasbro Children's Hospital; Assistant Professor, Warren Alpert School of Medicine at Brown University, Providence, Rhode Island

Leonardo Trasande, MD, MPP

School of Medicine, New York University, New York, New York

John K. Triedman, MD

Professor of Pediatrics, Harvard Medical School, Boston, Massachusetts

Megan M. Tschudy, MD, MPH

Assistant Professor, Pediatrics and Assistant Medical Director, Harriet Lane Clinic, Division of General Pediatrics and Adolescent Medicine, Johns Hopkins School of Medicine, Baltimore, Maryland

Jay Tureen, MD
Professor of Pediatrics and Infectious Diseases, University of California, San Francisco, San Francisco, California

Krishna K. Upadhya, MD, MPH
Assistant Professor of Pediatrics, Division of General Pediatrics and Adolescent Medicine, Johns Hopkins School of Medicine, Baltimore, Maryland

Elliott P. Vichinsky, MD
Medical Director, Hematology/Oncology, UCSF Benioff Children's Hospital; Oakland Professor of Pediatrics, University of California, San Francisco, San Francisco, California

Jennifer K. Walter, MD, PhD, MS
Assistant Professor of Pediatrics and Medical Ethics, University of Pennsylvania School of Medicine and Children's Hospital of Philadelphia, Philadelphia, Pennsylvania

John P. Welsh, PhD
Professor, Center for Integrative Brain Research, Seattle Children's Research Institute, University of Washington Autism Center, Seattle, Washington

Amy Whittle, MD
Assistant Clinical Professor, Department of Pediatrics, University of California, San Francisco, San Francisco, California

Ronald J. Wong
Senior Research Scientist, Department of Pediatrics, Division of Neonatal & Developmental Medicine, Stanford University School of Medicine, Stanford, California

Susan J. Woolford, MD, MPH
Medical Director, Pediatric Comprehensive Weight Management Center, C. S. Mott Children's Hospital; Co-Director, Program on Mobile Technology to Enhance Child Health, Child Health Evaluation and Research Unit, Department of Pediatrics, University of Michigan, Ann Arbor, Michigan

Hsi-Yang Wu, MD
Associate Professor of Urology, Stanford University Medical Center; Pediatric Urology Fellowship Program Director, Lucile Packard Children's Hospital, Stanford, California

H. Shonna Yin, MD, MS
Assistant Professor of Pediatrics and Population Health, Departments of Pediatrics and Population Health, New York University School of Medicine, New York, New York

Paul C. Young, MD
Professor of Pediatrics, University of Utah School of Medicine, Salt Lake City, Utah

Joseph A. Zenel, MD
Professor, Pediatrics, Sanford Children's Hospital, The Sanford School of Medicine, University of South Dakota, Vermillion, South Dakota

Barry Zuckerman, MD

Professor and Chair Emeritus, Boston University School of Medicine and Boston Medical Center, Boston, Massachusetts

Lonnie Zwaigenbaum, MD, MSC, FRCPC

Autism Research Centre, Glenrose Rehabilitation Hospital, Department of Pediatrics, University of Alberta, Alberta, Canada

Table of Contents

Journals Represented

Journals represented in this YEAR BOOK are listed below.

Acta Paediatrica
Academic Pediatrics
American Journal of Cardiology
Annals of Allergy, Asthma and Immunology
Appetite
Arthritis Care & Research
British Medical Journal
Clinical and Experimental Immunology
Clinical Pediatrics
European Journal of Clinical Nutrition
Journal of Adolescent Health
Journal of Allergy and Clinical Immunology
Journal of Pediatrics
Journal of Perinatology
Journal of the American Medical Association
Journal of the American Medical Association Dermatology
Journal of the American Medical Association Ophthalmology
Journal of the American Medical Association Pediatrics
Lancet
Medical Teacher
Neurology
New England Journal of Medicine
Pediatric Dermatology
Pediatrics
The British Journal of General Practice
Tobacco Control

STANDARD ABBREVIATIONS

The following terms are abbreviated in this edition: acquired immunodeficiency syndrome (AIDS), cardiopulmonary resuscitation (CPR), central nervous system (CNS), cerebrospinal fluid (CSF), computed tomography (CT), deoxyribonucleic acid (DNA), electrocardiography (ECG), health maintenance organization (HMO), human immunodeficiency virus (HIV), intensive care unit (ICU), intramuscular (IM), intravenous (IV), magnetic resonance (MR) imaging (MRI), ribonucleic acid (RNA), ultrasound (US), and ultraviolet (UV).

NOTE

The YEAR BOOK OF PEDIATRICS® is a literature survey service providing abstracts of articles published in the professional literature. Every effort is made to assure the accuracy of the information presented in these pages. Neither the editors nor the publisher of the YEAR BOOK OF PEDIATRICS® can be responsible for errors in the original materials. The editors' comments are their own opinions. Mention of specific products within this publication does not constitute endorsement.

To facilitate the use of the YEAR BOOK OF PEDIATRICS® as a reference tool, all illustrations and tables included in this publication are now identified as they appear in the original article. This change is meant to help the reader recognize that any illustration or table appearing in the YEAR BOOK OF PEDIATRICS® may be only one of many in the original article. For this reason, figure and table numbers will often appear to be out of sequence within the YEAR BOOK OF PEDIATRICS.®

Foreword

Some four decades ago, the government became concerned about the maldistribution of physicians and acted to place physicians in underserved areas. The creation of the National Health Service Corps is an example from that era. But getting doctors in underserved areas and keeping them there (and keeping them current) are different propositions. Physicians in rural areas in particular were disconnected from medical centers where advances were taking place and from medical libraries where the reports of such advances could be found. Even back then, having one or two subscriptions didn't seem enough, and there was little help available to identify and retrieve articles that could help isolated physicians care for specific patients. So the National Library of Medicine (NLM) created Grateful Med, a forerunner of Medline, on floppy disks that could be obtained and updated at no expense to the physician. Moreover, NLM added Lonesome Doc, a service by which any physician with a fax machine could request an article and have it delivered by return fax.

Now, of course, there is PubMed and the ability to search for articles easily—but "keeping up" is still a challenge and not just for physicians in remote areas but for all of us. The traditional advice given to many of us during our training years to read journals on a regular basis is not only difficult to fit into a busy lifestyle but also nearly impossible if one seeks to keep up with the ever-increasing number of journals. And online searches for specific information often generate an endless list of articles. How to know which ones are pertinent and worthwhile? An answer comes once a year, as it has for the past 80 years: YEAR BOOK OF PEDIATRICS. In the YEAR BOOK, editors from the time of Isaac Abt, not only the first editor of the YEAR BOOK OF PEDIATRICS but also the first president of the American Academy of Pediatrics, review multiple articles from multiple journals and add immense value with commentaries and humor.

As a resident in pediatrics, I preferred monthly journals to weekly ones, because, at the end of the year, I was only 12 issues behind, rather than 52. Then I discovered the YEAR BOOK. It was during Sydney Gellis' time as editor and, for me, a toss-up whether the greater reward was the identification and abstract of a notable article, the editorial commentary by an expert in the field, or Dr Gellis' remarks with what has been called his "wicked sense of humor." The baton was passed to Frank Oski, who continued the tradition of expert reviews and humorous comments, making the YEAR BOOK not only informative but fun. Then to Jim Stockman, who sprinkled what he calls "curious facts and curios" throughout the volumes he edited for 36 years. Jim's knowledge of trivia is likely unsurpassed but perhaps now challenged by the new editor, Michael Cabana, the only YEAR BOOK editor with the distinction of having won thousands of dollars as a contestant on *Jeopardy!* Dr Cabana promises to continue to bring the values of his predecessors, highlighting key articles with expert commentary. The YEAR BOOK is in good hands, and all of us in pediatrics are the beneficiaries. Bring on the 2015 edition, Michael!

Kenneth B. Roberts, MD

Introduction

On April 29, 1962, President John F. Kennedy hosted a dinner at the White House to honor a group of recent Nobel Prize winners. At the event, he welcomed the group by stating, "I think this is the most extraordinary collection of talent, of human knowledge, that has ever been gathered together at the White House, with the possible exception of when Thomas Jefferson dined alone." Kennedy was complimenting the many talents of Jefferson, who "could calculate an eclipse, survey an estate, tie an artery, plan an edifice, try a cause, break a horse, and dance the minuet."[1] Jefferson was not only a great leader, but a true Renaissance man. His talents and knowledge were both broad and diverse.

I can relate to this quote today because I have the honor of succeeding an editor whose talents and knowledge are also both broad and diverse. Over the last 36 years, Dr James Stockman has co-edited or edited the YEAR BOOK OF PEDIATRICS. In addition to his long tenure as editor, his ability to write every commentary on every topic from Allergy to Ophthalmology is also impressive. Commentaries have ranged from issues with chromosomal microarray for prenatal diagnosis to observations about sexting among young adults and everything in between. I suppose Dr Stockman might be able to write a commentary on how to "calculate an eclipse, survey an estate, tie an artery, or plan an edifice," as well.

I doubt if any new editor can match Dr Stockman's editorial range and ability to write commentaries on every article for the YEAR BOOK OF PEDIATRICS. As a result, I have assembled an "extraordinary collection of talent" for the 2015 edition of the YEAR BOOK OF PEDIATRICS. I am returning to a previous tradition of inviting selected experts to author the commentaries for each of the articles that we highlight in this book. You will recognize many of these names. Many issues in pediatric care are global, and there is much that we can learn from other health care systems. As a result, we are fortunate to have the comments and observations of experts from around the world. Furthermore, many of the current issues in pediatrics are multidisciplinary in nature. As a result, many commentaries are now authored by experts in specialties other than pediatrics, and even disciplines outside of medicine.

Over the last 80 years, each edition of the YEAR BOOK OF PEDIATRICS has served as a snapshot in time that documents the new knowledge that our field has accumulated with each passing year. Although no single book can document every advance, the YEAR BOOK OF PEDIATRICS helps capture some of this new knowledge in one resource. However, what sets this book apart is not really the knowledge contained in the collection of article summaries, but the wisdom that is shared in the expert commentaries. It is challenging for any clinician to stay up to date with the growing body of knowledge in pediatrics, but what is even more valuable is having an additional perspective or interpretation on how this new knowledge can be applied.

The poet T. S. Eliot (a 1948 Nobel Prize recipient) once asked, "Where is the wisdom we have lost in knowledge?"[2] It is my hope that these commentaries continue with the tradition of giving the reader that additional insight and wisdom, sometimes hidden within the knowledge of a new peer-reviewed journal article. After reading these commentaries, I have viewed the articles highlighted in this book with a different perspective, sometimes with new optimism, or caution, in applying these findings to my practice. As a result, I am deeply indebted to the many contributors to this 2015 edition of the YEAR BOOK OF PEDIATRICS, as well as the previous editors, Isaac Abt, Henry Poncher, Julius Richmond, Sydney Gellis, Frank Oski, and James Stockman, who have helped shape this publication and left a wonderful legacy.

Michael D. Cabana, MD, MPH
Editor, Year Book of Pediatrics

References

1. John F. Kennedy: "Remarks at a Dinner Honoring Nobel Prize Winners of the Western Hemisphere." April 29, 1962. Online by Gerhard Peters and John T. Woolley. The American Presidency Project. http://www.presidency.ucsb.edu/ws/?pid=8623. Accessed October 3, 2014.
2. Eliot TS. *Choruses from "the Rock"* in *The Complete Poems and Plays: 1909-1950*. Orlando, FL: Harcourt Brace and Company; 1980.

Dedication

This book is dedicated to the wonderful pediatricians and health care staff at 6840 S. Main Street in Downers Grove, IL and 404C W. Boughton Road in Bolingbrook, IL.

1 Adolescent Medicine

Marijuana-Using Drivers, Alcohol-Using Drivers, and Their Passengers: Prevalence and Risk Factors Among Underage College Students
Whitehill JM, Rivara FP, Moreno MA (Univ of Washington, Seattle; Univ of Washington School of Medicine, Seattle)
JAMA Pediatr 168:618-624, 2014

Importance.—Driving after marijuana use increases the risk of a motor vehicle crash. Understanding this behavior among young drivers and how it may differ from alcohol-related driving behaviors could inform prevention efforts.

Objective.—To describe the prevalence, sex differences, and risk factors associated with underage college students' driving after using marijuana, driving after drinking alcohol, or riding with a driver using these substances.

Design, Setting, and Participants.—Cross-sectional telephone survey of a random sample of 315 first-year college students (aged 18-20 years) from 2 large public universities, who were participating in an ongoing longitudinal study. At recruitment, 52.8% of eligible individuals consented to participate; retention was 93.2% one year later when data for this report were collected.

Main Outcomes and Measures.—Self-reported past-28-day driving after marijuana use, riding with a marijuana-using driver, driving after alcohol use, and riding with an alcohol-using driver.

Results.—In the prior month, 20.3% of students had used marijuana. Among marijuana-using students, 43.9% of male and 8.7% of female students drove after using marijuana ($P < .001$), and 51.2% of male and 34.8% of female students rode as a passenger with a marijuana-using driver ($P = .21$). Most students (65.1%) drank alcohol, and among this group 12.0% of male students and 2.7% of female students drove after drinking ($P = .01$), with 20.7% and 11.5% ($P = .07$), respectively, reporting riding with an alcohol-using driver. Controlling for demographics and substance use behaviors, driving after substance use was associated with at least a 2-fold increase in risk of being a passenger with another user; the reverse was also true. A 1% increase in the reported percentage of friends using marijuana was associated with a 2% increased risk of riding with a marijuana-using driver (95% CI, 1.01-1.03). Among students using any substances, past-28-day use of only marijuana was associated with a 6.24-fold increased risk of driving after substance use compared with using only alcohol (95% CI, 1.89-21.17).

Conclusions and Relevance.—Driving and riding after marijuana use is common among underage, marijuana-using college students. This is concerning given recent legislation that may increase marijuana availability.

▶ Cannabis (marijuana, pot) is a diverse amalgam of chemicals derived from the dioecious plant, *Cannabis sativa*, known to *Homo sapiens* for thousands of years. This annual flowering herb has been celebrated over the millennia for its effusive euphoric effects, making it an eidolon of substance use for many illicit drug consumers in the 21st century. It has become an eristic embranglement for many because the intense euphoric-inducing effects of its proactive ingredient, delta-9-tetrahydrocannabinol (THC), stimulate millions of humans to advocate for its legal and liberal use; this occurs even though the medical and mental adverse effects of cannabis make it an epinosic drug or nepenthe to smoke or consume as a comestible chemical.

Pressure is mounting in contemporary American society to ex post facto legalize this drug with the amaranthine argument that cannabis is a safe and natural plant providing countless medical benefits to humans. Just as the pressure mounted in the 20th century to withdraw prohibition for alcohol, apolaustic cannabis enthusiasts are mounting legal and fiscal pressure with bold statements based on skimble-skamble sciosophy to open similar flood gates for cannabis with the added caveat that cannabis is also "medicinal."

The scientific medical establishment must remind legislators and the public at large that much more carefully controlled research must be done to identify which if any of the more than 60 cannabinoids found in this plant may have positive medical benefits for specific medical disorders. If so, is the benefit-adverse effect ratio better than seen with Food and Drug Administration-approved medications for an identified condition? What we know now is that cannabis is a dangerous drug for adolescents to consume. The use of this drug with its Cadmean euphoria is linked to addiction, comorbid illegal drug consumption, adverse psychosocial and neurodevelopmental effects (including decreased attention span and problematic decision making), increased risk for psychosis as well as anxiety, among other concerns.[1,2] Cannabis use disorders are difficult to treat even with 21st-century psychopharmacologic agents and therapy.

The lifting of prohibition in the United States in 1933 resulted in countless traffic accidents and deaths from drivers who consumed alcohol. Teale and Marks were among the early researchers who alerted the scientific community to the similar link of persons driving a motor vehicle under the influence of cannabis.[3] Since then, many studies have been published establishing this louche link to injury and destruction in those who drive under the Icarian influence of cannabis.

This study by Whitehill et al yields some important results in this link in college students at a time when increased understanding of marijuana use could influence legislation aimed at increasing the availability of marijuana and diminishing the legal ramifications of marijuana use. The authors quickly point out that past research has documented that marijuana use increases automobile accidents and interweave data regarding both marijuana-using and alcohol-using underage college students to illustrate the seriousness of marijuana use in this population as well as the perception that marijuana use is not dangerous. The study is persuasive, succinct, and addresses a significant social concern that could ultimately help increase awareness of the dangers of marijuana use.

It was refreshing to see methodology that used ongoing longitudinal data of new college students because this is a time when cannabis use can dramatically increase for this population (also a result of this study). Because of these factors, this study helps debunk the myth that marijuana use is just a rite of passage for new college students and represents a dangerous and significant health hazard. The statistical analyses were also rigorous and fit the needs of the study.

Within the Results section, it was nice to see that 1 of the universities had a significant number of minority students, helping to make the results salient to more than just the European American population. The results were shocking, particularly for males, with regard to the high percentage of students who drove after using marijuana compared with a much lower percentage for driving after alcohol use (Table 2 in the original article). The authors used these data to illustrate that many young college students may have a perception that cannabis use is not dangerous.

This study did an excellent job of illustrating the significant health hazards of driving after using marijuana and, almost more important, by highlighting the idea that many young college students perceive driving after marijuana use to be safer than after alcohol use. This is a well-done study that can add to the existing literature, provide sound data, and also encourage ideas to help improve awareness of the seriousness of marijuana's oscitant effects, leading to impaired driving and potential death.

The literature on the serious adverse effects of cannabis use continues to grow. As we often do in pediatrics, we are left with the conclusion that prevention is best and, in this situation, that prevention of cannabis use by our youth should be emphasized as much as possible even in such a latitudinarian society as ours. Prevention of cannabis legalization may not be possible at this point but we must strive to continuously educate society about its many dangers including the increase in motor vehicle accident injuries and deaths due to cannabis consumption we unfortunately will see as this century progresses.

Pediatricians should teach their adolescent patients that one should not use cannabis and drive; that higher THC levels increases risk for motor vehicle accidents[4]; that combination of cannabis and alcohol increases THC levels more than using THC alone[5]; that cannabis levels are found in chronic smokers for at least 30 days after stopping its consumption[6]; that drivers under the influence of cannabis are often not aware they are impaired[7]; that one should never be a passenger in a motor vehicle operated by a driver who has consumed cannabis (acutely and/or chronically)[8]; that those under the influence of cannabis should take public transportation when leaving places of drug consumption[9]; that adequate public transportation at night should be available in all communities[9]; that those who consume cannabis must be taught never to drive or at lease wait several hours before driving[10]; and that cannabis consumption increases road rage in drivers.[11]

Although an abecedarian society is increasingly positive about the use of this myrmidon-inducing drug, education from health care advocates of children should a fortiori continue about the realities of this herb, which is an oubliette with its unforgiving Pied Piper effects on our children including dysfunctional neurocognition.[12]

"Pied Piper: I attract attention
Chiefly with a secret charm ...
Who doesn't know of the Pied Piper?
Alas, alas for Hamelin! ...
They wrote the story on a column,
And on the great church-window painted
The same, to make the world acquainted
How their children were stolen away ..."

The Pied Piper of Hamelin (Robert Browning: 1812—1889)

D. E. Greydanus, MD, Dr HC (Athens)

R. W. Apple, PhD

References

1. Greydanus DE, Hawver EK, Greydanus MM, Merrick J. Marijuana: current concepts. *Front Public Health*. 2013;1:42.
2. Farmer RF, Kosty DB, Seeley JR, Duncan SC, Lynskey MT, Rohde P. Natural course of cannabis use disorders. *Psychol Med*. 2014:1-10.
3. Teale D, Marks V. A fatal motor-car accident and cannabis use. Investigation by radioimmunoassay. *Lancet*. 1976;1:884-885.
4. Kuypers KP, Legrand SA, Ramaekers JG, Verstraete AG. A case-control study estimating accident risk for alcohol, medicines and illegal drugs. *PLoS One*. 2012;7:e43496.
5. Downey LA, King R, Papafotiou K, et al. The effects of cannabis and alcohol on simulated driving: influences of dose and experience. *Accid Anal Prev*. 2013;50: 879-886.
6. Bergamaschi MM, Karschner EL, Goodwin RS, et al. Impact of prolonged cannabinoid excretion in chronic daily cannabis smokers' blood on per se drugged driving laws. *Clin Chem*. 2013;59:519-526.
7. Penning R, Veldstra JL, Daamen AP, Olivier B, Verster JC. Drugs of abuse, driving and traffic safety. *Curr Drug Abuse Rev*. 2010;3:23-32.
8. Cartwright J, Asbridge M. Passengers' decisions to ride with a driver under the influence of either alcohol or cannabis. *J Stud Alcohol Drugs*. 2011;72:86-95.
9. Calafat A, Blay N, Juan M, et al. Traffic risk behaviors at nightlife: drinking, taking drugs, driving, and use of public transport by young people. *Traffic Inj Prev*. 2009;10:162-169.
10. Sewell RA, Poling J, Sofuoglu M. The effect of cannabis compared with alcohol on driving. *Am J Addict*. 2009;18:185-193.
11. Fierro I, Morales C, Alvarez FJ. Alcohol use, illicit drug use, and road rage. *J Stud Alcohol Drugs*. 2011;72:185-193.
12. Thames AD, Arbid N, Sayegh P. Cannabis use and neurocognitive functioning in a non-clinical sample of users. *Addict Behav*. 2014;39:994-999.

Sexting and Sexual Behavior Among Middle School Students

Rice E, Gibbs J, Winetrobe H, et al (Univ of Southern California, Los Angeles, CA; et al)
Pediatrics 134:e21-e28, 2014

Objective.—It is unknown if "sexting" (ie, sending/receiving sexually explicit cell phone text or picture messages) is associated with sexual activity and sexual risk behavior among early adolescents, as has been found for high school students. To date, no published data have examined these relationships exclusively among a probability sample of middle school students.

Methods.—A probability sample of 1285 students was collected along-side the 2012 Youth Risk Behavior Survey in Los Angeles middle schools. Logistic regressions assessed the correlates of sexting behavior and associations between sexting and sexual activity and risk behavior (ie, unprotected sex).

Results.—Twenty percent of students with text-capable cell phone access reported receiving a sext and 5% reported sending a sext. Students who text at least 100 times per day were more likely to report both receiving (odds ratio [OR]: 2.4) and sending (OR: 4.5) sexts and to be sexually active (OR: 4.1). Students who sent sexts (OR: 3.2) and students who received sexts (OR: 7.0) were more likely to report sexual activity. Compared with not being sexually active, excessive texting and receiving sexts were associated with both unprotected sex (ORs: 4.7 and 12.1, respectively) and with condom use (ORs: 3.7 and 5.5, respectively).

Conclusions.—Because early sexual debut is correlated with higher rates of sexually transmitted infections and teen pregnancies, pediatricians should discuss sexting with young adolescents because this may facilitate conversations about sexually transmitted infection and pregnancy prevention. Sexting and associated risks should be considered for inclusion in middle school sex education curricula.

▶ Sexting—sending or receiving sexually provocative images or words via cell phone text message—has received considerable attention in the media and some attention in social science research. Most previous work with adolescents has focused on the social or legal consequences of this behavior. For example, some adolescents have been charged with distributing child pornography after sending a nude image of an underage individual. In other cases, an individual who received an explicit photo shared it with others without the sender's consent, leading to embarrassment or distress. This study by Rice and colleagues is the first to examine the health implications of sexting in a probability sample of early adolescents.

Although there are exceptions (eg, Gorden-Messer[1]), the bulk of the previous literature documents an association between sexting and sexual activity—including activities that could be associated with risk (eg, multiple partners, unprotected sex). These studies were conducted with older adolescents or young adults (see Klettke et al for a review[2]). Rice and colleagues extend this work to a more vulnerable population: early adolescents (aged 10–15). The findings showed that most of these early adolescents (74%) had access to a cell phone capable of texting. Among these individuals, 1 in 5 had received a sext and 1 in 20 had sent a sext. For both sending and receiving a sext, an important predictor was overall texting activity—individuals who sent and received texts more often were more likely to engage in sexting. In addition, sexting was associated with being sexually active and with both protected and unprotected sex (broadly defined to include oral, vaginal, and anal sex).

There is an ongoing debate in the literature whether sexting is "normal" or problematic.[3,4] In reality, these are separate questions. Although there is a human tendency to believe that what is "normal" (typical, prevalent, ordinary) is also not problematic, this is not always the case. For example, according to the US Department of Health and Human Services,[5] at the height of tobacco's popularity in North America, about 1 in 2 adult Americans smoked cigarettes. Currently, approximately two-thirds of American adults are overweight or obese.[6] What is common can still be unhealthy.

A more important question is: "Is the association between sexting and sexual behavior causal?" For example, does sexting create more sexualized norms that promote sexual activity? Alternatively, is sexting merely a byproduct of an interest in sex, or a consequence of sexual activity (eg, intimate couples sharing intimate photos)? These questions cannot be answered by cross-sectional observational studies such as presented by Rice and colleagues (and most of the previous literature). Future longitudinal work may be able to shed light on this issue.

What the findings from this study do suggest, however, is that sexting is a potent marker of sexual activity in early adolescents. Sexual debut in early adolescence is associated with a variety of negative consequences, including sexually transmitted infections and unplanned pregnancy. Parents, pediatricians, teachers, and others may become aware of adolescents who are engaging in sexting. This awareness could lead to an opportunity to have a conversation about sexting, including the potential legal and social consequences of this behavior. It may also be an appropriate time to sensitively explore sexual activity and knowledge about behaviors that can reduce risk.

E. G. Benotsch, PhD

References

1. Gordon-Messer D, Bauermeister JA, Grodzinski A, Zimmerman M. Sexting among young adults. *J Adolesc Health*. 2013;52:301-306.
2. Klette B, Hallford DJ, Mellor DJ. Sexting prevalence and correlates: a systematic literature review. *Clin Psychol Rev*. 2014;34:44-53.
3. Levine D. Sexting: a terrifying health risk...or the new normal for young adults? *J Adolesc Health*. 2013;52:257-258.
4. Döring N. Consensual sexting among adolescents: Risk prevention through abstinence education or safer sexting? *J Psychosocial Research Cyberspace*. 2014;8.

5. National Center for Health Statistics. *Health, United States, 2013: with Special Feature on Prescription Drugs.* Hyattsville, MD: 2014.
6. U.S. Department of Health and Human Services. *The Health Consequences of Smoking—50 Years of Progress. A Report of the Surgeon General.* Atlanta, GA: U.S. Department of Health and Human Services, Centers for Disease Control and Prevention, National Center for Chronic Disease Prevention and Health Promotion, Office on Smoking and Health; 2014. Printed with corrections, January 2014.

Sexuality Talk During Adolescent Health Maintenance Visits

Alexander SC, Fortenberry JD, Pollak KI, et al (Duke Univ Med Ctr, Durham, NC; Indiana Univ School of Medicine, Indianapolis; Duke Cancer Inst, Durham, NC; et al)
JAMA Pediatr 168:163-169, 2014

Importance.—Physicians may be important sources of sexuality information and preventive services, and one-on-one confidential time during health maintenance visits is recommended to allow discussions of sexual development, behavior, and risk reduction. However, little is known about the occurrence and characteristics of physician-adolescent discussions about sexuality.

Objective.—To examine predictors of time spent discussing sexuality, level of adolescent participation, and physician and patient characteristics associated with sexuality discussions during health maintenance visits by early and middle adolescents.

Design, Setting, and Participants.—Observational study of audio-recorded conversations between 253 adolescents (mean age, 14.3 years; 53% female; 40% white; 47% African American) and 49 physicians (82% pediatricians; 84% white; 65% female; mean age, 40.9 years; mean [SD] duration in practice, 11.8 [8.7] years) coded for sexuality content at 11 clinics (3 academic and 8 community-based practices) located throughout the Raleigh/Durham, North Carolina, area.

Main Outcomes and Measures.—Total time per visit during which sexuality issues were discussed.

Results.—One hundred sixty-five (65%) of all visits had some sexual content within it. The average time of sexuality talk was 36 seconds (35% 0 seconds; 30% 1-35 seconds; and 35% ≥36 seconds). Ordinal logistic regression (outcome of duration: 0, 1-35, or ≥36 seconds), adjusted for clustering of patients within physicians, found that female patients (odds ratio [OR] = 2.58; 95% CI, 1.53-4.36), older patients (OR = 1.37; 95% CI, 1.13-1.65), conversations with explicit confidentiality discussions (OR = 4.33; 95% CI, 2.58-7.28), African American adolescents (OR = 1.58; 95% CI, 1.01-2.48), and longer overall visit (OR = 1.07; 95% CI, 1.03-1.11) were associated with more sexuality talk, and Asian physicians were associated with less sexuality talk (OR = 0.13; 95% CI, 0.08-0.20). In addition, the same significant associations between adolescent, physician, and visit characteristics were significantly associated with greater adolescent participation.

Conclusions and Relevance.—Our study may be the first to directly observe sexuality talk between physicians and adolescents. We found that one-third of all adolescents had annual visits without any mention of sexuality issues; when sexuality talk occurred, it was brief. Research is needed to identify successful strategies physicians can use to engage adolescents in discussions about sexuality to help promote healthy sexual development and decision making.

Trial Registration.—clinicaltrials.gov Identifier: NCT01040975.

▶ Adolescent and young adults' first sexual encounters frequently occur while they are still under the medical care of pediatricians. According to the Centers for Disease Control and Prevention Survey in 2011, 70% of youth report having had intercourse by age 19 years.[1] Although these data are consistent with our understanding that sexual activity is an expected component of adolescent development, epidemiologic data also show that negative outcomes are common. Young women aged 15 to 24 years have the highest rates of chlamydia and gonorrhea infection of any age group,[2] more than 700 000 teenagers become pregnant each year (the vast majority unintentionally),[3] and 1 in 4 of all new HIV infections occurs among youth aged 13 to 24 years.[4] Efforts to minimize risks of sexual activity are therefore critical. Unfortunately, the study by Alexander and colleagues described here suggests that physicians may not be contributing enough to those efforts.

The study reports that on average, 35 seconds of the adolescent preventive care visits were devoted to sexuality discussion (Table 2 in the original article). It is worth noting that the mean duration of visits in the study (23 minutes) was 5 minutes longer than the mean duration of all pediatric visits nationwide. That mean visit duration was reported to be 18 minutes on the most recent National Ambulatory Medical Care Survey.[5]

A unique strength of this study is the audio recording of visits. In addition to objectively documenting the duration of discussions in the visits, this method had the added advantage of recording whether the discussion was initiated by the adolescent or the provider. A key finding of this study was that sexuality discussions did not occur in any visits unless the provider initiated the discussion. Similarly, visits in which the provider discussed confidentiality were more likely to include discussions of sexuality. This finding reinforces the importance of having clear policies for confidentiality and discussing them with adolescents as part of preventive care visits.

There are several limitations of the study that might affect the generalizability of the findings. The adolescents in the study were all overweight (body mass index > 85%) and were recruited to participate in a study about how physicians communicate about healthy weight. Given the study sample, providers may have prioritized counseling about weight, leaving less time to address other preventive health topics. In addition, we cannot know if providers systematically view overweight teens differently and spend less time discussing sexual health topics with them compared with nonoverweight teens. However, recent data suggest that obese teens who are sexually active may engage in riskier behavior including using alcohol or drugs before sex.[6,7] It is vital that anticipatory guidance around sexual behavior occurs in this population.

The findings of this study are not surprising given prior evidence in the literature and recognition that pediatricians in practice may currently have less rather than more time on average to spend with their patients than occurred in this study. Given that time limitation, use of other tools to spark discussion and maximize opportunities for counseling may be needed.

A number of mechanisms can be used to facilitate sexual health discussions in the pediatric office. Use of previsit questionnaires either in electronic or paper form could help inform the adolescent that sexuality is a topic that the provider thinks is important to discuss during the visit. Sources of previsit questionnaires include Bright Futures[8] and The Rapid Assessment for Adolescent Preventive Services RAAPS.[9] Visit orientation for adolescents should also include information about the confidentiality they can expect and how that confidentiality will be maintained.[10] Information about making an office youth-friendly, including information about confidentiality, is available from the Centers for Disease Control and Prevention.[11]

Examples of ways to communicate with patients and families about confidentiality can be found online from sources such as the Adolescent Health Working Group based out of California[12] but must be adapted to reflect local laws on adolescent consent and confidentiality, which vary by state.[13] It is also important to remember that high-quality adolescent care necessitates giving the adolescent time alone in the visit to support their developing autonomy and need for privacy.[14] Finally, given that the common morbidities in adolescence revolve around behavioral health including sexuality, it may be that current visit lengths and reimbursement need to be increased to adequately meet the needs of this group.

Although health care providers are only 1 potential source of sexual health information, they are important gatekeepers of preventive care screening and service.[15] If we do not assess our patients' risks for pregnancy or sexually transmitted infections, we will miss the opportunities to screen them, provide contraception, and provide risk reduction counseling. Perhaps even more important, this study suggests that if we do not start the discussion with them about sexuality, we will lose the opportunity to give them the information and other tools they need to protect their health.

K. K. Upadhya, MD, MPH

G. S. Sucato, MD, MPH

References

1. Centers for Disease Control and Prevention. Sexual and reproductive health of persons aged 10–24 years—United States, 2002–2007. *MMWR Surveill Summ.* 2009;58:1-58.
2. Centers for Disease Control and Prevention. Fact Sheet: STD Trends in the United States 2011 National Data for Chlamydia, Gonorrhea, and Syphilis. http://www.cdc.gov/std/stats11/trends-2011.pdf. Accessed June 9, 2014.

3. Curtin SC, Abma JC, Ventura SJ, Henshaw SK. *Pregnancy Rates for U.S. Women Continue to Drop.* NCHS data brief, no 136. Hyattsville, MD: National Center for Health Statistics; 2013.
4. Centers for Disease Control and Prevention. HIV Among Youth. http://www.cdc.gov/hiv/risk/age/youth/index.html. Accessed June 9, 2014.
5. Cherry DK, Woodwell DA, Rechtsteiner EA. *National Ambulatory Medical Care Survey: 2005 Summary.* Advance data from vital and health statistics; no 387. Hyattsville, MD: National Center for Health Statistics; 2007.
6. Ratcliff MB, Jenkins TM, Reiter-Purtill J, Noll JG, Zeller MH. Risk-taking behaviors of adolescents with extreme obesity: normative or not? *Pediatrics.* 2011;127:827-834.
7. Leech TG, Dias JJ. Risky sexual behavior: a race-specific social consequence of obesity. *J Youth Adolesc.* 2012;41:41-52.
8. Bright Futures Tool and Resource Kit. http://brightfutures.aap.org/tool_and_resource_kit.html. Accessed September 26, 2014.
9. Rapid Assessment for Adolescent Preventive Services (RAAPS). https://www.raaps.org/. Accessed September 26, 2014.
10. American College of Obstetricians and Gynecologists. Tool Kit for Teen Care. 2nd ed: Confidentiality in Adolescent Health Care. http://www.acog.org/~/media/Departments/AdolescentHealthCare/TeenCarToolKit/ACOGConfidentiality.pdf?dmc=1&ts=20140609T1128427771. Accessed September 26, 2014.
11. Centers for Disease Control and Prevention. A teen-friendly reproductive health visit. http://www.cdc.gov/teenpregnancy/teenfriendlyhealthvisit.html. Accessed September 26, 2014.
12. Adolescent Health Working Group. AHWG's Provider Toolkit Series. http://www.ahwg.net/resources-for-providers.html. Accessed September 26, 2014.
13. Guttmacher Institute. U.S. Teenage Pregnancies, Births and Abortions, 2010: National and State Trends by Age, Race and Ethnicity. http://www.guttmacher.org/pubs/USTPtrends10.pdf. Accessed September 26, 2014.
14. Hagan JF, Shaw JS, Duncan PM, eds. Bright Futures: Guidelines for Health Supervision of Infants, Children, and Adolescents. 3rd ed. Elk Grove Village, IL: American Academy of Pediatrics; 2008:.
15. U.S. Preventive Services Task Force. Behavioral Counseling Interventions to Prevent Sexually Transmitted Infections: Draft Recommendation Statement. AHRQ Publication No. 13-05180-EF-2.

The Effect on Teenage Risky Driving of Feedback From a Safety Monitoring System: A Randomized Controlled Trial

Simons-Morton BG, Bingham CR, Ouimet MC, et al (Natl Insts of Health, Bethesda, MD; Univ of Michigan Transportation Res Inst, Ann Arbor; et al)
J Adolesc Health 53:21-26, 2013

Purpose.—Teenage risky driving may be due to teenagers not knowing what is risky, preferring risk, or the lack of consequences. Elevated gravitational-force (g-force) events, caused mainly by hard braking and sharp turns, provide a valid measure of risky driving and are the target of interventions using in-vehicle data recording and feedback devices. The effect of two forms of feedback about risky driving events to teenagers only or to teenagers and their parents was tested in a randomized controlled trial.

Methods.—Ninety parent-teen dyads were randomized to one of two groups: (1) immediate feedback to teens (Lights Only); or (2) immediate feedback to teens plus family access to event videos and ranking of the teen relative to other teenage drivers (Lights Plus). Participants' vehicles were instrumented with data recording devices and events exceeding .5 g were assessed for 2 weeks of baseline and 13 weeks of feedback.

Results.—Growth curve analysis with random slopes yielded a significant decrease in event rates for the Lights Plus group (slope = −.11, $p < .01$), but no change for the Lights Only group (slope = .05, $p = .67$) across the 15 weeks. A large effect size of 1.67 favored the Lights Plus group.

Conclusions.—Provision of feedback with possible consequences associated with parents being informed reduced risky driving, whereas immediate feedback only to teenagers did not.

▶ Injuries are the leading cause of mortality for adolescents in the United States. A large proportion is the result of motor vehicle crashes. By changing the driver licensing system to require many months of accompanied driving by teenagers before they begin driving on their own, we have substantially reduced this problem among novice drivers since the late 1990s. This period of accompanied driving gives adolescents the opportunity to learn from experience, while protected by the presence of an experienced co-driver, from the potentially catastrophic consequences of the errors that novice drivers inevitably make. Although the simple tasks involved in handling a vehicle can be learned quickly and relatively easily, the more subtle and important understanding that enables safe driving takes far longer to fully develop—perhaps as long as 3 years.

Unfortunately, crash rates remain inordinately high among young teenage drivers, and we continue to struggle in the search for policies, programs and other approaches to further reduce this problem. The many efforts to address adolescent driver risk that have been, and continue to be, widely embraced produce little or no measurable benefit. Nearly all educational activities, awareness campaigns, age-specific driving laws, and general admonitions to drive safely largely fail to engage the 2 primary causes of the high teenage driver crash rate—the fact that most teens are novices who have yet to develop a wealth of deeply ingrained wisdom about the complexities inherent in driving safely and the impulsiveness characteristic of adolescence. Experts on young driver behavior widely believe that the critical keys to reducing crash risk lie in 2 areas: providing more and more appropriate practical experience to beginners and ensuring parents (and other close family members) remain effectively engaged in the lives of teens as they begin driving on their own. The former addresses the lack of driving wisdom; the latter appears to be the best way to ameliorate the inevitable risks associated with adolescence.

The study by Simons-Morton and colleagues brings much-needed scientific rigor to the study of young driver risks and how they might be influenced. In the process it sheds some light—both intended and inadvertent—on the issues just mentioned. Experimentation (controlled trials) to study young driver issues is difficult. A number of studies use driving simulators to conduct experiments; however, the artificiality of simulated driving remains a serious drawback. Simons-Morton et al take advantage of modern technology to conduct a real-world experimental examination of whether and how a program that has reduced crashes among fleet vehicle drivers might also reduce young driver crashes.

This study addresses the key question of whether letting young drivers know they have executed a rough and possibly dangerous move (hard stop, hard turn) is alone sufficient to alter their behavior or whether more is needed. It turns out that merely alerting teens that certain behaviors are inappropriately excessive had little or no effect on their subsequent driving (ie, the "Lights Only" group). By contrast, making evidence of these actions available to the adolescent's parents (ie, the "Lights Plus" group) resulted in a fairly rapid and sustained improvement in driving behavior (Fig 2). So the issue seems to be more a matter of motivation to drive appropriately than the ability to do so.

As with any study, there are limitations to this one. It is important to bear in mind that rough driving, which is measured here, is not necessarily dangerous driving. A sustained pattern of such driving is associated with higher crash rates. The 2 are clearly related. Still, until interventions like that studied here are demonstrated to actually reduce crashes, and not simply influence driving actions that seem risky, we need to reserve judgment about their efficacy.

A serendipitous but important finding of this study is that it is difficult to engage parents in efforts to address their teenager's driving safety. With this study, and every other one of its type, recruiting families to participate has been a daunting challenge. This is partly because many parents feel that technologic monitoring violates a bond of trust between them and their children. Accordingly it is unlikely that many parents will ever put a camera or other monitoring device in their teen's vehicle. Nonetheless, it is clear from this study and others that are less scientifically rigorous that when novice teenage drivers

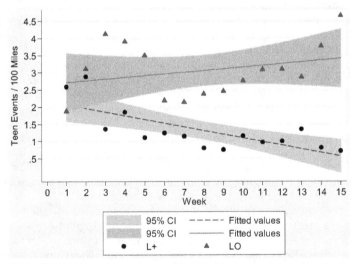

FIGURE 2.—Weekly observed rates of events/100 miles (shown as point prevalence) and predicted rates (shown as best fit lines) with 95% confidence intervals (shaded area) for Lights Only (LO; n = 43) and Lights Plus delayed feedback to family (L+; n = 45). (Reprinted from Simons-Morton BG, Bingham CR, Ouimet MC, et al. The effect on teenage risky driving of feedback from a safety monitoring system: a randomized controlled trial. *J Adolesc Health*. 2013;53:21-26, with permission from Elsevier.)

believe their behaviors may be known to parents, they drive in a more controlled or conscientious manner.

The general takeaway from this study is that if teenagers believe the adults in their lives may be paying attention to the teen's driving, they will generally be more controlled in their behavior. In essence, the camera in the vehicle allows parents to continue riding with the teenager "in spirit." It's a way of implementing the general principle that when individuals believe their behaviors are visible to others who matter, they are less likely to engage in actions that are generally considered inappropriate.

R. D. Foss, PhD

Risk Perceptions and Subsequent Sexual Behaviors After HPV Vaccination in Adolescents
Mayhew A, Mullins TLK, Ding L, et al (Univ of Cincinnati College of Medicine, OH; Cincinnati Children's Hosp Med Ctr, OH; et al)
Pediatrics 133:1-8, 2014

Objectives.—Concerns have been raised that human papillomavirus (HPV) vaccination could lead to altered risk perceptions and an increase in risky sexual behaviors among adolescents. The aim of this study was to assess whether adolescent risk perceptions after the first vaccine dose predicted subsequent sexual behaviors.

Methods.—Young women 13 to 21 years of age ($N = 339$) completed questionnaires immediately after HPV vaccination, and 2 and 6 months later, assessing demographic characteristics, knowledge/attitudes about HPV vaccination, risk perceptions, and sexual behaviors. Risk perceptions were measured by using 2 5-item scales assessing: (1) perceived risk of sexually transmitted infections (STI) other than HPV, and (2) perceived need for safer sexual behaviors after HPV vaccination. We assessed associations between risk perceptions at baseline and sexual behaviors over the next 6 months by using logistic regression, stratifying participants by sexual experience at baseline and age (13−15 vs 16−21 years).

Results.—Among all sexually inexperienced participants (42.5%), baseline risk perceptions were not associated with subsequent sexual initiation; in age-stratified analyses, girls 16 to 21 years of age who reported lower perceived risk for other STI (an inappropriate perception) were less likely to initiate sex (odds ratio [OR] 0.13, 95% confidence interval [CI] 0.03−0.69). Among all sexually experienced participants (57.5%) and in age-stratified analyses, baseline risk perceptions were not associated with subsequent number of sexual partners or condom use.

Conclusions.—Risk perceptions after HPV vaccination were not associated with riskier sexual behaviors over the subsequent 6 months in this study sample.

▶ Human papillomavirus (HPV) is the most common sexually transmitted infection (STI) in the United States. The vast majority of infections self-resolve, but persistent HPV can cause cervical cancer in females and other ano-genital cancers and genital warts in both females and males. Accordingly, the US Advisory Committee on Immunization Practices (ACIP) recommends the routine administration of either the quadrivalent HPV vaccine (introduced in 2006, for types 6, 11, 16, and 18) or the bivalent HPV vaccine (introduced in 2009, for types 16 and 18) for females 11 to 26 years of age. Despite the broad efforts to disseminate this information nationally, the actual uptake of the HPV vaccine remains low; recent Centers for Disease Control and Prevention (CDC) reports from 2010–2012 indicate that only half of females 13 to 17 years of age have received 1 dose, and only one-third have received all 3 doses.

Efficacy data are impressive, and yet vaccine acceptance has been compli-cated by parental and clinician concerns. Common concerns about longer-term efficacy and safety could apply to any newly introduced vaccine, but some barriers are related to the fact that HPV is an STI, and these concerns are unique compared with other vaccines. Parental concerns that we hear in clinical practice include the inaccurate perception that the vaccine is not neces-sary until onset of first sex, perceptions that the young patient will not become sexually active until a much older age, confusion over why the vaccine should be given to young adolescents, concern that administration of the vaccine will represent "permission" to engage in risky sexual behaviors, and preferences to "wait and see" before deciding. Clinicians themselves may also express similar concerns, which in turn influence the strength of their verbal recommendations to individual patients and parents. Clinicians' hesitancy is important because studies have shown that clinicians have significant influence on parents' deci-sions to receive HPV vaccine and parents place great trust in their regular clini-cians on this topic.

In this clinical context, Mayhew et al address the issues of whether female adolescents mistakenly think the vaccine minimizes the need to practice safer sex and whether they mistakenly think the vaccine decreases their risk for STIs other than HPV. The study asks whether adolescents with inaccurate per-ceptions then proceed to engage in riskier sex compared with those with a more accurate understanding. An important strength of the study is the prospective design that allows the observations over time, at the convenient vaccine administration intervals at the 2- and 6-month marks. The authors make the dis-tinction between mistaken perceptions and the actual translation of the percep-tions into worse sexual behaviors, which underscores the clinical significance of these perceptions. The risk perceptions were measured by 5-question scales, and it is reassuring that the majority of girls had correct perceptions that the vaccine did not change the need for safer sex or the risk for non-HPV STIs.

It is further reassuring that those with incorrect risk perceptions did not engage in riskier behaviors postvaccine compared with those with correct per-ceptions. The odds ratios for the associations between risk perceptions and sev-eral sexual behavior outcomes were nonsignificant. Furthermore, these odds ratios were estimated at both above and below 1, suggesting no clear trends in associations at all. In the stratified analyses, among the sexually inexper-ienced and older group (16- to 21-year-olds), those with mistaken perceptions of decreased risk afforded by the vaccine even had less risky sexual behaviors compared with those with correct perceptions. The authors emphasize that the decisions around sexual behaviors are complex and multifactorial, and receipt of the HPV vaccine does not appear to be a prominent factor.

This study about the effect of the vaccine on actual behaviors prompts some related questions. In a clinical visit, the salient question is whether the HPV vaccine is likely to change an individual person's risky behaviors postvaccine compared with prevaccine. However, the study did not directly address the phenomenon of behavioral change at the individual patient level. The current study separately considered the behaviors measured at the 3 time points. For example, it appears that group rates of condom use remained fairly stable at 59% to 63% across all time points but individual-level changes in a patient's condom use over time were not reported. It is likely that significant associations between risk perceptions and within-patient change would not have been found but this is not reported. Theoretically, another interesting study would be to randomize patients to receive or not receive the vaccine and compare the sexual behaviors of these 2 groups. However, such a study protocol would pose serious ethical issues given the known benefits of the vaccine and the current standard-of-care to administer the vaccine routinely.

In summary, this prospective study adds to the evidence to support the use of the HPV vaccine, beyond the most compelling reason that the vaccine is highly biologically efficacious. Parents and clinicians can feel reassured that incorrect perceptions of decreased risk postvaccine do not appear to translate into actual riskier behaviors. This type of information can be incorporated into clinical counseling for parents who express this concern and can further bolster clinicians to express strong recommendations for the HPV vaccine to adolescent girls.

L. Y. Hwang, MD

Association of Varying Number of Doses of Quadrivalent Human Papillomavirus Vaccine With Incidence of Condyloma
Herweijer E, Leval A, Ploner A, et al (Karolinska Institutet, Stockholm, Sweden; et al)
JAMA 311:597-603, 2014

Importance.—Determining vaccine dose-level protection is essential to minimize program costs and increase mass vaccination program feasibility. Currently, a 3-dose vaccination schedule is recommended for both the quadrivalent and bivalent human papillomavirus (HPV) vaccines. Although the primary goal of HPV vaccination programs is to prevent cervical cancer, condyloma related to HPV types 6 and 11 is also prevented with the quadrivalent vaccine and represents the earliest measurable preventable disease outcome for the HPV vaccine.

Objective.—To examine the association between quadrivalent HPV vaccination and first occurrence of condyloma in relation to vaccine dose in a population-based setting.

Design, Setting, and Participants.—An open cohort of all females aged 10 to 24 years living in Sweden (n = 1 045 165) was followed up between 2006 and 2010 for HPV vaccination and first occurrence of condyloma using the Swedish nationwide population-based health data registers.

Main Outcomes and Measures.—Incidence rate ratios (IRRs) and incidence rate differences (IRDs) of condyloma were estimated using Poisson regression with vaccine dose as a time-dependent exposure, adjusting for attained age and parental education, and stratified on age at first vaccination. To account for prevalent infections, models included a buffer period of delayed case counting.

Results.—A total of 20 383 incident cases of condyloma were identified during follow-up, including 322 cases after receipt of at least 1 dose of the vaccine. For individuals aged 10 to 16 years at first vaccination, receipt of 3 doses was associated with an IRR of 0.18 (95% CI, 0.15-0.22) for condyloma, whereas receipt of 2 doses was associated with an IRR of 0.29 (95% CI, 0.21-0.40). One dose was associated with an IRR of 0.31 (95% CI, 0.20-0.49), which corresponds to an IRD of 384 cases (95% CI, 305-464) per 100 000 person-years, compared with no vaccination. The corresponding IRDs for 2 doses were 400 cases (95% CI, 346-454) and for 3 doses, 459 cases (95% CI, 437-482). The number of prevented cases between 3 and 2 doses was 59 (95% CI, 2-117) per 100 000 person-years.

Conclusions and Relevance.—Although maximum reduction in condyloma risk was seen after receipt of 3 doses of quadrivalent HPV vaccine, receipt of 2 vaccine doses was also associated with a considerable reduction in condyloma risk. The implications of these findings for the relationship between number of vaccine doses and cervical cancer risk require further investigation.

▶ The industry-sponsored human papillomavirus (HPV) vaccine trials demonstrated the high efficacy of the vaccine in reducing abnormal cytology associated with the vaccine types and in reducing external lesions, specifically condyloma. Although the ultimate goal of the vaccine is to reduce cervical cancer, it was not realistic in the trials to use cancer outcomes because the rates of cervical cancer are too low in industrialized countries to power such studies.

The vaccine trials did demonstrate that overall efficacy rates were highest in younger women who were vaccinated and lowest in older women. This result is not surprising because the vaccine is considered preventive and not therapeutic. Once infected, the vaccine will not assist in prevention of disease to that HPV vaccine type. Acquisition of HPV is highly associated with number of sexual partners. Consequently, most countries target age groups that are most likely to not be sexually active to obtain the highest rates of efficacy. On the other hand, the vaccine trials included women already sexually active and showed high efficacy in this group. As a result, most countries also offer "catch-up" for women often up to 26 years of age.

Like most clinical trials, these initial studies are not likely to parallel real-life scenarios. First, the trials were limited to women with no more than 5 or 6 lifetime sexual partners, and second, compliance to 3 vaccinations was virtually 100%. Now that the vaccine has been implemented since 2007 in many countries, it is time to get a "real-life" look at vaccine efficacy. There are 2 vaccines on the market of which the quadrivalent vaccine has the lion's share in the United States. This vaccine includes the oncogenic HPV types 16 and 18 and also HPV 6 and 11, those associated with the development of genital warts (eg, condyloma). Hence, studies examining efficacy look for decreasing rates of condyloma or abnormal cytology. In the United States, these types of studies are difficult to conduct because there is no way to link vaccine histories and pathology registries on a large scale.

In the recent months, several studies have examined these "real-life" scenarios. Most studies come from countries that have large, countrywide registries that document vaccinations and disease outcomes. Herweijer et al reports on rates of condyloma in more than 1 million females aged 10 to 24 years of age followed up between 2006 and 2010. In 2007, Sweden had an opportunistic vaccine program for girls aged 13 to 17 years with an estimated 25% coverage rate, similar to the United States. In 2012, a school-based program was launched. Three registries were used in this study: a vaccine registry, a prescribed drug registry, and the patient registry. The latter 2 enabled the authors of this study to capture both prescriptions used for condyloma treatment and the documentation of the diagnosis of condyloma. As expected, many of the women did not complete the 3-dose series, so the study had the opportunity to examine efficacy in regards to number of doses, as well as age at first vaccination.

Not surprisingly, 3 doses of the vaccine begun at the younger age groups (10—13 years) had the greatest protection. The older the women at age of vaccination, the less protection observed. Although protection was seen among all the age groups and with any dose, 1 dose had least efficacy in all age groups (Table 2 in the original article).

Several articles have now been published with evidence that 1 and 2 doses results in some level of protection compared with no vaccination. This finding is likely not too surprising because several vaccines, such as those for hepatitis A and B, confer some protection with only 1 dose. The notion that 1 or 2 doses confers protection has already been embraced by many countries because the cost of vaccination is less in both purchasing price and scheduling. Although many agree that 1 or 2 doses results in some level of protection, the issue regarding durability remains the biggest controversy.

The durability of 3 doses looks excellent 7 to 9 years after vaccination. Much less is known about 1 or 2 doses. The consensus is that the mean interval between the first and second dose is likely critical for durability. The current regimen of 0-, 2-, and 6-month doses represents 2 vaccination doses with the third representing a booster for longer-term memory. Romanowski et al[1] found that a 0-, 2-month dose showed geometric mean antibody titers (GMT) for the bivalent vaccine that were inferior to a 0-, 6-month dose and the 0-, 6-month dose was similar to the three dose schedule. Age is also critical in that the younger the age of vaccination, the higher the antibody titer with 2 or 3 doses. This result is true not only immediately after vaccination but several years out. The mean interval in the Herweijer paper between doses 1 and 2 was 2.35 months (SD 1.44 months). Consequently, the long-term effect may not be as dramatic as the short-term effect.

The recent paper by Dobson et al[2] published in the *Journal of the American Medical Association*, directly compared 3 versus 2 doses (0, 6 months) in a randomized trial in girls aged 9 to 13 years. The GMT ratios for 2 versus 3 remained noninferior for all 4 vaccine genotypes at month 7 but not for HPV 18 by month 24 or HPV 6 at month 36. Many are not concerned because these titers are still much higher than that reported in natural infections and similar to those reported in women aged 16 to 26 years in the initial trials. The United Kingdom has just approved a 2-dose regimen for the quadrivalent vaccine for 9- to 13-year-olds with a mandate of a 6-month interval. If the interval is less than 6 months, it is recommended to give a third dose. If less than 3 doses is planned, it is also clear that age at vaccination will make a difference because the younger the age at vaccination, the higher the antibody titer is over time. A 3-dose regimen remains recommended for those 14 years and older. Two dose regimens are being used in other countries as well with the understanding that boosters may be required several years down the road.

It should be remembered that most condyloma are due to either HPV 6 or HPV 11, so efficacy is bound to appear higher than those calculated for abnormal cytology, which is due to many other HPV types not included in the current vaccines. Hence, efficacy rates for abnormal cytology is expected to look much lower for cytology and histology outcomes. Crowe et al[3] examined registry data from Australia, which has had a publicly funded HPV vaccine program implemented since 2007 in 12- to 17-year old girls in school and community catch-up phase for the 18- to 26-years-old. In this study, they focused on young women who had not started cervical cancer screening before the vaccination program. Completing 3 doses had an efficacy of 46% for high-grade disease and 2 doses, although lower, had an efficacy of 21%. Receiving only 1 dose in general did not show efficacy. As other studies, there was little no protection in women older than 22 years of age.

In summary, 3 doses of the HPV vaccine achieve the highest rates efficacy for condyloma and high-grade cervical disease. However, protection likely begins with the first dose and continues to increase with a second dose. If only 2 doses are to be recommended, long-term studies to examine durability will be essential. Meanwhile, we should make our best efforts to target the recommended age of 12 to 13 years with 3 doses of the vaccine to best protect our children's future risk for anogenital cancers.

A.-B. Moscicki, MD

References

1. Romanowski B, Schwarz TF, Ferguson LM, et al. Immunogenicity and safety of the HPV-16/18 AS04-adjuvanted vaccine administered as a 2-dose schedule compared with the licensed 3-dose schedule: results from a randomized study. *Hum Vaccin.* 2011;7:1374-1386.
2. Dobson SR, McNeil S, Dionne M, et al. Immunogenicity of 2 doses of HPV vaccine in younger adolescents vs 3 doses in young women: a randomized clinical trial. *JAMA.* 2013;309:1793-1802.
3. Crowe E, Pandeya N, Brotherton JM, et al. Effectiveness of quadrivalent human papillomavirus vaccine for the prevention of cervical abnormalities: case-control study nested within a population based screening programme in Australia. *BMJ.* 2014;348:1458.

Measuring School Health Center Impact on Access to and Quality of Primary Care

Gibson EJ, Santelli JS, Minguez M, et al (Columbia Univ Mailman School of Public Health, NY)
J Adolesc Health 53:699-705, 2013

Purpose.—School health centers (SHC) that provide comprehensive health care may improve access and quality of care for students; however, published impact data are limited.

Methods.—We evaluated access and quality of health services at an urban high school with a SHC compared with a school without a SHC, using a quasiexperimental research design. Data were collected at the beginning of the school year, using a paper and pencil classroom questionnaire (n = 2,076 students). We measured SHC impact in several ways including grade by school interaction terms.

Results.—Students at the SHC school were more likely to report having a regular healthcare provider, awareness of confidential services, support for health services in their school, and willingness to utilize those services. Students in the SHC school reported higher quality of care as measured by: respect for their health concerns, adequate time with the healthcare provider, understandable provider communications, and greater provider discussion at their last visit on topics such as sexual activity, birth control, emotions, future plans, diet, and exercise. Users of the SHC were also more likely to report higher quality of care, compared with either nonusers or students in the comparison school.

Conclusions.—Access to comprehensive health services via a SHC led to improved access to health care and improved quality of care. Impact was measureable on a school-wide basis but was greater among SHC users.

▶ Most schools in the United States provide health services, including medication delivery, therapy, and other services for children with special health care needs; identification and referral for common health problems; and health screenings. School health centers (SHCs) expand on these services by providing primary care, often including mental health and dental care, at the school. Approximately 2000 SHCs are operating in the United States and can be found in almost every state and territory. The Affordable Care Act acknowledged the role of SHCs in providing a health care safety net for underserved children and adolescents by allocating funds specifically for creating new SHCs and expanding services provided by existing SHCs.

Despite this support, SHCs face challenges related to financial sustainability and some pediatricians' concern that SHCs might fragment children's health care and threaten the medical home. Research on the role of SHCs in improving access to and quality of primary care has been limited by the challenges of coordinating between the school and health care systems, difficulty identifying the population to be studied (ie, determining who should be in the denominator), lack of data collection before implementation of SHCs, and lack of an adequate comparison or control group of students not exposed to SHCs.

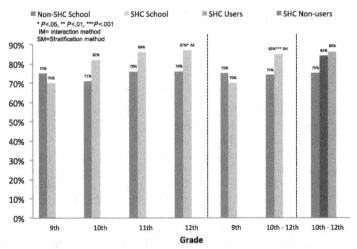

FIGURE 1.—Students reporting they have a regular provider or doctor to go to when they are sick. (Reprinted from Gibson EJ, Santelli JS, Minguez M, et al. Measuring school health center impact on access to and quality of primary care. *J Adolesc Health*. 2013;53:699-705, with permission from Society for Adolescent Health and Medicine.)

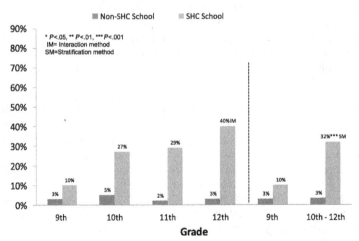

FIGURE 2.—Students who report using a school health center for medical care in the last 12 months. (Reprinted from Gibson EJ, Santelli JS, Minguez M, et al. Measuring school health center impact on access to and quality of primary care. *J Adolesc Health*. 2013;53:699-705, with permission from Society for Adolescent Health and Medicine.)

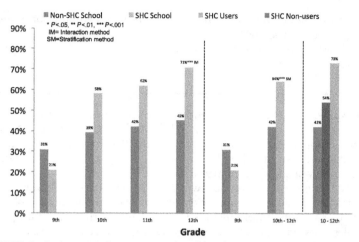

FIGURE 3.—Students reporting awareness of confidentiality in receiving adolescent health care. (Reprinted from Gibson EJ, Santelli JS, Minguez M, et al. Measuring school health center impact on access to and quality of primary care. *J Adolesc Health*. 2013;53:699-705, with permission from Society for Adolescent Health and Medicine.)

Gibson and colleagues overcame some of those challenges by working with the school system to identify a population of students in 1 school with an SHC and 1 school without an SHC. They compared ninth-grade students who did not have prior exposure to SHCs in the schools with and without a SHC and determined that the ninth-graders were not clinically or statistically different for key outcomes. These outcomes included identification of a regular doctor, awareness of confidentiality in receiving adolescent care, and measures of quality of care. The lack of difference in the 2 groups at the ninth-grade level strongly suggests that the later differences in outcomes between students in the school with and without a SHC seen at 10th through 12th grade are due to students' exposure to the SHC (Figs 1-3). By including more than 65% of the entire student population at each school, the investigators minimized concerns that students included in the study are somehow different from those who were not included in the study. In addition, the investigators were able to show that SHCs can have a schoolwide, population-based effect. The limitation of the study was that it was conducted in only 2 schools in 1 city with 1 SHC model; other populations and other SHC models may have different outcomes.

This study provides compelling evidence that SHCs can improve adolescents' access to high-quality primary care services. These findings should support efforts to fund expansion and maintenance of SHCs. In addition, at least for SHC models similar to that in this study, SHCs should not be seen as a threat to the medical home, but as a key player in the goal of providing a medical home for all adolescents.

M. A. Allison, MD, MSPH

Trends and Characteristics of Preventive Care Visits among Commercially Insured Adolescents, 2003-2010

Tsai Y, Zhou F, Wortley P, et al (Ctrs for Disease Control and Prevention (CDC), Atlanta, GA)
J Pediatr 164:625-630, 2014

Objective.—To examine preventive care visit patterns among commercially insured adolescents during 2003-2010. In 2005-2007, the Advisory Committee on Immunization Practices (ACIP) recommended 3 vaccines targeted at adolescents. We also investigate the relationship between preventive care visits and immunization.

Study Design.—Data were drawn from the MarketScan database. Adolescents aged 11-21 continuously enrolled in the same insurance plan during the calendar year were included. We calculated the annual proportion of adolescents with at least 1 preventive and 1 vaccination-related visit. Longitudinal analyses were conducted by following the 1992 birth cohort for 8 consecutive years.

Results.—The proportion of adolescents making at least 1 preventive visit increased from 24.6%-41.1% during 2003-2010. The rate of vaccination-related visits increased from 12.9%-26.3%. The magnitude of the increase in preventive and vaccination-related visits was greater during the years in which ACIP issued recommendations. The rates of preventive and vaccination-related visits were considerably higher among female and early adolescents and adolescents in managed care plans. Longitudinal analyses indicated that only 2.4% of adolescents had an annual preventive visit during the 8 years.

Conclusions.—Yearly improvements in preventive care visits by adolescents were substantial. ACIP recommendations may be associated with this improvement. However, ongoing efforts are needed to improve the use and delivery of preventive care services.

▶ It is very encouraging to see new vaccine recommendation as an effective strategy to bring adolescents to preventive visits. As the authors summarized succinctly, adolescents are underserved when it comes to the receipt of preventive care at a time when preventive counseling around high-risk behaviors are most needed.[1-3] When looking at the entire spectrum of health services utilized by adolescents, they have a higher tendency to use the emergency department (ED) as their usual source of care.[4] As pediatric/adolescent providers, we would love to see more adolescents come in to receive risk behavior counseling and to learn new skills to take care of their own health. Coming from a system's perspective, we also hope that adolescents would come in for preventive visits so that they could seek help through their pediatricians instead of the ED when an acute medical problem arises.

An interesting finding from this study is the reporting of longitudinal preventive visit rates of a cohort of adolescents in an 8-year span. It is concerning to see that a cohort of adolescents with 8 years of continued commercial insurance coverage have such a low preventive visit rate: only 2.4% of adolescents

TABLE 3.—Longitudinal Analysis on the Percentage of Adolescents Having at Least 1 Preventive Care Visit, 2003-2010 MarketScan Database

	Preventive Care Visits	
Having at Least 1 Visit	Male	Female
For 1 y	15.4	15.4
For 2 y	14.9	16.2
For 3 y	14.1	15.1
For 4 y	13.0	13.5
For 5 y	9.9	10.9
For 6 y	7.8	7.7
For 7 y	4.5	5.0
For 8 y	2.3	2.5
No visit during the 8 y	18.2	13.8
Mean number of visits	3.6	3.9

Adolescents included were those born in 1992 and enrolled in the same insurance plan for 8 years.

Reprinted from Journal Pediatrics. Tsai Y, Zhou F, Wortley P, et al. Trends and Characteristics of Preventive Care Visits among Commercially Insured Adolescents, 2003-2010. J Pediatr. 2014;164:625-630, Copyright 2014, with permission from Elsevier.

(2.3% for males; 2.5% for females) made at least 1 preventive visit each year throughout the 8-year study period (Table 3). By having stable commercial insurance coverage implied that these adolescents were from families not only with stable insurance coverage but also stable employment and income. A previous population study reported that adolescents who came from low-income families or who were uninsured had higher risk of not receiving preventive visits.[5] If only 2.4% had annual preventive visits for those with stable commercial insurance, what would the rate be for those who are uninsured, underinsured, or from a lower socioeconomic status?

The health policy landscape has changed significantly after this study period. The 2010 Affordable Care Act has strengthened the delivery of preventive care through both insurance coverage expansion and health plan benefit mandates (eg, no copayment for preventive care, expansion of covered preventive services).[2] Two Advisory Committee on Immunization Practices recommendations have been implemented since 2011: a quadrivalent meningococcal conjugate vaccine (Menactra) booster given after age 16 and human papillomavirus vaccine series for male adolescents starting at age 11.[6,7] It will be interesting to see if these policies facilitate further uptake of preventive visits among adolescents in the future.

J. S. Lau, MD

References

1. Irwin CE Jr. Clinical preventive services for adolescents: still a long way to go. *J Adolesc Health*. 2005;37:85-86.
2. Adams SH, Husting S, Zahnd E, Ozer EM. Adolescent preventive services: rates and disparities in preventive health topics covered during routine medical care in a California sample. *J Adolesc Health*. 2009;44:536-545.
3. Irwin CE Jr, Adams SH, Park MJ, Newacheck PW. Preventive care for adolescents: few get visits and fewer get services. *Pediatrics*. 2009;123:e565-e572.
4. Wilson KM, Klein JD. Adolescents who use the emergency department as their usual source of care. *Arch Pediatr Adolesc Med*. 2000;154:361-365.

5. English A. The patient protection and affordable care act of 2010: How does it help adolescents and young adults. Center for Adolescent Health and the Law. National Adolescent Health Information and Innovation Center [Internet]. August 2010. Accessed August 2, 2014.

6. Centers for Disease Control and Prevention (CDC). Recommendation of the Advisory Committee on Immunization Practices (ACIP) for use of quadrivalent meningococcal conjugate vaccine (MenACWY-D) among children aged 9 through 23 months at increased risk for invasive meningococcal disease. *MMWR Morb Mortal Wkly Rep*. 2011;60:1391-1392.

7. Centers for Disease Control and Prevention (CDC). Recommendations on the use of quadrivalent human papillomavirus vaccine in males—Advisory Committee on Immunization Practices (ACIP). *MMWR Morb Mortal Wkly Rep*. 2011;60: 1705-1708.

Lagging Behind or Not? Four Distinctive Social Participation Patterns Among Young Adults With Chronic Conditions

Sattoe JNT, Hilberink SR, van Staa A, et al (Rotterdam Univ, The Netherlands; et al)

J Adolesc Health 54:397-403, 2014

Purpose.—Typical childhood and adolescent development and acquiring self-management skills are crucial for a satisfying adult life and autonomy in social participation. The aims of this study were to identify patterns of autonomy in social participation and to explore differences between these patterns.

Methods.—Adolescents with various chronic conditions participating in a survey in 2006 (T0) were re-invited for a follow-up study (T1) in 2012. The young adults (18–25 years of age) assessed self management skills, their condition's impact on school or work, health-related quality of life (HRQoL), and social participation in various domains. Patterns were identified through cluster analysis. Differences between patterns were analyzed in bivariate and multivariate analyses.

Results.—Compared with healthy age-mates, our sample (n = 483) generally lagged behind in social participation. Four patterns emerged: typical developers, financially secure laggers, slow developers, and outgoing laggers. The patterns differed regarding gender, educational level, attending special education, having disability benefits, and degree of physical limitations. Groups with a higher level of autonomy in social participation did not necessarily have higher HRQoL but did report higher self-efficacy and independence at both measurements.

Conclusions.—Autonomy in some participation domains can coincide with a lack of autonomy in others. In addition, better social participation does not necessarily correlate with higher HRQoL, or vice versa. Yet, more social participation was associated with more self-efficacy and independence. Our results emphasize that there is no standardized approach. Clinicians should take care to address all life areas in clinical practice to screen patients' lived experiences and the need for social and self-management support.

▶ The many successes of modern pediatric medical care have meant that most youth with chronic conditions survive into adulthood. Although obviously necessary, survival alone is not a sufficient marker of success in our care of these patients. Those of us who care for this population all have stories of young adults who are living with childhood chronic conditions but are not thriving—the 30-year-old with sickle cell disease who spends more time in the hospital than at home, an 18-year-old with a liver transplant who never learned to read, a 25-year-old with diabetes who is so depressed, he stopped taking his insulin, for example. Stories like these remind us that our goal in adulthood for these youth is not only survival but also lives filled with happiness, friendships, and meaningful work and relationships.

Psychosocial engagement and achievement "in turn ... positively affect one's health and wellbeing."[1] For example, in the general US population, 25-year-olds with a bachelor's degree or higher have a life expectancy about 6 years longer than those without a high school diploma.[2] We would expect that youth with chronic conditions are likely to follow the same pattern as their peers in the general population.

Because psychosocial participation can be seen both as an outcome of youth development and as a predictor of future adult health outcomes, these aspects of patients' lives should be a central concern of medical providers who want to maximize the health of their patients. As these psychosocial outcomes span across childhood into young adulthood, a life course perspective is important for both pediatric and adult trained physicians.

In this study, the authors used a life course approach to understand psychosocial and health-related quality-of-life (HRQL) outcomes in young adults with chronic childhood conditions. They followed a Dutch cohort of youth with special health care needs to see how they had faired in terms of participation in adult life as well as HRQL, compared with age-matched control subjects. Furthermore, they wanted to understand how self-ratings of autonomy in the adolescent years correlated with independence in young adulthood. They tracked 483 youth with chronic conditions for 6 years, from 12 to 16 (at T0) to 18 to 24 years of age (mean age 20.6 years at T1).

The investigators measured different dimensions of autonomy in areas of social participation: financial, employment and education, housing, intimate relationships, and sexuality. They also looked at sociodemographic factors, as well as self-reported general independence during medical visits, and HRQL, among other ratings. Having multiple participation outcomes allowed them to create nuanced "patterns" of independence in young adults with chronic conditions.

The authors found that overall, this cohort had a lower level of autonomy than age-matched peers. Tellingly, they found that various social outcomes trended in different directions, and in fact, "full autonomy in one area of social participation can coincide with a total lack of autonomy in other areas."

TABLE 2.—Patterns Regarding Young Adults' Autonomy in Social Participation (% in Phase 3; n = 483)

Life areas patterns	Finances	Employment	Living	Relationships	Sexuality	Transportation	Leisure
1. Typical developers (n = 105)	100.0*	68.6	40.0	85.7*	78.1	96.2	55.2
2. Financially secure laggers (n = 109)	97.2*	55.0	.0*	.0*	22.9*	80.7	41.3
3. Slow developers (n = 96)	.0*	.0*	.0*	.0*	.0*	93.8	49.0
4. Outgoing laggers (n = 173)	.0*	.0*	28.3*	60.1	85.5	96.5	65.9
Total (n = 483)	43.7*	27.3*	18.8*	40.2*	52.8*	92.3	54.7
Reference group[a]	30.2[b]	63.3[c]	44.9[b]	64.0[d]	82.0[d]		
Post hoc[a]	1,2 > 3,4	1 > 2 > 3,4	1 > 4 > 2,3	1 > 4 > 2,3	1,2,4 > 3 1,4 > 2	1,3,4 >2 4> 2,3	1 > 2

[a]Chi-square post hoc test revealed that these differences were significant at $p < .05$.
[b]Reference group aged 20–25 years in 2011.
[c]Reference group aged 15–25 years in 2007.
[d]Data presented are from a report on Dutch youths (15–25 years of age) in 2005.
*$p < .001$ in binominal tests to test whether there are significant differences between our sample and Dutch age-mates.
Reprinted from Journal of Adolescent Health. Sattoe JNT, Hilberink SR, van Staa A, et al. Lagging Behind or Not? Four Distinctive Social Participation Patterns Among Young Adults With Chronic Conditions. J Adolesc Health. 2014;54:397-403, Copyright 2014, with permission from Society for Adolescent Health and Medicine.

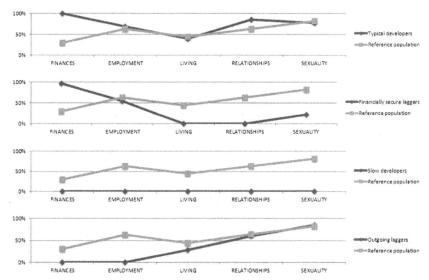

FIGURE 1.—Comparison of social participation between patterns and reference population. The x-axis represents the proportion of young adults in Phase 3, whereas the y-axis represents the life areas. (Reprinted from Sattoe JNT, Hilberink SR, van Staa A, et al. Lagging behind or not? Four distinctive social participation patterns among young adults with chronic conditions. *J Adolesc Health.* 2014;54:397-403, with permission from Society for Adolescent Health and Medicine.)

In post hoc analyses, the authors identified four common "patterns" of adult-like social participation: (1) "typical developers" were those who were most like the age-matched population, (2) "financially secure laggers" were less independent then peers in all areas except financial independence, (3) "slow developers" were the least fully independent across the board, and (4) "outgoing laggers" matched their peers in terms of social participation but were dependent on others in terms of income and employment (Table 2 and Fig 1).

The authors sought to identify if patterns of behavior and independence in adolescence were predictive of social outcomes and HRQL 6 years later. Self-efficacy at the baseline assessment was not associated with the future level of independence. Yet they did find that higher independence during consultations (medical visits) in adolescence was associated with a more age-typical developmental pattern at follow-up.

The patterns the authors describe are all based on post hoc data analysis, and as such it is difficult to determine directionality. Given this limitation in study design, the study might be best used for generating hypotheses for future inquiry. For example, in this cohort, those whose patterns of engagement were most similar to the population at large (ie, the "typical developers") had lower self-rated HRQL. The authors interpret this to suggest that being more active in society means these youth run into health-related barriers more than other youth, and this influences how they rate their HRQL. However, this group had a lower HRQL at baseline, a higher percentage receiving special education, and less educational attainment in young adulthood compared with the "slow developers" or "outgoing laggers." The typical developer group (along with the "financially secure laggers") also has a higher rate of receiving Wajong (a system that appears to be similar to Social Security Income for those with significant disabilities in the United States). If so, their lower HRQL in young adulthood is more a reflection on their overall health condition then their pattern of societal participation.

It is difficult to generalize the concept of "financially secure laggers" from the Dutch context. Certainly a financially independent young adult in the United States supporting himself or herself with his or her Social Security Income payment might be independent, but the word "secure" would not apply in that he or she is set on a path to poverty in adulthood if other financial support is not available. Likewise, patterns of social participation described in this study may not be transferrable to societies outside the Netherlands. It would be interesting to compare how youth with chronic conditions fare in different countries to better understand the role that social policies can play in societal engagement in adulthood.

A final limitation is that participants in this study were still relatively young at follow-up (mean age 20.6 years). The benefits of prolonged parental support are likely to continue into young adulthood. Though logistically challenging, seeing how this cohort of youth are fairing toward the end of their 20s might produce a more complete understanding of predictors of young adult outcomes.

With the expansion of insurance eligibility from the Affordable Care Act, more children are likely to qualify for ongoing insurance coverage into adulthood by the same payor (eg, by Medicaid and/or in private systems such as Kaiser). This long-term fiscal responsibility should help generate more interest and financial value in understanding these social determinants of health over the life course.

This study highlights the fact that adult psychosocial and societal participation outcomes are multifaceted, and studies looking at outcomes of the transition to adulthood will need to take that into account. There is no overall "level of independence" to be measured. As they note, an individual could be high in some aspects of independence in adulthood and quite low in other areas.

The study demonstrated how trajectories are delayed for some youth with chronic conditions (eg, the "slow developers" and "outgoing laggers"). Thus the loss of the multidisciplinary support that is common when youth move from pediatrics into adult medical care in the United States is especially harmful for these youth. It is important, then, to find ways to continue supportive, whole-person care through changes in the organization and funding of adult health care services. The emphasis on the patient-centered medical home within internal medicine is a potentially promising example of this.

This focus on psychosocial outcomes will require a change in educational curricula for the next generation of medical trainees. Providers will need to understand the importance of social determinants on health outcomes, and its developmental trajectories over the life course. It will not be enough to simply call the social worker or psychologist (especially given that these professionals are not present in many clinical practices). Physicians need to be able to do thorough assessments (beyond HEADSS) and know which recommendations or referrals are most likely to benefit the youth and his or her family. Medical providers need to know how to work as part of a multidisciplinary team, ideally with psychosocial professionals, and as a team identify appropriate resources to promote overall patient well-being.

There are questions for future research suggested by this study: How can education, vocation, and social participation be assessed effectively and efficiently within the medical setting? What kinds of interventions might best support youth to maximize adult independence and HRQL? Finally, how can team-based, holistic multidisciplinary care be organized and paid for in practice?

D. S. Lotstein, MD, MPH

References

1. Sattoe JN, et al. Lagging Behind or Not? Four Distinctive Social Participation Patterns Among Young Adults With Chronic Conditions. *Journal of Adolescent Health..* 2014;54:397-403.
2. Robert Wood Johnson Foundation Commission to Build a Healthier America. *More Education, Longer Life*. Princeton, NJ: 2008. Data: National Longitudinal Mortality Study, 1988-1998.

2 Allergy and Dermatology

Peanut, milk, and wheat intake during pregnancy is associated with reduced allergy and asthma in children
Bunyavanich S, Rifas-Shiman SL, Platts-Mills TA, et al (Icahn School of Medicine at Mount Sinai, NY; Harvard Pilgrim Health Care Inst, Boston, MA; Univ of Virginia Health System, Charlottesville; et al)
J Allergy Clin Immunol 133:1373-1382, 2014

Background.—Maternal diet during pregnancy may affect childhood allergy and asthma.

Objective.—We sought to examine the associations between maternal intake of common childhood food allergens during early pregnancy and childhood allergy and asthma.

Methods.—We studied 1277 mother-child pairs from a US prebirth cohort unselected for any disease. Using food frequency questionnaires administered during the first and second trimesters, we assessed maternal intake of common childhood food allergens during pregnancy. In mid-childhood (mean age, 7.9 years), we assessed food allergy, asthma, allergic rhinitis, and atopic dermatitis by questionnaire and serum-specific IgE levels. We examined the associations between maternal diet during pregnancy and childhood allergy and asthma. We also examined the cross-sectional associations between specific food allergies, asthma, and atopic conditions in mid-childhood.

Results.—Food allergy was common (5.6%) in mid-childhood, as was sensitization to at least 1 food allergen (28.0%). Higher maternal peanut intake (each additional z score) during the first trimester was associated with 47% reduced odds of peanut allergic reaction (odds ratio [OR], 0.53; 95% CI, 0.30-0.94). Higher milk intake during the first trimester was associated with reduced asthma (OR, 0.83; 95% CI, 0.69-0.99) and allergic rhinitis (OR, 0.85; 95% CI, 0.74-0.97). Higher maternal wheat intake during the second trimester was associated with reduced atopic dermatitis (OR, 0.64; 95% CI, 0.46-0.90). Peanut, wheat, and soy allergy were each cross-sectionally associated with increased childhood asthma, atopic dermatitis, and allergic rhinitis (ORs, 3.6 to 8.1).

Conclusion.—Higher maternal intake of peanut, milk, and wheat during early pregnancy was associated with reduced odds of mid-childhood allergy and asthma.

▶ "Doctor, I craved peanuts during my pregnancy, ate them all the time, and I am sure that is why my child has a peanut allergy."

It is human nature to look for causation in our personal experiences. Based on limited data, the American Academy of Pediatrics (AAP) in 2000 suggested that in the context of a family history of allergy, mothers should consider avoiding peanuts during pregnancy.[1] There has been somewhat of a knee-jerk assumption that if foods such as milk, egg, peanuts, nuts, and fish are notorious allergens, then avoiding them is a good idea. However, this approach has flaws. First, dietary proteins can cross the placenta, and it may be that such exposure provides an opportunity for development of tolerance. Second, foods are more than their proteins. For example, fish has omega-3 fatty acids that may reduce allergic immune responses.[2] The effect of food nutrients (vitamins, fats, antioxidants, etc) on immune responses may explain why different foods tracked with different allergy outcomes in the current study. In 2008, the AAP rescinded its suggestion about maternal avoidance of peanut during pregnancy.[3] This study adds evidence to the response that can be offered to the mother who is apt to put herself on a "guilt trip." We do not have evidence that her pregnancy diet caused this allergy. We have to admit, however, that we do not have definitive answers. This study is just 1 of a number on this topic. For example, different studies have come to different conclusions regarding the impact of ingesting peanut during pregnancy on peanut allergy outcomes.[4-6] The different conclusions drawn from the studies could reflect different study methods and the study populations, including selection for risk of allergy, geography, and diet. The current study evaluated a population from the United States that was not preselected for allergy risks, but the study population was from Massachusetts and had a high rate of peanut allergy (4.9%), which may affect generalizability.

Another aspect that was not evaluated in this study and is a confounding factor in any such work is the sum of all types of dietary and environmental exposures on the child after birth, in addition to genetic and epigenetic influences. Presumably, the maternal diet in early pregnancy may be associated with additional lifestyle factors of relevance, including numerous dietary and environmental exposures (eg, pets, infection) for the infant and child. For diet alone, the variables include breastfeeding, timing of introduction of whole proteins, including any infant formula, and the types of the foods selected.

It is worth noting that studies have increasingly supported the notion that extensive delays in introducing allergens such as peanut, egg, and milk are associated with increased rather than decreased risks of allergy.[7] A leading theory as to why this may be the case is that not eating the allergen prevents oral tolerance from ensuing during a period when the infant may be exposed to the food through sensitizing routes, such as the skin, especially if there is atopic dermatitis.[8]

Given the current state of knowledge, allergen-exclusion diets during pregnancy are not recommended, as supported by the study highlighted here;

breastfeeding is recommended; and a "healthy diet" that does not go out of the way to avoid any particular allergenic foods for otherwise healthy infants is probably the best advice.[3,9,10]

S. H. Sicherer, MD

References

1. American Academy of Pediatrics. Committee on Nutrition. Hypoallergenic infant formulas. *Pediatrics.* 2000;106:346-349.
2. Sausenthaler S, Koletzko S, Schaaf B, et al. Maternal diet during pregnancy in relation to eczema and allergic sensitization in the offspring at 2 y of age. *Am J Clin Nutr.* 2007;85:530-537.
3. Greer FR, Sicherer SH, Burks AW. Effects of early nutritional interventions on the development of atopic disease in infants and children: the role of maternal dietary restriction, breastfeeding, timing of introduction of complementary foods, and hydrolyzed formulas. *Pediatrics.* 2008;121:183-191.
4. Sicherer SH, Wood RA, Stablein D, et al. Maternal consumption of peanut during pregnancy is associated with peanut sensitization in atopic infants. *J Allergy Clin Immunol.* 2010;126:1191-1197.
5. Lack G, Fox D, Northstone K, Golding J. Factors associated with the development of peanut allergy in childhood. *N Engl J Med.* 2003;348:977-985.
6. Hsu JT, Missmer SA, Young MC, et al. Prenatal food allergen exposures and odds of childhood peanut, tree nut, or sesame seed sensitization. *Ann Allergy Asthma Immunol.* 2013;111:391-396.
7. Sicherer SH, Sampson HA. Food allergy: Epidemiology, pathogenesis, diagnosis, and treatment. *J Allergy Clin Immunol.* 2014;133:291-307.
8. Lack G. Update on risk factors for food allergy. *J Allergy Clin Immunol.* 2012; 129:1187-1197.
9. Muraro A, Halken S, Arshad SH, et al. EAACI food allergy and anaphylaxis guidelines. Primary prevention of food allergy. *Allergy.* 2014;69:590-601.
10. Fleischer DM, Spergel JM, Assa'ad AH, Pongracic JA. Primary prevention of allergic disease through nutritional interventions. *J Allergy Clin Immunol Pract.* 2013;1:29-36.

Prospective Study of Peripregnancy Consumption of Peanuts or Tree Nuts by Mothers and the Risk of Peanut or Tree Nut Allergy in Their Offspring

Frazier AL, Camargo CA Jr, Malspeis S, et al (Dana-Farber Children's Cancer Ctr, Boston, MA; Brigham and Women's Hosp and Harvard Med School, Boston, MA; et al)
JAMA Pediatr 168:156-162, 2014

Importance.—The etiology of the increasing childhood prevalence of peanut or tree nut (P/TN) allergy is unknown.

Objective.—To examine the association between peripregnancy consumption of P/TN by mothers and the risk of P/TN allergy in their offspring.

Design, Setting, and Participants.—Prospective cohort study. The 10 907 participants in the Growing Up Today Study 2, born between January 1, 1990, and December 31, 1994, are the offspring of women who previously reported their diet during, or shortly before or after, their pregnancy with this child as part of the ongoing Nurses' Health Study II. In 2006, the offspring reported physician-diagnosed food allergy. Mothers were asked to confirm the diagnosis and to provide available medical records and allergy test results. Two board-certified pediatricians, including a board-certified allergist/immunologist, independently reviewed each potential case and assigned a confirmation code (eg, likely food allergy) to each case. Unadjusted and multivariable logistic regression analyses were used to evaluate associations between peripregnancy consumption of P/TN by mothers and incident P/TN allergy in their offspring.

Exposure.—Peripregnancy consumption of P/TN.

Main Outcomes and Measures.—Physician-diagnosed P/TN allergy in offspring.

Results.—Among 8205 children, we identified 308 cases of food allergy (any food), including 140 cases of P/TN allergy. The incidence of P/TN allergy in the offspring was significantly lower among children of the 8059 nonallergic mothers who consumed more P/TN in their peripregnancy diet (≥ 5 times vs <1 time per month: odds ratio = 0.31; 95%CI, 0.13-0.75; $P_{trend} = .004$). By contrast, a nonsignificant positive association was observed between maternal peripregnancy P/TN consumption and risk of P/TN allergy in the offspring of 146 P/TN-allergic mothers ($P_{trend} = .12$). The interaction between maternal peripregnancy P/TN consumption and maternal P/TN allergy status was statistically significant ($P_{interaction} = .004$).

Conclusions and Relevance.—Among mothers without P/TN allergy, higher peripregnancy consumption of P/TN was associated with lower risk of P/TN allergy in their offspring. Our study supports the hypothesis that early allergen exposure increases tolerance and lowers risk of childhood food allergy.

▶ There is little question within the medical literature that the past 2 decades have seen an increased prevalence of peanut and tree-nut allergic children within the developed world. Because childhood immunoglobulin (Ig)E-mediated food allergy now affects almost 3% to 5% of the pediatric population, this issue extends well beyond the molecular interactions into the realm of public health and public policy. From the molecular immunologic standpoint, breast milk or formula is the first antigenic challenge a newborn infant faces. Undoubtedly, the first question for parents after a diagnosis of an IgE-mediated anaphylactic reaction is whether this could have been influenced by events during the pregnancy or nursing. Numerous studies, including the article by Frazier et al, attempt to shed light on this issue.

The article has several strengths, but an overlooked aspect is the comprehensive review of the animal model data and review of previous studies of the impact of allergenic food consumption during and after pregnancy. Furthermore, the discussion summarizes the background to the recent American Academy of Pediatrics Committee on Nutrition's statement regarding maternal dietary recommendations in regards to food allergy prevention and the respective changes in the recommendations.

Although the author's findings demonstrate no causal relationship between maternal nut consumption and development of food allergies in subsequent offspring, there remain numerous factors that cannot be fully accounted for. First, development of IgE-mediated food allergies probably revolve around the complex interaction of genetic, epigenetic, and environmental factors in both the in utero and ex utero phases, particularly through nursing and the development of the immunologically potent gut microbiome. Research is actively blossoming in this area but offers no better explanation at this time.

In addition, retrospective dietary studies can never fully delineate the complex interaction of food choices at crucial times of pregnancy and nursing. Maternal recall is always an issue, and many women may or may not be ingesting nut or allergenic foods without any knowledge. Currently, there is no consensus on sensitization dosages versus tolerance dosages of dietary antigen in early infancy and childhood.

As the authors note, demographics may have inadvertent effects of food allergy prevention such as the affect of higher antioxidant consumption in nut-ingesting mothers that could have a protective affect in this particular group. Mothers who have access to increased dietary nuts may also be avoiding other processed foods, which may have an impact on infant outcome. As many astute clinicians note, the demographics of this maternal cohort may also play a much larger role than the authors acknowledge. The maternal cohorts in the study are more than 95% white. Given the broader implications of the development of IgE-mediated food allergies and the increasing prevalence of atopic disease in minority populations, specifically African Americans, genetic differences may have a much larger role in the development of the clinical phenotype. The clinician can only assume that these findings are applicable to this white ethnic cohort and may not be appropriate to others.

What clinicians, and more importantly parents, are looking for is consistent evidence that dietary or other choices during pregnancy or afterward can have positive impacts on the prevention of IgE-mediated food allergies. Although this article does suggest that purposeful ingestion of nuts during pregnancy did not have a negative impact on outcomes, there remain large gaps in the general knowledge base and will likely change recommendations as the pendulum swings back. For now, eating a good healthy diet with variable sources of fresh, wholesome foods is still probably the best recommendation any pediatrician can offer an expectant parent to ensure the healthiest infant.

H. L. Leo, MD

Real-life experiences with omalizumab for the treatment of chronic urticaria

Sussman G, Hébert J, Barron C, et al (Univ of Toronto, Ontario, Canada; Laval Univ, Quebec, Canada)
Ann Allergy Asthma Immunol 112:170-174, 2014

Background.—Evidence has shown that omalizumab, a subcutaneous anti-IgE monoclonal antibody, is highly effective for the treatment of chronic urticaria.

Objective.—To evaluate omalizumab 150 mg/month in severe, difficult-to-treat, chronic urticaria in a real-life setting.

Methods.—This prospective open-label study evaluated of 150 mg of omalizumab in severe urticaria defined by a 7-day urticaria activity score (UAS-7) higher than 30, a history of oral glucocorticoid use, and by suboptimal response to previous treatments. Two subgroups of patients at different centers (Toronto and Quebec City, Canada) were included. The primary efficacy evaluation was a change in UAS-7 from baseline. A quantitative medication score assessed the use of other anti-urticarial medications.

Results.—Sixty-eight patients were included: 61 with chronic spontaneous urticaria, 6 with cold urticaria, and 1 with urticarial vasculitis. Patients were followed for up to 25 months. In Toronto, mean UAS-7 decreased from 32.2 at baseline to 5.7 after the last omalizumab treatment. Seventy-nine percent achieved complete remission during omalizumab therapy (UAS-7 0) and 6 (18%) showed improvement but never achieved complete remission. The most common maintenance dosing intervals were 1 to 3 months. In Quebec City, from baseline to 18 months, mean UAS-7 decreased from 24.4 to 2.2 and the quantitative medication score decreased from 13.3 to 3.0. All 6 patients with cold urticaria became symptom free, with a significant decrease of their cold stimulation tolerance test.

Conclusion.—Omalizumab 150 mg was effective in difficult to treat patients with severe, chronic urticaria refractory to recommended treatments who usually required prednisone. Omalizumab induced a longlasting positive response and was well tolerated without side effects.

▶ The era of biologics has arrived, and omalizumab, an anti-immunoglobulin (Ig)E monoclonal antibody, is the first to make headway in pediatric diseases. In this article, Sussman et al show that omalizumab can induce remission in adults with refractory chronic urticaria, and, most important, allows the subjects to come off glucocorticoids. This article has potential implications for pediatric patients.

Unlike its predecessors, this study showed the strength of omalizumab to treat patients with disease refractory to existing regimens. The phase III randomized double-blind placebo-controlled trial of omalizumab for chronic urticaria published in the *New England Journal of Medicine* included a much less sick patient population—subjects who failed first line-treatment, the approved doses of H1 blockers, and remained symptomatic.[1] The participants in the current study had failed much higher doses, second- and third-line regimens treatments, and had several rounds of steroids and remained symptomatic. Despite being a much sicker patient population, omalizumab still showed significant benefit.

The primary limitation of this study is the design—it is not randomized, blinded, or placebo controlled. It is open label and thus subject to bias by the investigators, the physicians evaluating the subjects, and the subjects themselves. The symptom reduction may be overestimated by both the subjects and the physicians. The control in the study was the individual participants' baseline symptoms before receiving omalizumab, not a placebo. These flaws, however, are characteristic of the real world of medicine, in which patients know what drugs they take and often have to pay for their medications out of pocket.

The current major barrier to the use of omalizumab is the cost. Sussman et al touched on this problem, noting that many of the subjects had to pay (Canadian) $700 per dose of omalizumab. Two studies done in the United States found omalizumab not to be cost-beneficial in adults with severe asthma, despite improvement in quality of life.[2,3] Similar studies have not been done in children, and the benefit of therapy early on in life may substantially reduce the long-term medical costs. Importantly, Sussman et al showed that patients with chronic urticaria responded to both fixed and on-demand dosing regimens; an on-demand dosing regimen may be less expensive and thus more cost-beneficial. More work is needed to determine the minimal, and thus least expensive, frequency and duration of omalizumab dosing in each given disease. Furthermore, if more widespread applicability is found with omalizumab, the cost will likely decrease.

Although this study was done in adults, the implications for children are enormous. The Inner-City Anti-IgE Therapy for Asthma (ICATA) study demonstrated that adding omalizumab to guidelines-based therapy dramatically reduced symptomatic days and the need for additional medications to control asthma.[4] The implication from Sussman et al is that these findings may be applicable to those with the most refractory disease, and omalizumab may spare children with refractory allergic diseases steroids and their associated lifelong consequences. Given the strong evidence supporting its use, the most recent guidelines from the National Asthma Education and Prevention Program recommend the use of omalizumab for children 12 years of age and older with moderate-to-severe asthma. Furthermore, the Food and Drug Administration has approved omalizumab for children 12 years of age and older with allergic asthma, while the European Union has approved its use for children as young as age 6 years.

Targeted use in patients at high risk for disease morbidity, and potential utility in even altering or modifying disease progression, development, or even onset may be the future. In the ICATA study, omalizumab was the most effective for those with sensitization and exposure to cockroach and dust mites. Other studies have looked for biomarkers, such as FeNO, eosinophilia, and periostin, to identify asthmatic patients that will respond to omalizumab, although using these markers for this purpose has not yet made it into clinical practice.[4-8] Furthermore, there are numerous trials on going examining omalizumab for other pediatric diseases, in particular atopic dermatitis and food allergy (NCT02062814, NCT01510626, NCT01157117, NCT00949078, NCT01781637, NCT02194530, NCT00968110, NCT01290913, NCT00932282). Phase I trials of omalizumab in atopic dermatitis have also shown promise.[9] More research is needed to determine if perhaps use of omalizumab may halt the atopic march in those most at risk. Nevertheless, until research evidence points toward lasting disease modification, omalizumab will likely be reserved for those with severe, refractory disease, like those included in this "real-life" study.

M. F. Huffaker, MD

W. Phipatanakul, MD, MS

References

1. Maurer M, Rosen K, Hsieh HJ, et al. Omalizumab for the treatment of chronic idiopathic or spontaneous urticaria. *N Engl J Med.* 2013;368:924-935.
2. Wu AC, Paltiel AD, Kuntz KM, Weiss ST, Fuhlbrigge AL. Cost-effectiveness of omalizumab in adults with severe asthma: results from the Asthma Policy Model. *J Allergy Clin Immunol.* 2007;120:1146-1152.
3. Campbell JD, Spackman DE, Sullivan SD. The costs and consequences of omalizumab in uncontrolled asthma from a USA payer perspective. *Allergy.* 2010;65: 1141-1148.
4. Busse WW, Morgan WJ, Gergen PJ, et al. Randomized trial of omalizumab (anti-IgE) for asthma in inner-city children. *N Engl J Med.* 2011;364:1005-1015.
5. Hanania NA, Wenzel S, Rosen K, et al. Exploring the effects of omalizumab in allergic asthma: an analysis of biomarkers in the EXTRA study. *Am J Respir Crit Care Med.* 2013;187:804-811.
6. Maselli DJ, Singh H, Diaz J, Peters JI. Efficacy of omalizumab in asthmatic patients with IgE levels above 700 IU/mL: a retrospective study. *Ann Allergy Asthma Immunol.* 2013;110:457-461.
7. Bousquet J, Wenzel S, Holgate S, Lumry W, Freeman P, Fox H. Predicting response to omalizumab, an anti-IgE antibody, in patients with allergic asthma. *Chest.* 2004;125:1378-1386.
8. Wahn U, Martin C, Freeman P, Blogg M, Jimenez P. Relationship between pre-treatment specific IgE and the response to omalizumab therapy. *Allergy.* 2009; 64:1780-1787.
9. Iyengar SR, Hoyte EG, Loza A, et al. Immunologic effects of omalizumab in children with severe refractory atopic dermatitis: a randomized, placebo-controlled clinical trial. *Int Arch Allergy Immunol.* 2013;162:89-93.

Six Children With Allergic Contact Dermatitis to Methylisothiazolinone in Wet Wipes (Baby Wipes)

Chang MW, Nakrani R (Univ of Connecticut School of Medicine, Farmington)
Pediatrics 133:e434-e438, 2014

Methylchloroisothiazolinone/methylisothiazolinone (MCI/MI) is a combination preservative used in personal care and household products and is a common cause of allergic contact dermatitis (ACD). Recently, MI alone, without MCI, has been increasingly used in consumer products in attempts to minimize allergic reactions. Wet wipes are extensively tested and traditionally believed to be innocuous. MI in wet wipes ("baby wipes") has not been previously reported to cause ACD in children in the United States. Only 1 previous report of ACD in a child in Belgium has been recently reported. We report 6 children with chronic, perianal/buttock, and facial eczematous dermatitis, refractory to multiple topical and oral antibiotics and corticosteroids. All tested positive to MCI/MI on patch testing. None wore diapers. All patients had been using wet wipes

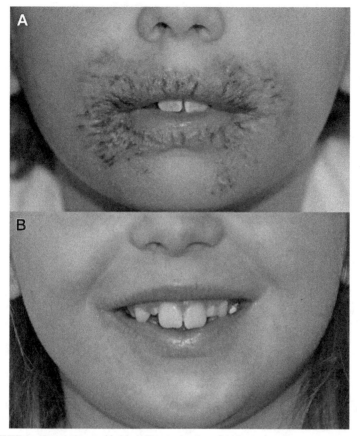

FIGURE 1.—Case 1, 8-year-old girl. A, On presentation, chronic, erythematous, eczematous patches and plaques with crusting and fissuring around mouth are noted. B, Rapid resolution occurred after discontinuation of offending wipes. (Reprinted from Chang MW, Nakrani R. Six children with allergic contact dermatitis to methylisothiazolinone in wet wipes (baby wipes). *Pediatrics.* 2014;133:e434-e438, with permission from the American Academy of Pediatrics.)

containing MI (without MCI) to affected areas. Discontinuation of wipes resulted in rapid and complete resolution. This is the first report of pediatric ACD to MI in wet wipes in the United States, and the largest series to date. ACD to MI in wet wipes is frequently misdiagnosed as eczema, impetigo, or psoriasis. Wet wipes are increasingly marketed in personal care products for all ages, and MI exposure and sensitization will likely increase. Dermatitis of the perianal, buttock, facial, and hand areas with a history of wet wipe use should raise suspicion of ACD to MI and prompt appropriate patch testing. Rapid resolution occurs after the allergen exposure is eliminated. All isothiozolinones should be avoided in personal care and household products for these patients.

▶ Flash! Baby wipes meant to prevent diaper rash cause diaper rash. What is a parent to do? Well for one thing, don't use the wipes if they contain

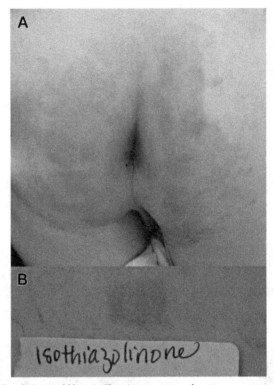

FIGURE 2.—Case 2, 6-year-old boy. A, Chronic, recurrent erythematous, eczematous patches and pla-ques on the perianal region. B, Patch test result displaying positive reaction to MCI/MI on day 3. (Reprin-ted from Chang MW, Nakrani R. Six children with allergic contact dermatitis to methylisothiazolinone in wet wipes (baby wipes). *Pediatrics*. 2014;133:e434-e438, with permission from the American Academy of Pediatrics.)

methylisothiazolinone (MI), particularly on older children who are no longer in diapers. When asked to write a commentary on a case series of 6 children who had contact dermatitis that resolved after discontinuing use of MI-containing wet wipes, I wondered what I could possibly add to the obvious statement, "Don't use MI-containing wet wipes." The answer came through investigative journalism.

For the clinician well versed in pattern recognition, skimming this article reveals specific cues such as "use of baby wipes" and "chronic eczematous rash," despite "treatment for the usual causes" with "the rash appearing around the mouth and perineum" (Figs 1 and 2). Acrodermatitis enteropathica readily comes to mind—but wait, the photos and Table 1 are of 6 children aged beyond their infant diaper years (3–8 years). One would think it would be rather obvious; signs of poor nutrition would probably appear before 6 months of age. Armed with the already-stated diagnosis given in the article title, plus the term "baby wipes," one cannot help but question why the baby wipes were being applied to older children, which is not the original intent of the product. The referenced case reports also involve children aged 4 years and 5 years. Time to investigate further.

TABLE 1.—Characteristics of Patients With ACD to MI in Wet Wipes (Baby Wipes)

	Patient 1	Patient 2	Patient 3	Patient 4	Patient 5	Patient 6
Age, y	8	6	4	4	4	3
Gender	Girl	Boy	Girl	Girl	Boy	Girl
Location	Perioral, perianal	Perioral, perianal	Anogenital	Perianal	Perianal	Perianal, trunk, extremities
Previous treatment	OA, TA, TCS	TCS	OA, TCS, TL	TCS	AF, OA, TCS, OCS	AF, TA, TCS
History of eczema	No	Yes	No	No	No	Yes
Patch test results on day 3 (T.R.U.E. Test)	++ MCI/MI	+MCI/MI	++ MCI/MI	++ MCI/MI +Cobalt	++ MCI/MI	+ MCI/MI + Nickel + Lanolin
Duration of symptoms before diagnosis	11 mo	12 mo	2 mo	1 mo	5 mo	6 mo
Brand of wipes used	Cottonelle Huggies	Huggies	Cottonelle	Cottonelle	Cottonelle	Cottonelle

Six children using wipes containing MI had positive patch test results and rapid resolution on discontinuation of offending wipes. Patch test interpretation (International Contact Dermatitis Research Group scoring): +/? (erythema), + (erythema + papule), ++ (erythema + papule + small vesicles), +++ (erythema + papule + bullae). AF, topical antifungal; OA, oral antibiotics; OCS, oral corticosteroids; TA, topical antibiotics; TCS, topical corticosteroids; TL, topical tacrolimus.

Reprinted from Chang MW, Nakrani R. Six children with allergic contact dermatitis to methylisothiazolinone in wet wipes (baby wipes). Pediatrics. 2014;133:e434-e438, with permission from the American Academy of Pediatrics.

After a brief investigation, I find that methylisothiazolinone is an isothiazolinone-derived preservative added to water-containing solutions to control microbial growth. Its presence in baby wipes is to prevent bacterial growth and "slime," a term describing the unorganized layer of extracellular material that bacteria produce to protect themselves from environmental dangers. (That must be why, back when I changed my children's diapers, those old wet wipes felt oily to touch. Bacteria must have been reproducing.) How much is MI used in wet wipes? A trip to the infant hygiene section in the local stores revealed that not a single wet wipe product contains MI, no matter which brand. A subsequent exploration of the website of the corporation responsible for manufacturing the baby wipes mentioned in the article disclosed the corporation's recent removal of MI from their baby-wipe product line. Apparently the corporation responded to media reports of MI skin sensitivity, perhaps spawned by this very article. Why bother writing a commentary on this article if MI is indeed removed from the market?

The answer is this: MI is still out there. A further Internet search finds MI used in other liquid hygiene products such as shampoo. (That must be why old shampoo feels slimy to me; it's not just due to drying-out liquid soap.) An important lesson learned.

Yet other questions remain. Why are there no case reports of diapered infants with allergic contact dermatitis due to MI? One reference at the end of the article describes the results of applying methylchloroisothiazolinone/methylisothiazolinone (MCI/MI) skin patches to children aged 5 months to 12 years, with resulting positive skin reactions; however, there are no case reports of diapered infants with allergic contact dermatitis due to MI. Before the MI removal, were there infants in diapers with persistent rashes due to MI-containing baby wipes? How many parents did not realize they were causing the rash with baby wipes? Or does MI skin sensitivity develop over years of exposure? What else are baby wipes used for, besides infants? Again an Internet search uncovers that baby wipes are being used for many tasks on people of all ages, including as facial makeup remover, stain remover, nasal tissue, skin cooler, hand wiper, hair "tamer," and toilet paper substitute.[1,2] We must remember that when we treat our patients for unexplainable signs and symptoms, our patients may be using a commercial product for unintended purposes.

My final comment is that this article reaffirms a case report's impact. It can uncover unintended use of a potential toxic substance. It can raise questions about a disease's etiology. It can motivate a large corporation to remove a potentially harmful substance from its product. And it can make a clinician think, speculate, and investigate.

J. A. Zenel, MD

References

1. 33 uses of 'baby' wipes that have nothing to do with babies! http://www.onegoodthingbyjillee.com/2012/08/7247.html. Accessed July 20, 2014.
2. Lewis S. 101 uses for baby wipes. http://blogs.babycenter.com/life_and_home/02242012-101-uses-for-baby-wipes/. Accessed July 20, 2014.

Breastfeeding Keratosis: This Frictional Keratosis of Newborns May Mimic Thrush

Kiat-Amnuay S, Bouquot J (Univ of Texas School of Dentistry at Houston)
Pediatrics 132:e775-e778, 2013

We report the first example, to our knowledge, of a frictional keratosis from exuberant sucking in a breastfeeding infant. A 2-month-old girl was referred for evaluation of a well-demarcated, nonsloughing white keratotic plaque of the lower lip mucosa, just inside the vermilion border. The plaque had a slightly irregular surface, had no surrounding erythema, and was the only such plaque in the mouth. It had been present for at least 3 weeks and had been unsuccessfully treated by her pediatrician via oral Mycostatin (nystatin). Her parents sought a second opinion when the infant was prescribed a full course of oral Diflucan (fluconazole). A cytopathology smear (Papanicolaou test) revealed abundant mature keratinocytes with no evidence of Candida. The mother admitted that the infant "worked hard" at sucking during breastfeeding and continued sucking long after feeding. The parents were unaware of any other habit or potential irritation of the lips. After 3 months of age the infant's sucking pattern became more "normal" and the keratosis disappeared; it did not recur during 3 years of follow-up. We propose the term "breastfeeding keratosis" for this entity (Table 1).

▶ When faced with a "white plaque" in the mouth of an infant, the diagnosis of thrush quickly comes to mind. Thrush is a common condition in infancy, with approximately 10% of infants estimated to have this condition during the first year of life.[1,2] Culture to confirm the diagnosis is rarely done, and empiric treatment has little risk. Many times, this strategy works. However, when empiric treatment does not work, even after confirming adherence to the medication regimen, it is important to consider a broader differential (Table 1).

There are 2 key points from this case report. First, Kiat-Amnuay et al now report and add a new entity to this list of white lesions in the mouth: breastfeeding keratosis. Vigorous infant sucking has been associated with frictional keratosis, which is essentially the development of a focal, hypertrophied, pink pad found on the lip. In contrast, breastfeeding keratosis is a white plaque (Figs 1 and 3 in the original article) on the lip mucosa. The etiology is irritation secondary to a habit of "pronounced" sucking. The condition resolves as the sucking becomes less vigorous over time.

The second key point from this case report is that it once again reaffirms the importance of a careful history. Beyond asking about the frequency and duration of breastfeeding, it is important to have the parent describe a typical breastfeeding session. The health care provider learned from the history that the "infant worked hard at sucking during breastfeeding." It is always important to return to the history and listen carefully, especially when the results of empiric treatment for an "easy" visual diagnostic case does not add up.

M. D. Cabana, MD, MPH

TABLE 1.—Keratotic, Nonsloughing Oral Mucosal Plaques and Macules in Infancy and Childhood

Diagnosis	Plaque or Macule?	Comment
Frictional keratosis	P	Smooth-surfaced, thick plaque of any mucosal surface from rubbing of mucosa by teeth or dental devices. Essentially equivalent to skin callus.
Linea alba	P	Thin, sometimes crenated, white linear plaque of buccal mucosa from rubbing teeth against the cheeks; usually bilateral.
Chronic cheek bite	P	Ragged white keratotic plaque of buccal mucosa along occlusal plane of the teeth; usually bilateral; from habit of chewing on cheeks (often during sleep). Also called morsicatio buccarum.
Chronic lip bite	P	Ragged white keratotic linear plaque of lower lip mucosa from habit of chewing on lower lip (often during sleep).
Tongue thrust habit	P	Ragged white keratotic linear plaque along lateral borders of tongue, often with indentations of tongue correlating to tooth contours; from habit of pushing tongue against teeth.
Breastfeeding keratosis	P	White, thick plaque of lip mucosa in breastfeeding infants; from habit of excess sucking; habit disappears naturally over time.
Migratory stomatitis	P	Serpiginous or circular thin white lines, often adjacent to red mucosa. Pattern of line changes on a daily or weekly schedule. Also called geographic mouth (geographic tongue if only the tongue is involved).
Lichen planus	P	White, intersecting "spider web" lines, perhaps on a red background. Usually on buccal and labial mucosa. Small potential for malignant transformation.
Lichenoid reaction	P	White, intersecting "spider web" lines on a red background. Usually on buccal mucosa. Hypersensitivity response to cinnamon- or peppermint-containing gum, candy, or to dental material.
Pachyonychia congenital	P	Leukoplakia-like white plaque of the dorsum of the tongue. Rare autosomal dominant disorder with abnormal nails and palmar/plantar keratosis.
Dyskeratosis congenital	P	Mucosal bullae and erosions, usually on the tongue and buccal mucosa, may develop into leukoplakia-like plaques. Rare, usually autosomal dominant disorder with hyperpigmentation of skin and dysplastic nails. Oral white lesions have a small risk of malignant transformation.
Leukoedema	M	Whitish-gray, diffuse macules of buccal mucosa, usually bilateral. Becomes more pronounced during childhood; more frequent in blacks.
White sponge nevus	M	Whitish-gray, diffuse, often corrugated macules of buccal mucosa, usually bilateral. Becomes more pronounced during childhood years. Familial disorder.
Witkop-Sallmann syndrome	M	Whitish-gray, diffuse macules of buccal mucosa, usually bilateral; ocular plaques may produce eventual blindness. Rare autosomal dominant disorder. Also called hereditary benign intraepithelial dyskeratosis. Caution: dyskeratotic epithelial cells may be misinterpreted as carcinoma.
Smokeless tobacco keratosis	M	Whitish-gray, diffuse macule of buccal and lower vestibular mucosa in area of chronic smokeless tobacco or snuff placement. Essentially a combined chemical burn and abrasion from the tobacco. Users usually start the habit at 8–13 years of age. Disappears completely with habit cessation. Small increased malignant transformation risk.
Listerine keratosis	M	Grayish-white macules of buccal mucosa, often bilateral, in persons who swish high-alcohol-content mouthwashes frequently throughout the day. Essentially a mild chemical burn.
Uremic stomatitis	M	Diffuse whitish-gray macules of the buccal and ventral lingual surfaces in terminal kidney failure; uremic oral odor often is present. Is transient in dialysis patients, disappearing completely immediately after a dialysis session, and then recurring before the next session.

None of the lesions are symptomatic except for occasional lichen planus and lichenoid reaction cases; geographic tongue may be sensitive to spicy or hot foods or may develop a burning sensation from secondary candidiasis.1–4 M, macule; P, plaque.

Reprinted from Kiat-Amnuay S, Bouquot J. Breastfeeding Keratosis: This Frictional Keratosis of Newborns May Mimic Thrush. Pediatrics. 2013;132:e775-e778. Copyright © 2013, by the American Academy of Pediatrics.

References

1. Bessa CF, Santos PJ, Aguiar MC, do Carmo MA. Prevalence of oral mucosal alterations in children from 0 to 12 years old. *J Oral Pathol Med.* 2004;33:17-22.
2. Yilmaz AE, Gorpelioglu C, Sarifakioglu E, Dogan DG, Bilici M, Celik N. Prevalence of oral mucosal lesions from birth to two years. *Niger J Clin Pract.* 2011; 14:349-353.

Cutaneous Findings Mistaken for Physical Abuse: Present but Not Pervasive

Schwartz KA, for the ExSTRA Investigators (Boston Med Ctr, MA; Seattle Children's Hosp, Washington; Seattle Children's Hosp and Univ of Washington; et al)

Pediatr Dermatol 31:146-155, 2014

Incorrect diagnoses during child abuse evaluations are serious. Because skin lesions are common in abuse, it is important to consider cutaneous mimics of physical abuse. The current study prospectively identified cutaneous mimics in a cohort of children evaluated for possible physical abuse. This is a secondary analysis of data from the Examining Siblings To Recognize Abuse research network's prospective, observational, cross-sectional study involving 20 U.S. child abuse teams. Subjects were younger than 10 years old and were evaluated by child abuse physicians (CAPs) for concerns of physical abuse. CAPs prospectively documented whether mimics were identified during their physical abuse evaluations. Details of each patient with cutaneous mimics were evaluated to determine the types of mimics, which part of the evaluations identified mimics, and the perceived abuse likelihood. Of 2,890 children evaluated for physical abuse, 137 had at least one mimic identified and 69 had some cutaneous mimic components. Although 985 of 2,753 (39%) subjects without mimics had high levels of abuse concern, only 9 of 137 (6%) children with mimics had high levels of abuse concern ($p < 0.001$). Of 69 children with cutaneous mimics, 56 (81%) were diagnosed by history and physical examination. Cutaneous abuse mimics were identified in 2.4% of children evaluated for physical abuse. Although it was eventually determined that there was little or no concern for abuse in 84% of children with cutaneous mimics, a small number were physically abused. CAP evaluation may be valuable in recognizing children with cutaneous mimics who also were abused.

▶ A child presents with a rash, or is it a bruise? Is it abuse, or just eczema? Is it a burn, or is it impetigo? The answers to these questions are not only often vexing for the general pediatrician but have significant ramifications. Making a report to child protective services for a common rash will alienate your patient's family and put them through a stressful and difficult investigation for no reason. Failure to recognize abuse places the child at risk for further injury and possible long-term morbidity and mortality. It's no wonder that only 250 pediatricians in the country are board-certified in child abuse pediatrics (CAP).

This article by the ExSTRA investigators helps shed some light on child abuse mimics and how often abuse actually occurs. Starting from a sample of high-risk children (siblings of abuse victims) being evaluated by a CAP, the authors focused on cutaneous findings noted during the evaluation that were mimics of abuse. These findings occurred relatively infrequently with 5% of the total sample of 2753 siblings being evaluated having any mimic and 2.5% having a cutaneous mimic.

The vast majority of children with a cutaneous mimic (96%) were not abused. The cutaneous mimics included congenital variants (congenital dermal melanosis, hemangiomas), dermatologic conditions (contact dermatitis, postinflammatory hyperpigmentation, atopic dermatitis, phytodermatitis), infections (impetigo, cellulitis, scalded skin, tinea) coagulopathies (idiopathic thrombocytopenic purpura, vonWillibrand disease [VWD]), and miscellaneous (clothing dye, neoplasm, Henoch–Schönlein purpura).

The variety of mimics may cause the general pediatrician to wonder if the CAP had some special testing or knowledge to make the diagnosis or rule out abuse. But this wasn't the case. Almost all of the mimics were identified by history and physical alone (81%) and adding simple coagulation tests lifted that percent to 88%. After careful evaluation, once a mimic is identified, there is still a possibility of concomitant abuse, but at least in this sample, the cases of abuse were not difficult to recognize.

The 4 cases concerning abuse included a 4-month-old with dermal melanosis but also multiple bruises; a 23-month-old with VWD and chronic subdural hematomas and an unexplained arm injury; a 28-month-old with a hemangioma, multiple bruises, and lower extremity injury with an inconsistent history; and a 24-month-old with tinea capitis and multiple facial bruises and petechiae. What is apparent from the 3 cases of cutaneous findings and concomitant abuse is that the cutaneous mimic had no resemblance to the injuries. In contrast, cases of impetigo, contact dermatitis, and many of the other skin conditions were thought to be abusive injuries. They just turned out not to be.

The bottom line is most skin mimics are just that—skin conditions. But know your available resources and contact your local CAP when in doubt.

S. D. Krugman, MD, MS

Eruptive Xanthomas Masquerading as Molluscum Contagiosum
Sorrell J, Salvaggio H, Garg A, et al (Northwestern Univ Feinberg School of Medicine, Chicago, IL; Univ of Texas Southwestern Med Ctr, Dallas; et al)
Pediatrics 134:e257-e260, 2014

Eruptive xanthomas are cutaneous manifestations of hyperlipidemias in which lipids accumulate in large foam cells within the skin. They classically present as crops of 1- to 4-mm yellow-orange papules and are often associated with extreme hypertriglyceridemia. We describe a 12-year-old boy with autism who was thought to have widespread molluscum contagiosum for a year before dermatologic consultation was obtained. Recognition of eruptive xanthomas led to the discovery of massive hypertriglyceridemia (serum triglycerides 6853 mg/dL) and diabetes mellitus. Through medical intervention, including insulin and fenofibrate therapy, and dietary modification with weight loss, the xanthomas cleared during the subsequent months, and his serum triglyceride levels nearly normalized.

▶ Recognizing the dermatologic manifestations of systemic disease facilitates timely diagnosis and institution of therapy. Eruptive xanthomas (Fig 1) are a skin sign of extreme hypertriglyceridemia—either primary or secondary—and other components of the metabolic syndrome including uncontrolled diabetes mellitus.[1] Early recognition of xanthomas prompts evaluation for hypertriglyceridemia and may prevent its potentially life-threatening downstream effect of acute pancreatitis. Unfortunately, as the prevalence of various childhood chronic diseases evolve, with increasing rates of type I and type 2 diabetes mellitus, as well as metabolic syndrome,[2] it is important for primary care providers to be alert for lesions potentially associated with these conditions.

The patient in the case described by Sorrell et al suffered a delay in diagnosis of nearly 2 years after onset of the eruption, misdiagnosed as molluscum contagiosum. Although molluscum (Fig 2) and eruptive xanthomas share some similarities (both are small, firm, dome-shaped papules) differentiating the 2 is critical and can be accomplished by observing key morphologic details of individual lesions, the eruption as a whole, and the overall clinical context.

Individual lesions of molluscum appear initially as flesh-colored or pink umbilicated papules clustered regionally or scattered widely on the body. Because molluscum is a viral infection cleared by immune activation, lesions in various stages will be observed in an individual patient due to evolving host response to the infection. Initial unaltered umbilicated papules will give way to various stages of inflammation manifest as erythema, edema, and ultimately a whitish or pustular appearance due to immune infiltration.

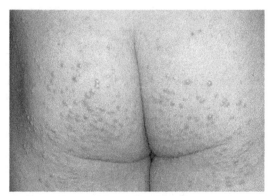

FIGURE 1.—Eruptive xanthomas. Discrete pink to yellow, smooth-surfaced, firm, monomorphous papules on the buttocks at presentation to our clinic. For Interpretation of the references to color in this figure legend, the reader is referred to web version of this article. (Reprinted from Sorrell J, Salvaggio H, Garg A, et al. Eruptive xanthomas masquerading as molluscum contagiosum. *Pediatrics.* 2014;134: e257-e260, with permission from the American Academy of Pediatrics.)

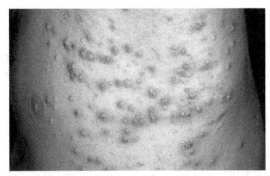

FIGURE 2.—Lesions in a severe case of molluscum contagiosum demonstrating the typical firm, domeshaped papules with central umbilication. (Reprinted from Sorrell J, Salvaggio H, Garg A, et al. Eruptive xanthomas masquerading as molluscum contagiosum. *Pediatrics*. 2014;134:e257-e260, with permission from the American Academy of Pediatrics.)

TABLE 1.—Clinical and Histologic Characteristics of Eruptive Xanthoma Versus Molluscum Contagiosum

	Eruptive Xanthoma	Molluscum Contagiosum
Cause	Hypertriglyceridemia	Poxvirus
Morphology	Firm, dome-shaped lipid-filled papules; Monomorphous	Firm, dome-shaped papules Not monomorphous
Usual size	1−4 mm	1−8 mm
Central core or umbilication	Occasional	Often
Confluence of papules	Occasional	Occasional
Color	Skin-colored to yellow-orange	Skin-colored to pink
Koebnerization	Yes	Yes
Inflammation	None	Often, including surrounding dermatitis
Histopathology	Lipidized dermal macrophages	Epidermal intracellular invasion with Henderson-Patterson bodies

Reprinted from Sorrell J, Salvaggio H, Garg A, et al. Eruptive xanthomas masquerading as molluscum contagiosum. Pediatrics. 2014;134:e257-e260, with permission from the American Academy of Pediatrics.

End-stage lesions will often be crusted or excoriated. The lesional stages are due to inflammation and represent the host response that precedes resolution. The acronym "BOTE" sign (beginning of the end) has been proposed to highlight the significance of inflammation as an expected variant in the evolution of molluscum immunity.[3] The eruption as a whole is not monotonous or monomorphic (except early in the course of infection); lesions in various stages will be observed, and this is a key differentiating point compared with eruptive xanthomas. Children with molluscum infection are often well; however, the overall course of infection can be prolonged, with crops of lesions occurring for up to and exceeding 2 years. If the diagnosis is in doubt, lesional contents can be mounted on a microscope slide for immediate confirmation upon recognition of viral inclusion bodies. Alternatively, a tissue biopsy, although often not necessary, is also diagnostic.

In contrast, individual lesions of eruptive xanthoma are often a distinctive yellow-orange color that derives from the lipid inclusions. Umbilication may be observed, but it is rare. Critically important for differentiating xanthomas from molluscum is that xanthomas are static; they do not trigger a host response and thus are not inflamed. Further, the overall eruption will be characteristically monomorphic (all lesions will look essentially the same in the same stage of development; Table 1). The clinical context may offer diagnostic clues—a family history of dyslipidemia or, in secondary cases, the use of certain medications, the presence of obesity, metabolic syndrome, diabetes, or abnormal laboratory parameters pointing to systemic illness.

In summary, the lesions of molluscum contagiosum and eruptive xanthoma may appear similar on the surface. However, a few basic morphologic features are all they share. Careful consideration of the details and subtle diagnostic clues of individual lesions, the eruption as a whole, and the clinical context should clarify the diagnosis and prompt the proper evaluation and management strategy.

K. M. Cordoro, MD

M. D. Cabana, MD, MPH

References

1. Loeckermann S, Braun-Falco M. Eruptive xanthomas in association with metabolic syndrome. *Clin Exp Dermatol.* 2010;35:565-566.
2. Dabelea D, Mayer-Davis EJ, Saydah S. Prevalence of type 1 and type 2 diabetes among children and adolescents from 2001 to 2009. *JAMA.* 2014;311:1778-1786.
3. Butala N, Siegfried E, Weissler A. Molluscum BOTE sign: a predictor of imminent resolution. *Pediatrics.* 2013;131:e1650-e1653.

High-Dose Isotretinoin Treatment and the Rate of Retrial, Relapse, and Adverse Effects in Patients With Acne Vulgaris

Blasiak RC, Stamey CR, Burkhart CN, et al (Univ of North Carolina at Chapel Hill)

JAMA Dermatol 149:1392-1398, 2013

Importance.—Isotretinoin is the most effective treatment for acne. The ideal dosing regimen is unknown.

Objective.—To determine the rates of relapse of acne vulgaris and retrial of isotretinoin after high cumulative-dose treatment and the changes to the adverse effect profile.

Design, Setting, and Participants.—A prospective, observational, intervention study was conducted from August 1, 2008, to August 31, 2010, in a single academic tertiary care center with multiple providers. A total of 180 patients with acne resistant to other treatments were enrolled. Of these, 116 participated in the 12-month follow-up survey, for a response rate of 64.4%.

Exposure.—Patients received isotretinoin, with dosing based on the providers' judgment. Patients were divided into 2 groups on the basis of cumulative dosing (<220 mg/kg and ≥220 mg/kg).

Main Outcomes and Measures.—Relapse (treatment with a prescription topical or oral acne medication after a course of isotretinoin) or retrial (retreatment with isotretinoin) at 12-month follow-up and adverse effects experienced during and after 12 months of treatment.

Results.—The mean age of the participants was 19.3 years, 51.9% were female, and 74.1% were white. At 12 months' follow-up, 97.4% of the patients reported that their acne was improved. Overall, acne in 32.7% of patients in the study relapsed at 12 months, and 1.72% of the patients required a retrial. In the lower-dose treatment group (<220 mg/kg), the relapse rate was 47.4% (95% CI, 32.3%-63.0%) compared with 26.9% (95% CI, 18.3%-37.8%) in the high-dose group ($P = .03$). Almost 100% of the patients in both treatment groups developed cheilitis and xerosis during treatment. Retinoid dermatitis was significantly more common in the high-dose treatment group (53.8% vs 31.6%; $P = .02$). None of the other adverse effects was significantly different between the 2 groups.

Conclusions and Relevance.—The dosing regimen used in the present study is considerably higher than that used in previous studies of isotretinoin. At 1 year after completion of isotretinoin treatment, we found that patients receiving 220 mg/kg or more had a significantly decreased risk of relapse. Rash was the only adverse effect that was significantly more common in the high-dose group during treatment. This study suggests that significantly higher doses of isotretinoin are effective for treating acne and decreasing relapse rates without increasing adverse effects.

▶ The introduction of isotretinoin provided a unique treatment with the capacity to induce complete or long-term remission of severe or recalcitrant acne, including nodulocystic acne, through a variety of mechanisms including suppressing sebum production, decreasing comedogenesis, and inhibiting colonization by *Propionibacterium acnes.*[1]

Isotretinoin has been shown to have tremendous effectiveness in affecting acne, with most patients being clear, or almost clear of acne at the conclusion of a course of therapy. The persistence of this effect varies; however, and the variation in long-term response has prompted investigation into how dosing regimens and treatment protocols may influence the disease course. The widely accepted goal for the cumulative dose of isotretinoin is 120 to 150 mg/kg, based on several studies.[2-5] In the study by Blasiak et al, 2 cumulative dosing end points (< 220 mg/kg and ≥220 mg/kg) were compared. It is important to note that because the participating physicians prescribed therapy until they observed no clinical lesions, the mean clinical dose for the lower dose study group was 170.8 mg/kg, which is higher than the accepted standard goal dose.[6]

Nearly all patients (96%–100%) experienced xerosis and cheilitis. Of all recorded side effects, only retinoid dermatitis was significantly elevated in the higher-dose group. The relapse rate was 47.4% in the lower-dose group compared with 26.9% in the higher-dose group; however, the only 2 patients requiring a repeat isotretinoin course were both in the higher-dose group. Although the difference was not significant, laboratory abnormalities were noted more frequently the higher dose group.

The striking part of the article is summarized in Table 5 of the original article, which shows adverse effects in both groups at the 12-month follow-up. Notably, both groups have a greater than expected percentage of patients with side effects 1 year after treatment (headaches in 12%, vision changes in 3%, muscle aches in 8%, joint aches in 7%, abdominal pain in 6%) with no significant differences between the 2 groups. Because no age-matched-control group was surveyed, it is difficult to deduce whether these side effects noted 1 year after treatment are secondary to the higher dose of isotretinoin. If they are related to isotretinoin, it implies that some significant side effects may be seen with higher dosing regimens, which both groups in this study used (> 120 mg/kg).

In our busy pediatric dermatology clinics, we have extensive experience with isotretinoin in the treatment of acne in preteens and adolescents and developed a standardized symptom survey that we use to analyze symptoms at the time that the patient is on the medication.[7] We typically use the highest tolerated "comfortable dose" during treatment (ie, the highest dose with minimal side effects and lab abnormalities), which is usually 0.5 to 1 mg/kg/day working up to the standard cumulative dose of 120 to 150 mg/kg. A lower daily dose does mean a longer duration of therapy to reach the same goal cumulative dose (1 mg/kg/day for 5–6 months vs 0.5 mg/kg/day for 9–10 months). Although we have not surveyed our patients 1 year later to assess the symptom complex, it is our sense that our rate of side effects during the course of isotretinoin, and certainly later, would be much lower with the standard dosing. We also have not noted such a high relapse rate, nearly 50% in this study, with our lower-dose treated patients.

As pointed out in the commentary on the article, this was a single-institution experience. Although it was a prospective study, the intervention was not controlled, and there was no randomization or blinding. The study suggests that higher dosing may lead to lower relapse rates with no significant increase in adverse effects. However, in our experience with lower-dose isotretinoin, we see equivalent to lower adverse effects while on treatment with lower relapse rates. We certainly do not see the high percentage of side effects 1 year after treatment. Further prospective studies comparing cumulative doses (< 150 mg/kg and ≥ 220 mg/kg) with a control group are needed.

S. Awasthi, MD

L. F. Eichenfield, MD

References

1. Eichenfield LF, Krakowski AC, Piggott C, et al. Evidence-based recommendations for the diagnosis and treatment of pediatric acne. *Pediatrics.* 2013;131 Suppl 3: S163-S186.
2. Cooper AJ. Treatment of acne with isotretinoin: recommendations based on Australian experience. *The Australasian journal of dermatology.* 2003;44(2):97-105.
3. Goldsmith LA, Bolognia JL, Callen JP, et al. American Academy of Dermatology Consensus Conference on the safe and optimal use of isotretinoin: summary and

recommendations. *Journal of the American Academy of Dermatology*. 2004;50(6): 900-906.

4. Kass F, Salamon I, Plutchik R, Hyman I. The assessment of depression: a model for quality review of emergency psychiatry. *The American journal of psychiatry*. 1978; 135(2):213-216.

5. Layton AM, Knaggs H, Taylor J, Cunliffe WJ. Isotretinoin for acne vulgaris— 10 years later: a safe and successful treatment. *The British journal of dermatology*. 1993;129(3):292-296.

6. Blasiak RC, Stamey CR, Burkhart CN, Lugo-Somolinos A, Morrell DS. High-dose isotretinoin treatment and the rate of retrial, relapse, and adverse effects in patients with acne vulgaris. *JAMA dermatology*. 2013;149(12):1392-1398.

7. Hodgkiss-Harlow CJ, Eichenfield LF, Dohil MA. Effective monitoring of isotretinoin safety in a pediatric dermatology population: a novel "patient symptom survey" approach. *Journal of the American Academy of Dermatology*. 2011;65(3): 517-524.

3 Blood

Hydroxyurea Is Associated With Lower Costs of Care of Young Children With Sickle Cell Anemia

Wang WC, for the BABY HUG Investigators (St Jude Children's Res Hosp, Memphis, TN; Montefiore Med Ctr, Bronx, NY; Clinical Trials & Surveys Corporation, Owings Mills, MD; et al)
Pediatrics 132:677-683, 2013

Background and Objective.—In the BABY HUG trial, young children with sickle cell anemia randomized to receive hydroxyurea had fewer episodes of pain, hospitalization, and transfusions. With anticipated broader use of hydroxyurea in this population, we sought to estimate medical costs of care in treated versus untreated children.

Methods.—The BABY HUG database was used to compare inpatient events in subjects receiving hydroxyurea with those receiving placebo. Unit costs were estimated from the 2009 MarketScan Multi-state Medicaid Database for children with sickle cell disease, aged 1 to 3 years. Inpatient costs were based on length of hospital stay, modified by the occurrence of acute chest syndrome, splenic sequestration, or transfusion. Outpatient expenses were based on the schedule required for BABY HUG and a "standard" schedule for 1- to 3-year-olds with sickle cell anemia.

Results.—There were 232 hospitalizations in the subjects receiving hydroxyurea and 324 in those on placebo; length of hospital stay was similar in the 2 groups. Estimated outpatient expenses were greater in those receiving hydroxyurea, but these were overshadowed by inpatient costs. The total estimated annual cost for those on hydroxyurea ($11 072) was 21% less than the cost of those on placebo ($13 962; $P = .038$).

Conclusions.—Savings on inpatient care resulted in a significantly lower overall estimated medical care cost for young children with sickle cell anemia who were receiving hydroxyurea compared with those receiving placebo. Because cost savings are likely to increase with age, these data provide additional support for broad use of hydroxyurea treatment in this population.

▶ A new era of hope was ushered in when the Multicenter Study of Hydroxyurea (MSH) in sickle cell disease (SCD) was published in 1995.[1] That study indicated that hydroxyurea could reduce hospitalizations, transfusions, and acute chest syndrome in adults (> 18 years old) with SCD. The BABY HUG study,[2] a randomized multicenter trial, essentially duplicated the findings in young patients with SCD (9—18 months old at enrollment) followed for 2 years.

Now the article by Wang et al assesses the cost savings of treatment of young children with SCD using standardized cost analysis methodology. The authors demonstrate the total estimated annual cost per patient for those on hydroxyurea, $11 072 ($9450 inpatient costs plus $1622 outpatient costs) was 21% less than the cost of those on placebo, $13 962 ($13 716 patient costs plus $246 outpatient costs). The difference was approximately $2890 per patient per year (Tables 2 and 3 in the original article). An estimate of cost savings by the MSH investigators of the original adult study[3] using local costs, not large databases, was $5210 (95% confidence interval: $−610 to $11 030; $P = .21$).

The importance of the cost analysis in the BABY HUG study is to demonstrate that even in the face of increased outpatient costs for monitoring children on hydroxyurea, the savings in health care costs on an annual basis favored treatment with hydroxyurea. In a health care system in which costs have clearly outstripped the ability of the government or private health insurance to keep up, "cost savings" may speak as loudly as clinical efficacy for a continuous therapy in a chronic disease.

One must take several important precautions in interpreting this study. The study assumes that the infrastructure for caring for children with SCD is as good across the United States as it is in the centers used for this trial. There is no indication that this is the case, and estimates of the costs of reproducing the infrastructure needed are not available. It is assumed, for instance, that all patients in this study were followed closely in the hospital and in the outpatient setting by board-certified pediatric hematologists.

The cost savings of $2890 annually could be wiped out by a single additional hospitalization per year (estimated in this analysis to be approximately $7700) in patients on hydroxyurea or by a prolonged length of stay of 1.5 days for each hospitalization for patients on the drug. Therefore, to maintain compliance and safety of the myelotoxic outpatient therapy and to carefully manage the children when they are hospitalized, these patients will likely need both a pediatric hematologist and a primary care physician.

Second, after being approved by the US Food and Drug Administration for individuals aged over 18 years, the percentage of adults currently on hydroxyurea is low (estimates range from 20% to 30%). The reasons for the lack of utilization are not entirely known but may include lack of access to the medication (eg, patients not followed regularly by a single physician), fear of perceived side effects of the drug (eg, cancer, sterility, congenital anomalies, loss of hair), discomfort of physicians using an anticancer drug for a nonmalignant disease, unwillingness of physicians to give the myelotoxic levels of the drug needed to produce favorable clinical outcomes, nonresponsiveness to or undertreatment with the drug, for example. Without knowledge of the precise causes of poor utilization in adults with SCD, can we expect parents and their children to be more willing to take the drug and be more compliant when they take it? Will hydroxyurea be as efficacious in children as it has not been in adults?

Third, SCD is a disorder in which ongoing cumulative organ damage may occur with relatively few clinical signs (eg, silent cerebral infarcts that lead to subtle but significantly decreased learning capacity, progressive infarction of the kidneys leading to renal failure, progressive pulmonary disease leading to pulmonary hypertension, autoinfarction of the spleen increasing susceptibility to infections). There are as yet no data to show that long-term silent organ damage will be prevented if children take hydroxyurea regularly. Although acute events may be decreased, will the effects of decreased organ damage lead to a healthier young adult after 18 years on hydroxyurea?

The lessons learned from the use of hydroxyurea to treat SCD adults over the past 19 years is that clinical efficacy as demonstrated by a blinded controlled clinical trial does not lead to effective therapy for patients in the real world of medicine. Whether the nonresearch setting for children with SCD offers more opportunity for effectiveness is untested and unknown.

G. J. Dover, MD

References

1. Charache S, Terrin ML, Moore R, et al. Effect of hydroxyurea on the frequency of painful crises in sickle cell anemia. Investigators of the multicenter study of hydroxyurea in sickle cell anemia. *N Engl J Med.* 1995;332:1317-1322.
2. Wang WC, Ware RE, Miller ST, et al. BABY HUG Investigators. Hydroxycarbamide in very young children with sickle cell anaemia: a multi-center, randomized controlled trial (BABY HUG). *Lancet.* 2011;377:1663-1667.
3. Moore RD, Charache S, Terrin ML, Ballas SK. Cost effectiveness of hydroxyurea in sickle cell anemia. Investigators of the multicenter study of hydroxyurea in sickle cell anemia. *Am J Hematol.* 2000;64:26-31.

Association of Hospital and Provider Types on Sickle Cell Disease Outcomes

Jan S, Slap G, Smith-Whitley K, et al (Perelman School of Medicine of the Univ of Pennsylvania, Philadelphia; The Children's Hosp of Philadelphia, PA)
Pediatrics 132:854-861, 2013

Objectives.—Adolescents and young adults (A/YA) with sickle cell disease (SCD) are hospitalized in both children's and general hospitals. We determined the effect of hospital type and provider specialty on outcomes of hospitalized A/YA with SCD and acute chest syndrome (ACS).

Methods.—This retrospective cohort study used the 2007–2009 Premier Database, a large multi-institutional database, to identify 1476 patients ages 16 to 25 years with 2299 admissions with SCD and ACS discharged from 256 US hospitals from 2007 to 2009. Multilevel logistic regression and zero-truncated negative binomial regression were performed after adjustment for patient demographic, clinical, and hospital characteristics to test the association of hospital type and provider specialty on death, endotracheal intubation, simple or exchange transfusion, length of stay (LOS), and 30-day readmission.

Results.—Of all admissions, 14 died and 45% were intubated. General hospitals had 13 deaths and were associated with higher intubation rates (predicted probability [PP], 48% [95% confidence interval (CI), 43%–52%]) and longer LOS (predicted mean LOS, 7.6 days [95% CI, 7.2–7.9]) compared with children's hospitals (PP of intubation, 24%

[95% CI, 5%—42%]; and predicted mean LOS, 6.8 days [95% CI, 5.6—5.8]). There was no difference by hospital type or provider specialty in PP of simple or exchange transfusion, or 30-day readmission.

Conclusions.—General hospitals carry higher intubation risks for A/YA with SCD and ACS compared with children's hospitals. We need to better understand the drivers of these differences, including the role of staff expertise, hospital volume, and quality of ongoing SCD care.

▶ Improving sickle cell disease (SCD)—related outcomes for adolescents and young adults (A/YA) continue to be of importance for the health care community. Understanding the complexity of care for this group, which Jan et al identifies as 16 to 25 years of age, is of particular significance because it is the age when transfer to adult care begins and when the most common reasons for hospitalizations, acute chest syndrome (ACS), becomes the leading cause of death. The stated purpose of this study was to assess the influence of provider and hospital type on outcomes of SCD, particularly ACS for A/YA.

The introduction gives a brief but balanced presentation of the history, diagnosis of SCD-ACS, the relative practice guidelines, and its relevance to patients 15 to 27 years old but does not provide a clear explanation as to why the authors specifically choose the age range of 16 to 25 years. It was not clear in the article whether there are any physiologic differences across the life span of persons with SCD. An explanation of the developmental and maturational differences within this age range would have provided a better understanding of the specific differences that influence outcomes of sickle cell disease. In addition, a brief explanation of the typical disease progression would allow for a better understanding by the non-SCD specialist, about the condition's natural history and complication such as ACS.

It is evident that this article contains a well-thought-out methodology and a robust analysis. The findings substantiate the study's hypothesis that hospital and practitioner type influences the quality of care received and affects the length of stay and health outcomes of A/YA with sickle cell disease that present with ACS.

Two noted limitations of the study were the lumping of pediatricians, internists, hospitalists, and family medicine practitioners into 1 category of practitioners, and as noted by the authors, the deficiency of information as to which hospitals are SCD centers. It is likely that differences in specialty type could have accounted for the variation in training relating to general intubation practices as well as intubation practices related to sickle cell disease.

Further questions remain about how to improve outcomes. What should a hospitalist, generalist, internist, administrator, or medical director from a general hospital do with these findings? The discussion provided a sound system-level recommendation for regionalization of general hospitals but did not provide a prioritized set of recommendations to address the disparities in treatment and outcomes between pediatric and general hospitals. Suggestions included "minimizing insurance lapses, training more adult providers in SCD care, and developing policies that improve care coordination as A/YA transition to adult care."

With limited resources, prioritized recommendations for providers and health care administrators would have strengthened the article.

These limitations do not negate the importance of this article for clinical practice and administrative policy. Micro-level (individual) and macro-level (access, provision of care) influences outcomes in SCD are recognized and discussed. The bottom line is that every hospital wants to decrease the length of stay, readmission, and morbidity and mortality rates for chronic disease patients. Thus, this work confirms the public health perspective that person and place influences health outcomes that influence hospital admissions/readmissions and length of stay. The study findings open the door to initiate discussion about additional training in residency and beyond for internists, family practitioners, pediatricians, and other specialists that treat A/YA with sickle cell disease in general hospital settings. The fact is, such training can bridge public health and medicine by incorporating the socioenvironmental and cultural aspects of SCD and their implications on outcomes in general hospital settings.

Transition into adulthood, along with the type of care facility and provider, continues to influence continuity and quality of care for adolescents and young adults with chronic conditions such as SCD. Fragmented care leads to higher morbidity and increased hospitalizations with additional medical complications for not only the patients but also the hospital responsible for care. The clinical and administrative implications of these findings highlight the importance of regionalization and coordination of care for chronic conditions within general hospitals. Coordination between children's and general hospitals to facilitate a smooth transition is vital to minimizing complicated clinical presentations at general hospitals, increase inpatient and ambulatory quality of care, and reduce length of stay for adolescent and young adult patients with SCD. This article, irrespective of its limitations, contributes to our understanding of the challenges faced by A/YA with SCD.

J. Telfair, DrPH, MSW, MPH

Intravenous Magnesium Sulfate for Vaso-occlusive Episodes in Sickle Cell Disease
Goldman RD, Mounstephen W, Kirby-Allen M, et al (BC Children's Hosp, Vancouver, Canada; Univ of Toronto, Ontario, Canada)
Pediatrics 132:e1634-e1641, 2013

Background and Objective.—Vaso-occlusive episodes (VOEs) are the most common complication of sickle cell disease in children. Treatment with magnesium seems to improve cellular hydration and may result in reduced vaso-occlusion. This study aimed to determine if intravenous (IV) magnesium sulfate ($MgSO_4$) reduces length of stay (LOS) in hospital, pain scores, and cumulative analgesia when compared with placebo.

Methods.—Randomized, double-blind, placebo-controlled trial in children aged 4 to 18 years requiring admission to hospital with a sickle cell disease VOE requiring IV analgesia. Participating children received IV $MgSO_4$ (100 mg/kg) every 8 hours or placebo in addition to standard therapy. We used a t test or Mann-Whitney test (continuous variables), Fisher's exact test, or χ^2 test (frequencies). P values were considered significant if <.05, and 95% confidence intervals were calculated for the difference between groups.

Results.—One hundred six children were randomly assigned to the study, and 104 were included. Fifty-one (49%) received $MgSO_4$. Children's mean age was 12.4 years (range: 4–18 years; SD: 3.8 years), and 56 (54%) were females. There was no significant difference in the primary outcome measure, LOS in hospital, with a mean of 132.6 and 117.7 hours in the $MgSO_4$ and placebo groups, respectively ($P = .41$). Therewas no significant difference between groups for the secondary outcomes of mean pain scores (4.9 ± 2.6 vs 4.8 ± 2.6, respectively; $P = .92$) or analgesic requirements (continuous morphine infusion [$P = .928$], boluses of IV morphine [$P = .82$], acetaminophen [$P = .34$], ibuprofen [$P = .15$], naproxen [$P = .10$]). Only minor adverse events were recorded in both groups. Pain at the infusion site was more common in the $MgSO_4$ group.

Conclusions.—IV $MgSO_4$ was well tolerated but had no effect on the LOS in hospital, pain scores, or cumulative analgesia use in admitted children with a VOE.

▶ Sickle cell disease is a worldwide health problem that affects millions of patients and more than 400 000 annual births. Recent advances in understanding the complex pathophysiology of sickle cell disease has led to the development of several promising therapeutic options of pathophysiology of sickling. These therapeutic interventions attack the sickle cell pathology at several biologic points from the initial primary mutation to its many downstream effects.

One of the first key downstream effects of the primary mutation is the intracellular sickle cell polymer formation, which results in decreased red cell deformability and leads to membrane damage. Drugs that increase fetal hemoglobin such as hydroxyurea may slow polymerization. Once the membrane is damaged, the phospholipid phosphatidylserine is exposed, and this induces red cell destruction, elevated free plasma hemoglobin, and nitric oxide depletion. These abnormalities lead to a marked increase in inflammatory cytokines, pro-coagulants, and reactive oxygen species. The cumulative effects of these changes are endothelial dysfunction, cellular adhesion to endothelium, and vaso-occlusion. This process is amplified by a hypoxia-induced ischemia reperfusion injury.

Several new therapeutic strategies that alter 1 or more aspects of this pathologic sequence are under clinical trial. Patients need both preventative and acute therapy. Preventative therapy is more likely to have a beneficial effect. However, acute therapies are needed to augment the beneficial effects of chronic therapy. Daily hydroxyurea increases fetal hemoglobin and improves the overall pathophysiology of sickle cell disease, but patients continue to have ongoing acute events and chronic organ dysfunction. There is a great need for therapies that are beneficial in the acute setting.

Studying the efficacy of magnesium in acute events makes sense. Magnesium improves cellular hydration by inhibiting efflux of potassium and loss of cellular water. In addition, magnesium is a known vasodilator. Furthermore, there are pilot studies indicating efficacy and safety. Unfortunately, this study of magnesium for acute painful events showed no benefit. The benefit may not be observed because of the limitations of the study, which should be corrected in a large multicenter ongoing trial.[1] The intravenous magnesium in sickle cell vaso-occlusive crisis (MAGIC) trial is being conducted by the Pediatric Emergency Care Applied Research Network (PECARN).[2] However, many promising therapeutic agents have not been beneficial in sickle cell disease. Drugs have been studied that increase cellular hydration in sickle cell disease but have not decreased painful events. A phase 3 trial of Senicapoc, a novel Gardos channel inhibitor, increased hemoglobin levels and improved red cell deformability but increased painful events.[3] Sickle cell patients have multiple clinical phenotypes. Very anemic patients have limited painful events but ongoing ischemic injury such as stroke. High hemoglobin patients have increased painful events but decreased chronic organ ischemic injury. Senicapoc likely increased the hemoglobin, which resulted in increased viscosity and painful events.

Magnesium may benefit sickle cell patients but not necessarily decrease painful events. The vasodilator effect of magnesium may be beneficial in improving tissue perfusion; however, magnesium's vasodilator effect is significantly dependent on endothelial release of nitric oxide. Because sickle cell patients are nitric oxide—deficient, particularly during acute events, this benefit may be minimized. We recently demonstrated that arginine therapy was beneficial in the treatment of sickle cell painful events and may also amplify the actions of hydroxyurea.[4] Perhaps magnesium therapy with coadministration of arginine should be studied.

The present drug development approach to sickle cell disease is searching for a single agent that dramatically alters the clinical course of patients. There have been several drugs that already demonstrated some benefit in sickle cell disease. However, because its beneficial effect has not been characterized as a magic bullet, its further development is often stopped or abandoned. In my opinion, this approach is wrong. Therapeutic trials in sickle cell disease should be based on the pediatric cancer model. In this model, combination drug therapy acting on different pathways synergistically has resulted in a dramatic improvement in survival and quality of life. This approach is largely driven by pharmaceutical requirements, which can only be modified if the National Institutes of Health and other funding agencies support more combination chemotherapy trials.

E. P. Vichinsky, MD

References

1. Vichinsky EP, ed. Emerging Therapies Targeting the Pathophysiology of Sickle Cell Disease. 2014/03/05 ed. Philadelphia, PA: Elsevier, Inc.; 2014.
2. Badaki-Makun O, Scott JP, et al. Pediatric Emergency Care Applied Research Network Magnesium in Sickle Cell Crisis Study, G. Intravenous magnesium for pediatric sickle cell vaso-occlusive crisis: methodological issues of a randomized controlled trial. *Pediatr Blood Cancer.* 2014;61:1049-1054.

3. Castro OL, Gordeuk VR, Gladwin MT, Steinberg MH. Senicapoc trial results support the existence of different sub-phenotypes of sickle cell disease with possible drug-induced phenotypic shifts. *Br J Haematol.* 2011;155:636-638.
4. Morris CR, Kuypers FA, Lavrisha L, et al. A randomized, placebo-controlled trial of arginine therapy for the treatment of children with sickle cell disease hospitalized with vaso-occlusive pain episodes. *Haematologica.* 2013;98:1375-1382.

Hemostatic Abnormalities in Noonan Syndrome

Artoni A, Selicorni A, Passamonti SM, et al (A. Bianchi Bonomi Hemophilia and Thrombosis Ctr, Milan, Italy; San Gerardo Hosp, Monza, Italy; et al)
Pediatrics 133:e1299-e1304, 2014

Background.—A bleeding diathesis is a common feature of Noonan syndrome, and various coagulation abnormalities have been reported. Platelet function has never been carefully investigated.

Methods.—The degree of bleeding diathesis in a cohort of patients with Noonan syndrome was evaluated by a validated bleeding score and investigated with coagulation and platelet function tests. If ratios of prothrombin time and/or activated partial thromboplastin time were prolonged, the activity of clotting factors was measured. Individuals with no history of bleeding formed the control group.

Results.—The study population included 39 patients and 28 controls. Bleeding score was ≥ 2 (ie, suggestive of a moderate bleeding diathesis) in 15 patients (38.5%) and ≥ 4 (ie, suggestive of a severe bleeding diathesis) in 7 (17.9%). Abnormal coagulation and/or platelet function tests were found in 14 patients with bleeding score ≥ 2 (93.3%) but also in 21 (87.5%) of those with bleeding score <2. The prothrombin time and activated partial thromboplastin time were prolonged in 18 patients (46%) and partial deficiency of factor VII, alone or in combination with the deficiency of other vitamin K–dependent factors, was the most frequent coagulation abnormality. Moreover, platelet aggregation and secretion were reduced in 29 of 35 patients (82.9%, $P < .01$ for all aggregating agents).

Conclusions.—Nearly 40% of patients with the Noonan syndrome had a bleeding diathesis and >90% of them had platelet function and/or coagulation abnormalities. Results of these tests should be taken into account in the management of bleeding or invasive procedures in these patients.

▶ Noonan syndrome is a relatively common multisystem developmental disorder that can cause significant long-term morbidity. Recent molecular advances have led to the identification of causative mutations in several genes, each of which results in hyperactivation of a single signaling pathway important in many cell types. This aberrant signaling produces a range of clinical features, including characteristic facial features, cardiac anomalies, growth problems, and cognitive delays.

Many of these patients also have a bleeding diathesis—in some reports, close to 90% of Noonan's patients have abnormal bleeding symptoms.[1] However, the etiology of the bleeding diathesis associated with Noonan syndrome is not clear. Previous studies have described patients with a variety of clotting-factor deficiencies, including Factors II, V, VII, VIII, IX, and XI.[2-6] Smaller case series have also described patients with abnormal von Willebrand testing[2-4] and abnormalities in platelet function.[4] Neither etiology nor severity of bleeding phenotype has been correlated with genotype, demonstrating how little we understand about mechanisms influencing phenotypic expression of the underlying molecular lesion.[1]

This study is one of the largest series to date evaluating the etiology of the bleeding diathesis seen in patients with Noonan syndrome. Similar to previous studies, Artoni et al identified laboratory abnormalities in close to 90% of their cohort (Table 5 in the original article). The authors found that a significant number of patients had deficiencies in Factor VII and other vitamin K—dependent coagulation factors, which responded to vitamin K supplementation. The nutritional status of these patients was not reported. Because feeding difficulties and growth issues are frequently seen in Noonan's patients, they may be more prone to intermittent vitamin K deficiency. It is also important to note that not all laboratory abnormalities identified in this article result in an increased bleeding propensity. For example, 3 patients were identified as having Factor XII deficiency, which prolongs the partial thromboplastin time but is not associated with an increased bleeding phenotype.

In addition to these clotting factor deficiencies, Artoni et al also evaluated platelet function in 35 patients. Platelet activation in vivo is a multistep process, influenced by many factors including localized shear forces, endothelial damage, and internal signaling responses to outside agonists. Distilling all of these factors into a reproducible in vitro assay that is truly reflective of platelet function is technically challenging. Although a large percentage (82.9%) of Noonan's patients showed platelet dysfunction on platelet aggregometry, a quarter of the control patients also had abnormalities on this assay despite having no bleeding symptoms. A practical consideration is that platelet aggregometry generally cannot be completed before 1 year of age because of the amount of blood that must be phlebotomized. Because many patients with Noonan syndrome have cardiac anomalies needing intervention in the neonatal period, this evaluation may not be completed prior to major surgical intervention. Treatment of excessive bleeding in the meantime may require empiric treatment.

Currently, the American Academy of Pediatrics recommends that all patients with Noonan syndrome undergo evaluation for a bleeding diathesis by a hematologist.[7] This study confirms that most patients will likely need an extensive workup. Because a third of patients had platelet dysfunction in addition to other laboratory abnormalities, it will be challenging to develop a stepwise approach to the workup. In addition, laboratory abnormalities were identified in a large number of patients regardless of bleeding score. The use of bleeding scores is problematic in pediatric patients because younger patients have had fewer hemostatic challenges than adult patients. Moreover, in this report, it appears that there is no correlation between the bleeding score and the likelihood of having a laboratory abnormality. However, we note that 80% (4 of

5) of those patients who had surgery with a bleeding score of 4 or greater had bleeding complications, and 66% (10 of 15) who had surgery and did not bleed had a bleeding score of less than 2. This finding suggests that a good history may still be a better predictor of surgical bleeding than laboratory testing in this cohort of patients.

Ultimately, this study confirms that a bleeding diathesis is prevalent in Noonan syndrome patients. As in other studies, the etiology of the bleeding diathesis is variable and, in many cases, multifactorial. This series found a particularly high percentage of patients with platelet dysfunction. However, abnormal platelet function testing was not necessarily predictive of bleeding. For patients who do bleed, treatment with general hemostatic agents and even platelet transfusion may be warranted.

T. Q. Huang, MD

J. N. Huang, MD

References

1. Briggs BJ, Dickerman JD. Bleeding disorders in Noonan syndrome. *Pediatr Blood Cancer.* 2012;58:167-172.
2. Massarano AA, Wood A, Tait RC, Stevens R, Super M. Noonan syndrome: coagulation and clinical aspects. *Acta Paediatr.* 1996;85:1181-1185.
3. Bertola DR, Carneiro JDA, D'Amico EA, et al. Hematological findings in Noonan Syndrome. *Rev Hosp Clin Fac Med Sao Paulo.* 2003;58:5-8.
4. Witt DR, McGillvray BC, Allanson JE, et al. Bleeding diathesis in Noonan syndrome: a common association. *Am J Med Genet.* 1988;31:305-317.
5. Sharland M, Patton MA, Talbot S, Chitolie A, Bevan DH. Coagulation − factor deficiencies and abnormal bleeding in Noonan's syndrome. *Lancet.* 1992;339:19-21.
6. Kitchens CS, Alexander JA. Partial deficiency of coagulation factor XI as newly recognized feature of Noonan syndrome. *J Pediatr.* 1983;102:224-227.
7. Romano AA, Allanson JE, Dahlgren J, et al. Noonan syndrome: clinical features, diagnosis, and management guidelines. *Pediatrics.* 2010;126:746-759.

4 Child Development/ Behavior

The Familial Risk of Autism
Sandin S, Lichtenstein P, Kuja-Halkola R, et al (Karolinska Institutet, Stockholm, Sweden; et al)
JAMA 311:1770-1777, 2014

Importance.—Autism spectrum disorder (ASD) aggregates in families, but the individual risk and to what extent this is caused by genetic factors or shared or nonshared environmental factors remains unresolved.

Objective.—To provide estimates of familial aggregation and heritability of ASD.

Design, Setting, and Participants.—A population-based cohort including 2 049 973 Swedish children born 1982 through 2006. We identified 37 570 twin pairs, 2 642 064 full sibling pairs, 432 281 maternal and 445 531 paternal half sibling pairs, and 5 799 875 cousin pairs. Diagnoses of ASD to December 31, 2009 were ascertained.

Main Outcomes and Measures.—The relative recurrence risk (RRR) measures familial aggregation of disease. The RRR is the relative risk of autism in a participant with a sibling or cousin who has the diagnosis (exposed) compared with the risk in a participant with no diagnosed family member (unexposed). We calculated RRR for both ASD and autistic disorder adjusting for age, birth year, sex, parental psychiatric history, and parental age. We estimated how much of the probability of developing ASD can be related to genetic (additive and dominant) and environmental (shared and nonshared) factors.

Results.—In the sample, 14 516 children were diagnosed with ASD, of whom 5689 had autistic disorder. The RRR and rate per 100 000 person-years for ASD among monozygotic twins was estimated to be 153.0 (95% CI, 56.7-412.8; rate, 6274 for exposed vs 27 for unexposed); for dizygotic twins, 8.2 (95% CI, 3.7-18.1; rate, 805 for exposed vs 55 for unexposed); for full siblings, 10.3 (95% CI, 9.4-11.3; rate, 829 for exposed vs 49 for unexposed); for maternal half siblings, 3.3 (95% CI, 2.6-4.2; rate, 492 for exposed vs 94 for unexposed); for paternal half siblings, 2.9 (95% CI, 2.2-3.7; rate, 371 for exposed vs 85 for unexposed); and for cousins, 2.0 (95% CI, 1.8-2.2; rate, 155 for exposed vs 49 for unexposed). The RRR pattern was similar for autistic disorder but of slightly higher magnitude. We found support for a disease etiology including only additive genetic and nonshared environmental effects. The ASD heritability was estimated to be 0.50 (95% CI, 0.45-0.56) and the autistic disorder heritability was estimated to 0.54 (95% CI, 0.44-0.64).

Conclusions and Relevance.—Among children born in Sweden, the individual risk of ASD and autistic disorder increased with increasing genetic relatedness. Heritability of ASD and autistic disorder were estimated to be approximately 50%. These findings may inform the counseling of families with affected children.

▶ After a child is diagnosed with autism spectrum disorder (ASD), among the first questions that parents ask are "what caused this?" and "how likely is it that my next child will have ASD?" This article includes useful information on ASD recurrence risk as well as provocative conclusions regarding the potential causes of the disorder.

This study is one of the largest studies on familial risk of ASD ever reported and includes data from a broad range of family relationships (ie, twins, siblings, half-siblings, and cousins) that will serve as a useful reference for clinicians.

ASD is diagnosed much more commonly in the general community than it was 30 years ago, so it is surprising to find that recurrence rates have not increased to a greater degree. However, the rates reported in this article are consistent with those from other recent population-based studies in Denmark and California. That said, the risk of ASD in siblings (in this study, 12.9%) is substantial (Fig 1 in the original article).

However, it is also important to note that heritability estimates apply at a population level and do not have a straightforward interpretation for individual families, particularly with respect to etiologically diverse conditions such as ASD. Indeed, the segregation models used in this article to estimate genetic and environmental contributions may not be suitable for ASD, given current knowledge on etiologic mechanisms. For example, recent research highlights the importance of rare, de novo genomic variants, which would not be shared by affected relatives and thus not modeled as "genetic."

In addition, "nonshared environment" is essentially residual variance in the model used to account for how risk varies by degree of relatedness (ie, risk to cotwins, vs siblings, vs cousins). For example, prematurity is a known risk factor for ASD, so if gestational age varied between siblings, this could inflate the apparent role of "nonshared environment." This does not correspond to how the public generally views environment (eg, in relation to toxic exposures), so families should be cautioned in how this aspect of the article is interpreted.

Nevertheless, many siblings are reported to have related challenges (eg, language delays, anxiety, obsessive traits) that are subthreshold for ASD, but still have a significant impact on day-to-day functioning. The siblings of children with ASD should genuinely be considered to be "high risk" and in need of careful developmental surveillance.

L. Zwaigenbaum, MD, PhD

Patches of Disorganization in the Neocortex of Children with Autism

Stoner R, Chow ML, Boyle MP, et al (Univ of California, San Diego, La Jolla; et al)

N Engl J Med 370:1209-1219, 2014

Background.—Autism involves early brain overgrowth and dysfunction, which is most strongly evident in the prefrontal cortex. As assessed on pathological analysis, an excess of neurons in the prefrontal cortex among children with autism signals a disturbance in prenatal development and may be concomitant with abnormal cell type and laminar development.

Methods.—To systematically examine neocortical architecture during the early years after the onset of autism, we used RNA in situ hybridization with a panel of layer- and cell-type—specific molecular markers to phenotype cortical microstructure. We assayed markers for neurons and glia, along with genes that have been implicated in the risk of autism, in prefrontal, temporal, and occipital neocortical tissue from postmortem samples obtained from children with autism and unaffected children between the ages of 2 and 15 years.

Results.—We observed focal patches of abnormal laminar cytoarchitecture and cortical disorganization of neurons, but not glia, in prefrontal and temporal cortical tissue from 10 of 11 children with autism and from 1 of 11 unaffected children. We observed heterogeneity between cases with respect to cell types that were most abnormal in the patches and the layers that were most affected by the pathological features. No cortical layer was uniformly spared, with the clearest signs of abnormal expression in layers 4 and 5. Three-dimensional reconstruction of layer markers confirmed the focal geometry and size of patches.

Conclusions.—In this small, explorative study, we found focal disruption of cortical laminar architecture in the cortexes of a majority of young children with autism. Our data support a probable dysregulation of layer formation and layer-specific neuronal differentiation at prenatal developmental stages. (Funded by the Simons Foundation and others.)

▶ There has been consensus for more than a decade that autism spectrum disorder (ASD), a prevalent developmental disorder affecting social interaction and communication, has a strong genetic component that affects brain development and function. The earliest neuroanatomic studies—elegantly simple by today's standards—carefully measured head circumference and brain volume during early development to conclude that autism was associated with altered perinatal growth of the cerebrum. Early brain enlargement was found to be prominent in the frontal lobe, but changes in brain volume were also observed in the temporal lobe and cerebellum, as well as subcortical nuclei, and most regressed with aging into adolescence.

More recent genetic experiments over the past decade reinforced the early anatomic studies when they identified alterations in the expression of whole families of genes that code for proteins involved in neuronal migration, neuronal wiring, and synaptic transmission. The unexpected breadth of the genetic alterations affecting such a wide range of neuronal operations has revealed a bewildering complexity in brain dysfunction in ASD. Indeed, no single gene defect, no single brain regional disturbance, and no single neurophysiological process gone awry underlies ASD.

Although a high degree of biological heterogeneity mirrors an equally heterogeneous degree of clinically expressed functional impairment, the common outcome is that all children with ASD are confronted with myriad, often-subtle sensory and cognitive impairments interacting to significantly alter sociability and communication. Our current understanding of this biological heterogeneity has belied an earlier (naive) hope that ASD might be treated by addressing a single gene defect or by delivering a single drug. The tremendous accumulation of behavioral and biological data has indicated that understanding the developmental and physiological pathways altered in ASD will have tremendous clinical importance by revealing early biomarkers that can help efforts to understand etiologic mechanisms and direct treatment. Thus, current scientific focus is to use high-resolution mapping of brain dysfunction to understand heterogeneity of ASD symptom expression.

Stoner et al take a bold step by providing the first high-resolution images of how gene expression is altered within the cerebral cortex of children with ASD. Using postmortem brain samples from children with ASD and typically developing controls, obtained from 4 tissue banks, the experiment quantified the regional alterations in gene expression in neocortex at the cellular level. Gene expression was measured by quantifying the expression of a series of RNA transcripts that were judiciously chosen to probe the laminar distribution of the neocortical gray matter (Fig 1 in the original article).

At first glance, the experiments demonstrated the presence of layer-specific alterations in gene expression in ASD. However, more detailed examination using serial reconstruction and 3-dimensional computer rendering (Fig 3 in the original article) revealed that the alterations in gene expression were not uniform, but rather always occurred in 5- to 7-mm diameter "patches" that extended deep into the gray matter through all cortical layers. Although the specific genes affected were different between cases, the patch organization of the phenomenon was invariant, perhaps pointing to a common underlying process involved in ASD. Of note was that the impairments in gene expression were not accompanied by a loss of neurons or the laminar organization of the neocortex, indicating that the gene expression deficits may be the consequence of altered neuronal migration and affect the functioning of the neuronal network within the patch.

The study appears to indicate that the neocortical pathophysiology of ASD is modular. At a macroscopic level, modularity is observed by the regional presence of the patches of disorganized gene expression in frontal and temporal lobes but not in the occipital lobe. At a microscopic level, modularity is observed by the apparently random occurrence of discrete patches of disorganized gene expression embedded within large expanses of normal neocortex that appear to be spared.

It will be important to replicate the findings of Stoner et al and, thereafter, to identify the factors that so precisely define the borders of this susceptibility. What causes any given patch to be present where it is found, and why is adjacent tissue not similarly affected? There is ample precedence for physiologic and neurochemical modularity within the brain orthogonal to the lamination axis in layered brain structures. Although revealing the modularity of brain has often proved more challenging than observing laminar cytology, nonlaminar modularity at a histologic level has been long recognized in Brodmann's areas. The search for the factors that define these much smaller patch locations and specify their spatial extent may provide significant insight into neocortical function and its susceptibility for disruption in ASD.

S. R. Dager, MD

D. W. Shaw, MD

J. P. Welsh, PhD

Validation of the Modified Checklist for Autism in Toddlers, Revised With Follow-up (M-CHAT-R/F)

Robins DL, Casagrande K, Barton M, et al (Georgia State Univ, Atlanta; Univ of Connecticut, Storrs)
Pediatrics 133:37-45, 2014

Objective.—This study validates the Modified Checklist for Autism in Toddlers, Revised with Follow-up (M-CHAT-R/F), a screening tool for low-risk toddlers, and demonstrates improved utility compared with the original M-CHAT.

Methods.—Toddlers ($N = 16\,071$) were screened during 18- and 24-month well-child care visits in metropolitan Atlanta and Connecticut. Parents of toddlers at risk on M-CHAT-R completed follow-up; those who continued to show risk were evaluated.

Results.—The reliability and validity of the M-CHAT-R/F were demonstrated, and optimal scoring was determined by using receiver operating characteristic curves. Children whose total score was ≥ 3 initially and ≥ 2 after follow-up had a 47.5% risk of being diagnosed with autism spectrum disorder (ASD; confidence interval [95% CI]: 0.41−0.54) and a 94.6% risk of any developmental delay or concern (95% CI: 0.92−0.98). Total score was more effective than alternative scores. An algorithm based on 3 risk levels is recommended to maximize clinical utility and to reduce age of diagnosis and onset of early intervention. The M-CHAT-R detects ASD at a higher rate compared with the M-CHAT while also reducing the number of children needing the follow-up. Children in the current study were diagnosed 2 years younger than the national median age of diagnosis.

Conclusions.—The M-CHAT-R/F detects many cases of ASD in toddlers; physicians using the 2-stage screener can be confident that most screen-positive cases warrant evaluation and referral for early intervention. Widespread implementation of universal screening can lower the age of ASD diagnosis by 2 years compared with recent surveillance findings, increasing time available for early intervention.

▶ Over the past decade, we have seen improved developmental surveillance and screening in pediatric practice, with a simultaneous rise in the identification of autism. However, the age of diagnosis for autism spectrum disorders (ASD) remains over 4 years of age, despite the availability of evidence-based early intervention treatments for children under 3 years. With this revision of the Modified Checklist for Autism in Toddlers (the M-CHAT-R/F), we are ushered into a new era for both developmental screening and early identification of ASD. The revised M-CHAT-R/F has improved on its predecessor both for detection of ASD and for implementation in the pediatric office setting, hopefully leading to earlier identification and treatment of affected children.

With the M-CHAT-R/F, its authors have shortened the parent-completed questionnaire to 20 questions while carefully simplifying its scoring and interpretation, mindfully thinking of its implementation in the primary medical home setting. The test's total score now places a child into a low-, medium-, or high-risk category (Fig 3 in the original article). The low risk child (score < 3) follows the usual schedule for ongoing surveillance and screening, whereas those at high risk (≥8) are recommended for immediate referral for diagnostic evaluation and intervention. It is for those described as at medium risk that the major improvements have been obtained, reducing the overidentification and high false positivity of the M-CHAT. When a child tests in this category (score 3–7), a 5- to 10-minute follow-up interview that is well-suited for the performance by the health care provider or office staff is advised as a second stage. For those scoring ≥2 on interview, diagnostic referral and intervention are recommended.

Using this methodology in a large screening study of more than 15 000 children in Atlanta and Connecticut, the investigators achieved high levels of sensitivity and specificity (0.94 and 0.83, respectively; Fig 2 in the original article). All 75 children in the high-risk group had a developmental disorder, including 44 with ASD. In the medium risk group (n = 105), nearly half (47.5%) had ASD, and all but 5% had another developmental disorder or concern (positive predictive value 0.95). On the other hand, 9 children with ASD who were of concern to the pediatrician through surveillance screened negatively (low risk).

This article suggests that use of the M-CHAT-R/F may result in earlier identification of ASD as well as other developmental disorders if implemented in this new risk categorization and 2-stage procedure. At the same time, it also forces a reconsideration of the methods used for developmental screening. Prior models for developmental screening used a broad screening for multiple poorly defined developmental conditions ("developmental delay"). However, the M-CHAT screens for a specific developmental disorder, autism, akin to the paradigm of other pediatric screening initiatives such as screening for newborn metabolic disorders and early hearing detection.

From this example and experience, a shift away from general developmental screening toward targeted screening for specific conditions, particularly those of greatest severity with highest need for short- and long-term child and family intervention and assistance such as the neuromotor disorders, intellectual disability and non-ASD language impairments, must be considered.

The new 2-stage process also requires reconsideration of the current guidelines of the American Academy of Pediatrics (AAP). This trial conforms to the recommended 18- and 24-month ASD screening ages, with demonstrated reliability and validity. However, its risk categorization and algorithm for diagnosis and referral differs from the 2006 AAP guidelines, in which referral for diagnosis and intervention would be called for in those children screening in both the moderate- and high-risk groups. By introducing the second step, with its improved sensitivity, specificity, and positive predictive value, the primary care pediatrician can feel more confident in the test results and better able to counsel families. At the same time, the ongoing use of developmental surveillance is supported by missed cases in screening. Continued use of the M-CHAT-R/F, including its use in high-risk samples, will further clarify its strengths and weaknesses in identifying ASD as well as other related conditions. In the meantime, it is time to use this revised test for autism and developmental surveillance and screening in the pediatric primary care setting.

P. H. Lipkin, MD

Preventing Early Infant Sleep and Crying Problems and Postnatal Depression: A Randomized Trial
Hiscock H, Cook F, Bayer J, et al (The Royal Children's Hosp, Parkville, Australia; The Royal Children's Hosp, Melbourne, Australia; et al)
Pediatrics 133:e346-e354, 2014

Objective.—To evaluate a prevention program for infant sleep and cry problems and postnatal depression.

Methods.—Randomized controlled trial with 781 infants born at 32 weeks or later in 42 well-child centers, Melbourne, Australia. Follow-up occurred at infant age 4 and 6 months. The intervention including supplying information about normal infant sleep and cry patterns, settling techniques, medical causes of crying and parent self-care, delivered via booklet and DVD (at infant age 4 weeks), telephone consultation (8 weeks), and parent group (13 weeks) versus well-child care. Outcomes included caregiver-reported infant night sleep problem (primary outcome), infant daytime sleep, cry and feeding problems, crying and sleep duration, caregiver depression symptoms, attendance at night wakings, and formula changes.

Results.—Infant outcomes were similar between groups. Relative to control caregivers, intervention caregivers at 6 months were less likely to score >9 on the Edinburgh Postnatal Depression Scale (7.9%, vs 12.9%, adjusted odds ratio [OR] 0.57, 95% confidence interval [CI] 0.34 to 0.94), spend >20 minutes attending infant wakings (41% vs 51%, adjusted OR 0.66, 95% CI 0.46 to 0.95), or change formula (13% vs 23%, $P < .05$). Infant frequent feeders (>11 feeds/24 hours) in the intervention group were less likely to have daytime sleep (OR 0.13, 95% CI 0.03 to 0.54) or cry problems (OR 0.27, 95% CI 0.08 to 0.86) at 4 months.

Conclusions.—An education program reduces postnatal depression symptoms, as well as sleep and cry problems in infants who are frequent feeders. The program may be best targeted to frequent feeders.

▶ Low-cost universal interventions to prevent child health and developmental problems are greatly needed. Hiscock and colleagues made an effort to address this need by performing a well-designed randomized, controlled trial of a community-based intervention meant to prevent infant crying and sleep problems and resulting maternal psychological distress. They recruited 770 families—quite a large sample size compared to existing literature—who were receiving postpartum nurse home visits in Melbourne, Australia. Intervention-arm parents received a booklet and DVD that was both informational (eg, teaching parents about normal infant behaviors) and skill-based (eg, how to read infant cues, demonstrating settling techniques). Intervention parents were also offered support by telephone at 6 to 8 weeks and at an in-person support meeting at 12 weeks' postpartum, both staffed by trained psychologists and nurses. Control participants received usual well child care.

The investigators should be applauded for crafting and carrying out such a large yet methodologically sound community-based intervention. They were also prudent to study multiple outcome measures because it is never clear at the outset which outcome will be most sensitive to the intervention. In this case, they found no differences between intervention and control arms on their primary outcome: parent report of sleep, crying, or feeding problems at 4 or 6 months. This is not surprising, given the wide variability of infant crying and sleep behaviors and the factors influencing whether they are experienced as problems by their parents.

Despite this lack of effect on infant behaviors, parent outcomes were improved at 6 months: intervention group caregivers were significantly less likely to have clinically significant depression symptoms, had fewer doubts about how to manage their infant's sleep, and reported fewer maladaptive infant care behaviors such as excessive time attending to the child overnight, changing the infant's formula in response to crying, or having difficulty setting limits. This result is remarkable and truly demonstrates the power of improving parent self-efficacy and coping skills with regard to infant distress in both improving parent mental health and adherence with recommended infant care practices. We propose that although this intervention may not have changed infant behavior, it changed parent perception of that behavior as stressful and therefore improved the dyad's goodness of fit. This in turn supported parents' sense of efficacy in adjusting to their new parenting role.

Improvements in parental mental health have important implications for child developmental and health outcomes. Young children of depressed mothers have higher rates of developmental delay, social-emotional problems, behavioral and sleep dysregulation, and early academic difficulties. However, as Hiscock and colleagues understand, the relationship between parent mental health and infant behavior is bidirectional: difficult or fussy babies, particularly those who cannot self-soothe, may precipitate anxiety and depression symptoms in their caregivers, leading to a transactional cycle of difficulties with parent—child interactions, coregulation, more negative child outcomes, parent dissatisfaction, and so on.

This transactional relationship is illustrated in this study's stratified analyses. Babies designated as frequent feeders (a proxy for an infant with self-regulation problems or parents who are unsure how else to soothe their infant) benefited differentially from this intervention. Frequent-feeder intervention infants had 87% lower odds of having daytime sleep problems (OR 0.13, 95% confidence interval [CI] 0.03—0.54) and 73% lower odds of crying problems at 4 months (OR 0.27, 95% CI 0.08—0.86), suggesting that the skills taught through the intervention materials and clinical encounters were helping parents adapt to the extremes of infant behavior. It would have been interesting to examine whether the parents of these improved infants showed even lower rates of post-partum depression symptoms or maladaptive infant care behaviors.

Although the intervention evaluated in this trial recognizes that new parents need developmental guidance and concrete skills training to help them feel efficacious and less stressed, it largely puts the parent in a passive learning role. By expecting parents to watch a DVD or read a pamphlet given to them in the first few weeks of being a new parent—a particularly sleep-deprived and exhausted stage of parents' lives—many parents may not have accessed the materials optimally. Only half of parents took advantage of the in-person support session at 13 weeks, which speaks to how difficult it might be to engage parents during this time.

How can large-scale interventions engage parents in a more active and personalized learning role? Programs such as the Fussy Baby Network specifically work to engage parents by tailoring the therapeutic process to the needs of the dyad, empowering parents to understand and respond to their infants individually, rather than using a "top-down" educational approach. However, such dyad-centered interventions are difficult to craft on a community scale. We suggest that new mobile technology-based interventions may hold more promise for engaging new parents than booklets or videos. Brief, digestible, and practical doses of visual information, informed by the parent's concerns and infant's temperament and developmental status, can be sent to parents at weekly intervals instead of a large "information dump" all in 1 sitting, much of which may not be retained or returned to in times of need. This approach also holds promise for engaging more parents from lower socioeconomic strata, who were underrepresented in this trial yet have a higher risk of both maternal depression and infant regulatory problems. Finally, such interventions might be even less costly—and more effective—if fully integrated into the existing health infrastructure or trusted medical home, rather than delivered in parallel.

J. S. Radesky, MD
B. S. Zuckerman, MD

Antidepressants and Suicide Attempts in Children

Cooper WO, Callahan ST, Shintani A, et al (Vanderbilt Univ School of Medicine, Nashville, TN; et al)
Pediatrics 133:204-210, 2014

Objectives.—Recent data showing possible increased risk for suicidal behavior among children and adolescents treated with selective serotonin reuptake inhibitors (SSRIs) and serotonin-norepinephrine reuptake inhibitors (SNRIs) antidepressants have created significant concern among patients, families, and providers, including concerns about the risk of individual antidepressants. This study was designed to compare the risk for medically treated suicide attempts among new users of sertraline, paroxetine, citalopram, escitalopram, and venlafaxine to risk for new users of fluoxetine.

Methods.—A retrospective cohort study included 36 842 children aged 6 to 18 years enrolled in Tennessee Medicaid between 1995 and 2006 who were new users of 1 of the antidepressant medications of interest (defined as filling no prescriptions for antidepressants in the preceding 365 days). Medically treated suicide attempts were identified from Medicaid files and vital records and confirmed with medical record review.

Results.—Four hundred nineteen cohort members had a medically treated suicide attempt with explicit or inferred attempt to die confirmed through medical record review, including 4 who completed suicide. The rate of confirmed suicide attempts for the study drugs ranged from 24.0 per 1000 person-years to 29.1 per 1000 person-years. The adjusted rate of suicide attempts did not differ significantly among current users of SSRI and SNRI antidepressants compared with current users of fluoxetine. Users of multiple antidepressants concomitantly had increased risk for suicide attempt.

Conclusions.—In this population-based study of children recently initiating an antidepressant, there was no evidence that risk of suicide attempts differed for commonly prescribed SSRI and SNRI antidepressants.

► Concerns over the risks and benefits of new antidepressant medications for children and adolescents have created a quandary for many prescribers, families, and pediatric patients. There may not be 1 best (or worst) medication in this group of antidepressants in terms of potential harm and risk of suicide. This study by Cooper et al is significant and examines previous data further and in relation to the regulatory warnings that created considerable controversy. Although this research was not designed to answer some of the other important questions regarding long-term outcomes of medications or comparisons to cognitive behavioral therapy, it does provide some useful additional evidence.

The 2004 Food and Drug Administration (FDA) black box warnings for selective serotonin reuptake inhibitors (SSRIs) and the newer classes of antidepressants were confusing for physicians, parents, and patients alike. This action was a culmination of other international bodies, regulatory organizations, and pharmaceutical notices about specific antidepressants (paroxetine, venlafaxine, and others).[1] The FDA action was rooted in efforts to promote safety and disclose potential issues. Yet the decision to post a safety alert and ask providers to conduct close follow-up surveillance when starting new antidepressants was based on limited data, and all of the medications listed in the safety alert were grouped together broadly. Research reports showed changes in prescription trends for specific antidepressants during the decade of the 2000s after the warning.[2] A few reports, albeit based on limited ecological data, even speculated that a 2004 increase in adolescent suicide rates could potentially have been connected to the FDA warning.[3]

These results may temper the suggestion that some medications are more "safe" than the others and allow providers to focus on other considerations in selecting therapy and discussing treatment selection with teens and families. Although no single medication was statistically distinct in the analyses of new prescriptions, it is notable that multiple concurrent medications are associated with an increased risk of suicide attempts when compared with monotherapy (Table 2 in the original article). The practice of polypharmacy has been growing for mental health disorders. These prescribing practices include the use of antidepressants with stimulants, antipsychotics, and others. The authors note it is not clear whether association is related to the antidepressant treatment or use of multiple antidepressants is merely a proxy for more severe or complex mental health disorder in children. It is readily apparent that pediatric patients on multiple psychotropic medications are a high-risk group deserving close attention.

Cooper et al demonstrate the value of large data sets and partnerships with insurance payers such as Medicaid to review prescription records and link these with outcomes. Clinical trials may provide data on medication effectiveness, but secondary analyses can provide the robust power to examine relatively rare potential harms (suicidality was between 24.0 and 29.1 incidents per 1000 person-years on treatment with only 4 completed suicides) and the ability to subanalyze specific medications separately. Health services research can provide evidence that is a vital supplement to clinical observations, pharmaceutical figures, patient anecdotes, or regulatory communications.

It is important that clinicians understand the purpose and focus of this study, along with the important remaining questions surrounding antidepressant prescriptions and treatment decisions. These results are based on comparisons of new antidepressant prescriptions to fluoxetine as a standard. The design is focused on medications and not on the role of counseling and psychotherapy, which may be equal or favorable to medications for some children and adolescents with depression. The study has sound exclusion criteria and design. However, the larger question still remains: what is the risk of suicide while starting an antidepressant versus the potential positive effects from treatment in reducing depressive symptoms and preventing suicide as the ultimate outcome of interest?

Although this analysis cannot answer a key question on the long-term outcomes versus potential harms of antidepressants, we do know that most depressive disorders go untreated or undertreated. For many patients, medications may play an important role. The stakes are high—suicide is third leading diagnosis in terms of US adolescent-age mortality, and depression is the leading cause of global disability among adolescents. Thus, we need more studies of this nature to understand risks and outcomes of psychopharmacological treatment. Ultimately, physicians and providers face a daunting task to weigh limited evidence on potential benefits and risks in management of pediatric depressive disorders and the often complicating comorbid conditions. Treatment must be individualized and carefully communicated amid the breadth of information on the Internet, in the media, and from other sources.

J. L. Rushton, MD, MPH

References

1. Busch SH, Barry CL. Pediatric Antidepressant Use After The Black-Box Warning. *Health Aff.* 2009;28(3):724-733.
2. Libby AM, Brent DA, Morrato EH, Orton HD, Allen R, Valuck RJ. Decline in treatment of pediatric depression after FDA advisory on risk of suicidality with SSRIs. *Am J Psychiatry.* 2007;164(6):884-891.
3. Gibbons RD, Brown CH, Hur K, et al. Early Evidence on the Effects of Regulators' Suicidality Warnings on SSRI Prescriptions and Suicide in Children and Adolescents. *Am J Psychiatry.* 2007;164:1356-1363.

Effects of Child Development Accounts on Early Social-Emotional Development: An Experimental Test
Huang J, Sherraden M, Kim Y, et al (Saint Louis Univ, St Louis, MO; Washington Univ in St Louis, MO; Virginia Commonwealth Univ, Richmond)
JAMA Pediatr 168:265-271, 2014

Importance.—This study, based on Oklahoma's statewide Child Development Accounts (CDAs) program, presents findings from the first experimental test of the hypothesis that creating lifelong savings accounts for children at birth promotes their long-term well-being.

Objective.—To examine the effects of CDAs, an innovative social policy to encourage lifelong saving and asset building for long-term development, on parent-reported social-emotional development in early childhood.

Design, Setting, and Participants.—A statewide randomized experiment of CDAs was conducted in 2008, drawing a probability sample of 7328 children from all infants born in two 3-month periods in Oklahoma (April 1 through June 30 and August 1 through October 31, 2007). After agreeing to participate in the experiment, caregivers of 2704 infants completed a baseline survey and were randomly assigned to treatment (n = 1358) and control groups (n = 1346). Approximately 84% of participants completed a follow-up survey in the spring of 2011.

Interventions.—The intervention offered CDAs, built on the existing Oklahoma 529 college-savings plan, to treatment participants. It also provided additional financial incentives and information.

Main Outcomes and Measures.—The primary outcome—child social-emotional development—is measured by scores from a 17-item version of the Ages and Stages Questionnaire: Social-Emotional. Caregivers completed it in the 3-year follow-up survey. Lower scores indicate better functioning.

Results.—The CDAs have positive effects on social-emotional development for children at approximately age 4 years. The nonweighted treatment-control difference is −1.56 (90% CI, −2.87 to −0.22; $P = .06$), but the weighted difference is nonsignificant. The effects appear to be greater for disadvantaged subsamples, such as low-income households (weighted mean difference, −2.21; 90% CI, −4.01 to −0.42; $P = .04$).

Conclusions and Relevance.—As a complement to other early education and health interventions, CDAs may improve social-emotional development in early childhood. Their effects may be explained as a mediating process that influences parents. Child Development Accounts may influence parental attitudes, behaviors, expectations, and involvement; in turn, these may affect child development.

▶ Although it may not be apparent to the typical reader, this study represents the culmination of almost a quarter century of social science surrounding the putative importance of assets (ie, wealth as opposed to income) to children's lives and well-being. Particularly interesting is the fact that the interest in assets really started with the publication by Michael Sherraden of his landmark, but largely theoretical, book, *Assets and the Poor.*[1] And here is Sherraden again, along with colleagues, Huang, Kim, and Clancy, 22 years later with the empirical culmination of much intervening research.

The theory is deceptively simple: income is a flow, and assets (ie, savings) are a stock. They serve different functions in a family. Income takes care of everyday expenses, whereas assets are the stuff of which upward mobility is made. Big human capital investments—like a college education—are not made out of a weekly paycheck. Rather, an asset reserve is what communicates to a child that college is a possibility. Or that home ownership is just around the corner. Or even that job loss will not mean eviction.

The theory was given a boost by my own work[2] and that of other scholars who showed parental assets to be the second most powerful predictor of children's educational success (after parental education). This work, done during the late 1990s, laid the groundwork for a series of experimental evaluations, the most ambitious of which is presented here, Oklahoma's OK SEED. Although the results were certainly less stronger (as may be expected) than the observational studies, the significant impact of account holding for disadvantaged families is certainly promising.

We must keep in mind that the treatment—a $1000 educational account held by the state in the child's name along with matching funds for mothers to open their own college savings accounts—was a modest, almost symbolic, intervention, given the cost of higher education today. So it remains all the more remarkable that the researchers found that the socioemotional development of 4-year-olds (far from college age when the monies could be accessed) was improved compared with the control group. Far from being the final work, this article should serve as the pilot study for an experiment in which the treatment is an order of magnitude larger (ie, at least $10 000). Then we can start to truly assess the social-psychological impact of assets for the poor.

D. Conley, PhD

References

1. Sherraden MW. *Assets and the Poor.* (M.E. Sharpe, Inc; Armonk, NY). 1991.
2. Conley D. *Being Black, Living in the Red: Race, Wealth and Social Policy in America.* (University of California Press: Berkeley, CA). 1999.

5 Dentistry and Otolaryngology (ENT)

Large cohort study finds a statistically significant association between excessive crying in early infancy and subsequent ear symptoms
Hestbaek L, Sannes MM, Lous J (Univ of Southern Denmark, Odense, Denmark; Kiropraktorklinikken, Horten, Norway)
Acta Paediatr 103:e206-e211, 2014

Aim.—The diagnosis of infantile colic is based on excessive crying. However, several causal factors can account for this disconcerting, nonspecific symptom. The main aim of this study was to investigate a possible association between excessive crying during the first 6 months of life and subsequent ear problems.

Methods.—Data from a cohort study of 26 983 Danish children were used. Mothers participated in four telephone interviews and one questionnaire and provided information on crying in the first 6 months of life and ear symptoms at the ages of 6 months, 18 months and 7 years.

Results.—There was a statistically significant association between excessive crying in infancy and subsequent ear symptoms. A gradual increase in subsequent ear problems was seen with increasing crying time at all the data collection times.

Conclusion.—The results of this study suggest a possible link between excessive crying and ear infections. Whether such a link is causal or due to common underlying factors is still unknown. We recommend thorough ear examinations in children with symptoms compatible with infantile colic.

▶ Working out what causes infant colic and how best to manage it has been occupying researchers for the better part of a century. Colic (ie, excessive crying occurring more than 3 hours per day, for more than 3 days per week, for more than 3 weeks) causes great distress to families and is costly given that it is one of the most common reasons parents present to health professionals in the first months of an infant's life. This article is therefore of interest because it looks at a possible cause of infant colic. For the first time, researchers have looked at early infant crying and later child ear infections, antibiotic use, and

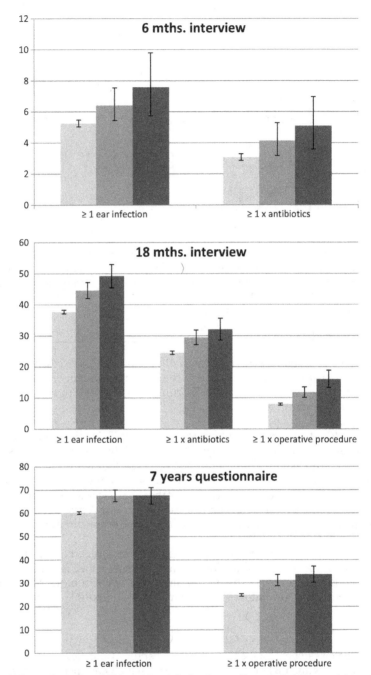

FIGURE 1.—Proportion of children with ear infections (reported by mother), children receiving antibiotic treatment and children having operative procedures (myringotomy and/or tympanostomy) at three different time points in relation to three mutually excessive groups of crying. Error bars indicate 95% confidence intervals. Results for operative procedures are left out at 6 months because <1% of babies had this. Use of antibiotics was not recorded at the age of 7 years. □ Normal crying, n~24,800 ▓ Excessive crying, n~1470 ■ Extremely excessive crying, n~700. (Reprinted from Hestbaek L, Sannes MM, Lous J. Large cohort study finds a statistically significant association between excessive crying in early infancy and subsequent ear symptoms. *Acta Paediatr.* 2014;103:e206-e211, with permission from Foundation Acta Pædiatrica.)

insertion of tympanostomy tubes in a large, longitudinal, population-based cohort.

I won't be changing my practice just yet. The authors describe an association between excessive infant crying and ear infections and antibiotic use at ages 6 and 18 months (Fig 1). They suggest that clinicians seeing infants with colic should examine the infants' ears but also acknowledge that to do this would require pneumatic otoscopy and tympanometry as simply looking in infants' ears to make a diagnosis of otitis media is unreliable. Putting aside the practicality of making a reliable diagnosis of otitis media in an infant, there are a number of other issues that need to be considered.

Mothers were asked about ear infections and crying when the infant was 6 months old. Infants who cry excessively are more likely to be taken to the doctor, who in turn, may be more likely to diagnose a medical cause of crying such as otitis media and prescribe antibiotics. Thus, this help-seeking behavior may explain the relationship between "otitis media" and excessive crying rather than any ear infection per se. Ear infections as a cause of true colic would be unlikely. After 3 weeks an ear infection would either have resolved (in which case the infant's crying would decrease) or worsened. If it worsened, you would expect the infant to develop other signs and symptoms such as fever, dehydration, or poor weight gain, and these are not issues seen in infant colic in which a baby is typically well despite the crying.

Another issue is that parents who had an infant who cried excessively may be more likely to see their child as potentially vulnerable to infections over time. They may be more likely to ascribe a diagnosis of ear infection in a toddler who is grizzly with an upper respiratory tract infection and may be more likely to attend a doctor and get antibiotics as a result. Relying on parent report of an ear infection rather than a clinical diagnosis makes this possibility even greater.

Finally, parents who remained in this cohort were of higher socioeconomic status than those who dropped out of the study. Again, more affluent parents may be more likely to seek health care for their children than those who are less well off. Children of affluent parents may be more likely to receive antibiotics and undergo operations to manage recurrent "otitis media."

Thus, the authors' conclusion that we should do a "thorough ear examination as part of the routine examination of excessively crying infants" seems premature. Further research such as case-control studies with blinded assessment of ear infection in infants with and without colic are needed before we change practice. The natural history of ear infections in infants also needs to be documented because ear infections in older children are often self-limiting and do not require antibiotics.[1] Although searching for a possible cause of infant colic remains commendable, examining ears and prescribing antibiotics is not a route we want to go down yet.

H. Hiscock, MBBS, FRACP, MD

Reference

1. The Royal Children's Hospital, Melbourne. Acute Otitis Media Clinical Practice Guideline. http://www.rch.org.au/clinicalguide/guideline_index/Acute_Otitis_Media. Accessed May 18, 2014.

Xylitol Syrup for the Prevention of Acute Otitis Media

Vernacchio L, Corwin MJ, Vezina RM, et al (Pediatric Physician's Organization at Children's, Brookline, MA; Boston Univ, MA; et al)
Pediatrics 133:289-295, 2014

Background.—Acute otitis media (AOM) is a common childhood illness and the leading indication for antibiotic prescriptions for US children. Xylitol, a naturally occurring sugar alcohol, can reduce AOM when given 5 times per day as a gum or syrup, but a more convenient dosing regimen is needed for widespread adoption.

Methods.—We designed a pragmatic practice-based randomized controlled trial to determine if viscous xylitol solution at a dose of 5 g 3 times per day could reduce the occurrence of clinically diagnosed AOM among otitis-prone children 6 months through 5 years of age.

Results.—A total of 326 subjects were enrolled, with 160 allocated to xylitol and 166 to placebo. In the primary analysis of time to first clinically diagnosed AOM episode, the hazard ratio for xylitol versus placebo recipients was 0.88 (95% confidence interval [CI] 0.61 to 1.3). In secondary analyses, the incidence of AOM was 0.53 episodes per 90 days in the xylitol group versus 0.59 in the placebo group (difference 0.06; 95% CI −0.25 to 0.13); total antibiotic use was 6.8 days per 90 days in the xylitol group versus 6.4 in the placebo group (difference 0.4; 95% CI −1.8 to 2.7). The lack of effectiveness was not explained by nonadherence to treatment, as the hazard ratio for those taking nearly all assigned xylitol compared with those taking none was 0.93 (95% CI 0.56 to 1.57).

Conclusions.—Viscous xylitol solution in a dose of 5 g 3 times per day was ineffective in reducing clinically diagnosed AOM among otitis-prone children.

▶ Acute otitis media (AOM) is one of the most common diseases of childhood. Almost half of all pediatric antibiotic prescriptions are written for otitis media, and an excess of $100 is spent per episode. Despite this, 80% of AOM episodes resolve spontaneously within 3 days. Beginning in the 1990s in Western Europe and later in the 2000s in the United States, concern grew over antibiotic resistance and treatment side effects. In 2004, the American Academy of Family Physicians and the American Academy of Pediatrics published recommendations highlighting initial watchful waiting in children with otitis media.[1] Seeing a persistence of symptoms, many families seek alternative modes of treatment and prevention.

Xylitol is a natural sugar found in many fruits and used as a sweetener in chewing gum. It has been well studied by several randomized controlled trials and thought to have preventative properties in otitis media. Xylitol inhibits the growth of *Streptococcus pneumoniae* and inhibits the attachment of both *S pneumoniae* and *Haemophilus influenzae* to nasopharyngeal cells.[2] Kurola et al in 2009 offered a possible explanation for this: exposure to xylitol lowered cpsB (pneumococcal capsular locus) gene expression, which changes the ultrastructure of the pneumococcal capsule.[3]

Unfortunately most reports thus far showing efficacy have prescribed a regimen of daily dosing 5 times per day and usually include the gum as opposed to the syrup. Adherence to regimens greater than 3 times a day is difficult to achieve. In addition, for small children, who are most prone to otitis, gum is impractical. This study attempts to find another avenue for prevention: viscous xylitol solution 5 grams given 3 times daily. Unfortunately this regimen did not seem to be preventative (Fig 2 in the original article). In a previous report,[4] Vernacchio et al highlighted the optimal dose of xylitol, 5 grams delivered 3 times daily in infants as young as 6 months of age, which is higher than most other published reports. In this current study, even this higher, optimal dosage did not seem to lead to prevention.

One potential reason for the negative results is that the investigators included children who had known middle-ear fluid at the start of the study, unlike many other studies. These patients, described as "otitis-prone," are more likely to be heavily colonized with bacteria associated with AOM. As a result, xylitol may be less effective for these particular children. I do believe they are correct in including these patients in their study and asserting this importance because this study population better reflects actual patients. If previous studies had included these patients as well, I wonder if the efficacy would have been so pronounced. Clearly the search continues for more practical, effective means for preventing otitis media.

J. R. Levi, MD

References

1. American Academy of Pediatrics Subcommittee on Management of Acute Otitis Media. Diagnosis and management of acute otitis media. *Pediatrics.* 2004;113: 1451-1465.
2. Uhari M, Tapianen T, Kontiokari T. Xylitol in preventing acute otitis media. *Vaccine.* 2000;19:S144-S147.
3. Kurola P, Tapainen T, Kaijalaninen T, Uhari M, Saukkoriipi A. Xylitol and capsular gene expression in Streptococcus pneumonia. *J Med Microbiol.* 2009;58: 1470-1473.
4. Vernacchio L, Vezina RM, Mitchell AA. Tolerability of oral xylitol solution in young children: implications for otitis media prophylaxis. *Int J Pediatr Otorhinolaryngol.* 2007;71:89-94.

A Trial of Treatment for Acute Otorrhea in Children with Tympanostomy Tubes

van Dongen TMA, van der Heijden GJMG, Venekamp RP, et al (Univ Med Ctr Utrecht, the Netherlands)

N Engl J Med 370:723-733, 2014

Background.—Recent guidance for the management of acute otorrhea in children with tympanostomy tubes is based on limited evidence from trials comparing oral antibiotic agents with topical antibiotics.

Methods.—In this open-label, pragmatic trial, we randomly assigned 230 children, 1 to 10 years of age, who had acute tympanostomy-tube otorrhea to receive hydrocortisone—bacitracin—colistin eardrops (76 children) or oral amoxicillin—clavulanate suspension (77) or to undergo initial observation (77). The primary outcome was the presence of otorrhea, as assessed otoscopically, 2 weeks after study-group assignment. Secondary outcomes were the duration of the initial otorrhea episode, the total number of days of otorrhea and the number of otorrhea recurrences during 6 months of follow-up, quality of life, complications, and treatment-related adverse events.

Results.—Antibiotic—glucocorticoid eardrops were superior to oral antibiotics and initial observation for all outcomes. At 2 weeks, 5% of children treated with antibiotic—glucocorticoid eardrops had otorrhea, as compared with 44% of those treated with oral antibiotics (risk difference, −39 percentage points; 95% confidence interval [CI], −51 to −26) and 55% of those treated with initial observation (risk difference, −49 percentage points; 95% CI, −62 to −37). The median duration of the initial episode of otorrhea was 4 days for children treated with antibiotic—glucocorticoid eardrops versus 5 days for those treated with oral antibiotics ($P < 0.001$) and 12 days for those who were assigned to initial observation ($P < 0.001$). Treatment-related adverse events were mild, and no complications of otitis media, including local cellulitis, perichondritis, mastoiditis, and intracranial complications, were reported at 2 weeks.

Conclusions.—Antibiotic—glucocorticoid eardrops were more effective than oral antibiotics and initial observation in children with tympanostomy tubes who had uncomplicated acute otorrhea. (Funded by the Netherlands Organization for Health Research and Development; Netherlands Trial Register number, NTR1481.)

▶ Acute otitis media (AOM) is "bread-and-butter" general pediatrics and has been associated with lower quality-of-life scores for both the affected child and his or her caregivers.[1,2] Therefore, it is not terribly surprising that tympanostomy tube placement is the most commonly performed pediatric ambulatory surgery. Approximately 667 000 pediatric outpatients undergo myringotomy and tube placement annually with usual indications of recurrent AOM or recurrent/persistent otitis media with effusion (OME).[3] Tympanostomy tube otorrhea (TTO) is a common complication of tympanostomy tube placement; 25% of patients develop late-onset TTO, drainage occurring 2 or more weeks after tube placement.[4] Late-onset TTO is most often caused by acute otitis media with typical respiratory pathogens (bacterial—nontypable *Haemophilus influenza, Streptococcus pneumonia,* and *Moraxella catarrhalis*—as well as viral pathogens). Children resistant to treatment may have TTO secondary to *Staphylococcus aureus* or *Pseudomonas aeruginosa,* particularly when history of water contamination is present. Although tympanostomy tube placement has been shown to improve quality-of-life scores, TTO is predictive of lower quality-of-life scores postoperatively.[5]

Effective and efficient treatment of TTO can minimize this burden. The randomized controlled trial of van Dongen et al out of the Netherlands compared TTO treatment options in afebrile children 1 to 10 years of age. Topical therapy with hydrocortisone—bacitracin—colistin otic drops was compared against low-dose amoxicillin—clavulanic acid (30-7.5 mg/kg divided 3 times daily) and initial observation. Both treatment arms had comparable 3 times daily dosing schedules for a 7-day treatment course. Enrollment included examination by a study physician to confirm the presence of otorrhea before patients were randomized by block with age stratification to 1 of the 3 study arms. In addition to parental symptom diaries, follow-up examinations were performed at 2 weeks and 6 months posttreatment. At the 2-week follow-up visit, only 5% of children treated with the otic drops had persistent otorrhea compared with 44% on oral amoxicillin—clavulanate and 55% who did not receive treatment. This represents a number needed to treat of 3 for the otic drops compared with oral amoxicillin—clavulanate. Duration of symptoms was also 1 day shorter (4 vs 5 days) in the otic drops group compared with the amoxicillin—clavulanate treatment group, a statistically significant difference. An interesting additional finding is that although there was a lower rate of persistent otorrhea at 2 weeks for the children treated with amoxicillin—clavulanate compared with no treatment, this difference was not statistically significant.

Some limitations exist for this study. First, cultures of the otorrhea showed high rates of *Pseudomonas* and *S aureus,* likely because of the broad age range of subjects. *Pseudomonas* is resistant to amoxicillin—clavulanate, and *S aureus* also has higher resistance rates to amoxicillin—clavulanate. Generalizability to a population in the United States is also limited because of higher resistance rates overall compared with Europe, including for *S pneumoniae,* for which a higher dose of amoxicillin—clavulanate is often used (40—45 mg/kg/day of amoxicillin for low dose, increasing to 80—90 mg/kg/day for treatment failures). Additionally, the otic drop studied is not available in the United States.

Nonetheless, these findings confirm the American Academy of Otolaryngology-Head and Neck Surgery's clinical practice guidelines to treat otorrhea with otic drops alone.[6] If the hydrocortisone—bacitracin—colistin otic drop becomes available in the United States, additional studies comparing different antibiotic-corticosteroid drops may be needed. In the meantime, ciprofloxacin-dexamethasone is generally recommended. It has also been found to be superior to oral antibiotics and results in earlier resolution of symptoms (day 4 vs 5) compared with ciprofloxacin alone, although both have similar rates of treatment success at 14 days.[7,8]

K. A. M. Nackers, MD

J. G. Frohna, MD, MPH

References

1. Blank SJ, Grindler DJ, Schulz KA, Witsell DL, Lieu JE. Caregiver quality of life Is related to severity of otitis media in children. *Otolaryngol Head Neck Surg.* 2014; 151:348-353.
2. Grindler DJ, Blank SJ, Schulz KA, Witsell DL, Lieu JE. Impact of otitis media severity on children's quality of life. *Otolaryngol Head Neck Surg.* 2014;151: 333-340.
3. Cullen KA, Hall MJ, Golosinskiy A. Ambulatory surgery in the United States, 2006. *Natl Health Stat Report.* 2009;(11):1-25.
4. Kay DJ, Nelson M, Rosenfeld RM. Meta-analysis of tympanostomy tube sequelae. *Otolaryngol Head Neck Surg.* 2001;124:374-380.
5. Rosenfeld RM, Bhaya MH, Bower CM, et al. Impact of tympanostomy tubes on child quality of life. *Arch Otolaryngol Head Neck Surg.* 2000;126:585-592.
6. Rosenfeld RM, Schwartz SR, Pynnonen MA, et al. Clinical practice guideline: tympanostomy tubes in children. *Otolaryngol Head Neck Surg.* 2013;149:S1-S35.
7. Dohar J, Giles W, Roland P, et al. Topical ciprofloxacin/dexamethasone superior to oral amoxicillin/clavulanic acid in acute otitis media with otorrhea through tympanostomy tubes. *Pediatrics.* 2006;118:e561-e569.
8. Roland PS, Anon JB, Moe RD, et al. Topical ciprofloxacin/dexamethasone is superior to ciprofloxacin alone in pediatric patients with acute otitis media and otorrhea through tympanostomy tubes. *Laryngoscope.* 2003;113:2116-2122.

Academic Achievement of Children and Adolescents With Oral Clefts

Wehby GL, Collet B, Barron S, et al (Univ of Iowa; Univ of Washington, Seattle)
Pediatrics 133:785-792, 2014

Background and Objective.—Previous studies of academic achievement of children with oral clefts have mostly relied on small, clinic-based samples prone to ascertainment bias. In the first study in the United States to use a population-based sample with direct assessment, we evaluated the academic achievement of children with oral clefts relative to their classmates.

Methods.—Children born with isolated oral clefts in Iowa from 1983 to 2003 were identified from the Iowa Registry for Congenital and Inherited Disorders and matched to unaffected classmates by gender, school/school district, and month and year of birth. Academic achievement was assessed by using standardized tests of academic progress developed by the Iowa Testing Programs. Iowa Testing Programs data were linked to birth certificates for all children. Regression models controlled for household demographic and socioeconomic factors. The analytical sample included 588 children with clefts contributing 3735 child-grade observations and 1874 classmates contributing 13 159 child-grade observations.

Results.—Children with oral clefts had lower scores than their classmates across all domains and school levels, with a 5-percentile difference in the overall composite score. Children with clefts were approximately one-half grade level behind their classmates and had higher rates of academic underachievement and use of special education services by 8 percentage points. Group differences were slightly lower but remained large and significant after adjusting for many background characteristics.

Conclusions.—Children with oral clefts underperformed across all academic areas and grade levels compared with their classmates. The results support a model of early testing and intervention among affected children to identify and reduce academic deficits.

▶ As pediatricians, we want more for our patients than longer and healthier lives. Another goal of our practice is that our patients grow into adults capable of achieving their ambitions and contributing productively to society. As such, research that identifies an association between health and academic achievement influences how we practice medicine.

We don't yet know why children with oral clefts have lower test scores and higher chances of placement in special education. But knowledge of the association allows for earlier identification of academic problems and implementation of relevant interventions. A history of an isolated, corrected, oral cleft joins a sizable list of health conditions associated with lower academic achievement and/or cognitive deficits. This list includes premature birth, low birth weight, congenital heart disease, cerebral palsy, and in utero exposure to tobacco, alcohol, drugs, and toxins. Noncongenital conditions include a history of childhood hypoglycemia, cancer, child abuse and other stresses, concussion, and exposure to toxins more commonly found in impoverished neighborhoods. Is it feasible and desirable for all children with these medical histories to receive psychological assessments before school entry?

The answer is likely not, which is why Wehby et al refer to the concepts of "response to intervention" and of universal screening.[1] These are contemporary educational terms that are worthy of pediatricians' attention and understanding. Adjustments in federal special education laws now guide schools to conduct benchmark assessments of all students in general education. Children whose reading, math, or behavior is found to lag behind their peers may then receive smaller group instruction or instruction of greater intensity, within the general education system. This subset of children requires continuing progress monitoring (eg, biweekly or bimonthly), and children whose rate of learning growth fails to improve with these interventions will be referred on to receive comprehensive psychological, language, and other assessments. Depending on the outcome of these, some will be placed in special education with an individualized educational program (IEP).

There are understandable reasons for school districts across the nation to be notoriously unequal in their progress toward this model. For one, it goes against the grain of a deeply embedded educational culture, and it takes time to steer the ship in a new direction. Second, this model is far more complex to put into practice than meets the eye. For example, even children with the same inherent learning difficulty can present with seemingly widely different severities of deficits because of confounding factors, such as variations in the classroom environment, the teacher, stresses in the child's life, and difficulty of the learning material. Moreover, having the data from serial classroom-assessments does not necessarily mean that the educational system knows yet how to best utilize that information. For instance, if a child does well and catches up to his or her peers after a period of intensive instruction, should the system halt the intervention to see how the student does with regular intensity? Or should the intensive intervention continue because it has been successful? Some would even argue that success indicates an even further increase in the intensity of instruction. Answers to these unknowns are the subjects of research in universities with academic departments that focus on learning and special educational interventions.

Pediatricians play an important role in the "response to intervention" process because several health-related factors can contribute to a child's cognitive abilities and academic performance. In the case of oral clefts, for example, it could be obstructive sleep apnea underlying some learning problems (because even after successful surgical correction, sleep apnea is more common among children with a history of oral clefts). Pediatricians have access to information, and they can influence many educationally relevant health factors. Effects of medication, family stress or dysfunction, attention-related and other psychiatric disorders, and comorbidities are examples of health issues that contribute to learning difficulties or underachievement.

When students with medical or psychiatric problem do not fit well into a classroom of "regular" children, teachers must not rely on doctors to treat them medically until they do fit in. Likewise, doctors must not pass the buck to the educational system with the expectation that if our schools would only modify educational programs with boundless plasticity, our patients' academic and school behavioral problems would be addressed. The authors of this article promote continuing collaboration between medical teams and schools—and this is exactly what children need.

H. Taras, MD, MPH

Reference

1. Fuchs D, Fuchs LS. Introduction to Response to Intervention: What, why, and how valid is it? *Reading Research Quarterly.* 2006;41:93-99.

6 Endocrinology

Effect of sugars in solutions on subjective appetite and short-term food intake in 9- to 14-year-old normal weight boys
Van Engelen M, Khodabandeh S, Akhavan T, et al (Mount Saint Vincent Univ, Halifax, Nova Scotia, Canada; Ryerson Univ, Toronto, Ontario, Canada)
Eur J Clin Nutr 68:773-777, 2014

Background and Objective.—The role of sugars in solutions on subjective appetite and food intake (FI) has received little investigation in children. Therefore, we examined the effect of isocaloric solutions (200 kcal/ 250 ml) of sugars including sucrose, high-fructose corn syrup-55 (HFCS) or glucose, compared with a non-caloric sucralose control, on subjective appetite and FI in 9- to 14-year-old normal weight (NW) boys.
Participants and Methods.—NW boys (n = 15) received each of the test solutions, in random order, 60 min before an *ad libitum* pizza meal. Subjective appetite was measured at baseline (0 min), and 15, 30, 45 and 60 min.
Results.—Only glucose ($P = 0.003$), but neither sucrose nor HFCS, reduced FI compared with the sucralose control. This led to a higher cumulative energy intake, compared with sucralose, after sucrose ($P = 0.009$) and HFCS ($P = 0.01$), but not after glucose. In all treatment sessions, subjective average appetite increased from baseline to 60 min, but change from baseline average appetite was the highest after sucrose ($P < 0.005$). Furthermore, sucrose ($r = -0.59$, $P = 0.02$) and HFCS ($r = -0.56$, $P = 0.03$), but not glucose, were inversely associated with test meal FI when the treatment dose (200 kcal) was expressed on a body weight (kg) basis.
Conclusions.—Change from baseline subjective average appetite was the highest after sucrose, but only the glucose solution suppressed FI at the test meal 60 min later in NW boys.

▶ What can be said about sugar-sweetened beverages (SSBs) that hasn't been said before? Depends on whom you ask. For instance, Liz Applegate, a sports nutritionist and spokesperson for the American Beverage Association states, "The human body does not differentiate between naturally occurring sugars from fruit versus sugars added to foods (sweetened beverages, cakes or candy). The notion that liquid sugar has a different impact on the body (such as negatively affecting the liver and pancreas) compared to "solid sugar" is not supported by the totality of scientific research."[1]

Yet concern has been raised that sugar is a primary factor in the pathogenesis of obesity and metabolic syndrome, due to 3 inherent properties: 1) generation of liver fat and insulin resistance, 2) promotion of cellular aging, and 3) effects on the reward center leading to excessive consumption.[2] Furthermore, SSBs generate even greater concern because they 4) do not suppress the hunger hormone ghrelin, 5) are even more rapidly absorbed than added sugar in food, and 6) have a higher caloric density.[3]

In the past year, 4 notable clinical papers have examined the connection among SSBs, consumption, and obesity. Each looks at the issue in a slightly different way. Each alone has inherent strengths and weaknesses; but taken together, it's a case of "the preponderance of the evidence."

First, the global health burden: De Vogli et al, using data obtained from the 37 countries of the Organization for Economic Cooperation and Development, examined the relationship between fast-food transactions and the rates of weight gain over a 10-year period in adults[4] and found a remarkably strong positive correlation. This article has the disadvantage of pooled rather than individual data; thus some might dismiss this as "ecological" data, which is thought to be of low quality. Yet it has the advantage of time series—that is, looking at the rate of change of individual populations over time and factoring out confounders, which is known as "econometric analysis," a much more robust method of examination.

As you might expect, "economic freedom" (ie, disposable income) was 1 major factor driving fast-food transactions, and therefore weight gain. In addition, the investigators had the individual purchase data, and they were able to examine the contributions of individual foodstuffs purchased to the body mass index (BMI) increase. Neither total calories nor animal fat explained the association; rather, the association between fast food and BMI change over time was mediated specifically by SSB consumption. Adjusting for these other variables did not weaken the SSB effect.

Second, the epidemiology in children: De Boer et al, using the Early Childhood Longitudinal Survey—Birth Cohort, examined the association between SSB consumption and obesity in preschoolers.[5] They showed that at age 2, there was no association, but by age 4, the frequency of SSB consumption correlated with BMI z-score, even when adjusted for race/ethnicity, socioeconomic status, mother's BMI, and television viewing. Although similar results have been reported previously, this article is unique in that it provides both cross-sectional and longitudinal data to support a specific effect of SSBs on weight gain. However, the study cannot categorically state whether the effect is specific to SSBs or due to effects on total calories ingested.

Third, an examination of mechanism: Van Engelen et al performed a clinical research study[6] in which children were randomly fed beverages containing glucose, high-fructose corn syrup (HFCS), sucrose, or sucralose (diet sweetener) control and then allowed to gorge on a meal of pizza. Appetite was measured at baseline and every 15 minutes for an hour. Only glucose reduced food intake compared with the sucralose control, suggesting that the brain in some fashion compensated for the energy in the glucose drink. Neither sucrose nor HFCS suppressed appetite; in fact, when the dose of either sweetener was expressed as a function of body weight, there was a positive correlation between SSB ingestion and subjective appetite. Unfortunately, there was no water control (important as sucralose may increase insulin release on its own,[7] which may change appetite), and there was no measurement of effect on energy expenditure or weight change. Although the biochemical mechanisms of this effect cannot be determined from this study, it certainly argues that "all sugars are not the same" and that sugar drives excessive consumption, at least acutely.

Finally, the question of conflicts of interest in elaborating the data. Do SSBs cause obesity? Again, it depends on who you ask. Bes-Rastollo et al performed a meta-analysis of 18 studies regressing SSB consumption against BMI increase in adults.[8] Their independent variable was food-company sponsorship of the study. Of the 6 studies sponsored by the food industry, 5 showed no effect of SSBs on BMI. Yet of the 12 studies that were independently funded, 10 demonstrated a significant association between SSB consumption and BMI increase. Those reviews with conflicts of interest were 5 times more likely to present a conclusion of no positive association than those without conflicts of interest (relative risk: 5.0, 95% confidence interval [CI]: 1.3–19.3). Of course, the authors could not rule out the existence of publication bias among those studies not declaring conflicts of interest.

Each study is valuable but inherently flawed. That's human research for you— especially when it's about diet. Randomized controlled trials cannot be done; they would be too long, too expensive, impossible to control, impossible to monitor, immoral, and illegal. So we are forced to use clinical research studies with surrogate end points for short-term effects and natural history studies to examine long-term effects. Again, it's about the preponderance of the evidence—and the evidence is more and more apparent. Sugar is a problem. Liquid sugar is a bigger problem. And the food industry is doing its best to sugar-coat the message.

R. H. Lustig, MD, MSL

References

1. Applegate L. Viewpoints: Soda labeling bill is based on misleading statements. The Sacramento Bee. http://www.sacbee.com/2014/07/02/6527186/viewpoints-soda-labeling-bill.html. Accessed August 5, 2014.
2. Weiss R, Bremer AA, Lustig RH. What is metabolic syndrome, and why are children getting it? *Ann N Y Acad Sci.* 2013;1281:123-140.
3. Bremer AA, Lustig RH. Effects of sugar-sweetened beverages on children. *Pediatr Ann.* 2012;41:26-30.
4. De Vogli R, Kouvonen A, Gimeno D. The influence of market deregulation on fast food consumption and body mass index: a cross-national time series analysis. *Bull World Health Organ.* 2014;92:99-107.
5. DeBoer MD, Scharf RJ, Demmer RT. Sugar-sweetened beverages and weight gain in 2- to 5-year-old children. *Pediatrics.* 2013;132:413-420.
6. Van Engelen M, Khodabandeh S, Akhavan T, Agarwal J, Gladanac B, Bellissimo N. Effect of sugars in solutions on subjective appetite and short-term food intake in 9- to 14-year-old normal weight boys. *Eur J Clin Nutr.* 2014;68: 773-777.
7. Pepino MY, Tiemann CD, Patterson BW, Wice BM, Klein S. Sucralose affects glycemic and hormonal responses to an oral glucose load. *Diabetes Care.* 2013;36: 2530-2535.
8. Bes-Rastrollo M, Schulze MB, Ruiz-Canela M, Martinez-Gonzalez MA. Financial conflicts of interest and reporting bias regarding the association between sugar-sweetened beverages and weight gain: a systematic review of systematic reviews. *PLoS Med.* 2013;10:e1001578.

Preterm Birth and Random Plasma Insulin Levels at Birth and in Early Childhood

Wang G, Divall S, Radovick S, et al (Johns Hopkins Univ Bloomberg School of Public Health, Baltimore, MD; Johns Hopkins Univ School of Medicine, Baltimore, MD; et al)
JAMA 311:587-596, 2014

Importance.—Although previous reports have linked preterm birth with insulin resistance in children and adults, it is not known whether altered insulin homeostasis is detectable at birth and tracks from birth through childhood.

Objective.—To investigate whether preterm birth is associated with elevated plasma insulin levels at birth and whether this association persists into early childhood.

Design, Setting, and Participants.—A prospective birth cohort of 1358 children recruited at birth from 1998 to 2010 and followed-up with prospectively from 2005 to 2012 at the Boston Medical Center in Massachusetts.

Main Outcomes and Measures.—Random plasma insulin levels were measured at 2 time points: at birth (cord blood) and in early childhood (venous blood). The median age was 1.4 years (interquartile range [IQR], 0.8-3.3) among 4 gestational age groups: full term (≥39 wk), early term (37-38 wk), late preterm (34-36 wk), and early preterm (<34 wk).

Results.—The geometric mean of insulin levels at birth were 9.2 µIU/mL (95% CI, 8.4-10.0) for full term; 10.3 µIU/mL (95% CI, 9.3-11.5) for early term; 13.2 µIU/mL (95% CI, 11.8-14.8) for late preterm; and 18.9 µIU/mL (95% CI, 16.6-21.4) for early preterm. In early childhood, these levels were 11.2 µIU/mL (95% CI, 10.3-12.0) for full term; 12.4 µIU/mL (95% CI, 11.3-13.6) for early term; 13.3 µIU/mL (95% CI, 11.9-14.8) for late preterm; and 14.6 µIU/mL (95% CI, 12.6-16.9) for early preterm. Insulin levels at birth were higher by 1.13-fold (95% CI, 0.97-1.28) for early term, 1.45-fold (95% CI, 1.25-1.65) for late preterm, and 2.05-fold (95% CI, 1.69-2.42) for early preterm than for those born full term. In early childhood, random plasma insulin levels were 1.12-fold (95% CI, 0.99-1.25) higher for early term, 1.19-fold (95% CI, 1.02-1.35) for late preterm, and 1.31-fold (95% CI, 1.10-1.52) for early preterm than those born full term. The association was attenuated after adjustment for postnatal weight gain and was not significant after adjustment for insulin levels at birth. Infants ranked in the top insulin tertile at birth were more likely to remain in the top tertile (41.2%) compared with children ranked in the lowest tertile (28.6%) in early childhood.

Conclusions and Relevance.—There was an inverse association between gestational age and elevated plasma insulin levels at birth and in early childhood. The implications for future development of insulin resistance and type 2 diabetes warrant further investigation.

▶ It is now generally accepted that perinatal adversity is associated with a higher risk of adult diseases, particularly those associated with the metabolic syndrome. These diseases all feature insulin resistance, which with compensatory hyperinsulinism, is seen as intimately involved in their development. The link between early insulin resistance and later adult disease has been well established in term, small for gestational age (SGA) survivors who have a marked (~40%) reduction in insulin sensitivity in childhood that tracks into adult life. The data about preterm survivors have been less clear, but most studies have shown a similar pattern with a reduction in peripheral insulin sensitivity in children, youth, and adults approaching middle age.

This study by Wang et al, with its extremely large sample size, has confirmed previous evidence linking preterm birth with a reduction in insulin sensitivity and is the most important paper to come out in this area over the past year. Moreover, the data have a number of other novel findings. First, they indicate that the changes in insulin sensitivity begin before delivery with cord insulin levels being elevated in the more preterm survivors (Table 1 in the original article). It has previously been hypothesized that the reduction in insulin sensitivity observed in this group was secondary to postnatal insults from early environmental adversity, especially abnormal early postnatal nutrition. However, Wang et al are suggesting that alterations in insulin sensitivity occur before delivery and may reflect physiologic stress or other alterations in the fetus that indeed may have resulted in them being born preterm.

The study also confirms that insulin sensitivity tracks throughout early childhood (Fig 3 in the original article), especially in those who gain weight more rapidly. Rapid weight gain not surprisingly was much more common in those born preterm. This finding is important because it is similar to data from term SGA studies, suggesting later adult disease is much more likely when there is both early life adversity and rapid early weight gain that progresses to adult obesity.

Finally, Wang et al have elegantly demonstrated that insulin levels do depend on whether infants are small, appropriate or large for gestational age. This most likely reflects relative leanness and needs to be considered when assessing insulin sensitivity in children born preterm. Of note, however, the insulin levels in all 3 groups were higher with progressively lower gestational age.

The study is well designed and by far the largest study to date examining insulin sensitivity in preterm infants. Its major weakness is using random insulin levels to assess insulin sensitivity. However, the sample size makes this less of an issue. Glucose levels are not required to assess insulin sensitivity in children because they are rarely abnormal. Most experts would agree that fasting insulin is a reasonable measure of insulin sensitivity at this age. As the authors concede, however, fasting insulin is a better measure of hepatic insulin sensitivity, and at least 2 previous studies have suggested that preterm children have reductions in peripheral insulin sensitivity using gold standard assessments of insulin sensitivity (eg, intravenous glucose tolerance test and minimal model software) with no changes seen in fasting insulin. In this context, random insulin levels may have been better than fasting insulin and explain why associations were observed.

This study has highlighted that reductions in insulin sensitivity occur in preterm survivors even before birth and track with time. These data will need confirmation, but if these changes occur before birth, the focus of management may need to be antenatal rather than trying to prevent insulin resistance by altering neonatal care. From a public health perspective, it suggests that all those preterm born (approximately 10% of births) are at higher risk of metabolic syndrome morbidities in later life. However, there is a large window to act to prevent this occurring. Reduced weight gain, a healthy lifestyle, and preventing adult obesity would seem to be the most likely factors to minimize long-term sequelae.

P. L. Hofman, FRACP

A Randomized Trial of Hyperglycemic Control in Pediatric Intensive Care

Macrae D, for the CHiP Investigators (Royal Brompton and Harefield NHS Foundation Trust, London, UK; et al)
N Engl J Med 370:107-118, 2014

Background.—Whether an insulin infusion should be used for tight control of hyperglycemia in critically ill children remains unclear.

Methods.—We randomly assigned children ($\leq$16 years of age) who were admitted to the pediatric intensive care unit (ICU) and were expected to require mechanical ventilation and vasoactive drugs for at least 12 hours to either tight glycemic control, with a target blood glucose range of 72 to 126 mg per deciliter (4.0 to 7.0 mmol per liter), or conventional glycemic control, with a target level below 216 mg per deciliter (12.0 mmol per liter). The primary outcome was the number of days alive and free from mechanical ventilation at 30 days after randomization. The main prespecified subgroup analysis compared children who had undergone cardiac surgery with those who had not. We also assessed costs of hospital and community health services.

Results.—A total of 1369 patients at 13 centers in England underwent randomization: 694 to tight glycemic control and 675 to conventional glycemic control; 60% had undergone cardiac surgery. The mean between-group difference in the number of days alive and free from mechanical ventilation at 30 days was 0.36 days (95% confidence interval [CI], −0.42 to 1.14); the effects did not differ according to subgroup. Severe hypoglycemia (blood glucose, <36 mg per deciliter [2.0 mmol per liter]) occurred in a higher proportion of children in the tight-glycemic-control group than in the conventionalglycemic-control group (7.3% vs. 1.5%, $P < 0.001$). Overall, the mean 12-month costs were lower in the tight-glycemic-control group than in the conventional-glycemiccontrol group. The mean 12-month costs were similar in the two groups in the cardiac-surgery subgroup, but in the subgroup that had not undergone cardiac surgery, the mean cost was significantly lower in the tight-glycemic-control group than in the conventional-glycemic-control group: −$13,120 (95% CI, −$24,682 to −$1,559).

Conclusions.—This multicenter, randomized trial showed that tight glycemic control in critically ill children had no significant effect on major clinical outcomes, although the incidence of hypoglycemia was higher with tight glucose control than with conventional glucose control. (Funded by the National Institute for Health Research, Health Technology Assessment Program, U.K. National Health Service; CHiP Current Controlled Trials number, ISRCTN61735247.)

▶ Understanding hyperglycemia, from etiology to optimal management, remains a major challenge in pediatric critical care. Several important clinical trials directly addressing the relevance and impact of hyperglycemia have emerged in recent years, noting that aggressive treatment likely improves mortality and morbidities in select groups.

This landmark study by Macrae and colleagues from the CHiP trial (Control Hyperglycemia in Pediatric Intensive Care) engaged more than a dozen intensive care units across the United Kingdom and randomized more than 1300 patients into 2 tiers of glycemic control. The largest and most diverse study yet to address this question in the pediatric population demonstrated that survival and ventilator-free days were similar between groups. Subgroup analysis revealed that noncardiac patients with tight glycemic control had substantially shorter length of stay, received less renal replacement therapy, and generated less total cost than those in the conventional management arm, which permitted moderate, but not unchecked, hyperglycemia (up to 216 mg/dL). Hypoglycemia remained a concern, with an increased incidence of severe hypoglycemia in the tight glycemic control group.

Fortunately, technologic refinements may limit the risk of hypoglycemia as more sensitive computerized feedback systems emerge for the clinical market, although the implementation of these systems remains somewhat costly and a drain on nursing resources.

This study has deservedly attracted broad attention, from therapeutic nihilists that consider aggressive treatment unwarranted and potentially dangerous, to those who avidly support tighter glycemic controls. Despite the large number of patients, the study was one of glycemic targeting rather than the approach to achieve such control; thus, not all the patients in either arm received directed insulin therapy, nor was the hyperglycemia the result of a single etiology. There were several divergences from other clinical studies that focused either on insulin therapy (treatment vs no treatment), involved few centers or fewer patients, used different target ranges for glycemic control, or used different subpopulations, including or excluding the more homogenous cardiac patients. Despite the herculean efforts from these clinical trials, the jury is still out on the approach to, and definition of, optimal glycemic control in pediatric critical illness. Pundits will continue to offer this study to defend their viewpoint, negative or positive, and it is unlikely that a larger study of similar structure will reveal radically new understanding. A large, ongoing trial in the United States, the HALF-PINT study (Heart and Lung Failure—Pediatric Insulin Titration Trial), involving 30 centers and 1800 patients, employs state-of-the-art glucose monitoring and even tighter definitions for tight and standard glycemic control (clinicaltrials.gov; NCT01565941). Perhaps the study will offer new insights into the subgroups that will benefit from tight glycemic control, but more likely the results will affirm that our ability to recognize and intervene on hyperglycemia exceeds our understanding of the etiologies for the hyperglycemia.

Far from a being a homogenous entity, hyperglycemia may result from the compensatory/counterregulatory stress response, which may be adaptive or maladaptive depending on the circumstance and the duration. Furthermore, we have only a rudimentary clinical understanding of the mitochondrial derangements and metabolic uncoupling that results from and during critical illness. Mitochondrial dysfunction may be transient, after a discrete stimulus such as cardiopulmonary bypass (witness the self-resolving type B hyperlactemia), or it may be the result of unchecked inflammation, such as may occur during sepsis or SIRS (the systemic inflammatory response syndrome). We now understand that injury from reactive oxygen moieties, ongoing tissue hypoxia, global energy failure, and evolving tissue death are both a result of and a manifestation of mitochondrial dysfunction. The past decade has seen an exponential rise in our understanding of mitochondrial biology. We have diverged from a simplistic viewpoint, that the mitochondrial is "the source of robust adenosine triphosphate generation," into a broader recognition that mitochondria are central signaling organelles, coordinating environmental stress responses, integrating events occurring at the plasma membrane, sensing and managing reactive oxygen species, and responding to inflammation and that they serve as active participants in transcriptome and epigenetic regulation. Insulin therapy, far from simply correcting hypoglycemia, is a direct and pivotal player in the anabolic to catabolic switch that defines critical illness, thus extensively modulating both tissue energy utilization and mitochondrial function. However, alterations in insulin levels alone may not address nor alter the underlying derangements of the host.

As always, the clinical application of knowledge lags behind our understanding at the bench. Perhaps the greatest truth is that we have yet to conduct a clinical trial focusing on the etiology of hyperglycemia, directing supportive care at the reversible causes, and then monitoring the systemic response. Placing endogenous insulin levels and mitochondrial dysfunction at the forefront of the debate could radically alter the discussion surrounding the negative impact of hyperglycemia. Instead of grouping patients into larger, tighter, or more homogenous clinical groups, a trial that segregates appropriate "stress-response" hyperglycemic states from the pathologic may well reveal a central truth, that the hyperglycemia is a symptom of the problem rather than the problem. Perhaps the patients that improved with tight control had mitochondrial dysfunction that was self-resolving or responsive to supportive care, and those that failed to improve manifested different etiologies. Perhaps supplemental insulin therapy alone is sufficient to reverse selective derangements in catabolism and yet fails to adequately reverse the complex compensatory/maladaptive milieu in other states. Without greater clarity into the biology of tissue and organs and the integrative means to easily determine mitochondrial health, such as suitable systemic biomarkers, we will continue to struggle to distinguish the maladaptive from the protective, the causal from the associated, and we will continue to focus our considerable energy into clinical trials that in some fashion attempt to overcome the "limitations" of those that have come before.

Yes, we should continue to study our care, and strive to improve the outcome for our most vulnerable patients. Yet when large, well-constructed and well-controlled trials fail to meet our expectations, we need to remember to ask what it is we don't understand rather than only designing and implementing a larger, better constructed, better controlled trial to parse out the slivers of truth. If there was ever a time when a translational approach is needed, it could well be the question of critical-illness associated hyperglycemia; is it the problem, or is it but a sign of the profound and complex biochemical response of the host experiencing a critical illness?

C. L. Epting, MD

Risedronate in children with osteogenesis imperfecta: a randomised, double-blind, placebo-controlled trial

Bishop N, Adami S, Ahmed SF, et al (Univ of Sheffield, UK; Univ of Verona, Italy; Univ of Glasgow, UK; et al)
Lancet 382:1424-1432, 2013

Background.—Children with osteogenesis imperfecta are often treated with intravenous bisphosphonates. We aimed to assess the safety and efficacy of risedronate, an orally administered third-generation bisphosphonate, in children with the disease.

Methods.—In this multicentre, randomised, parallel, double-blind, placebo-controlled trial, children aged 4—15 years with osteogenesis imperfecta and increased fracture risk were randomly assigned by telephone randomisation system in a 2:1 ratio to receive either daily risedronate ($2 \cdot 5$ or 5 mg) or placebo for 1 year. Study treatment was masked from patients, investigators, and study centre personnel. Thereafter, all children received risedronate for 2 additional years in an open-label extension. The primary efficacy endpoint was percentage change in lumbar spine areal bone mineral density (BMD) at 1 year. The primary efficacy analysis was done by ANCOVA, with treatment, age group, and pooled centre as fixed effects, and baseline as covariate. Analyses were based on the intention-to-treat population, which included all patients who were randomly assigned and took at least one dose of assigned study treatment. The trial is registered with ClinicalTrials.gov, number NCT00106028.

Findings.—Of 147 patients, 97 were randomly assigned to the risedronate group and 50 to the placebo group. Three patients from the risedronate group and one from the placebo group did not receive study treatment, leaving 94 and 49 in the intention-to-treat population, respectively. The mean increase in lumbar spine areal BMD after 1 year was $16 \cdot 3\%$ in the risedronate group and $7 \cdot 6\%$ in the placebo group (difference $8 \cdot 7\%$, 95% CI $5 \cdot 7$—$11 \cdot 7$; $p < 0 \cdot 0001$). After 1 year, clinical fractures had occurred in 29 (31%) of 94 patients in the risedronate group and 24 (49%) of 49 patients in the placebo group ($p = 0 \cdot 0446$). During years 2 and 3 (open-label phase), clinical fractures were reported in 46 (53%) of 87 patients in the group that had received risedronate since the start of the study, and 32 (65%) of 49 patients in the group that had been given placebo during the first year. Adverse event profiles were otherwise similar between the two groups, including frequencies of reported upper-gastrointestinal and selected musculoskeletal adverse events.

Interpretation.—Oral risedronate increased areal BMD and reduced the risk of first and recurrent clinical fractures in children with osteogenesis imperfecta, and the drug was generally well tolerated. Risedronate should be regarded as a treatment option for children with osteogenesis imperfecta.

▶ Osteogenesis imperfecta (OI) is an inherited condition affecting approximately 1 in 10000 persons. The phenotypic hallmark is brittle bones with subsequent increased fracture rates. Other clinical features are variable and can include blue sclerae, dentinogenesis imperfecta, hearing loss, growth impairment, blood vessel fragility, and ligamentous laxity. Most cases are due to mutations in type 1 collagen, although recently other genetic causes have been elucidated. Types of OI range from mild disease (type I) with an increased fracture rate and low bone mineral density (BMD) but little bone deformity, through moderate types (types III/IV), to lethal forms (type II) with severe bone pathology and respiratory failure.

It is well-established that for moderate to severe cases, the OI bone disease can be partially ameliorated using intravenous bisphosphonate therapy, predominately pamidronate given over 3 days every 2 to 4 months. Bisphosphonates primarily decrease bone resorption, attenuating the high bone turnover found in bone with an abnormal collagen matrix. The first case reports using intravenous bisphosphonate for types III/IV OI appeared in the late 1980s. Since then, multiple treatment regimens have shown success in improving BMD, reducing fracture rates and improving quality of life in this population.

However, bisphosphonate treatment is not curative, nor, for a variety of reasons, is it routinely employed for persons with more mild forms of OI, who also suffer from fracture and bony pain. Most reported treatment regimens require intravenous access, which is sometimes difficult in these patients and carry the high costs associated with hospital admissions and/or infusion center access. Additionally, evidence is lacking that the benefits of bisphosphonate therapy in those with the mildest forms of OI outweigh the risks. Also, persons with mild OI have lower fracture rates than more severely affected persons, necessitating that studies are done over long treatment periods in larger populations to prove that a regimen significantly affects fracture rates. Before this report, other studies failed to show consistent benefits, perhaps because of inadequate power or inadequate drug dose, limiting enthusiasm for oral therapy. The only prior large, randomized, placebo-controlled multisite study using low-dose alendronate did not decrease fractures in this population. Another study of oral risedronate treatment in 26 children with mild OI also failed to show an improvement in fracture rate. Therefore, several questions have remained unanswered, including questions regarding the efficacy of oral forms of bisphosphonate and whether more mild OI cases should receive bisphosphonates.

This article by Bishop et al in *The Lancet* provides important evidence in support of using oral risedronate therapy in children with mild OI. This large, international, randomized, parallel, double-blind, placebo controlled trial randomized 97 subjects to risedronate and 50 patients to placebo for 1 year followed by an open-label 2-year extension phase in which all subjects received risedronate. This is a robust study with a rigorous study design and the largest studied cohort of its kind. Importantly, this cohort consisted of mostly of individuals with mild

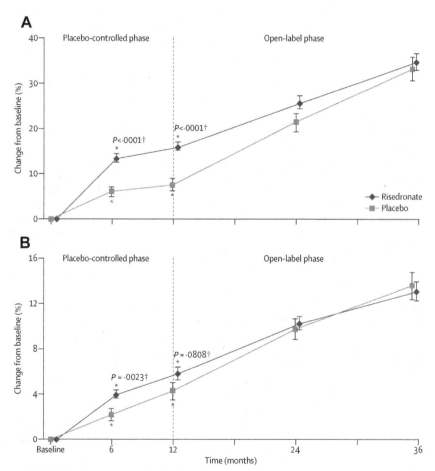

FIGURE 2.—Changes in areal bone mineral density. Data are least-squares mean percentage changes in areal bone mineral density from baseline for lumbar spine (A) and total body (B). Error bars show standard error. *Indicates significant difference from baseline, as assessed from 95% CI s unadjusted for multiple comparisons. †*p* values indicates difference from placebo as assessed from the ANCOVA model with fixed effects for age group, treatment, and pooled centre, with baseline as covariate. (Reprinted from Bishop N, Adami S, Ahmed SF, et al. Risedronate in children with osteogenesis imperfecta: a randomised, double-blind, placebo-controlled trial. *Lancet*. 2013;382:1424-1432; with permission.)

OI—86% of the risedronate-treated group and 82% of the placebo-treated group. In this study, an 8.7% greater annual increase in lumbar spine areal bone mineral density (BMD) was seen in the risedronate-treated subjects compared with the placebo-treated persons. Greater increases were also seen in total body BMD measures. Furthermore, both cohorts showed continued BMD gains in the 2-year extension phase (Fig 2). Most important, both first and recurrent fractures were significantly attenuated; during the first year, they occurred in 49% of the placebo-treated patients and only 31% of the patients receiving risedronate. Risedronate was well tolerated as the frequency of adverse events, including gastrointestinal events typical of bisphosphonate use, was similar between the risedronate and placebo treated groups.

Oral risedronate may be an optimal bisphosphonate treatment option for children with mild OI. Several questions persist, however. First, this study did not compare the effectiveness of risedronate to pamidronate, the most commonly used intravenous therapy for more severe OI. Additionally, risedronate-treated subjects had a trend toward a greater likelihood of a vertebral collapse on radiographs, although this is likely due to improved ability to visualize the mineralized vertebrae endplates with bisphosphonate therapy rather than worsening spinal disease. Additional unanswered questions include how this therapy would affect subjects with more severe forms of OI and whether the side effect profile would be worse in these persons who have a greater likelihood of gastrointestinal issues due in part to chest wall and spinal deformity. Finally, an improvement in pain and ambulation was not found in this study as it has been in studies of IV bisphosphonates, although this mild population studied by Bishop et al likely had less pain and fewer ambulatory difficulties than other study cohorts.

The newer intravenous bisphosphonate, zoledronic acid, may be the bisphosphonate treatment of the future, particularly for severe OI, because it may be dosed once or twice a year with infusions taking under an hour, decreasing costs and time away from daily activities for families with OI. Studies with this drug are ongoing. Novel therapies will also likely soon emerge, which target the pathophysiology of OI more precisely. The recent description of excess transforming growth factor (TGF)-beta as part of the OI phenotype is paving the way for use of anti-TGF-beta therapies in clinical trials. However, these therapies will first need be tested in more severe forms of the disease and will likely be associated with high costs. Oral bisphosphonate therapy still has the advantages of current availability and convenient, affordable dosing. Notably, this article is the first to show significant improvement in fracture rates with oral bisphosphonate in a large cohort of mild OI subjects, and should lead to expanded use of this therapy for this population in need.

M. M. Fisher, MD

L. A. DiMeglio, MD, MPH

Milk Consumption During Teenage Years and Risk of Hip Fractures in Older Adults

Feskanich D, Bischoff-Ferrari HA, Frazier AL, et al (Harvard Univ, Boston, MA; Univ of Zurich, Switzerland)

JAMA Pediatr 168:54-60, 2014

Importance.—Milk consumption during adolescence is recommended to promote peak bone mass and thereby reduce fracture risk in later life. However, its role in hip fracture prevention is not established and high consumption may adversely influence risk by increasing height.

Objectives.—To determine whether milk consumption during teenage years influences risk of hip fracture in older adults and to investigate the role of attained height in this association.

Design, Setting, and Participants.—Prospective cohort study over 22 years of follow-up in more than 96 000 white postmenopausal women from the Nurses' Health Study and men aged 50 years and older from the Health Professionals Follow-up Study in the United States.

Exposures.—Frequency of consumption of milk and other foods during ages 13 to 18 years and attained height were reported at baseline. Current diet, weight, smoking, physical activity, medication use, and other risk factors for hip fractures were reported on biennial questionnaires.

Main Outcomes and Measures.—Cox proportional hazards models were used to calculate relative risks (RRs) of first incidence of hip fracture from low-trauma events per glass (8 fl oz or 240 mL) of milk consumed per day during teenage years.

Results.—During follow-up, 1226 hip fractures were identified in women and 490 in men. After controlling for known risk factors and current milk consumption, each additional glass of milk per day during teenage years was associated with a significant 9% higher risk of hip fracture in men (RR = 1.09; 95% CI, 1.01-1.17). The association was attenuated when height was added to the model (RR = 1.06; 95% CI, 0.98-1.14). Teenage milk consumption was not associated with hip fractures in women (RR = 1.00 per glass per day; 95% CI, 0.95-1.05).

Conclusions and Relevance.—Greater milk consumption during teenage years was not associated with a lower risk of hip fracture in older adults. The positive association observed in men was partially mediated through attained height.

▶ Is taller stature an acceptable trade-off for a slightly increased risk of hip fracture?

Is the slogan "Milk does a body good" untrue?

In a large, well-designed retrospective study, Feskanich et al report that risk of hip fracture was higher among men who recalled drinking more milk during adolescence, in part mediated by the association between increased stature and hip fracture. The authors also found that milk consumption was associated with taller stature, with an average of nearly 2 cm height increase in those who drank more than 4 glasses of milk each day compared with those who consumed less than 2 glasses per week. The authors reported an increased risk of hip fracture (4.5% in men and 5.0% in women) for each additional centimeter of height.

The 2010 dietary guidelines for Americans recommend consuming fat-free or low-fat milk products because milk and dairy are often significant sources of dietary calcium and protein in the American diet, which are needed to achieve optimal bone mass during adolescence and young adulthood.[1] In 2010, the Food and Nutrition Board of the Institute of Medicine issued new guidelines for nutrients of importance to bone health.[2] The adequate intake (AI) of 1300 mg of calcium for adolescents is equivalent to 4 daily servings of milk. Multiple trials have demonstrated a positive association between dairy intake and bone mineral density with the assumption that increasing bone density and strength will reduce the risks of osteoporosis and fracture that occur in older age.[3,4]

So why did this study find an increased risk of fracture in men who drink more milk? As the authors note, this study is limited by the retrospective reporting of adolescent milk consumption. The reporting occurred many decades after the events and may not accurately reflect milk intake. Additionally, the greatest benefits of calcium intake, including milk consumption, may be strongest during late childhood and preadolescence, years that were not examined in this study. Understanding the role of milk and dairy intake during childhood and early adolescence is important to pursue in future studies.

Increased milk consumption as a risk factor for hip fracture was only observed in men, although the majority of hip fractures (71.4%) described in the study occurred in women, similar to other studies. The sexual dimorphism of these findings is interesting and may be related to the higher risk of hip fracture among women. Was the positive association between milk intake and fracture only identified in men because women are, at baseline, at a much higher risk of hip fracture, and the impact of milk consumption and height is therefore minimal?

In addition to milk consumption, it would be interesting to consider the roles of total dairy intake, total protein intake, and overall nutrition because multiple dietary components contribute to linear growth and bone health. The value of milk for bone health and overall health is in part dependent on the quality of the diet without milk. The authors described that those who consumed at least 4 glasses of milk per day as teenagers were the most active; had higher intakes of cheese, fruits and vegetables, and meat and fish; and were most likely to take a multivitamin. Weight-bearing exercise and consuming a healthy diet are also associated with increased bone strength and density, and therefore, it is even more surprising that the men with recall of the greatest overall nutrition were those most likely to experience hip fractures. It would be important to see these findings replicated in other populations with more accurate or real-time collection of dietary history.

Because this study excluded participants who were of nonwhite race/ethnicity, the results cannot be generalized to a broader population. Ninety-two percent of the reported milk consumption was whole milk, which is different from the current recommendations for consumption of nonfat or low-fat milk and dairy. Because optimal vitamin D and accompanying calcium absorption may occur with lower fat versus whole milk, the results from this study could have been affected by the high rate of whole-fat milk consumption.

This report brings up stimulating questions about the role of height and linear growth on bone mineral density and fracture risk. Further research is needed to examine the relationship between milk consumption and adult height to determine whether the relationship is solely related to milk, or if it also affected by total dairy and/or total protein consumption. What is it about increased height that raises the fracture risk? Considerations include differences in bone geometry and taller stature, the impact of falling from a higher center of gravity, or differences in risk of falling based on height.

In summary, milk and other dairy products provide convenient and reliable sources of calcium, vitamin D, and protein intake. For those with poor-quality diets, achieving good overall nutrition may be compromised with reduced milk intake. Therefore, we will continue to recommend 3 cups of milk per day for adolescents to provide nutrients that are essential for good bone health. However, this article provides important "food for thought" and hopefully will generate more research into the relationships between childhood and adolescent dairy intake and later fracture risk during adulthood.

L. S. Topor, MD, MMSc

C. M. Gordon, MD, MSc

References

1. United States Department of Agriculture and the United States Department of Health and Human Services. Dietary Guidelines for Americans, 2010. http://www.health.gov/dietaryguidelines/dga2010/DietaryGuidelines2010.pdf. Accessed July 1, 2014.
2. Institute of Medicine (IOM). *Dietary Reference Intakes for Calcium and Vitamin D*. Washington, DC: The National Academies Press; 2011.
3. Sahni S, Tucker KL, Kiel DP, Quach L, Casey VA, Hannan MT. Milk and yogurt consumption are linked with higher bone mineral density but not with hip fracture: the Framingham Offspring Study. *Arch Osteoporos*. 2013;8:119.
4. Rizzoli R. Dairy products, yogurts, and bone health. *Am J Clin Nutr*. 2014;99:1256S-1262S.

7 Gastroenterology

Outcome after Discontinuation of Immunosuppression in Children with Autoimmune Hepatitis: A Population-Based Study
Deneau M, Book LS, Guthery SL, et al (Univ of Manitoba, Winnipeg, Canada; Univ of Utah, Salt Lake City)
J Pediatr 164:714-719, 2014

Objective.—To assess sustained immunosuppression-free remission (SIFR) in children with autoimmune hepatitis (AIH).

Study Design.—We retrospectively reviewed all children with AIH in the region between 1986 and 2011 using a population-based methodology.

Results.—We identified 56 children with AIH (62.5% females; median age, 11.1 years [IQR, 5.7-14.4 years], followed for a median of 5.6 years [IQR, 2.8-8.6 years]). Liver disease was characterized by type II AIH in 8.9%, cirrhosis in 14.0%, and primary sclerosing cholangitis in 21.4%. Coexisting nonhepatic immune-mediated diseases occurred in 37.5%. Biochemical remission on immunosuppressive therapy was achieved in 76.4% of all patients with AIH at a median of 1.2 years (IQR, 0.4-3.6 years); 23.1% of these patients experienced a subsequent relapse. Discontinuation of all immunosuppressive medications was attempted in 16 patients and was successful in 14 patients (87.5%) with type 1 AIH (median age at discontinuation, 8.9 years [IQR, 3.5-17.9 years], treated for a median of 2.0 years [IQR, 1.3-3.5 years] after diagnosis), with SIFR occurring at a median of 3.4 years (IQR, 2.6-5.8 years) of follow-up. Excluding patients with inflammatory bowel disease who received immunosuppressive therapy independent of their liver disease, the probability of achieving SIFR within 5 years of diagnosis of AIH was 41.6% (95% CI, 25.3%-62.9%). Baseline patient characteristics associated with an inability to achieve biochemical remission on immunosuppression or SIFR were elevated international normalized ratio, positive antineutrophil cytoplasmic antibody titer, cirrhosis, and a nonhepatic autoimmune disorder.

Conclusion.—We found a high rate of successful discontinuation of all immunosuppressive medications in carefully selected patients with AIH in a population-based cohort. SIFR is an achievable goal for children with AIH, particularly those with type I disease in stable biochemical remission on immunosuppressive therapy.

▶ When a patient is presented with the diagnosis of autoimmune hepatitis (AIH), the initial jolt is the diagnosis itself, but the persistent battle is the realization that the illness bears with it a lifetime of immunosuppressant medications

103

and associated side effects. Children tend to have more severe disease at presentation, with cirrhosis reported in 40% to 80% at diagnosis.[1] The milder forms of disease described in adults, where decision to treat may be individualized, are typically not seen in children.

With prompt initiation of immunosuppressive treatment, 80% of patients will achieve remission and long-term survival.[2] However, deleterious effects of long-term steroids on linear growth, bone development, and physical appearance can be problematic in a growing child. In fact, 80% of patients will experience these side effects after 2 years of steroid treatment regardless of the regimen.[3] Although azathioprine and 6-mercaptopurine are used as steroid sparing agents, these bring with them their own side effects such as cytopenia requiring blood draws for monitoring, pancreatitis, and hepatotoxicity.[3] Consequently, adults are generally given the opportunity to withdraw immunosuppression after sustained normalization of lab indices on treatment along with histological confirmation of remission. However, in children treatment withdrawal is more problematic, especially during puberty when there is increased risk of relapse. According to previous studies, only about 20% of AIH type 1 pediatric patients have been able to discontinue therapy successfully.[1]

The study by Deneau et al represents an important advance in our understanding of factors that predict whether a patient is an appropriate candidate for complete withdrawal of immunosuppressive medication. This carefully conducted study is unique in that not only is it one of the few population based cohorts of AIH patients, but it is also the largest pediatric cohort reported to date.

However there are a number of limitations. The population studied, located in the western United States, is more homogeneous than in the rest of the country. Prior studies have shown that African American, Arabian, and Asian patients are more likely than Caucasian patients to present with cirrhosis, have cholestatic features, and are less likely to respond to standard immunosuppression.[3] All of these features were identified in the Deneau study as poor prognostic factors of sustained immunosuppression-free remission (SIFR). It is possible that the relatively high percentage of patients able to achieve SIFR in the study was higher than previously published results due to there being a larger proportion of an ethnic group that was predisposed to succeed. It is important to note that although the study identified a relatively high probability of 41.6% of achieving SIFR, this number is somewhat misleading because it is a cumulative probability that could be misinterpreted by the reader as a raw percentage. In dissecting the actual numbers, there were only 16 highly selected patients in whom withdrawal of immunosuppression was attempted out of 56 in the whole population.

Furthermore, the inclusion of patients with autoimmune sclerosing cholangitis (ASC) in the calculations related to the outcomes is problematic because ASC and AIH are 2 entities that are similar but also different in prognosis and relapse rates. Recently, the normal range of alanine aminotransferase (ALT) in pediatric patients has been brought to question by Molleston et al,[4] and it would have been helpful to know what values of ALT were used to define "normalization" in the study. In addition, although cirrhosis was identified as an important baseline factor, it seems that there was no single centralized review of histology. Lastly, it would have been helpful to know the doses of the medications used.

Upon completion of the article, the reader is left with a glimmer of hope for those patients who are fortunate to fall under the category of the "carefully selected" few. However, for the other portion of patients with the identified factors such as elevated international normalized ratio, positive antinuclear cytoplasmic antibody, and/or cirrhosis at diagnosis we should have a lower threshold for considering evaluation for liver transplant. The Deneau study also underscores the importance of screening all children with AIH for nonhepatic autoimmune diseases—a practice that is yet to be universally incorporated, but, once done, could be an invaluable piece of the puzzle for determining future SIFR potential in pediatric patients.

E. Shin, MD

K. B. Schwarz, MD

References

1. Mieli-Vergani G. Autoimmune Hepatitis in Children: what is Different from Adult AIH? *Seminars in Liver Disease.* 2009;29:297-306.
2. Mieli-Vergani G, et al. Paediatric autoimmune liver disease. *Arch Dis Child.* 2013; 98:1012-1017.
3. Manns M, et al. Diagnosis and management of Autoimmune Hepatitis, AASLD Practice Guidelines. *Hepatology.* 2010; Vol.51, No.6.
4. Molleston J, Schwimmer J, et al. Histological Abnormalities in Children with Nonalcoholic Fatty Liver Disease and Normal or Mildly Elevated Alanine Aminotransferase levels. *J Pediatr.* 2014;164:707-713.

Use of Corticosteroids After Hepatoportoenterostomy for Bile Drainage in Infants With Biliary Atresia: The START Randomized Clinical Trial

Bezerra JA, for the Childhood Liver Disease Research and Education Network (ChiLDREN) (Cincinnati Children's Hosp Med Ctr, OH; et al)
JAMA 311:1750-1759, 2014

Importance.—Biliary atresia is the most common cause of end-stage liver disease in children. Controversy exists as to whether use of steroids after hepatoportoenterostomy improves clinical outcome.

Objective.—To determine whether the addition of high-dose corticosteroids after hepatoportoenterostomy is superior to surgery alone in improving biliary drainage and survival with the native liver.

Design, Setting, and Patients.—The multicenter, double-blind Steroids in Biliary Atresia Randomized Trial (START) was conducted in 140 infants (mean age, 2.3 months) between September 2005 and February 2011 in the United States; follow-up ended in January 2013.

Interventions.—Participants were randomized to receive intravenous methylprednisolone (4 mg/kg/d for 2 weeks) and oral prednisolone (2 mg/ kg/d for 2 weeks) followed by a tapering protocol for 9 weeks (n = 70) or placebo (n = 70) initiated within 72 hours of hepatoportoenterostomy.

Main Outcomes and Measures.—The primary end point (powered to detect a 25% absolute treatment difference)was the percentage of participants with a serum total bilirubin level of less than 1.5 mg/dL with his/her native liver at 6 months posthepatoportoenterostomy. Secondary outcomes included survival with native liver at 24 months of age and serious adverse events.

Results.—The proportion of participants with improved bile drainage was not statistically significantly improved by steroids at 6 months posthepatoportoenterostomy (58.6% [41/70] of steroids group vs 48.6% [34/70] of placebo group; adjusted relative risk, 1.14 [95% CI, 0.83 to 1.57]; $P=.43$). The adjusted absolute risk difference was 8.7% (95% CI, −10.4% to 27.7%). Transplant-free survival was 58.7% in the steroids group vs 59.4% in the placebo group (adjusted hazard ratio, 1.0 [95% CI, 0.6 to 1.8]; $P=.99$) at 24 months of age. The percentage of participants with serious adverse events was 81.4% [57/70] of the steroids group and 80.0% [56/70] of the placebo group ($P>.99$); however, participants receiving steroids had an earlier time of onset of their first serious adverse event by 30 days posthepatoportoenterostomy (37.2% [95% CI, 26.9% to 50.0%] of steroids group vs 19.0% [95% CI, 11.5% to 30.4%] of placebo group; $P=.008$).

Conclusions and Relevance.—Among infants with biliary atresia who have undergone hepatoportoenterostomy, high-dose steroid therapy following surgery did not result in statistically significant treatment differences in bile drainage at 6 months, although a small clinical benefit could not be excluded. Steroid treatment was associated with earlier onset of serious adverse events in children with biliary atresia.

Trial Registration.—clinicaltrials.gov Identifier: NCT00294684.

▶ As a pediatric hepatologist, I am grasping for anything that can improve surgical outcomes after a Kasai portoenterostomy. When parents of biliary atresia infants ask me about outcomes, I frequently quote surgical outcomes as a "rule of thirds." A third will drain their bile but need a liver transplant in childhood due to complications of cirrhosis. The second third drain bile and do not need a liver transplant until adolescence or early adulthood. The final third will never drain their bile and will ultimately require a liver transplant in the first 1 to 2 years of life to survive. At the time of surgery, I cannot predict what group their child is in, and I have no medications to shift that child into a different outcome group. Because biliary atresia is still the most common indication for pediatric liver transplant, there has been significant focus on medical therapy to improve surgical outcomes. This study is important because the researchers are trying to decrease the "bottom third" that will need early transplant.

Biliary atresia has always been thought to be both inflammatory and fibrotic. If we fix the inflammation in the biliary tree, will this prevent fibrosis and improve outcomes? Several very small, open-label studies using corticosteroids after portoenterostomy have shown some promise. However, a larger randomized study in the United Kingdom (with lower doses of steroids than this study) showed faster improvement in bilirubin but no difference in percentage of children needing liver transplant at 2 years of age.[1] Bottom line: the bilirubin dropped, but it did not change the percentage of early liver transplant.

This study by Bezerra and colleagues is similar to the UK study but unique in several areas. First, the sample size is much larger (140 vs 71). Given that this is a rare condition, the ability to include this many patients is remarkable. Second, the dose of corticosteroids was much higher to start (4 mg/kg/day) and the taper was far longer (14 weeks) than the UK study. These high doses of steroids are closer to the doses used in some favorable studies in Japan.

Unfortunately, after 2 years of follow-up, the study did not demonstrate a significant change in bilirubin at 6 months or transplantation at 2 years. In addition, serious adverse events appeared even earlier than in infants receiving placebo. Maybe steroids are actually harmful?

There is only 1 limitation that is worth discussing. The biggest concern about a multicenter study that evaluates a surgical procedure is whether the levels of surgical skill are equal across centers. Data have shown that experienced centers may have improved outcomes, leading to certain countries centralizing the operation to a handful of hospitals.[2] This is not the case in the United States, and this study included more than 10 surgeons. Could surgical technique alter the outcome? The authors specifically address this question, stating that patients were randomized by site and postoperative protocols were standardized, therefore limiting surgeon skill as a variable.

In conclusion, I think this study will put the steroids discussion to rest. Small changes in bilirubin may be present, but this therapy does not appear to help the bottom line: decreased transplants under the age of 2. Therefore, I would not recommend steroids for my patients with biliary atresia.

S. A. Elisofon, MD

References

1. Davenport M, Stringer MD, Tizzard SA, McClean P, Mieli-Vergani G, Hadzic N. Randomized, double-blind, placebo-controlled trial of corticosteroids after Kasai portoenterostomy for biliary atresia. *Hepatology.* 2007;46(6):1821-1827.
2. Davenport M, De Ville de Goyet J, Stringer MD, et al. Seamless management of biliary atresia in England and Wales (1999-2002). *Lancet.* 2004;363(9418): 1354-1357.

Effectiveness of Anti-TNFα for Crohn Disease: Research in a Pediatric Learning Health System

Forrest CB, Crandall WV, Bailey LC, et al (The Children's Hosp of Philadelphia, PA; Univ of Pennsylvania, Philadelphia; et al)

Pediatrics 134:37-44, 2014

Objectives.—ImproveCareNow (ICN) is the largest pediatric learning health system in the nation and started as a quality improvement collaborative. To test the feasibility and validity of using ICN data for clinical research, we evaluated the effectiveness of anti-tumor necrosis factor-α (anti-TNFα) agents in the management of pediatric Crohn disease (CD).

Methods.—Data were collected in 35 pediatric gastroenterology practices (April 2007 to March 2012) and analyzed as a sequence of non-randomized trials. Patients who had moderate to severe CD were classified as initiators or non-initiators of anti-TNFα therapy. Among 4130 patients who had pediatric CD, 603 were new users and 1211 were receiving anti-TNFα therapy on entry into ICN.

Results.—During a 26-week follow-up period, rate ratios obtained from Cox proportional hazards models, adjusting for patient and disease characteristics and concurrent medications, were 1.53 (95% confidence interval [CI], 1.20—1.96) for clinical remission and 1.74 (95% CI, 1.33—2.29) for corticosteroid-free remission. The rate ratio for corticosteroid-free remission was comparable to the estimate produced by the adult SONIC study, which was a randomized controlled trial on the efficacy of anti-TNFα therapy. The number needed to treat was 5.2 (95% CI, 3.4—11.1) for clinical remission and 5.0 (95% CI, 3.4—10.0) for corticosteroid-free remission.

Conclusions.—In routine pediatric gastroenterology practice settings, anti-TNFα therapy was effective at achieving clinical and corticosteroid-free remission for patients who had Crohn disease. Using data from the ICN learning health system for the purpose of observational research is feasible and produces valuable new knowledge.

▶ Pediatric clinical trials are essential; however, their conduct may be impeded by ethical concerns, limited funding, and inadequate patient numbers to provide sufficient power. Thus, alternative clinical research approaches are needed. This relevant and timely study examines a clinical question using a unique methodology: analyzing data collected from a learning health system for the purpose of observational research.

In a learning health system, data collected from clinical practice inspires scientific investigation. In turn, scientific evidence influences clinical practice. This cycle continues, leading to improvements in the quality of care of patients. The ImproveCareNow Network is a learning health system comprising 35 pediatric gastroenterology practices. Importantly, Forrest et al demonstrated that prospectively collected data in large pediatric learning health system may be used for the purpose of observational research to examine important clinical questions.

In this study, investigators used a learning health system to evaluate the effectiveness of antitumor necrosis factor-α (anti-TNFα) agents in managing pediatric Crohn disease. Although adult studies demonstrate that anti-TNFα agents are efficacious over placebo in induction and maintenance of remission of moderate-to-severe Crohn disease, pediatric efficacy studies are lacking. The ImproveCareNow learning health system the authors used "examines observational registry data as a sequence of non-randomized trials," utilizing sample sizes at least 6 to 10 times larger than current prospective pediatric data on anti-TNFα agent utility. This methodology enables the authors to increase the power of the study by allowing each patient to potentially contribute more than 1 trial to the data analysis.

This ability to use large sample sizes can facilitate further comparative effectiveness studies on drug efficacy in pediatric inflammatory bowel disease, as well as more specific questions (eg, therapeutic drug monitoring, premedications, effects of medications on statural growth and bone health, as well as effects on additional clinical outcomes, and risk stratification).

In this study, the authors highlighted the benefits of treatment with anti-TNFα agents, achieving similar results to pediatric single-group efficacy studies and adult controlled clinical trials. In pediatric gastroenterology practices, those children with Crohn disease prescribed anti-TNFα therapy (initiators) were more likely to achieve clinical and corticosteroid-free remission compared with those children who were not prescribed such therapy (noninitiators) (Table 2 in the original article).

The authors clearly outlined the limitations of their study and the impact on the interpretation of their findings. They addressed the effects of missing data, unmeasured confounders, and loss to follow-up. There are also other potential biases, similar to those associated with open-label trials, such as the potential of reporting bias of adverse events.[1] In addition, although both the initiator and noninitiator groups were fairly similar (Table 1 in the original article), there is the potential of a bias in which patients were selected for treatment. Although there were statistically significant differences between the initiator and noninitiator groups in the Physician Global Assessment, this difference was not clinically significant.

Despite these limitations, this article has important implications for future study. Forrest et al effectively assesses the efficacy of anti-TNFα agents in managing pediatric inflammatory bowel disease—a relatively understudied area that accounts for practice variability among pediatric gastroenterologists. Most important, this study highlights a novel methodology (learning health systems) that overcomes some barriers to performing pediatric clinical trials. Learning health systems such as ImproveCareNow are a promising methodology for not only expanding the body of knowledge by examining questions asked in previous efficacy studies but also for studying the myriad unanswered clinical questions in pediatric inflammatory bowel disease and medical practice in general. Studies using this methodology will lead to improvements in our caring of patients and generate data that will further stimulate scientific investigation.

A. I. Srinath, MD

N. Gupta, MD, MAS

Reference

1. Juni P, Altman DG, Egger M. Systematic reviews in health care: assessing the quality of controlled clinical trials. *BMJ*. 2001;323:42-46.

Effect of Thalidomide on Clinical Remission in Children and Adolescents With Refractory Crohn Disease: A Randomized Clinical Trial

Lazzerini M, Martelossi S, Magazzù G, et al (Inst for Maternal and Child Health IRCCS "Burlo Garofolo," Trieste, Italy; Univ of Messina, Italy; et al)
JAMA 310:2164-2173, 2013

Importance.—Pediatric-onset Crohn disease is more aggressive than adult-onset disease, has high rates of resistance to existing drugs, and can lead to permanent impairments. Few trials have evaluated new drugs for refractory Crohn disease in children.

Objective.—To determine whether thalidomide is effective in inducing remission in refractory pediatric Crohn disease.

Design, Setting, and Patients.—Multicenter, double-blind, placebo-controlled, randomized clinical trial of 56 children with active Crohn disease despite immunosuppressive treatment, conducted August 2008—September 2012 in 6 pediatric tertiary care centers in Italy.

Interventions.—Thalidomide, 1.5 to 2.5 mg/kg per day, or placebo once daily for 8 weeks. In an open-label extension, nonresponders to placebo received thalidomide for an additional 8 weeks. All responders continued to receive thalidomide for an additional minimum 52 weeks.

Main Outcomes and Measures.—Primary outcomes were clinical remission at week 8, measured by Pediatric Crohn Disease Activity Index (PCDAI) score and reduction in PCDAI by $\geq 25\%$ or $\geq 75\%$ at weeks 4 and 8. Primary outcomes during the open-label follow-up were clinical remission and 75% response.

Results.—Twenty-eight children were randomized to thalidomide and 26 to placebo. Clinical remission was achieved by significantly more children treated with thalidomide (13/28 [46.4%] vs 3/26 [11.5%]; risk ratio [RR], 4.0 [95% CI, 1.2-12.5]; $P = .01$; number needed to treat [NNT], 2.86). Responses were not different at 4 weeks, but greater improvement was observed at 8 weeks in the thalidomide group (75% response, 13/28 [46.4%] vs 3/26 [11.5%]; RR, 4.0 [95% CI, 1.2-12.5]; NNT = 2.86; $P = .01$; and 25% response, 18/28 [64.2%] vs 8/26 [30.8%]; RR, 2.1 [95% CI, 1.1-3.9]; NNT = 2.99; $P = .01$). Of the nonresponders to placebo who began receiving thalidomide, 11 of 21 (52.4%) subsequently reached remission at week 8 (RR, 4.5 [95% CI, 1.4-14.1]; NNT = 2.45; $P = .01$). Overall, 31 of 49 children treated with thalidomide (63.3%) achieved clinical remission, and 32 of 49 (65.3%) achieved 75% response. Mean duration of clinical remission in the thalidomide group was 181.1 weeks (95% CI, 144.53-217.76) vs 6.3 weeks (95% CI, 3.51-9.15) in the placebo group ($P < .001$). Cumulative incidence of severe adverse events was 2.1 per 1000 patient-weeks, with peripheral neuropathy the most frequent severe adverse event.

Conclusions and Relevance.—In children and adolescents with refractory Crohn disease, thalidomide compared with placebo resulted in improved clinical remission at 8 weeks of treatment and longer-term maintenance of remission in an open-label follow-up. These findings require replication to definitively determine clinical utility of this treatment. *Trial Registration.*—clinicaltrials.gov Identifier: NCT00720538.

▶ When most people hear about the drug thalidomide, the first thought that comes to mind is usually the serious fetal malformations that were noted when it was used as treatment for morning sickness during pregnancy in the 1950s and 1960s.[1] However, thalidomide has recently been making a therapeutic comeback in the management of inflammatory skin lesions caused by leprosy, systemic lupus erythematosus, and Behcet disease, as well as in multiple myeloma. Uncontrolled studies of thalidomide have also reported encouraging results in the treatment of Crohn disease, a chronic inflammatory intestinal disorder that currently has no cure and is increasing in incidence in the pediatric population.

With their study, Lazzerini et al have further turned our attention to thalidomide as being efficacious in inducing and maintaining remission in Crohn disease for children who have failed standard first- and second-line immune therapies. This is the first clinical trial (in adults or children) evaluating thalidomide treatment for Crohn disease. It is also only one of a handful of therapeutic trials in pediatric Crohn disease, and the fact that it is placebo-controlled makes it even more unique.

Thalidomide is an immunomodulatory medication that is known to inhibit tumor necrosis factor alpha (TNFα), a key cytokine involved in systemic inflammation. Since the late 1990s, biologic agents with anti-TNFα properties, such as infliximab, have revolutionized the management of Crohn disease for both children and adults and have significantly changed the treatment paradigm. However, up to 30% of patients may not respond to these TNFα antagonists, and a significant number who do will lose response over time. Additionally, patients who have failed one TNFα antagonist have significantly decreased response rates when treated with a second TNFα antagonist. Interestingly, although thalidomide also downregulates TNFα, it also has independent inhibitory effects on angiogenesis, as well as on NFkB and interleukin-12 activities, which can also decrease the inflammatory response associated with Crohn disease. This may explain why children in this study who had been previously refractory to infliximab still responded well to thalidomide.

Thalidomide's toxicity will remain a significant concern for patients and clinical providers. In addition to the well-known teratogenic effects, peripheral neuropathy has been found to be a limiting side effect for long-term use. However, thalidomide use is regulated by a standardized distribution system that aims to minimize the risk of teratogenicity while allowing it to be used as a therapeutic agent. If the controlled data in Lazzerini et al's study can be replicated and is found to hold true, then thalidomide may become a feasible option for patients with resistant Crohn disease.

M. Oliva-Hemker, MD

Treating infant colic with the probiotic *Lactobacillus reuteri*: double blind, placebo controlled randomised trial

Sung V, Hiscock H, Tang MLK, et al (Royal Children's Hosp, Parkville, Victoria, Australia; et al)

BMJ 348:g2107, 2014

Objective.—To determine whether the probiotic *Lactobacillus reuteri* DSM 17938 reduces crying or fussing in a broad community based sample of breastfed infants and formula fed infants with colic aged less than 3 months.

Design.—Double blind, placebo controlled randomised trial.

Setting.—Community based sample (primary and secondary level care centres) in Melbourne, Australia.

Participants.—167 breastfed infants or formula fed infants aged less than 3 months meeting Wessel's criteria for crying or fussing: 85 were randomised to receive probiotic and 82 to receive placebo.

Interventions.—Oral daily *L reuteri* (1×10^8 colony forming units) versus placebo for one month.

Main Outcomes Measures.—The primary outcome was daily duration of cry or fuss at 1 month. Secondary outcomes were duration of cry or fuss; number of cry or fuss episodes; sleep duration of infant at 7, 14, and 21 days, and 1 and 6 months; maternal mental health (Edinburgh postnatal depression subscale); family functioning (paediatric quality of life inventory), parent quality adjusted life years (assessment of quality of life) at 1 and 6 months; infant functioning (paediatric quality of life inventory) at 6 months; infant faecal microbiota (microbial diversity, colonisation with *Escherichia coli*), and calprotectin levels at 1 month. In intention to treat analyses the two groups were compared using regression models adjusted for potential confounders.

Results.—Of 167 infants randomised from August 2011 to August 2012, 127 (76%) were retained to primary outcome; of these, a subset was analysed for faecal microbial diversity, *E coli* colonisation, and calprotectin levels. Adherence was high. Mean daily cry or fuss time fell steadily in both groups. At 1 month, the probiotic group cried or fussed 49 minutes more than the placebo group (95% confidence interval 8 to 90 minutes, $P = 0.02$); this mainly reflected more fussing, especially for formula fed infants. The groups were similar on all secondary outcomes. No study related adverse events occurred.

Conclusions.—*L reuteri* DSM 17938 did not benefit a community sample of breastfed infants and formula fed infants with colic. These findings differ from previous smaller trials of selected populations and do not support a general recommendation for the use of probiotics to treat colic in infants.

Trial Registration.—Current Controlled Trials ISRCTN95287767 (Fig 2).

▶ The description "7-week-old infant with colic" on a morning clinic schedule will inevitably trigger a sigh from any provider. Right now, there are no known

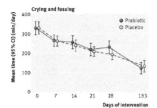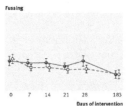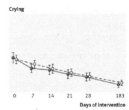

FIGURE 2.—Daily duration of cry or fuss over study period and at 6 month follow-up. Day 28 = 1 month; day 183 = 6 months. (Reprinted from Sung V, Hiscock H, Tang MLK, et al. Treating infant colic with the probiotic *Lactobacillus reuteri*: double blind, placebo controlled randomised trial. *BMJ*. 2014;348:g2107, with permission from the BMJ Publishing Group Ltd.)

effective treatments for colic. In the end, the combination of a careful history, a thorough examination, attentive listening, and calm reassurance is the best intervention that pediatricians can offer. Although colic eventually self-resolves, the condition can be impressively disruptive for families. In addition, colic is relatively common. Colic is typically defined as inconsolable crying for greater than 3 hours per day, for more than 3 days per week in an infant, who is otherwise healthy and well fed and between the ages of 3 weeks and 3 months. It is estimated that the cumulative incidence rates of colic are between 5% to 19% in the community.[1]

As a result, the publication of this study by Sung et al was eagerly awaited. Two previous randomized controlled trials (RCTs) evaluated the effectiveness of *Lactobacillus reuteri* (DSM 17938) in the treatment of infantile colic and both were "positive" studies. The first RCT, conducted at the University of Turin (Regina Margherita Children Hospital) and published in 2010, included 50 breastfed infants (2–16 weeks of age) with colic. A positive response (defined as a 50% reduction in crying time from baseline) was more common in the infants given *L reuteri* throughout the 21-day intervention period (*P* < .05).[2] The second study, published in 2013, was conducted at the Medical University of Warsaw and included 80 infants less than 5 months of age with colic. Once again, the rate of responders was significantly higher in the group supplemented with *L reuteri* compared with the placebo group during the 28-day intervention.[3]

Sung et al enrolled 167 infants aged less than 13 weeks with colic in this study from the Royal Children's Hospital in Melbourne, Australia. Unlike the previous 2 studies, the results from this study by Sung et al were negative. At the end of the 1-month intervention, there were no differences in crying time (Fig 2). In addition, the investigators also measured the frequency of "fussing," which was not different between the 2 groups.

All the studies used the same regimen and the same probiotic, *L reuteri* DSM17398, a very feasible and accessible intervention for parents; however, there is no consistent result. How can pediatric providers reconcile the results of these 3 well-done and rigorous studies?

One issue is that a specific mechanism of action for the probiotic *L reuteri* on colic has not been fully elucidated. For example, there are potential effects of *L reuteri* on gut motility, colonic sensory nerves, or colon contractile activity.[4]

In addition, *L reuteri* may influence the overall bacterial community dynamics, given that several studies have noted that the gut microbiota between infants with colic is different from the microbiota of those infants without colic.[5-7]

Focusing on factors that may affect the infant gut microbiota, there are potential differences in the inclusion and exclusion criteria that may affect the results. Unlike previous studies, the study by Sung et al did not exclude those infants with gastroesophageal reflux. In addition, some infants had been exposed to proton pump inhibitors. Changes in gastric pH may affect the intestinal microbiota.[8] In addition, the Sung study included infants who were formula-fed, and less than half were exclusively breastfed, compared with the study by Savino et al, which only included breastfed infants. Finally, as the authors note, it is possible that the baseline gut microbiota of infants born in Australia may differ from the microbiota of European infants.

With the high costs of randomized, double-blind, placebo-controlled trials, another approach is for investigators to standardize outcomes and methods to allow for easier cross-comparison of results. In addition, with close collaboration, it is potentially possible to combine data from individual clinical trials in an individual participant data meta-analysis (IPDMA), which can allow subgroup analysis to help identify which types of patients may benefit from specific interventions.[9] This work toward an IPDMA on this topic is currently ongoing,[10] and the results will be of even greater interest to clinicians.

In the meantime, the use of *L reuteri* DSM 17938 for colic is still promising. There were few, if any, serious adverse events reported in the 3 RCTs thus far. Factors that may influence the success of *L reuteri* DSM 17938 may include a history of gastroesophageal reflux disease, as well as exposure to a proton-pump inhibitor and lack of breastfeeding. For the next infant who presents with colic, after a careful history, a thorough examination, attentive listening, and calm reassurance, you might still be willing to consider a probiotic supplement, *L reuteri* DSM 17938.

M. D. Cabana, MD, MPH

References

1. Lucassen PL, Assendelft WJ, van Eijk JT, Gubbels JW, Douwes AC, van Geldrop WJ. Systematic review of the occurrence of infantile colic in the community. *Arch Dis Child*. 2001;84:398-403.
2. Savino F, Cordisco L, Tarasco V, et al. *Lactobacillus reuteri* DSM 17938 in infantile colic: a randomized, double-blind, placebo-controlled trial. *Pediatrics*. 2010; 126:e526-e533.
3. Szajewska H, Gyrczuk E, Horvath A. *Lactobacillus reuteri* DSM 17938 for the management of infantile colic in breastfed infants: a randomized, double-blind, placebo-controlled trial. *J Pediatr*. 2013;162:257-262.
4. Savino F, Tarasco V. New treatments for infant colic. *Curr Opin Pediatr*. 2010; 22:791-797.
5. de Weerth C, Fuentes S, Puylaert P, de Vos WM. Intestinal microbiota of infants with colic: development and specific signatures. *Pediatrics*. 2013;131:e550-e558.
6. Lehtonen L, Korvenranta H, Eerola E. Intestinal microflora in colicky and non-colicky infants: bacterial cultures and gas-liquid chromatography. *J Pediatr Gastroenterol Nutr*. 1994;19:310-314.

7. Mentula S, Tuure T, Koskenala R, Korpela R, Kononen E. Microbial composition and fecal fermentation end products from colicky infants—a probiotic supplementation pilot. *Microb Ecol Health Dis.* 2008;20:37-47.
8. Garcia-Mazcorro JF, Suchodolski JS, Jones KR, et al. Effect of the proton pump inhibitor omeprazole on the gastrointestinal bacterial microbiota of healthy dogs. *FEMS Microbiol Ecol.* 2012;80:624-636.
9. Riley RD, Lambert PC, Abo-Zaid G. Meta-analysis of individual participant data: rationale, conduct, and reporting. *BMJ.* 2010;340:c221.
10. PROSPERO International prospective register of systematic reviews. *Lactobacillus reuteri* DSM 17938 for managing infant colic: protocol for an individual participant data meta-analysis. http://www.crd.york.ac.uk/PROSPERO/display_record.asp?ID=CRD42014013210#.U__4ath0zIU. Accessed August 28, 2014.

Prophylactic Use of a Probiotic in the Prevention of Colic, Regurgitation, and Functional Constipation: A Randomized Clinical Trial

Indrio F, Di Mauro A, Riezzo G, et al (Moro Univ of Bari, Italy; Natl Inst for Digestive Diseases, IRCCS "Saverio de Bellis," Castellana Grotte, Italy)
JAMA Pediatr 168:228-233, 2014

Importance.—Infantile colic, gastroesophageal reflux, and constipation are the most common functional gastrointestinal disorders that lead to referral to a pediatrician during the first 6 months of life and are often responsible for hospitalization, feeding changes, use of drugs, parental anxiety, and loss of parental working days with relevant social consequences.

Objective.—To investigate whether oral supplementation with Lactobacillus reuteri DSM 17938 during the first 3 months of life can reduce the onset of colic, gastroesophageal reflux, and constipation in term newborns and thereby reduce the socioeconomic impact of these conditions.

Design.—A prospective, multicenter, double-masked, placebo-controlled randomized clinical trial was performed on term newborns (age <1 week) born at 9 different neonatal units in Italy between September 1, 2010, and October 30, 2012.

Setting.—Parents were asked to record in a structured diary the number of episodes of regurgitation, duration of inconsolable crying (minutes per day), number of evacuations per day, number of visits to pediatricians, feeding changes, hospitalizations, visits to a pediatric emergency department for a perceived health emergency, pharmacologic interventions, and loss of parental working days.

Participants.—In total, 589 infants were randomly allocated to receive L reuteri DSM 17938 or placebo daily for 90 days.

Interventions.—Prophylactic use of probiotic.

Main Outcomes and Measures.—Reduction of daily crying time, regurgitation, and constipation during the first 3 months of life. Cost-benefit analysis of the probiotic supplementation.

Results.—At 3 months of age, the mean duration of crying time (38 vs 71 minutes; $P < .01$), the mean number of regurgitations per day (2.9 vs 4.6; $P < .01$), and the mean number of evacuations per day (4.2 vs 3.6; $P < .01$) for the L *reuteri* DSM 17938 and placebo groups, respectively, were significantly different. The use of *L reuteri* DSM 17938 resulted in an estimated mean savings per patient of €88 (US $118.71) for the family and an additional €104 (US $140.30) for the community.

Conclusions and Relevance.—Prophylactic use of *L reuteri* DSM 17938 during the first 3 months of life reduced the onset of functional gastrointestinal disorders and reduced private and public costs for the management of this condition.

Trial Registration.—clinicaltrials.gov Identifier: NCT01235884.

▶ Functional gastrointestinal disorders are common in children and have substantial public health and economic consequences. Thus, there is interest in reducing this burden.

Evidence suggests that gut microbiota play a role in the development of functional gastrointestinal disorders and that the gut microbiota in subjects with these disorders differ from those in an unaffected population. If so, it is logical to assume that manipulation of the gut microbiota could be a preventive measure in the evolution of these disorders and also may play a therapeutic role.

Indrio et al are to be praised for making an important contribution by evaluating the effectiveness of one of the best-studied probiotics, *Lactobacillus reuteri* DSM 17938, in preventing infant functional gastrointestinal disorders. The choice of probiotic was well substantiated because at the time of the planning of the study, *L reuteri* DSM 17938 had been shown to be effective for the treatment of some of these disorders, such as infantile colic. Two independent randomized controlled trials (RCTs) showed that *L reuteri* DSM 17938 is likely to reduce crying times in infants with infantile colic, at least in exclusively or predominantly exclusively breastfed infants. However, another recent study that also involved formula-fed infants did not confirm this effect.

The trial by Indrio et al was well designed and conducted. The strengths of the study include appropriate randomization, allocation concealment, and blinding as well as the use of a true placebo. Data were reported based on intention-to-treat analysis. The study was adequately powered. The primary outcomes were infantile colic (defined by the duration of inconsolable crying in minutes per day), reflux (regurgitation episodes per day), and constipation (measured by stool frequency). One limitation is that crying was not assessed in an objective way. The investigators relied on parents' reports of the duration of crying recorded in diaries. The precision and validity of such reporting may be questioned. Moreover, symptoms such as irritability and fussing might have been difficult to isolate from crying.

Perhaps the most interesting data are those related to infantile colic. This is usually a self-limited condition, typically resolving by 4 to 5 months of age. However, it may be distressing to parents, and any safe and effective preventive and/or therapeutic measures would be desirable. In the probiotic group compared with the placebo group, a reduction of crying time by approximately 51 minutes per day at 1 month and 33 minutes per day at 3 months is not only statistically significant, but it is also clinically relevant.

In contrast, one may question the clinical relevance of the effect of *L reuteri* DSM 17938 on regurgitation. Uncomplicated regurgitation in an otherwise healthy infant is not a disease; it is a normal developmental issue that does not require treatment. In the probiotic group compared with the placebo group, a reduction of regurgitation by 1.7 episodes per day at 3 months is unlikely to be clinically important.

Similarly, one may question the clinical importance of the results regarding the difference in stool frequency between the 2 groups (1.2 stools per day at 1 month and 0.6 stool per day at 3 months). By the way, the title of the article is misleading with respect to functional constipation because this outcome was not assessed.

One important question is, should we be preventing functional gastrointestinal disorders such as infantile colic at all? As pointed out in the article discussion, "an unselected general population was recruited, and the possible risk of over-treating normal neonates cannot be excluded." On the other hand, some evidence suggests that childhood functional gastrointestinal disorders are being linked to those occurring later in life. For example, it has been suggested that colic during infancy increases the susceptibility to recurrent abdominal pain, allergic diseases, and psychological disorders in childhood. A recent systematic review suggests a link to migraine. In the study by Indrio et al, the follow-up period was 3 months. Thus, one cannot tell whether *L reuteri* DSM 17938 provides a permanent protection against the development of functional gastrointestinal disorders or whether it only delays the onset of symptoms. The jury is still out.

As is common nowadays, the investigators considered not only the clinical impact of the intervention aimed at preventing functional gastrointestinal disorders, but also the financial impact. Although it has been shown that the treatment provides a cost-saving benefit to the families and health care system, the limitation is that this economic evaluation could not be easily extrapolated from one setting to another.

In conclusion, it was documented for the first time in an RCT that *L reuteri* DSM 17938 was effective for preventing common functional gastrointestinal disorders in infants, particularly infantile colic, in both breastfed and formula-fed infants. Given the lack of effective therapy for infantile colic, these new data are welcome. Nonetheless, even if the results are encouraging, I agree with the authors that repeat studies are needed.

H. Szajewska, MD

Efficacy and Safety of *Saccharomyces boulardii* for Acute Diarrhea
Feizizadeh S, Salehi-Abargouei A, Akbari V (Isfahan Univ of Med Sciences, Iran; Shahid Sadoughi Univ of Med Sciences, Yazd, Iran)
Pediatrics 134:e176-e191, 2014

Background and Objective.—The efficacy of *Saccharomyces boulardii* for treatment of childhood diarrhea remains unclear. Our objective was to systematically review data on the effect of *S. boulardii* on acute childhood diarrhea.

Methods.—Our data sources included Medline, Embase, CINAHL, Scopus, and The Cochrane Library up to September 2013 without language restrictions. Randomized controlled trials and non-randomized trials that evaluated effectiveness of *S. boulardii* for treatment of acute diarrhea in children were included. Two reviewers independently evaluated studies for eligibility and quality and extracted the data.

Results.—In total, 1248 articles were identified, of which 22 met the inclusion criteria. Pooling data from trials showed that *S. boulardii* significantly reduced the duration of diarrhea (mean difference [MD], −19.7 hours; 95% confidence interval [CI], −26.05 to −13.34), stool frequency on day 2 (MD, −0.74; 95% CI, −1.38 to −0.10) and day 3 (MD, −1.24; 95% CI, −2.13 to −0.35), the risk for diarrhea on day 3 (risk ratio [RR], 0.41; 95% CI, 0.27 to 0.60) and day 4 (RR, 0.38; 95% CI, 0.24 to 0.59) after intervention compared with control. The studies included in this review were varied in the definition of diarrhea, the termination of diarrhea, inclusion and exclusion criteria, and their methodological quality.

Conclusions.—This review and meta-analysis show that *S. boulardii* is safe and has clear beneficial effects in children who have acute diarrhea. However, additional studies using head-to-head comparisons are needed to define the best dosage of *S. boulardii* for diarrhea with different causes.

▶ Probiotics are live microorganisms, which when administered in adequate amounts confer a health benefit on the host.[1] Probiotics have shown benefits in treatment and prevention of varied diseases, including respiratory infections, irritable bowel syndrome, necrotizing enterocolitis (NEC), and allergies. Patients regularly use probiotics as supplements or in their food intake. Physicians are also regularly recommending probiotics to patients. As demonstrated by the recent interest in fecal transplant to treat *Clostridium difficile*, physicians are comfortable using bacteria to treat diarrhea or other diseases.[2] However, one of the interesting points of this meta-analysis is that not all probiotics are bacterial. This well-conducted meta-analysis is for the yeast *Saccharomyces boulardii*. As the authors demonstrate, quite a few studies have been conducted with *S boulardii*.

Meta-analysis has the potential to truly change practice more than single trials.[3] This meta-analysis addresses but also highlights some of the major issues with probiotics as treatments. The authors included 22 studies in their final analysis; no studies were conducted in the United States and only 2 in Europe. Diarrhea in the developing world is a very different disease than what we often witness in our clinics. So although I believe their outcome of 20 fewer hours is clinically relevant, one cannot be sure how that relates to our patients.

The authors also only included studies of *S boulardii*. One of the major complaints about probiotic meta-analysis is that often many strains of probiotics are combined. The data for probiotic usage in NEC is overwhelming; however, it is difficult for neonatologists to know which strain to use because almost all of the studies have been different strains. This is not the case for diarrhea; the authors demonstrate that there is a large literature base for using *S boulardii* in diarrhea treatment.

The authors used 4 quality measures to evaluate methodological quality: sequence generation, allocation concealment, blinding, and follow-up. Many others such as funding source, CONSORT usage, and registration, among others, could have also been included. However, using only their 4 criteria, only 1 study was determined to be adequate for all 4 criteria. For overall quality on all 4 parameters, 4 studies were rated as good, 13 as fair, and 5 as poor. Additionally, as expected, there were many causes of diarrhea. Although the data are supportive of the usage of *S boulardii*, there are many limitations of these studies that cause concerns. This analysis clearly calls for more studies conducted by nonindustry support.

Patients do not often think of adverse events when taking supplements. The literature supporting the safety of orally supplemented probiotics in a variety of disease states is robust, and in general patients need not be worried. However, there is a potential for sepsis when consuming probiotics. The authors report good safety measures for *S boulardii*; however, as discussed, there are many limitations of the studies they reviewed. Bacterial sepsis is much easier to treat than fungal sepsis. Precaution needs to be taken for very ill or immunocompromised children and until there is further research, I will recommend bacterial probiotics for children who are severely ill.

In conclusion, more studies are needed, in different populations and with high levels of quality measures. But for the majority of the kids we see with diarrhea or who are at risk of diarrhea from antibiotics or travel, *S boulardii* is a reasonable option for us to recommend.

D. Merenstein, MD

References

1. Health and Nutritional Properties of Probiotics in Food Including Powder Milk with Live Lactic Acid Bacteria. In: Report of a Joint FAO/WHO Expert Consultation on Evaluation of Health and Nutritional Properties of Probiotics in Food Including Powder Milk with Live Lactic Acid Bacteria. Food and Agriculture Organization of the United Nations and World Health Organization. Córdoba, Argentina.
2. LoVecchio A, Cohen MB. Fecal microbiota transplantation for Clostridium difficile infection: benefits and barriers. *Curr Opin Gastroenterol.* 2014;30:47-53.
3. Murad MH, Montori VM, Ioannidis JP. How to read a systematic review and meta-analysis and apply the results to patient care: users' guides to the medical literature. *JAMA.* 2014;312:171-179.

Usefulness of Symptoms to Screen for Celiac Disease

Rosén A, Sandström O, Carlsson A, et al (Umeå Univ, Sweden; Lund Univ, Sweden; et al)
Pediatrics 133:211-218, 2014

Objective.—To describe the frequency of symptoms and associated conditions among screening-detected celiac disease (CD) cases and non-CD children and to evaluate questionnaire-based case-finding targeting the general population.

Methods.—In a population-based CD screening of 12-year-olds, children and their parents completed questionnaires on CD-associated symptoms and conditions before knowledge of CD status. Questionnaire data for those who had their CD detected in the screening ($n = 153$) were compared with those of children with normal levels of CD markers ($n = 7016$). Hypothetical case-finding strategies were also evaluated. Questionnaires were returned by 7054 (98%) of the children and by 6294 (88%) of their parents.

Results.—Symptoms were as common among screening-detected CD cases as among non-CD children. The frequency of children with screening-detected CD was similar when comparing the groups with and without any CD-related symptoms (2.1% vs 2.1%; $P = .930$) or CD-associated conditions (3.6% vs 2.1%; $P = .07$). Case-finding by asking for CD-associated symptoms and/or conditions would have identified 52 cases (38% of all cases) at a cost of analyzing blood samples for 2282 children (37%) in the study population.

Conclusions.—The current recommended guidelines for finding undiagnosed CD cases, so-called active case-finding, fail to identify the majority of previously undiagnosed cases if applied in the general population of Swedish 12-year-olds. Our results warrant further studies on the effectiveness of CD case-finding in the pediatric population, both at the clinical and population-based levels.

▶ The now available and widespread use of specific and sensitive serologic markers for celiac disease (CD) has allowed for remarkable advances in our understanding of the true prevalence of CD and the apparent increase in its prevalence over the past few decades. Currently the diagnosis of celiac disease is based on positive serologic markers with confirmation through classic intestinal biopsy histology findings obtained through endoscopy.

Although in the past the diagnosis was more frequent in patients with typical symptoms (such as diarrhea, steatorrhea, failure to thrive, or vitamin deficiencies), increasing awareness of the condition has resulted in the recognition that there is also a growing population of patients presenting without these classic features of malabsorption. Such patients would be missed if only classical symptoms were sought for further testing. Identifying a set of symptoms and/or conditions within the pediatric population that could single out patients at highest risk for celiac disease would likely help to limit unnecessary blood testing and or biopsies and greatly enhance the efficiency of care, cost-effectiveness, and patient quality of life and satisfaction.

This study is important and stands out because it appears to be among the first to evaluate which possible symptoms and/or conditions related to CD may help to better identify which pediatric patients are at highest risk for CD and warrant further blood screening and biopsies.

The study looked at a large ($N = 10\,041$), population-based cohort of 12-year-old children in Sweden, without previously diagnosed CD to determine whether screening practices for CD could be driven by positive questionnaire testing for symptoms and/or conditions felt to be related to celiac disease.

This investigation was an excellent follow-up to the recent study looking at the relationship between symptoms and CD-screening results in adults, which failed to show a correlation.[1] Quite unexpectedly, this study failed to show a correlation between a symptom or symptoms and/or conditions and positive testing for celiac disease (Tables 1 and 2 in the original article).

A potential flaw of the study was the age of participants enrolled. In fact, despite the fact that the median age for the diagnosis of CD in Sweden in 6.8 years,[2] 12-year-old subjects were enrolled in the study. Thus, a large percentage of subjects, roughly 90% of patients with CD (which is equal to 0.9% of the general population) from the start have been excluded from the analysis, which may have ultimately skewed the findings, resulting in a lack of clinical significance. By excluding these patients from analysis, the study design potentially creates the problem of "spectrum" bias, which is a bias that is created if the subjects for a study of a diagnostic test or screening tool did not have a reasonable spectrum of the condition being tested.[3] Considering that the prevalence of CD in the general population in Europe is around 1%,[4] this clearly removed a large proportion of positive subjects from the pool from the start, possibly altering the outcomes.

Additionally, although the 2012 European Society for Pediatric Gastroenterology, Hepatology and Nutrition guidelines list diarrhea, chronic constipation, abdominal distention/bloating, vomiting, failure to thrive, stunted growth, and possibly abdominal pain (although a generic complaint) as the most common CD-related symptoms and type I diabetes mellitus, Down syndrome, Turner syndrome, Williams syndrome, immunoglobulin (Ig)A deficiency, IgA nephropathy, autoimmune thyroid and liver disease, and juvenile chronic arthritis as the most common CD-associated conditions,[5] the study failed to include vomiting, failure to thrive, short stature, autoimmune liver disease, IgA deficiency, and IgA nephropathy in its questionnaires.

The study ultimately concluded that CD-associated symptoms and conditions were as common among detected CD cases as among non-CD children when reported before knowledge of their CD status. The use of symptoms alone or in combination with other patient conditions such as a screening tool were not sufficiently accurate for predicting CD. The authors also found that in this group, there was no difference in CD prevalence among symptomatic and asymptomatic children and that CD case finding conducted by elicitation of symptoms and conditions had poor diagnostic accuracy. It is quite possible that the inclusion of these other well-recognized symptoms and conditions would have increased the positive predictive value of their questionnaire and resulted in statistically significant findings as well.

That being said, identification of a screening questionnaire to pinpoint those at highest risk for CD is of utmost importance and again would help to drastically reduce unnecessary testing, health care costs, and undue stress and procedures on patients. Repeating this study in a younger population and with a more inclusive set of symptoms and conditions in the questionnaires may unmask symptoms or conditions that could better guide which patients do and do not warrant additional screening labs and biopsies in the future.

S. Guandalini, MD

H. Jericho, MD

References

1. Katz KD, Rashtak S, Lahr BD, et al. Screening for celiac disease in a North American population: sequential serology and gastrointestinal symptoms. *Am J Gastroenterol.* 2011;106:1333-1339.
2. Namatovu F, Sandstrom O, Olsson C, Lindkvist M, Ivarsson A. Celiac disease risk varies between birth cohorts, generating hypotheses about causality: evidence from 36 years of population-based follow-up. *BMC Gastroenterol.* 2014;14:59.
3. Newman T, Kohn M. *Evidence Based Diagnosis.* Chapter 5 of Critical appraisal of studies of diagnostic tests. New York, NY: Cambridge University Press; 2009.
4. Mustalahti K, Catassi C, Reunanen A, et al. The prevalence of celiac disease in Europe: results of a centralized, international mass screening project. *Ann Med.* 2010;42:587-595.
5. Husby S, Koletzko S, Korponay-Szabo IR, et al. European Society for Pediatric Gastroenterology, Hepatology, and Nutrition guidelines for the diagnosis of coeliac disease. *J Pediatr Gastroenterol Nutr.* 2012;54:136-160.

Pediatric Abdominal Radiograph Use, Constipation, and Significant Misdiagnoses

Freedman SB, Thull-Freedman J, Manson D, et al (Univ of Toronto, Ontario, Canada)
J Pediatr 164:83-88, 2014

Objective.—To determine the proportion of children diagnosed with constipation assigned a significant alternative diagnosis within 7 days (misdiagnosis), if there is an association between abdominal radiograph (AXR) performance and misdiagnosis, and features that might identify children with misdiagnoses.

Study Design.—We conducted a retrospective cohort study of consecutive children <18 years who presented to a pediatric emergency department in Toronto, between 2008 and 2010. Children assigned an *International Statistical Classification of Diseases and Related Health Problems 10th Revision* code consistent with constipation were eligible. Misdiagnosis was defined as an alternative diagnosis during the subsequent 7 days that resulted in hospitalization or an outpatient procedure that included a surgical or radiologic intervention. Constipation severity was classified employing text word categorization and the Leech score.

Results.—3685 eligible visits were identified. Mean age was 6.6 ± 4.4 years. AXR was performed in 46% (1693/3685). Twenty misdiagnoses (0.5%; 95% CI 0.4, 0.8) were identified (appendicitis [7%], intussusception [2%, bowel obstruction [2%], other [9%]). AXR was performed more frequently in misdiagnosed children (75% vs 46%; $P = .01$). These children more often had abdominal pain (70% vs 49%; $P = .04$) and tenderness (60% vs 32%; $P = .01$). Children in both groups had similar amounts of stool on AXR ($P = .38$) and mean Leech scores (misdiagnosed $= 7.9 \pm 3.4$; not misdiagnosed $= 7.7 \pm 2.9$; $P = .85$).

Conclusions.—Misdiagnoses in children with constipation are more frequent in those in whom an AXR was performed and those with abdominal pain and tenderness. The performance of an AXR may indicate diagnostic uncertainty; in such cases, the presence of stool on AXR does not rule out an alternative diagnosis.

▶ The first principle in Sir Zachary Cope's classic approach to abdominal pain is "that of the necessity of making a serious and thorough attempt at diagnosis, usually predominantly by means of history and physical examination."[1] This article presents a case study illustrating the timelessness of Cope's 1921 classic, through the use of chart abstraction of an emergency department's electronic health record (EHR) to explore the frequency of and factors associated with clinically significant misdiagnoses of constipation among children seen in a pediatric emergency department.

From the authors' primary analysis, we learn that clinically significant misdiagnoses represent a small proportion (0.5%) of those discharged with constipation. Although this is a small proportion, given the ubiquity of the constipation diagnosis—with US estimates of 400 000 emergency department visits annually by children 0 to 17 years for constipation (2009–2011)—this represents 2000 cases erroneously diagnosed as constipation that turned out to have clinically significant diagnoses.[2]

In their secondary analysis, the authors explore characteristics of the initial visit associated with significant misdiagnosis, identifying a chief complaint of abdominal pain, the presence of abdominal tenderness, and the ordering of an abdominal radiograph (AXR) as the 3 factors more common among those misdiagnosed.

An important contribution of these findings lies in characterizing the value of EHR-derived data in measuring—and ultimately mitigating—diagnostic errors. Cope himself stresses the importance of exploring root causes of diagnostic error: "one often, if not always, learns more by analyzing the process of, and detecting the fallacy of, an incorrect diagnosis then by taking unction to oneself when the diagnosis proves correct." In exploring potential root causes, the authors characterize 3 diagnostic errors as responsible for the misdiagnoses: 1) failure to perform an adequate history and physical examination, 2) ordering the wrong diagnostic test (ie, the AXR, which the authors characterize as being ordered to "confirm" the diagnosis), and 3) incorrectly interpreting the test. Let's consider each error in the context of what we—as clinicians, researchers, and quality improvement stakeholders—would need to implement to measure and mitigate it, including potential unintended consequences that might result from such efforts.[3,4]

The first diagnostic error relies on the authors' assessment of the adequacy of the history and exam based on data extracted from unstructured fields in the EHR. They cite the higher rate of abdominal pain and tenderness among those with misdiagnosis. It is impossible to determine from the EHR whether the true predictor of misdiagnosis was more complete documentation of pain and tenderness or failure to consider the presence of these findings in decision making. Although EHRs have the potential to provide detailed patient-level data about the care being provided and health outcomes, the authors' laborious methods for data extraction illustrate data quality issues arising from the lack of standardization of EHR data structure and difficulty of extraction.[5] In facing the challenge of using the EHR to distinguish quality of care from quality of documentation, we would need to consider the trade-off between the efficiency and clinical utility of unstructured text and the data quality of standardized, structured fields.[6]

The second diagnostic error relies on the assumption that ordering an AXR "to 'confirm' a diagnosis" of constipation is erroneous. This illustrates 2 pitfalls in measuring quality. One involves Monday-morning quarterbacking: as the ultimate discharge diagnosis is not known at the time the provider orders the AXR, classification based on the discharge diagnosis cannot be used to assess the quality of that decision. Because patients without a diagnosis of constipation were excluded, it is not known whether providers may have ordered AXRs appropriately—say, on patients who had 1 of the 5 features (prior abdominal surgery, foreign body ingestion, abnormal bowel sounds, abdominal distention, or peritoneal signs) found to be predictive of major abdominal disease on AXR.[7] Of these 5 features, only 1, abdominal distention, is included among the factors abstracted—and notably is 1 of the predictors of misdiagnosis. The EHR cannot tell us about confounding—perhaps providers ordered more AXRs precisely because of distention. To address this pitfall, we would need to reframe any quality measurement related to constipation misdiagnosis so that it better reflects the decisions as faced by providers in real time.

The other pitfall illustrated by this error is the importance of assessing the quality of the evidence for a recommendation thought to be relevant to an adverse outcome.[8] Although the authors cite studies showing the limited value of AXRs in diagnosing constipation, the recommendations in the medical literature are not consistent; for example, the American College of Radiology and Society for Pediatric Radiology's practice guideline includes constipation as an indication for AXR performance.[9] One approach to addressing this pitfall would be performing a systematic review of evidence relevant to the real world decision of the provider.

In exploring the third diagnostic error (AXR misinterpretation), the authors focus on individual health provider factors commonly implicated in diagnostic errors: cognitive biases, in this case, arising from heuristics.[10] The AXR-interpretation error may exemplify 2 of the most common cognitive errors: anchoring bias (the failure to continue considering reasonable alternatives after an AXR confirms the presence of stool) and confirmation bias (the tendency to interpret AXRs in a way that confirms their preconceived diagnosis).

Contextualized in the cognitive psychology framework of Dual Process Theory, the described heuristics associated with AXR use are key components of the "System 1" mode of diagnostic thinking, which is instantaneous, intuitive, effortless, and often correct.[11] With good reason, clinicians practicing in the study setting—an emergency department—rely especially extensively on System 1 thinking.[12] Evidence about the role of AXRs in assessing abdominal pain would inform the "System 2" mode of diagnostic thinking, which refers to the more conscious, deliberate, systematic, and analytical process that clinicians use to synthesize medical evidence. Although System 2 processing is typically effective and correct, it is slower and more laborious than System 1. Given the efficiency of System 1 thinking, overreliance on System 2 thinking might have the unintended consequence of slowing patient triage in an acute-care setting. Indeed, a review of the evidence related to diagnostic errors finds little evidence that System 1 thinking is primarily to blame, given the complexity of individual and systemic determinants involved in clinical decision-making.[13]

The 3 errors cited thus highlight the complex and diverse determinants of health care provider decision making, as well as some of the challenges inherent in designing EHR-based metrics aimed at mitigating these errors.[8] Rigorous characterization of the diagnostic error itself and diverse determinants of provider practice—including provider heuristics and guideline-utility—can help advance our understanding of clinical decision making, and ultimately enhance the value and quality of patient care.

The findings also return us to Cope's first principle: to focus careful attention on the history and physical examination in diagnosing the source of abdominal pain. Although AXRs still have a role in the evaluation of abdominal pain, the article is a reminder to use an AXR finding of stool as an opportunity to pause to consider what alternative diagnoses we may be missing.

M. R. Sills, MD, MPH

References

1. Silen W, Cope Z. *Cope's early diagnosis of the acute abdomen.* 22nd ed. Oxford, UK; New York: Oxford University Press; 2010.
2. Quality AfHRa. HCUPNet. National Statistics on All ED Visits 2009-2011. http://hcupnet.ahrq.gov. Accessed July 18, 2014.
3. Bardach NS, Cabana MD. The unintended consequences of quality improvement. *Curr Opin Pediatr.* 2009;21:777-782.
4. Pines JM, Isserman JA, Hinfey PB. The measurement of time to first antibiotic dose for pneumonia in the emergency department: a white paper and position statement prepared for the American Academy of Emergency Medicine. *J Emerg Med.* 2009;37:335-340.
5. Walker JM, Carayon P. From tasks to processes: the case for changing health information technology to improve health care. *Health Aff (Millwood).* 2009; 28:467-477.
6. Torda PT. Aldo Achieving the Promise of Electronic Health Record-enabled Quality Measurement: a Measure Developer's Perspective. eGEMs (Generating Evidence & Methods to improve patient outcomes). 2013;1.
7. Rothrock SG, Green SM, Hummel CB. Plain abdominal radiography in the detection of major disease in children: a prospective analysis. *Ann Emerg Med.* 1992; 21:1423-1429.
8. Flottorp SA, Oxman AD, Krause J, et al. A checklist for identifying determinants of practice: a systematic review and synthesis of frameworks and taxonomies of factors that prevent or enable improvements in healthcare professional practice. *Implement Sci.* 2013;8:35.
9. American College of Radiology. ACR—SPR Practice guideline for the performance of abdominal radiography. 2011. http://www.acr.org/.~/media/ACR/Documents/PGTS/guidelines/Abdominal_Radiography.pdf. Accessed August 25, 2014.

10. Croskerry P. From mindless to mindful practice — cognitive bias and clinical decision making. *N Engl J Med.* 2013;368:2445-2448.
11. Croskerry P. Clinical cognition and diagnostic error: applications of a dual process model of reasoning. *Adv Health Sci Educ Theory Pract.* 2009;14:27-35.
12. Croskerry P. Achieving quality in clinical decision making: cognitive strategies and detection of bias. *Acad Emerg Med.* 2002;9:1184-1204.
13. Norman GR, Eva KW. Diagnostic error and clinical reasoning. *Med Educ.* 2010; 44:94-100.

Magnetic Foreign Body Injuries: A Large Pediatric Hospital Experience

Strickland M, Rosenfield D, Fecteau A (Univ of Toronto, Ontario, Canada)
J Pediatr 165:332-335, 2014

Objective.—To examine trends in magnet-related injuries and hypothesize that changes are a result of new neodymium-iron-boron magnets that are smaller, stronger, and commonly sold in sets.

Study Design.—In this retrospective chart review, we searched our institution's electronic patient record for patients less than 18 years old who were diagnosed with magnetic foreign body ingestion between 2002 and 2012. Cases were analyzed for patient, magnetic foreign body, and management characteristics. Incidence rates and case characteristics were compared between the first 8 years of the study period and the last 3.

Results.—We identified 94 patients who met our search criteria. Of confirmed ingestions, the median age was 4.5 years and 65% were male. The incidence of visits increased between the 2002-2009 period and the 2010-2012 period by a factor of 2.94 (95% CI, 1.84-4.70), whereas the incidence of injuries involving multiple magnets increased by a factor of 8.40 (95% CI, 3.44-20.56). The volume of the magnets decreased from 878.6 mm^3 to 259.8 mm^3. Six cases required surgical removal of the magnets because of intra-abdominal sepsis or concern for imminent bowel perforation.

Conclusions.—Since 2002, there has been a significant increase in the incidence of magnetic foreign body injuries. These injuries have increasingly involved multiple, smaller magnets and required operative intervention.

▶ As an interventional pediatric gastroenterologist, I love cool toys and gadgets. "Buckyballs," "Zen magnets," "Nanodots," and the like are just that: very cool toys. These 200-plus sets of small (5 mm), round, bright, colorful magnets look like candy and are great fun to play with no matter what your age. So how did such a hip new toy become one of our most significant child safety hazards?

Consider this: to toddlers, these magnets look like candy. So, of course, they try and eat them (Fig 1). To tweens and teens, these strong magnets can mimic tongue, lip, and cheek piercings. So guess what? They try it. No manufacturer ever meant them to be swallowed, but that's exactly what happens; it is a tale of unintended consequences. Once in the gastrointestinal tract, the impressive power of these magnets attract each other across a loop of bowel and voila, impending disaster beckons.

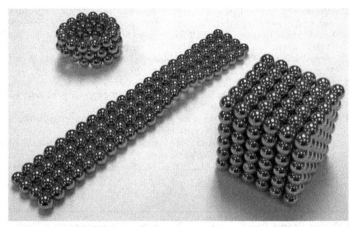

FIGURE 1.—Tiny, rare-earth magnets. From the US Consumer Product Safety Commission (CPSC) web site. Available at http://www.cpsc.gov/onsafety/2011/11/magnet-dangers/. Accessed October 30, 2014.

In this article, Strickland et al. emphasize several points. (1) The incidence of multiple magnet ingestions has significantly increased since 2010, coincident with the appearance of the toys in the marketplace. (2) The frequency and severity of intestinal injury has increased. (3) The frequency of surgical intervention has increased. Interestingly, although their study is limited by being a single-center study, their results coincide with the published findings across North America.[1,2]

The US Consumer Product Safety Commission (CPSC) and their Canadian counterpart, Health Canada, responded dramatically and appropriately by issuing product recalls.[3,4] Indeed, the Health Canada mandatory product recall in 2013 was the first in Canadian history, emphasizing the magnitude and serious nature of child health risk. The CPSC has been subjected to vigorous criticism, suggesting the banning of these toys is an outrageous infringement of personal civil liberty.[5]

So be it. As pediatricians, our first and foremost concern is child safety. We have recognized the problem, sounded the alarm, and established appropriate plan of care, but we cannot rest.[6] Although high-powered magnets have been taken off the market, we must remain vigilant about the ongoing risk for injuries. As emphasized by Strickland et al, these high-powered magnet toys remain in households across America, so we must remain diligent in our efforts to educate the public and health care practitioners about the unsuspected danger of these toys.

M. A. Gilger, MD

References

1. Abbas M, Oliva-Hemker M, Choi J, Lustik M, Gilger M, Noel A. Magnet ingestions in children presenting to US emergency departments, 2002—2011. *J Pediatr Gastroenterol Nutr.* 2013;57:18-22.

2. Silverman J, Brown J, Willis M, Ebel B. Increase in pediatric magnet-related foreign bodies requiring emergency care. *Ann Emerg Med.* 2013;62:604-689.
3. United States Consumer Product Safety Commission. Buckyballs and Buckycubes High-Powered Magnet Sets Recalled Due to Ingestion Hazard. http://www.cpsc.gov/en/Newsroom/News-Releases/2014/Buckyballs-and-Buckycubes-High-Powered-Magnet-Sets-Recalled/. Accessed August 16, 2014.
4. Healthy Canadians. Health Canada orders NeoMagnetic Gadgets Inc. to recall magnet sets. http://healthycanadians.gc.ca/recall-alert-rappel-avis/hc-sc/2013/34263r-eng.php. Accessed August 16, 2014.
5. 33 Charts. Children and Magnets: a Fatal Attraction. http://33charts.com/2012/07/magnets.html. Accessed August 16, 2014.
6. American Academy of Pediatrics. AAP Alerts Pediatricians to Dangers of Magnet Ingestions. http://www.aap.org/en-us/advocacy-and-policy/federal-advocacy/Pages/AAP-Alerts-Pediatricians-to-Dangers-of-Magnet-Ingestions.aspx. Accessed August 16, 2014.

Use of White Blood Cell Count and Negative Appendectomy Rate

Bates MF, Khander A, Steigman SA, et al (Alpert Med School of Brown Univ, Providence, RI)
Pediatrics 133:e39-e44, 2014

Background.—Despite increased utilization of laboratory, radiologic imaging, and scoring systems, negative appendectomy (NA) rates in children remain above 3% nationwide. We reviewed the clinical data of patients undergoing appendectomy to further reduce our NA rate.

Methods.—A retrospective review was conducted of all appendectomies performed for suspected appendicitis at a tertiary children's hospital during a 42-month period. Preoperative clinical, laboratory, and radiographic data were collected. Variables absent or normal in more than half of NAs were further analyzed. Receiver operating characteristic curves were constructed for continuous variables by using appropriate cutoff points to determine sensitivity and false-positive rates. The results were validated by analyzing the 12 months immediately after the establishment of these rules.

Results.—Of 847 appendectomies performed, 22 (2.6%) had a pathologically normal appendix. The only variables found to be normal in more than half of NAs were white blood cell (WBC) count (89%) and neutrophil count (79%). A receiver operating characteristic curve indicates that using WBC cutoffs of 9000 and 8000 per μL yielded sensitivities of 92% and 95%, respectively, and reduction in NA rates by 77% and 36%, respectively. Results observed in the subsequent 12 months confirmed these expected sensitivities and specificities.

Conclusions.—Absence of an elevated WBC count is a risk factor for NA. Withholding appendectomy for WBC counts <9000 and 8000 per μL reduces the NA rate to 0.6% and 1.2%, respectively. Missed true appendicitis in patients with normal WBC counts can be mitigated by a trial of observation in those presenting with early symptom onset.

▶ Acute appendicitis in the pediatric population represents the most common emergent abdominal surgery. Surgeons are often faced with a constellation of symptoms, physical examination findings, laboratory values, and imaging findings from which we base our decision to operate on or observe the patient. Over the past several decades, the diagnostic accuracy in acute appendicitis has improved significantly, providing appropriate decreases in morbidity and mortality. The next reasonable step to further refine the care in appendicitis is try to decrease the rate of negative appendectomy, which remains 3% to 5% nationwide. We now need to focus on specific information obtained in the diagnostic algorithm that may help improve the sensitivity and specificity around the diagnosis of acute appendicitis.

The authors focus on white blood cell count (WBC) as an important value that may help decrease negative appendectomy rates. Their recent experience suggests that withholding appendectomy for those patients with WBC counts <9000 and <8000 per µL reduced negative appendectomy rates to 0.6% and 1.2%, respectively. However by using this cutoff, it also decreases the sensitivity of the WBC count to 92%, leading to a higher false-negative rate or missed appendicitis.

This article is 1 among a series of other studies that have looked into how we may enhance the efficiency of our workup in pediatric appendicitis. However, we must caution clinicians not to rely too heavily on 1 piece of data rather than considering the entire spectrum of the child's presentation, especially key elements of the history and physical exam. Closer evaluations of data elements involved in the diagnosis of pediatric appendicitis must be carefully studied and examined in an effort to improve the care we provide for children who present with abdominal pain. Information from this study and others in the future will hopefully rectify the overuse of potentially damaging computed tomography scans.

R. T. Russell, MD, MPH
M. K. Chen, MD

Effect of Hispanic Ethnicity and Language Barriers on Appendiceal Perforation Rates and Imaging in Children
Levas MN, for the Pediatric Emergency Medicine Collaborative Research Committee of the American Academy of Pediatrics (Med College of Wisconsin, Milwaukee; et al)
J Pediatr 164:1286-1291, 2014

Objective.—To determine the association between Hispanic ethnicity and limited English proficiency (LEP) and the rates of appendiceal perforation and advanced radiologic imaging (computed tomography and ultrasound) in children with abdominal pain.

Study Design.—We performed a secondary analysis of a prospective, cross-sectional, multicenter study of children aged 3-18 years presenting with abdominal pain concerning for appendicitis between March 2009 and April 2010 at 10 tertiary care pediatric emergency departments in the US. Appendiceal perforation and advanced imaging rates were compared between ethnic and language proficiency groups using simple and multivariate regression models.

Results.—Of 2590 patients enrolled, 1001 (38%) had appendicitis, including 36% of non-Hispanics and 44% of Hispanics. In multivariate modeling, Hispanics with LEP had a significantly greater odds of appendiceal perforation (OR, 1.44; 95% CI, 1.20-1.74). Hispanics with LEP with appendiceal perforation of moderate clinical severity were less likely to undergo advanced imaging compared with English-speaking non-Hispanics (OR, 0.64; 95% CI, 0.43-0.95).

Conclusion.—Hispanic ethnicity with LEP is an important risk factor for appendiceal perforation in pediatric patients brought to the emergency department with possible appendicitis. Among patients with moderate clinical severity, Hispanic ethnicity with LEP appears to be associated with lower imaging rates. This effect of English proficiency and Hispanic ethnicity warrants further investigation to understand and overcome barriers, which may lead to increased appendiceal perforation rates and differential diagnostic evaluation.

▶ Even in the age of sophisticated diagnostic technology, communication between patient and physician remains fundamentally important. For patients and families who do not speak English well, this critical component of medical practice is often compromised. More than 25 million people in the United States have limited English proficiency (LEP).[1] LEP patients and children with LEP parents experience disparities in health care quality and patient safety. When LEP patients and families have access to bilingual providers or trained professional interpreters, they have improved health communication, patient satisfaction, and health care outcomes and safer care.[2] However, as the article by Levas et al demonstrates, language barriers still contribute to harm and worse health care outcomes for children in LEP families.

The findings by Levas et al add to the large body of literature demonstrating the adverse effects of language barriers on health care quality and outcomes. Their focus on appendiceal perforation is especially timely and relevant to the current health care delivery policy environment. Current policies and public interest in a more transparent view of health care quality has contributed to using appendiceal perforation as a measure of health care delivery system quality. Appendicitis is the most common surgical emergency in children, and perforation can be avoided with timely diagnosis and treatment. The article by Levas et al references data that perforation rates remain greater than 20%, and disparities exist in perforation rates among minority children and those with public health insurance.

In this study, Levas et al found that 34% of Hispanic children with LEP parents with appendicitis had a perforation compared with 25% of non-Hispanic children whose parents reported English as the primary home language. Although not highlighted in the abstract or paper, there was in impressive difference in rates of appendicitis among children enrolled in the study. Of the Hispanic children with a language barrier in the study, 48% had appendicitis, whereas only 36% of non-Hispanic children without a language barrier had appendicitis—a difference that was statistically significant. This finding demonstrates that children with LEP parents may experience barriers to the timely diagnosis of appendicitis before presentation to the emergency department, reduced access to care due to language, or both.

Pediatric primary care practitioners often perform initial evaluations of children with acute abdominal pain. Prompt recognition in the primary care office of the signs and symptoms of appendicitis could hasten definitive diagnosis and treatment. However, appropriate management of language barriers remains a challenge for pediatricians. A study that compared pediatricians' self-reported use of formal interpreters in 2004 and 2010 found that reports of interpreter use increased only modestly in that time period with 50% of pediatricians reporting that they used interpreters with LEP patients in 2004 and 56% reporting use in 2010.[3] Suboptimal management of language barriers in primary care likely is a contributing factor to the higher rates of appendicitis and appendiceal perforation among children in LEP families found in the Levas et al study.

Reducing health care disparities due to language requires improvement in identification of the language need and use of appropriate language services. Identification of a patients and families who need or want their health care communication to be in a language other than English is more complex than it would seem. In the Levas et al study, they categorized families that stated they spoke a language other than English at home as "LEP." The actual definition of LEP is that of people who speak a language other than English at home and report that they speak English less than "very well," when responding to the question, "How well do you speak English?" The Levas et al study actually identified children in non-English primary language households. Among children in such households, there are some children whose parents may speak English very well and experience no language barriers in health care. The imprecision of the LEP definition in the Levas et al study would have biased their to the null and so does not change the overall message.

The importance of making this distinction, however, lies in the fact that it is one of several terms to consider when attempting to identify patients and families who need language services and that varying definitions make tracking outcomes across studies and health systems difficult. Several entities, notably the Institute of Medicine and the Joint Commission, recommend that health care systems ask patients or caregivers about their preferred health care language. Once health systems standardize the way in which they identify a language need, the next important, but often not straightforward, step is where to document this in the medical record to effectively alert providers across the continuum of care that language services may be needed. Preferred health care language documentation is among the "meaningful use" criteria for demographics documentation to receive federal monies for electronic health record implementation. However, where this is documented is not assessed by "meaningful use." This lack of a consistent location for preferred language documentation in the medical record may result in this information being recorded in a manner that is not useful to providers and that does not result in the desired patient care impact.

Once a language need has been identified, federal mandates based on Title VI of the Civil Rights Acts require health care organizations to provide meaningful access to language services. The current standards are to use a bilingual provider or a trained, professional interpreter to communicate with LEP patients and caregivers. The demand for bilingual providers far exceeds supply, but the supply of providers who speak some Spanish is much greater because it is a common language taught in schools. This has led to the dangerous practice of some clinicians using their limited Spanish skills to "get by" during patient encounters. Patients may also "get by" on their limited English skills. There are numerous examples of medical errors or diagnostic delay when providers or patients "get by."

To ensure providers have sufficient skills for communication in a language other than English, providers' language proficiency should be evaluated. Commercial tests exist for this purpose, although adoption of language proficiency certification for physician providers certainly is not yet universally employed. Similarly, trained professional interpreters are not always used for health care encounters. Staff members who are not trained in interpretation are often asked to provide "ad hoc" interpretation, and patient's family members are commonly used as interpreters. In the study of pediatricians referenced here, use of either of these modalities was reported by at least half of pediatricians. When trained, professional interpreters are not used, there is a greater likelihood of translation errors or incomplete information transfer.[2,4]

The study by Levas et al stated that language services varied according to individual hospital policies. Larger health systems and clinics, those in urban settings, and academic medical centers tend to have a greater supply of interpreters and more robust language services policies.[3,5] This could mean that the disparities identified by Levas et al are not as bad as they could be if smaller, more rural, and nonacademic emergency departments were evaluated. However, because language services use was not standardized in the study, there was likely variation in practice across hospitals and individual patient encounters, making their findings generalizable to many health care systems across the United States.

In summary, Levas et al provide a clear message that children in families who experience language barriers in health care are at risk for worse health care outcomes. This is unacceptable. Although not perfect, there are ways to mitigate the potential negative effects of language barriers and improve health care quality and safety for LEP patients and families. Suboptimal identification of patients with language needs and underutilization of appropriate language services continue due to a lack of funding and often a lack of accountability for lower quality health care or quality-of-care disparities. The burden on health systems for improving overall quality and reducing disparities is increasing. Having current evidence that demonstrates clear quality gaps using a metric that is in use among policy makers is the kind of study that may be most helpful in convincing health system administrators and policy makers that language services in health care need concerted attention and financial support. For pediatricians who work with children in LEP families, these are not new issues, and the findings by Levas et al are not surprising. There is hope, however, that having new data in a more accountable health care policy climate will finally spur meaningful change.

L. R. DeCamp, MD, MSPH

References

1. United States Census Bureau. Selected social characteristics in the United States. 2012 American Community Survey 1-year estimates. http://factfinder2. census.gov/faces/tableservices/jsf/pages/productview.xhtml?pid=ACS_12_1YR_ DP02&prodType=table. Accessed July 18, 2014.
2. Karliner LS, Jacobs EA, Chen AH, Mutha S. Do professional interpreters improve clinical care for patients with limited English proficiency? A systematic review of the literature. *Health Serv Res.* 2007;42:727-754.
3. DeCamp LR, Kuo DZ, Flores G, O'Connor K, Minkovitz CS. Changes in language services use by US Pediatricians. *Pediatrics.* 2013;132:e396-e406.
4. Flores G, Abreu M, Barone CP, Bachur R, Lin H. Errors of medical interpretation and their potential clinical consequences:a comparison of professional versus adhoc versus no Interpreters. *Ann Emerg Med.* 2012;60:545-553.
5. Diamond LC, Wilson-Stronks A, Jacobs EA. Do hospitals measure up to the national culturally and linguistically appropriate services standards? *Med Care.* 2010;48:1080-1087.

8 Genitourinary Tract

Rates of Adverse Events Associated With Male Circumcision in US Medical Settings, 2001 to 2010
El Bcheraoui C, Zhang X, Cooper CS, et al (Ctrs for Disease Control and Prevention, Atlanta, GA; The Univ of Iowa)
JAMA Pediatr 168:625-634, 2014

Importance.—Approximately 1.4 million male circumcisions (MCs) are performed annually in US medical settings. However, population-based estimates of MC-associated adverse events (AEs) are lacking.

Objectives.—To estimate the incidence rate of MC-associated AEs and to assess whether AE rates differed by age at circumcision.

Design.—We selected 41 possible MC AEs based on a literature review and on medical billing codes. We estimated a likely risk window for the incidence calculation for each MC AE based on pathogenesis. We used 2001 to 2010 data from SDI Health, a large administrative claims data set, to conduct a retrospective cohort study.

Setting and Participants.—SDI Health provided administrative claims data from inpatient and outpatient US medical settings.

Main Outcomes and Measures.—For each AE, we calculated the incidence per million MCs. We compared the incidence risk ratio and the incidence rate difference for circumcised vs uncircumcised newborn males and for males circumcised at younger than 1 year, age 1 to 9 years, or 10 years or older. An AE was considered probably related to MC if the incidence risk ratio significantly exceeded 1 at $P < .05$ or occurred only in circumcised males.

Results.—Records were available for 1 400 920 circumcised males, 93.3% as newborns. Of 41 possible MC AEs, 16 (39.0%) were probable. The incidence of total MC AEs was slightly less than 0.5%. Rates of potentially serious MC AEs ranged from 0.76 (95% CI, 0.10-5.43) per million MCs for stricture of male genital organs to 703.23 (95% CI, 659.22-750.18) per million MCs for repair of incomplete circumcision. Compared with boys circumcised at younger than 1 year, the incidences of probable AEs were approximately 20-fold and 10-fold greater for males circumcised at age 1 to 9 years and at 10 years or older, respectively.

Conclusions and Relevance.—Male circumcision had a low incidence of AEs overall, especially if the procedure was performed during the first year of life, but rose 10-fold to 20-fold when performed after infancy.

▶ With the 2012 change in American Academy of Pediatrics (AAP) guidelines regarding circumcision[1] the controversy regarding neonatal circumcision continues to revolve around whether the medical benefits of prevention of sexually transmitted diseases and urinary tract infection outweigh the risks of circumcision. A separate issue of autonomy—namely, if the choice to undergo a circumcision is a medical decision that should be made by parents for their infant son—also remains.

This article is the largest series to date, evaluating 1.4 million boys in the United States who underwent circumcision between 2001 and 2010. Ninety-five percent underwent circumcision as infants, 2% between 1 and 9 years, and 3% at 10 years or older. It found a complication rate of less than 0.5% and a very low rate of devastating injuries, such as amputation, in 4 of 1 million cases. Urethral strictures were not increased in the circumcision group. Bleeding occurred in 1% of patients, and subsequent revisions for excess foreskin and adhesions occurred in 2% of patients. These findings are in line with complication rates found in smaller studies.

The large size of the study allowed the authors to break down the complications by age groups. They found that complications occurred in 0.4% of the infants, 9% of the 1- to 9-year-olds, and 5% of those aged 10 years and older. The 1- to 9-year-old boys required more division of penile adhesions and skin bridges. The boys aged 10 and older had more inflammation after surgery and unfortunately were at highest risk for penile amputation. These findings are understandable because the penis does not lengthen significantly between ages 2 and 9 even though boys are growing in weight, which predisposes the shaft skin to stick to the glans after the circumcision. As boys approach puberty, the increased blood flow to the shaft skin results in more postoperative edema and inflammation. There is room for improvement in preventing these complications if parents are given postoperative instructions to retract the foreskin to prevent adhesions and skin bridges, along with judicious use of nonsteroidal anti-inflammatory drugs.

As with all administrative database papers, the lack of clinical detail in the data makes some findings difficult to interpret. For example, the authors surmise that the 4 penile amputations in uncircumcised boys may have been miscoded, had a circumcision in a nonmedical setting, or were complications of surgery for rare urologic conditions such as exstrophy. Because the overall complication rate is similar to previous studies, this data appear to be generalizable to the US population.

What we can draw from this article is that circumcision in the United States is safe, and if parents are considering circumcision for their son, it is best performed during the newborn period. The problem with disseminating this information is that parents usually make up their mind about circumcision before speaking to the pediatrician taking care of the newborn boy. As reviewed in the AAP policy statement, 80% of parents have decided whether their son will be circumcised before speaking to any medical professional. Reasons for deciding for circumcision included hygiene in 50%, having the boy appear similar to his father or brothers in 25%, and religious reasons in 12%. Obstetricians and family practitioners will likely have a larger impact on informing parents of the risks and benefits of circumcision than pediatricians. Although this paper does not address the concerns of those who oppose neonatal circumcision

on grounds of autonomy, it does provide us solid evidence on the safety of circumcision as practiced in medical settings in the United States.

H.-Y. Wu, MD

Reference

1. American Academy of Pediatrics Task Force on Circumcision. Male Circumcision. *Pediatrics.* 2012;130:e756-e785.

Discovery of Hypospadias during Newborn Circumcision Should Not Preclude Completion of the Procedure

Chalmers D, Wiedel CA, Siparsky GL, et al (Children's Hosp Colorado, Aurora; Univ of Colorado School of Medicine, Aurora)
J Pediatr 164:1171-1174, 2014

Objective.—To test the hypothesis that completion of newborn circumcision does not complicate hypospadias repair, and that circumcision will
minimize future operations.

Study Design.—Children referred for distal hypospadias over a 5-year
period were grouped by presentation. Children with an aborted circumcision owing to concerns for hypospadias were subdivided into patients who
underwent hypospadias repair (group 1a) and those who underwent circumcision (group 1b). Group 2 consisted of patients with a completed

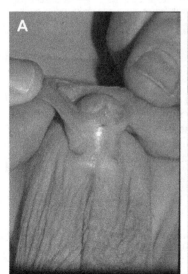
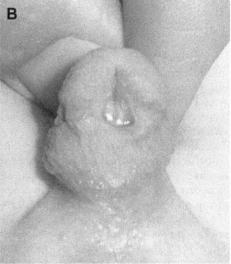

FIGURE 1.—A, Distal hypospadias with incomplete prepuce/dorsal hood. B, Megameatus appearance after circumcision of the intact prepuce. (Photo courtesy of Lawrence Baskin.) (Reprinted from Chalmers D, Wiedel CA, Siparsky GL, et al. Discovery of hypospadias during newborn circumcision should not pre- clude completion of the procedure. *J Pediatr.* 2014;164:1171-1174, with permission from Elsevier.)

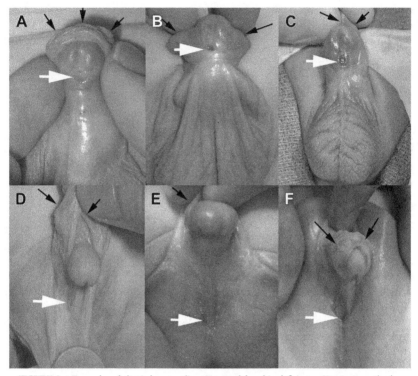

FIGURE 2.—Examples of classic hypospadias: 1) ventral foreskin deficiency. 2) ectopic urethral meatus and 3) penile curvature. A-C. Distal shaft hypospadias with failure of ventral foreskin fusion resulting in a dorsal hooded prepuce. D-F. Severe hypospadias with foreskin abnormalities and associated penile curvature. (Black arrows denote abnormal dorsal hooded foreskin, white arrows ectopic urethral meatus.)

circumcision who underwent hypospadias repair. Children with traditionally recognized distal hypospadias served as controls.

Results.—A total of 93 newborns had an aborted newborn circumcision. Of these, 28 underwent hypospadias repair (group 1a), and 47 underwent circumcision completion under general anesthesia (group 1b). The remaining 18 either deferred surgery or underwent in-office circumcision. Ten patients with hypospadias and an intact prepuce had a completed circumcision and subsequently underwent repair (group 2). The control group comprised 151 patients. No patients with a completed circumcision experienced complications after hypospadias repair, whereas the control group had a 5.3% rate of complications.

Conclusion.—Performing circumcision in newborns with hypospadias and an intact prepuce did not affect repair or the risk of complications. These findings, along with previous results, demonstrate that newborn circumcision can be safely completed in children with an intact prepuce. Furthermore, aborting a newborn circumcision after dorsal slit will expose a

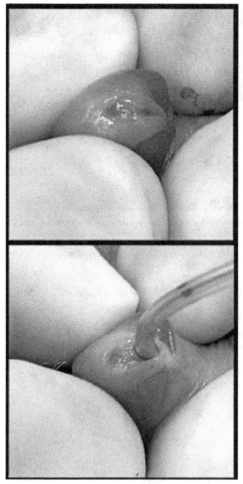

FIGURE 3.—Example of "concealed hypospadias" with mild urethral abnormality (with feeding tube) and dorsally located blind urethra pit.

substantial number of children to additional procedures under general anesthesia.

▶ Classic teaching is that all patients with hypospadias should not undergo neonatal circumcision secondary to the possible need for the foreskin for future reconstruction. This point is certainly true for patients who have "classic hypospadias," which is characterized by 3 features: (1) the ventral foreskin not fusing in the midline and the majority of the foreskin remaining on the dorsal aspect of the penis; (2) abnormal urethral meatus location and associated abortive urethra spongiosum located in an ectopic position on the penis such as the proximal glans, coronal margin, anywhere along the shaft of the penis,

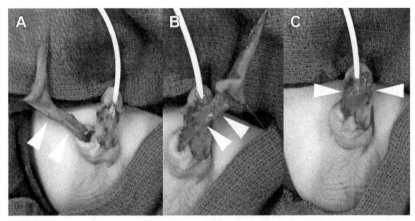

FIGURE 4.—De-epithelized foreskin flap to cover the reconstructed urethra in classic hypospadias repair thereby reducing the incidence of fistula formation. A. Vascularized foreskin flap based on the blood supply of the prepuce dissected free. B. Flap placed on top of reconstructed urethra. C. Foreskin removed from flap (de-epithelized) and sutured on top of reconstructed urethra (white arrowheads denote flap).

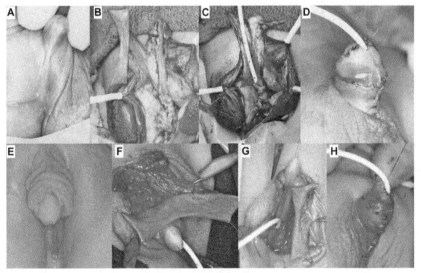

FIGURE 5.—Foreskin vascularized pedicle flap used for urethral reconstruction in classic hypospadias. Preoperative photographs of severe classic hypospadias A, E. Corresponding operative photographs of the prepared foreskin flap (onlay island flap) and urethral reconstruction B, C and F, G. Panels D and H show the completed repair.

scrotum, or perineum; and (3) penile curvature, most often associated with severe forms of hypospadias (Fig 2).

In contrast, a small subset of patients has a variant of hypospadias (concealed hypospadias) that is not apparent until the time of circumcision. In these patients, the foreskin is not abnormal and the glans and urethral meatus is only visualized after taking down the physiologic adhesions between the inner foreskin and the glans at the time of neonatal circumcision (Fig 1B in Chalmers et al and Fig 3).

Chalmers et al are to be commended for emphasizing this important fact concerning "concealed hypospadias" and bringing this issue to our attention in their retrospective review of 93 newborns, who had an aborted newborn circumcision secondary to the possibility of hypospadias. What Chalmers et al have clearly shown is that hypospadias with an intact prepuce can be repaired successfully without the need for the foreskin (secondary deepithelized foreskin flap).

Why is this the case, and should this change our management when concealed hypospadias is revealed at the time of circumcision? In classic hypospadias (Fig 2), the aborted foreskin is typically used as a secondary layer to cover the reconstructed urethra with a vascularized pedicle flap of deepithelized subcutaneous tissue based on the foreskin arteries (Fig 4). This flap allows a barrier between the reconstructed urethra and the reconstructed skin, providing essentially a watertight seal, which has been shown to reduce the incidents of postoperative fistula formation. In more severe hypospadias, the skin of the abnormal prepuce on its vascular pedicle can be used itself to reconstruct the urethra (Fig 5).

These two reconstructive scenarios are not germane for concealed hypospadias, in which the foreskin is circumferential and the urethral abnormality is located on the glans. In this case, reconstruction, if deemed necessary, focuses on reconstructing a normal glans along with a smaller urethroplasty. There is simply little room within the glans to place an extra layer of tissue (secondary deepithelized foreskin flap) over the reconstructed urethra and, as noted by Chalmers et al, this tissue is not necessary for a successful repair.

In concealed hypospadias and, for that matter, mild classic hypospadias, often parental concerns are focused on removing the excess foreskin with little concern about the glandular urethra. When the urethra is abnormal, it may be quite mild, requiring essentially connecting the normal urethra with a blind ending urethral pit (Fig 3). One variant found in "concealed hypospadias" is the so-called megameatus intact prepuce (Fig 1B in Chalmers et al). In this case, the glandular urethra is quite wide and, as documented by Chalmers et al, can be successfully repaired without the need for excess tissue from the foreskin.

Therefore, the classic dogma that circumcision should not be completed if "concealed hypospadias" is discovered should no longer be taught. What should be emphasized, however, is that if indeed the patient has classic hypospadias upon examination, as pointed out by the authors, neonatal circumcision should not be attempted because the classic Plastibell or Gomco techniques are not amenable when there is an asymmetric or abnormally formed foreskin secondary to a higher risk of possible urethral or glandular injury. In contrast, when the foreskin is normally formed, if hypospadias is noted after beginning the circumcision, there appears to be no reason why the circumcision cannot be completed. In fact, many of these patients will require no further surgery as pointed out in the study because the residual defect may be minor and not in need of formal repair. Chalmers and colleagues are to be commended for an outstanding study concerning circumcision in concealed hypospadias where previous dogma was incorrect.

L. S. Baskin, MD

Antimicrobial Prophylaxis for Children with Vesicoureteral Reflux

The RIVUR Trial Investigators (Univ of Pittsburgh Med Ctr, PA; Women and Children's Hosp of Buffalo, NY; Wayne State Univ School of Medicine, Detroit; et al)
N Engl J Med 370:2367-2376, 2014

Background.—Children with febrile urinary tract infection commonly have vesicoureteral reflux. Because trial results have been limited and inconsistent, the use of antimicrobial prophylaxis to prevent recurrences in children with reflux remains controversial.

Methods.—In this 2-year, multisite, randomized, placebo-controlled trial involving 607 children with vesicoureteral reflux that was diagnosed after a first or second febrile or symptomatic urinary tract infection, we evaluated the efficacy of trimethoprim–sulfamethoxazole prophylaxis in preventing recurrences (primary outcome). Secondary outcomes were renal scarring, treatment failure (a composite of recurrences and scarring), and antimicrobial resistance.

Results.—Recurrent urinary tract infection developed in 39 of 302 children who received prophylaxis as compared with 72 of 305 children who received placebo (relative risk, 0.55; 95% confidence interval [CI], 0.38 to 0.78). Prophylaxis reduced the risk of recurrences by 50% (hazard ratio, 0.50; 95% CI, 0.34 to 0.74) and was particularly effective in children whose index infection was febrile (hazard ratio, 0.41; 95% CI, 0.26 to 0.64) and in those with baseline bladder and bowel dysfunction (hazard ratio, 0.21; 95% CI, 0.08 to 0.58). The occurrence of renal scarring did not differ significantly between the prophylaxis and placebo groups (11.9% and 10.2%, respectively). Among 87 children with a first recurrence caused by Escherichia coli, the proportion of isolates that were resistant to trimethoprim–sulfamethoxazole was 63% in the prophylaxis group and 19% in the placebo group.

Conclusions.—Among children with vesicoureteral reflux after urinary tract infection, antimicrobial prophylaxis was associated with a substantially reduced risk of recurrence but not of renal scarring. (Funded by the National Institute of Diabetes and Digestive and Kidney Diseases and others; RIVUR ClinicalTrials.gov number, NCT00405704.) (Fig 2, Table 2)

▶ Over the past few decades in the pediatric urinary tract infection (UTI) literature, the prophylactic antibiotics pendulum has swung back and forth with vigor. Although the use of daily antibiotics for children with vesicoureteral reflux (VUR) was recommended by the American Academy of Pediatrics (AAP) in the 1999 UTI practice parameter,[1] a series of subsequent trials suggested that

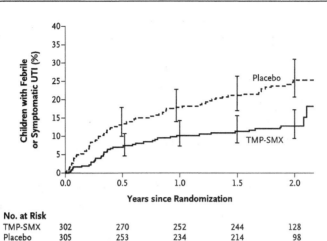

FIGURE 2.—Time to first recurrent febrile or symptomatic UTI. Shown are Kaplan–Meier estimates of the cumulative percentage of children who had a recurrent febrile or symptomatic UTI according to study group. Fewer children assigned to TMP-SMX prophylaxis had a UTI than children assigned to placebo (*P* < 0.001 by log-rank test). I bars indicate 95% confidence intervals. (Reprinted from The RIVUR Trial Investigators. Antimicrobial prophylaxis for children with vesicoureteral reflux. *N Engl J Med.* 2014;370:2367-2376, with permission from Massachusetts Medical Society.)

prophylactic antibiotics were not only ineffective in preventing recurrent UTI but also led to resistant organisms.[2-5] However, these trials were criticized for being underpowered and having insufficient blinding.[6]

In 2009, a well-designed trial (PRIVENT) involving 576 children with a first-time UTI demonstrated that daily trimethoprim-sulfamethoxazole (TMP-SMX) for 1 year did in fact reduce recurrence risk, with a number-needed-to-treat (NNT) of approximately 14.[7] However, this reduced UTI risk was not accompanied by a reduction in renal scarring on dimercaptosuccinic acid (DMSA) scanning at 1 year. In short, 14 children needed to be treated daily for 1 year to prevent 1 child from needing antibiotics for ~1 week, a trade-off that did not appear to support the routine use of prophylactic antibiotics.[8]

But uncertainty lingered. The PRIVENT trial included children with and without VUR, and only a fraction of the children actually underwent the 1-year DMSA scan. Perhaps an impact on scarring would be detectable if a larger group of children with VUR was studied. With this possibility in mind, many eagerly awaited publication of the Randomized Intervention for VUR (RIVUR) study. In this well-designed study, children with VUR were randomized to daily TMP-SMX versus placebo for 2 years and underwent a DMSA scan at the end of the study period.[9]

The primary outcome in the RIVUR study, recurrent UTI within 2 years, was less common in the daily antibiotic arm (15% vs 27%, relative risk 0.54, 95% confidence interval 0.38—0.77) (Fig 2).[9] The NNT was 8, less than that found in PRIVENT because the study period was twice as long. In fact, the number of doses of antibiotics needed to prevent 1 recurrent UTI was actually higher in RIVUR (5840 doses) than it was in PRIVENT (5110 doses). In both

TABLE 2.—Clinical Outcomes According to Study Group

| Outcome | Trimethoprim−Sulfamethoxazole | Placebo | Absolute Difference in Risk (95% CI) |
	no. of children/total no. (%)		percentage points
Recurrent febrile or symptomatic UTI*			
Children with missing 2-yr data classified as having had an event (intention-to-treat analysis)	77/302 (25.5)	114/305 (37.4)[†]	11.9 (4.6 to 19.2)
Children with missing 2-yr data classified as not having had an event (intention-to-treat analysis)[‡]	39/302 (12.8)	72/305 (25.4)[§]	12.6 (6.1 to 19.0)
Children with missing 2-yr data omitted	39/264 (14.8)	72/263 (27.4)[§]	12.6 (5.7 to 19.5)
Treatment failure[‡¶]	14/302 (5.0)	27/305 (9.6)[‖]	4.5 (0.2 to 8.8)
Renal scarring**			
Overall	27/227 (11.9)	24/235 (10.2)	−1.7 (−7.4 to 4.0)
Severe[††]	9/227 (4.0)	6/235 (2.6)	−1.4 (−4.7 to 1.8)
New[‡‡]	18/220 (8.2)	19/227 (8.4)	0.2 (−4.9 to 5.3)
Any cortical defect	29/227 (12.8)	25/235 (10.6)	−2.1 (−8.0 to 3.7)
Antimicrobial resistance			
Resistant *Escherichia coli* in stool	56/203 (27.6)	41/210 (19.5)	−8.1 (−16.2 to 0.1)
First recurrent febrile or symptomatic UTI with resistant *E. coli*	19/30 (63.3)[§§]	11/57 (19.3)	−44.0 (−64.1 to −24.0)
First recurrent febrile or symptomatic UTI with any resistant pathogen	26/38 (68.4)[§§]	17/69 (24.6)	−43.8 (−61.7 to −25.8)

*Included are 7 children (3 in the trimethoprim−sulfamethoxazole group and 4 in the placebo group) with febrile or symptomatic UTIs that occurred before a missed 2-year visit. Imputation was applied to 38 children in the trimethoprim−sulfamethoxazole group and 42 children in the placebo group.

[†]$P = 0.002$ by log-rank test stratified according to five core sites.

[‡]Percentages are based on Kaplan−Meier 2-year estimates.

[§]$P < 0.001$ by the log-rank test stratified according to five core sites.

[¶]Treatment failure was defined as the occurrence of two febrile UTIs (28 children), one febrile UTI and three symptomatic UTIs (2 children), four symptomatic UTIs (2 children), or new or worsening renal scarring (9 children).

[‖]$P = 0.04$ by the log-rank test stratified according to five core sites.

**Renal scarring was defined as a decreased uptake of tracer that was associated with loss of contours or the presence of cortical thinning.

[††]Severe renal scarring was defined as scarring in more than 4 of 12 segments in at least one kidney or global atrophy characterized by a diffusely scarred and shrunken kidney.

[‡‡]New renal scarring was defined as scarring on the outcome renal scan with technetium-99m−labeled dimercaptosuccinic acid that was not present at baseline.

[§§]$P < 0.001$ by the Cochran−Mantel−Haenszel test stratified according to five core sites.

Reprinted from The RIVUR Trial Investigators. Antimicrobial prophylaxis for children with vesicoureteral reflux. N Engl J Med. 2014;370:2367-2376, with permission from Massachusetts Medical Society.

studies, prophylactic antibiotics increased the risk of resistant organisms (Table 2).

Is it worth giving > 5000 doses of antibiotics to prevent 1 UTI, even if this comes at the expense of increased antibiotic resistance? Perhaps yes, if other complications associated with recurrent UTI, such as renal scarring, are prevented. However, despite the reduction in recurrent UTI risk in the treatment arm, there was no difference in scarring rates between groups in the RIVUR study (12% in prophylaxis group vs 10% in placebo group, $P = .55$). The authors suggest that the lack of impact on scarring (and the overall low rate of scarring) might be explained by the fact that "parents, who were instructed to be vigilant, sought early medical attention."[9] However, this explanation belies findings from multiple prior investigations,[10-14] including a study performed by the RIVUR study's lead author,[14] where the duration of symptoms before UTI presentation was not associated with the risk of scarring.

How will the RIVUR results affect our management of children with a UTI? The lack of impact of prophylactic antibiotics on renal scarring in children with VUR, despite the reduction in UTI risk, brings up several pivotal questions. One, what is the true nature of the association between UTI, scarring and, ultimately, chronic kidney disease in children with VUR? The causal pathway for this association is poorly understood,[15] and the RIVUR results suggest that the risk of chronic kidney disease is unlikely to be affected by UTI prevention. Second, do the RIVUR results support aggressively pursuing the diagnosis of VUR? The authors suggest that yes, they do, and that the 2011 AAP UTI guidelines recommendation to defer routine voiding cystourethrogram (VCUG) on children with a first febrile UTI[16] should be reconsidered.[9]

If prophylactic antibiotics prevent recurrent UTIs in children with VUR, then it must be important to perform routine VCUGs to find those children who will benefit, right? Wrong. There is simply no evidence that the presence of VUR in any way affects the efficacy of prophylactic antibiotics. More antibiotic doses were needed to prevent a UTI in the RIVUR trial, where all children had VUR, than in the PRIVENT trial, where only 43% of the children were known to have VUR. Furthermore, there was no difference in the efficacy of prophylactic antibiotics in children with and without VUR in PRIVENT. Therefore, the benefit of diagnosing VUR is even less clear now than it was before. Furthermore, especially given that approximately 24 VCUGs need to be done to identify 1 child with VUR who would benefit from prophylactic antibiotics (assuming NNT of 8 and prevalence of VUR in children with UTI of ~33%),[16] there is clearly a cost, both financial and medical.[17]

Of course one could also skip the VCUG and put every child with a first-time UTI on prophylactic antibiotics. However, at a cost of more than 5000 doses of antibiotics to prevent 1 UTI, increased antibiotic resistance, and the potential for rare but serious adverse effects such as Stevens-Johnson syndrome that may not be detectable in trials of this size, it is way too high a price to pay.

A. R. Schroeder, MD

T. B. Newman, MD, MPH

References

1. American Academy of Pediatrics, Steering Committee on Quality Improvement and Management, Roberts KB. Urinary tract infection: clinical practice guideline for the diagnosis and management of the initial UTI in febrile infants and children 2 to 24 months. *Pediatrics.* 2011;128:595-610.
2. Garin EH, Olavarria F, Garcia Nieto V, Valenciano B, Campos A, Young L. Clinical significance of primary vesicoureteral reflux and urinary antibiotic prophylaxis after acute pyelonephritis: a multicenter, randomized, controlled study. *Pediatrics.* 2006;117:626-632.
3. Montini G, Rigon L, Zucchetta P, et al. Prophylaxis after first febrile urinary tract infection in children? A multicenter, randomized, controlled, noninferiority trial. *Pediatrics.* 2008;122:1064-1071.

4. Pennesi M, Travan L, Peratoner L, et al. Is antibiotic prophylaxis in children with vesicoureteral reflux effective in preventing pyelonephritis and renal scars? A randomized, controlled trial. *Pediatrics.* 2008;121:e1489-e1494.

5. Roussey-Kesler G, Gadjos V, Idres N, et al. Antibiotic prophylaxis for the prevention of recurrent urinary tract infection in children with low grade vesicoureteral reflux: results from a prospective randomized study. *J Urol.* 2008;179:674-679.

6. Hoberman A, Keren R. Antimicrobial prophylaxis for urinary tract infection in children. *N Engl J Med.* 2009;361:1804-1806.

7. Craig JC, Simpson JM, Williams GJ, et al. Antibiotic prophylaxis and recurrent urinary tract infection in children. *N Engl J Med.* 2009;361:1748-1759.

8. Newman TB. The new American Academy of Pediatrics urinary tract infection guideline. *Pediatrics.* 2011;128(3):572-575.

9. Antimicrobial prophylaxis for children with vesicoureteral reflux. *N Engl J Med.* 2014.

10. Benador D, Neuhaus TJ, Papazyan JP, et al. Randomised controlled trial of three day versus 10 day intravenous antibiotics in acute pyelonephritis: effect on renal scarring. *Arch Dis Child.* 2001;84:241-246.

11. Doganis D, Siafas K, Mavrikou M, et al. Does early treatment of urinary tract infection prevent renal damage? *Pediatrics.* 2007;120:e922-e928.

12. Fernandez-Menendez JM, Malaga S, Matesanz JL, Solís G, Alonso S, Pérez-Méndez C. Risk factors in the development of early technetium-99m dimercaptosuccinic acid renal scintigraphy lesions during first urinary tract infection in children. *Acta Paediatr.* 2003;92:21-26.

13. Hewitt IK, Zucchetta P, Rigon L, et al. Early treatment of acute pyelonephritis in children fails to reduce renal scarring: data from the Italian Renal Infection Study Trials. *Pediatrics.* 2008;122:486-490.

14. Hoberman A, Wald ER, Hickey RW, et al. Oral versus initial intravenous therapy for urinary tract infections in young febrile children. *Pediatrics.* 1999;104:79-86.

15. Craig JC, Williams GJ. Denominators do matter: it's a myth—urinary tract infection does not cause chronic kidney disease. *Pediatrics.* 2011;128:984-985.

16. Roberts KB. Urinary tract infection: clinical practice guideline for the diagnosis and management of the initial UTI in febrile infants and children 2 to 24 months. *Pediatrics.* 2011;128:595-610.

17. Schroeder AR, Abidari JM, Kirpekar R, et al. Impact of a more restrictive approach to urinary tract imaging after febrile urinary tract infection. *Arch Pediatr Adolesc Med.* 2011;165:1027-1032.

Continuous renal replacement therapy in neonates and small infants: development and first-in-human use of a miniaturised machine (CARPEDIEM)

Ronco C, Garzotto F, Brendolan A, et al (San Bortolo Hosp, Vicenza, Italy; et al)
Lancet 383:1807-1813, 2014

Background.—Peritoneal dialysis is the renal replacement therapy of choice for acute kidney injury in neonates, but in some cases is not feasible or effective. Continuous renal replacement therapy (CRRT) machines are used off label in infants smaller than 15 kg and are not designed specifically for small infants. We aimed to design and create a CRRT machine specifically for neonates and small infants.

Methods.—We prospectively planned a 5-year project to conceive, design, and create a miniaturised Cardio-Renal Pediatric Dialysis Emergency Machine (CARPEDIEM), specifically for neonates and small infants. We created the new device and assessed it with in-vitro laboratory tests, completed its development to meet regulatory requirements, and obtained a licence for human use. Once approved, we used the machine to treat a critically ill neonate.

Findings.—The main characteristics of CARPEDIEM are the low priming volume of the circuit (less than 30 mL), miniaturised roller pumps, and accurate ultrafiltration control via calibrated scales with a precision of 1 g. In-vitro tests confirmed that both hardware and software met the specifications. We treated a 2·9 kg neonate with haemorrhagic shock, multiple organ dysfunction, and severe fluid overload for more than 400 h with the CARPEDIEM, using continuous venovenous haemofiltration, single-pass albumin dialysis, blood exchange, and plasma exchange. The patient's 65% fluid overload, raised creatinine and bilirubin concentrations, and severe acidosis were all managed safely and effectively. Despite the severity of the illness, organ function was restored and the neonate survived and was discharged from hospital with only mild renal insufficiency that did not require renal replacement therapy.

Interpretation.—The CARPEDIEM CRRT machine can be used to provide various treatment modalities and support for multiple organ dysfunction in neonates and small infants. The CARPEDIEM could reduce the range of indications for peritoneal dialysis, widen the range of indications for CRRT, make the use of CRRT less traumatic, and expand its use as supportive therapy even when complete renal replacement therapy is not indicated.

▶ The recent article by Ronco and colleagues identifies a major breakthrough in the use of renal replacement therapy (RRT) in infants. Throughout the world, peritoneal dialysis (PD) is the mainstay for RRT in the neonatal and infantpopulation.[1] Within the United States, no continuous RRT machine is approved for use in infants. In fact, the smallest extracorporeal circuit in United States is roughly about 90 mL, which for a 3-kg child would still represent roughly 30% of extracorporeal blood.

Ronco and colleagues have manufactured and reported the use of a new machine called Cardio-Renal Pediatric Dialysis Emergency Machine (CARPE-DIEM), which is a 27-mL extracorporeal circuit for use in RRT in infants. This is a new device that is yet to be tested in the United States. It has been used as a single case reported as described in this article, yet this device has been used in other infants throughout Europe.

The advantage of this device is that it is a small extracorporeal circuit, and it is easy to use. The disadvantage of this device is similar to that of all areas of continuous RRT: it requires vascular access as well as specialized dialysate or replacement solutions. Additionally, intensive training of neonatal intensive care unit nursing staff is needed for maintenance of this machinery during treatments.

This case study also points out other issues related to acute kidney injury (AKI) in infants. The case described here was markedly volume-overloaded and infected infant who had gone from a baseline weight of 2.7 kg to 5.5 kg before initiation RRT. Therefore, attention to fluid management is paramount in terms of care of such infants before the need for RRT.[2]

Over the past 15 years, work by our group as well as others has identified non-RRT techniques for AKI in infants.[3] These also need to be discussed as part of an armamentarium, as an alternative treatment of these highly difficult-to-treat infants.

The hope is that this new device will have a significant impact on the survival ability of children requiring RRT in this population. Like all devices, CARPE-DIEM will be adapted and improved on with time to be able to fulfill varying needs. This device also requires more work by industry biomedical engineers as well as by clinicians in medical systems to improve issues related to vascular access, solutions, and anticoagulation techniques for children in need of renal replacement therapy.

This device should not be seen as panacea for improvement of AKI therapy but as a significant breakthrough of materialization of RRT in these small and high-risk children.

T. E. Bunchman, MD

References

1. Bonilla-Félix M. Peritoneal dialysis in the pediatric intensive care unit setting: techniques, quantitations and outcomes. *Blood Purif.* 2013;35:77-80.
2. Golstein SL, Somers MJ, Baum MA, et al. Pediatric patients with multi-organ dysfunction syndrome receiving continuous renal replacement therapy. *Kidney Int.* 2005;67:653-658.
3. Hobbs DJ, Steinke JM, Chung JY, et al. Rasburicase improves hyperuricemia in infants with acute kidney injury. *Pediatr Nephrol.* 2010;25:305-309.

9   Heart and Blood Vessels

Echocardiography Screening of Siblings of Children With Bicuspid Aortic Valve
Hales AR, Mahle WT (Emory Univ School of Medicine, Atlanta, GA)
Pediatrics 133:e1212-e1217, 2014

Background and Objective.—Left heart defects, such as bicuspid aortic valve (BAV), are heritable. Consensus guidelines have recommended echocardiographic screening of first-degree relatives. The utility of this approach in siblings of children with BAV is not known. The objective of this study is to evaluate the yield of routine screening of siblings of children with BAV and undertake an economic analysis of this practice.

Methods.—Siblings of children with BAV who underwent echocardiographic screening in a single pediatric cardiology practice were identified. The anatomic features and hemodynamics of siblings newly diagnosed with BAV were recorded. A Markov model was constructed to determine cost-effectiveness ratios, and sensitivity analyses were performed.

Results.—There were 207 screened siblings of 181 children with BAV. The median age at screening was 7 years. BAV was identified in 21 (10.1%) of siblings screened. The median peak Doppler gradient was 18 mm Hg. Aortic insufficiency was mild or less in all. The mean cost to diagnose BAV in a sibling was $2109 per new case found. The estimated mean cost to avert a single aortic dissection in the third or fourth decade of life was $363 911. The estimated cost per life-year saved was $74 884 and ranged from $17 461 to $1 136 536 in sensitivity analysis.

Conclusions.—Echo screening among siblings of those with BAV is effective and inexpensive and may lower the risk of the complications of such as dissection, although it comes at a moderate cost relative to benefits gained. Screening of siblings should be incorporated into clinical care.

▶ This article is an excellent addition to the growing literature on the incidence and risk of bicuspid aortic valve (BAV). Specifically this article highlights that routine echocardiographic screening of siblings of children of BAV is an accurate and cost-effective means of diagnosing BAV and aortopathies. The article includes a good summary of the current state of knowledge about the overall incidence of BAV and the reasons behind current consensus guidelines recommending screening of first-degree relatives. In addition, this article is the first to assess the cost-effectiveness of screening echocardiography.

The authors demonstrate that echocardiographic screening meets the criteria of an effective screening program in that BAV and aortic dissection is a significant health problem, there is a benefit from early detection, the screening test is accurate, safe, widely available, and cost-effective, as well as the fact that early diagnosis makes a difference in outcomes including potentially decreasing catastrophic events such as aortic dissection. The 10% incidence of BAV in siblings is consistent with previously published data and highlights the high heritability of this lesion.

A unique and valuable contribution of this study is the cost analysis (Fig 1 in the original article). Based on my experience, I feel the authors were conservative in their assumptions on the accuracy of echocardiography to correctly diagnose BAV as well as in their estimates of the dissection rate per 1000 patient years. I feel that the accuracy rate of the echocardiography is greater than 80% and that emerging data from the Genetically Triggered Thoracic Aortic Aneurysms and Cardiovascular Conditions (GenTAC) registry and other adult registries show a higher risk of dissection. These will make screening echocardiography an even more cost-effective tool.

In addition to the societal/economic cost of the screening program, there is, of course, an unquantifiable but extremely important individual benefit of preventing an acute dissection and/or sudden death. A limitation of this study is that not all siblings of the patients were screened, which raises concerns for a selection bias. Another limitation is that the racial breakdown of the patients screened was not discussed, because there are different dissection rates and response to treatment by race.[1]

The risk of ascending aorta dissection or development of aortic valve regurgitation discussed in this article highlight the need for excellent transitions in care from pediatricians to adult caregivers. Screening programs will increase the diagnosis of BAV in childhood; however, the greatest time of risk is during adulthood. Aortic dissection and other aortic disease are the second most common cause of cardiovascular death after coronary artery disease. Aortic dissection has become such a risk that the National Heart, Lung, and Blood Institute is now sponsoring GenTAC, a multisite registry of patients with dilated aortas, dissections, BAVs, and other aortic disease.[2] An extension of this article is how important it is for the primary care givers as well as cardiologists to ensure that their patients and families know the need for continued follow-up during adulthood. Another important point for all caregivers is that the number of siblings screened was below what would be expected. It becomes important for the primary caregiver to follow-up with the family and stress the importance of ensuring that all the siblings are evaluated.

I recommend a close reading of this article because there are a number of additional important points enclosed as well. The article summarizes that overall incidence of BAV (at least 1%–2%) is as high as traditional teaching for all congenital heart disease and then add to this figure the marked, 5- to 10-fold increase risk in siblings. The inability to reliably screen patients by physical examination with only 50% being heard in routine clinical practice and 67% with an experienced pediatric cardiologist shows the need for referral and echocardiography regardless of physical exam findings. Although it is not necessary to memorize all of these num-bers, it is critical for everyone who takes care of children to know about the impor-tance of screening echocardiograms for siblings of patients with BAV and, in the affected patients, the need for long-term care.

W. J. Ravekes, MD

References

1. Bossone E, Pyeritz RE, O'Gara P, et al. Acute aortic dissection in blacks: insights from the International Registry of Acute Aortic Dissection. *Am J Med.* 2013;126: 909-915.
2. Eagle KA, LaMarie SA, Volguina I, et al. Rationale and design of the National Registry of Genetically Triggered Thoracic Aortic Aneurysms and Cardiovascular Conditions (GenTAC). *Am Heart J.* 2009;157:319-326.

Natural History of Wolff-Parkinson-White Syndrome Diagnosed in Childhood
Cain N, Irving C, Webber S, et al (Med Univ of South Carolina, Charleston; Freeman Hosp, Newcastle-upon-Tyne, UK; Vanderbilt Univ, Nashville, TN)
Am J Cardiol 112:961-965, 2013

Wolff-Parkinson-White (WPW) syndrome carries a risk for symptomatic arrhythmias and sudden death. The aim of this study was to examine the natural history of patients with Wolff-Parkinson-White syndrome diag-nosed in childhood followed longitudinally at a single institution. The study population consisted of 446 patients. The median age of diagnosis was 7 years, and 61% were male. Associated heart disease was present in 40 patients (9%). Modes of presentation included supraventricular tachycardia (38%), palpitations (22%), chest pain (5%), syncope (4%), atrial fibrillation (0.4%), sudden death (0.2%), and incidental findings (26%); data were unavailable in 4%. During the study period, a total of 243 patients (54%) had supraventricular tachycardia, and 7 patients (1.6%) had atrial fibrillation. Of patients who presented at ≤3 months of age, 35% had resolution of manifest preexcitation compared with 5.8% who presented at >3 months of age ($p < 0.0001$). There were 6 sud-den deaths (1.3%), with an incidence of 2.8 per 1,000 patient-years. Two of these patients had structurally normal hearts (incidence 1.1 per 1,000 patient-years). Four of these patients had associated heart disease (inci-dence 27 per 1,000 patient-years) ($p < 0.01$). In conclusion, in a large pop-ulation of patients with Wolff-Parkinson-White syndrome diagnosed in childhood, 64% had symptoms at presentation, and an additional 20% developed symptoms during follow-up. There were 6 sudden deaths (1.3%), with an overall incidence of 1.1 per 1,000 patient-years in patients with structurally normal hearts and 27 per 1,000 patient-years in patients with associated heart disease.

▶ Of all the monsters that hide under the bed in pediatric medicine, the fear of having a child die suddenly and unexpectedly from an undiagnosed cardiac condition is certainly one of the scariest. It has long been recognized that Wolff-Parkinson-White (WPW) syndrome (commonly known as WPW) is one of the handful of cardiac diseases that has the rare but nonetheless real potential to result in this catastrophic outcome. Recent changes in practice have underlined the importance of having accurate and modern data on the frequency with which dangerous arrhythmia occurs in patients who have ventricular preexcitation on electrocardiogram, the cardinal sign of WPW.

The first change is the now widespread use of the electrocardiogram (ECG) for screening healthy children, on a community basis, before participation in sports, or before prescription of noncardiac medications such as stimulant and psychotropic agents. This practice of ECG screening identifies increasing numbers of patients with electrocardiographic changes of WPW but without symptoms. A second change is the wide availability and use of catheter ablation

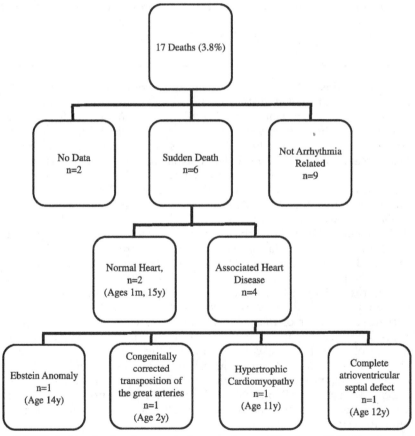

FIGURE 6.—Mortality data. Seventeen deaths occurred among 446 patients with WPW syndrome, 6 of which were arrhythmia related. Four patients with sudden death had associated heart disease. (Reprinted from Cain N, Irving C, Webber S, et al. Natural history of Wolff-Parkinson-white syndrome diagnosed in childhood. *Am J Cardiol.* 2013;112:961-965, with permission from Elsevier.)

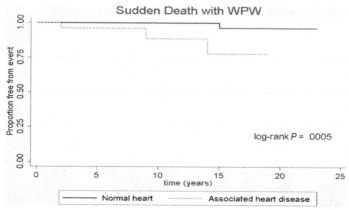

FIGURE 7.—Kaplan-Meier curve for sudden death. Patients with associated heart disease were significantly more likely to experience sudden death compared with patients with structurally normal hearts. (Reprinted from Cain N, Irving C, Webber S, et al. Natural history of Wolff-Parkinson-white syndrome diagnosed in childhood. *Am J Cardiol.* 2013;112:961-965, with permission from Elsevier.)

procedures to treat this syndrome. These procedures identify and target the actual myocardial fiber, which causes WPW, historically known as the bundle of Kent. Highly successful, this procedure effectively eliminates the risk of dangerous arrhythmias but in turn introduces new costs, concerns, and risks for iatrogenic injury into the management of these patients.

The current article by Cain and colleagues is an important addition to our expanding knowledge of the outcomes of patients with WPW, collected over many years during which its diagnosis and management has evolved (Figs 6 and 7).

For a disease in which the outcome may present decades after diagnosis, follow-up over such long periods is crucial, and few institutions have the ability to track as many patients over such an extended time. This work will help us to refine our understanding of the risks associated with WPW. By helping us to better quantify those risks, in the future we will be more able to identify those patients who may benefit most from invasive procedures to treat this problem.

J. K. Triedman, MD

Postural Orthostatic Tachycardia Syndrome (POTS) and Vitamin B$_{12}$ Deficiency in Adolescents
Öner T, Guven B, Tavli V, et al (Dr. Behçet Uz Children's Hosp, Alsancak, Izmir, Turkey)
Pediatrics 133:e138-e142, 2014

Objective.—Vitamin B$_{12}$ is involved in the production of adrenaline from noradrenaline. It is the cofactor involved in catecholamine degradation and plays a role in myelin synthesis. The current study aimed to investigate the association between vitamin B_{12} levels and postural orthostatic tachycardia syndrome (POTS) during adolescence when accelerated myelin synthesis increases the vitamin B_{12} need.

Methods.—One hundred twenty-five patients (mean age 11.1 ± 2.3 years; 60% female) reporting short-term loss of consciousness and diagnosed with vasovagal syncope based on anamnesis with a normal distribution and 50 control subjects (mean age 10.94 ± 2.5 years, 62% female) were included in this study. Serum vitamin B_{12}, folic acid, and ferritin levels were measured prospectively in addition to other tests. We defined vitamin B_{12} deficiency as a serum level <300 pg/mL.

Results.—Vitamin B_{12} levels were significantly lower in the patient group compared with the control group (47.2% vs 18%, $P < .001$). In the patient group, children with the POTS pattern had significantly lower vitamin B_{12} levels compared with children without the POTS response ($P = .03$).

Conclusions.—Vitamin B_{12} deficiency in patients with POTS may lead to sympathetic nervous system baroreceptor dysfunction.

▶ Öner and colleagues have provided a good service in making postural orthostatic tachycardia syndrome (POTS) more widely known. POTS affects up to 1% of adolescents, causing chronic fatigue, dizziness, nausea, and pains.[1,2] It is often associated with significant comorbidities[3] and can be debilitating.

Unfortunately, POTS is still incompletely recognized and inadequately understood. Although POTS has troubled patients for generations, it was first described as a specific entity in 1993[4] and first reported in an adolescent in 1999.[5] Today, predisposing features, helpful diagnostic measures, and useful therapeutic modalities are increasingly available. As well noted by Öner and colleagues, POTS and "chronic fatigue syndrome" often have overlapping presentations.

Descriptive studies reveal that POTS is more common in females than males and in whites than in blacks. High-achieving adolescents, especially those with physical hypermobility, seem to be preferentially affected. Adolescent POTS usually begins near or soon after the onset of pubertal changes and often follows an illness (such as mononucleosis) or an injury. There is some evidence that both iron deficiency (as evidenced by a low ferritin level, even without anemia) and hypovitaminosis D are associated with POTS,[6,7] but the pathophysiology of the condition has not been elucidated.

There are anecdotal reports that vitamin B_{12} deficiency may be associated with POTS. Öner and colleagues have added some scientific rigor to link B_{12} deficiency with POTS-like findings, and they have postulated plausible mechanisms through which B_{12} might act in the pathogenesis of POTS.

Although Öner and colleagues found more B_{12} deficiency in their POTS-like group of patients, it is not clear just how their findings should be applied. Details of the patient populations, testing measures, and data interpretation may limit the application and usefulness of the work.

POTS is usually diagnosed based on the finding of excessive postural tachycardia in a patient with symptoms suggestive of autonomic dysfunction (chronic fatigue, postural dizziness, often nausea) who does not have evidence of a different cause of the findings (with deconditioning, dehydration, and anxiety sometimes masquerading as POTS). Some investigators have proposed that fainting and/or orthostatic hypotension represent separate diagnostic considerations and preclude a diagnosis of POTS.[8]

Who were the subjects in this study? They were all being evaluated for syncope, and it is not reported whether they had chronic fatigue, r frequent postural dizziness, or other symptoms. Öner and colleagues excluded patients with "neurologic, psychiatric, and cardiovascular disorders." Most people consider POTS to be a form of autonomic dysfunction, which is a neurologic disorder, and most people consider syncope to be a cardiovascular condition. Furthermore, anxiety, a "psychiatric disorder," is a frequent comorbidity with POTS. It is thus not clear from Öner's article just who the patients were and how they might relate to other patients; they all had syncope, but it is not clear that any really had POTS. Also, nutritional status and conditioning are unmentioned confounders.

In addition, the subjects in this study ranged in age from 5 to 16 years with a median age of 11 years. POTS is a problem of adolescents, not preadolescents, so it seems that at least half of the syncopal subjects would not have even been candidates for a diagnosis of POTS. Normative data for tilt tests are not available for young children.

The diagnostic measures used are also worth reviewing. Tilt-table tests for POTS are best done with the patient relaxed; inserting venous and arterial catheters tends to create anxiety that can alter results. (It is true, however, that infusing medication can be useful when tilting patients to find non-POTS causes of syncope.) Typically, a 10-minute tilt is considered adequate; many normal healthy subjects become presyncopal and/or faint when subjected to longer tilting. Öner is accurate in saying that his 20-minute tilts (at 85 degrees instead of the standard 60–70 degrees) had "adequate sensitivity rates," but it is likely that this steep prolonged tilt was not adequately specific because it would have provoked symptomatic changes in vital signs in many normal subjects.

In recent years, studies in normal populations have shown that healthy adolescents can have up to a 40-beat-per-minute change in heart rate with positional challenge (both with standing[9] and with controlled tilting[10]). The current criteria for a diagnosis of POTS include postural tachycardia of at least 40 beats per minute for adolescents; Öner and colleagues used the "adult" criteria of 30 beats per minute in the children and adolescents they studied.

It is difficult to know what represents a "normal" level of vitamin B_{12}. Öner and colleagues used 300 pg/mL as a lower limit of "normal"; most other researchers use 200 pg/mL.[11] One of Öner's subgroups did have lower levels of B_{12} than another group, but it is not clear that any of the patients were truly vitamin B_{12} deficient.

Finally, the results may have been overextended. Finding a "POTS pattern" (presumably postural tachycardia of $\geq 30+$ beats per minute) was taken as an indication of the patient having POTS; however, it is not clear that the subjects actually qualified for a diagnosis of POTS (when, in fact, they are not reported to have had chronic symptoms of POTS, age-appropriate excesses of postural tachycardia, or exclusion of confounding conditions). The concluding sentence of the article claims that the study "shows the association between the etiopathogenesis of POTS and vitamin B_{12} deficiency-induced sympathetic nervous system baroreceptor dysfunction." In fact, the study showed an association between lower B_{12} levels and higher postural heart rates between subgroups of a population of children and adolescents with syncope. The authors did not specifically study POTS patients (by current definitions), and they did not do any baroreceptor testing; similarly, they only looked at an association without any testing of either the etiology of POTS or the pathogenesis of POTS or B_{12} deficiency.

A. E. Jones, MD

P. R. Fischer, MD

References

1. Kizilbash SJ, Ahrens SP, Bruce BK, et al. Adolescent fatigue, POTS, and recovery: a guide for clinicians. *Curr Probl Pediatr Adolesc Health Care.* 2014;44:108-133.
2. Johnson JN, Mack KJ, Kuntz NL, Brands CK, Porter CJ, Fischer PR. Postural orthostatic tachycardia syndrome : a clinical review. *Pediatr Neurol.* 2010;42: 77-85.
3. Ojha A, Chelimsky TC, Chelimsky G. Comorbidities in pediatric patients with postural orthostatic tachycardia syndrome. *J Pediatr.* 2011;158:20-23.
4. Schondorf R, Low PA. Idiopathic postural orthostatic tachycardia syndrome: an attenuated form of acute pandysautonomia? *Neurology.* 1993;43:132-137.
5. Sumiyoshi M, Nakata Y, Mineda Y, Yasuda M, Nakazato Y, Yamaguchi H. Analysis of heart rate variability during head-up tilt testing in a patient with idiopathic postural orthostatic tachycardia syndrome (POTS). *Jpn Circ J.* 1999;63:496-498.
6. Antiel RM, Caudill JS, Burkhardt BE, Brands CK, Fischer PR. Iron insufficiency and hypovitaminosis D in adolescents with chronic fatigue and orthostatic intolerance. *South Med J.* 2011;104:609-611.
7. Jarjour IT, Jarjour LK. Low iron storage and mild anemia in postural tachycardia syndrome in adolescents. *Clin Auton Res.* 2013;23:175-179.
8. Raj SR. Postural tachycardia syndrome (POTS). *Circulation.* 2013;127: 2336-2342.
9. Skinner JE, Driscoll SW, Porter CB, et al. Orthostatic heart rate and blood pressure in adolescents: reference ranges. *J Child Neurol.* 2010;25:1210-1215.
10. Singer W, Sletten DM, Opfer-Gehrking TL, Brands CK, Fischer PR, Low PA. Postural tachycardia in children and adolescents: what is normal? *J Pediatr.* 2012; 160:222-226.
11. Centers for Disease Control and Prevention. Vitamin B12 deficiency. http://www.cdc.gov/ncbddd/b12/detection.html. Accessed July 2, 2014.

Clinical Features and Follow-Up in Patients with 22q11.2 Deletion Syndrome

Cancrini C, on behalf of the Italian Network for Primary Immunodeficiencies (IPINet) (Bambino Gesù Children's Hosp and Tor Vergata Univ, Rome, Italy; et al)
J Pediatr 164:1475-1480, 2014

Objective.—To investigate the clinical manifestations at diagnosis and during follow-up in patients with 22q11.2 deletion syndrome to better define the natural history of the disease.

Study Design.—A retrospective and prospective multicenter study was conducted with 228 patients in the context of the Italian Network for Primary Immunodeficiencies. Clinical diagnosis was confirmed by cytogenetic or molecular analysis.

Results.—The cohort consisted of 112 males and 116 females; median age at diagnosis was 4 months (range 0 to 36 years 10 months). The diagnosis was made before 2 years of age in 71% of patients, predominantly related to the presence of heart anomalies and neonatal hypocalcemia. In patients diagnosed after 2 years of age, clinical features such as speech and language impairment, developmental delay, minor cardiac defects, recurrent infections, and facial features were the main elements leading to diagnosis. During follow-up (available for 172 patients), the frequency of autoimmune manifestations ($P = .015$) and speech disorders ($P = .002$) increased. After a median follow-up of 43 months, the survival probability was 0.92 at 15 years from diagnosis.

Conclusions.—Our data show a delay in the diagnosis of 22q11.2 deletion syndrome with noncardiac symptoms. This study provides guidelines for pediatricians and specialists for early identification of cases that can be confirmed by genetic testing, which would permit the provision of appropriate clinical management.

▶ Perhaps no syndrome causes more confusion than the 22q11 deletion syndrome (22DS) because no syndrome has more names: velocardiofacial syndrome (VCFS), Sedlackova syndrome, Cayler syndrome, conotruncal anomaly face syndrome, and of course DiGeorge syndrome (DGS). Even experienced pediatric specialists become understandably confused. "My patient with a 22q11 deletion just presented with hypocalcemia, and we now come to find she has a submucous cleft—does she still have DGS, or does she have VCFS?" It obviously does not matter which term you use. What matters is that the child be evaluated and monitored for the myriad (more than 200) potential abnormalities that have been reported associated with 22DS.

TABLE 1.—Clinical Features Suggesting the Diagnosis of the 22q11.2DS in 127 Infants and in 59 Children ≥2 Years Old

	<2 y Old		≥2 y Old		Total	
	n	%	n	%	N	%
Patients evaluable	127		59		186	
Clinical features						
Cardiac defects	90	71	13	22	103	55
Neonatal hypocalcemia	29	23	8	14	37	20
Infections	12	9	10	17	22	12
Autoimmune manifestations	0	0	4	7	4	2
Otorhinolaryngologic manifestations	4	3	6	10	10	5
Neuropsychological manifestations	5	4	17	29	22	12
Typical features	12	9	19	32	31	17
Not known	35		7		42	

The study by Cancrini and colleagues draws attention to the variability of 22DS but also highlights how a patient's presenting finding(s) affect(s) the timing of diagnosis and even subsequent management (Table 1). Clinical geneticists know that many patients with 22DS may go undiagnosed when they lack one of the major malformations associated with this syndrome. This experience is highlighted in this study because those with a heart defect were diagnosed far earlier than those without this common, but not universal, finding.

The authors acknowledge that their method of ascertainment through a network of immunodeficiency centers likely results in an underestimation of certain findings that are more prevalent in other studies, such as palatal defects. Also, they recognize that they may have detected a higher prevalence of neuropsychiatric disorders, common and serious finding(s) in 22DS, if they had surveyed an older population. However, these are minor complaints because this is an excellent study in its thoroughness and scope. Rather, these limitations reflect a common theme that can be found in almost any study of 22DS.

Like the blind men and the elephant, the way any group of researchers portrays 22DS is typically dependent on the perspective of the specialty. To immunologists, 22DS is a T-cell immunodeficiency; to behavioral patricians, it is a specific pattern of developmental learning deficits; to speech and language professionals, it is a variety of palatal and speech defects.

This study encourages a holistic view of 22DS through at least 2 points. First, classic findings such as heart defects, cleft palate, hypocalcemia, and immunodeficiency are seen in many but by no means all cases of 22DS. Second, the other, more consistent features such as typical facies, speech patterns, and behavioral and learning differences, are far more subtle and may be unrecognized by inexperienced clinicians. This study's finding that 100% of patients were reported to have the characteristic facial appearance when examined by a clinical geneticist illustrates this point. Appreciation of the range of potential presenting findings, not just the "classic" clinical picture will hopefully lead to earlier and more appropriate intervention and accurate genetic counseling.

Another consequence of the wide variability associated with 22DS is that it is easily overdiagnosed based solely on clinical findings, and this too has dangers. Today, 22DS is most commonly diagnosed by array comparative genome hybridization (aCGH) or fluorescence in situ hybridization (FISH). However, a negative test for either does not exclude other genetic causes for the abnormalities frequently associated with this disorder. Many identifiable genetic conditions, such as Alagille syndrome or Noonan syndrome, are also characterized by congenital heart defects and would never be detected by DS22 FISH testing and only rarely by aCGH. Although recognizing the signs of DS22 may be the first step in making the diagnosis, ruling out this diagnosis by no means suggests that the workup is complete.

One final point to be drawn from this article and from many others that have investigated 22DS is that these patients are best served in a multidisciplinary clinic or center that can provide the diverse resources that are required to serve these patients. The specialties involved in the care of patients with 22DS are as varied as the disorder itself. In addition to routine pediatric care, these children often need the services of a diverse group of medical and surgical subspecialists, various therapists, and behavioral-developmental professionals to maximize their potential. Coordinating this level of care is a daunting task that typically falls to the primary care pediatrician but can be more easily achieved through access to multidisciplinary clinics. However, the first step toward delivery of appropriate care is making the diagnosis, and raising awareness of the many diverse presentations of 22DS will aid practitioners of all fields in recognizing this common disorder.

N. H. Robin, MD

J. A. Hamm, MD

Asymmetric Crying Facies in the 22q11.2 Deletion Syndrome: Implications for Future Screening

Pasick C, McDonald-McGinn DM, Simbolon C, et al (Univ of Pennsylvania, Philadelphia; Children's Hosp of Philadelphia, PA)
Clin Pediatr 52:1144-1148, 2013

Objective.—Asymmetric crying facies (ACF) is congenital hypoplasia of the depressor anguli oris muscle characterized by asymmetry of lower lip depression during crying. This has an overall incidence of 0.6%. This study determines the incidence of ACF in a large population of patients with 22q11.2 deletion.

Patients and Methods.—A retrospective review of medical records on patients with a confirmed 22q11.2 deletion was undertaken.

Results.—A total of 836 records were reviewed. Of these, 117 (14%) were noted to have ACF on physical examination. Within this latter group, palatal anomalies were common (77%), as was congenital heart disease (78%); however, these numbers did not differ significantly from their known prevalence in the 22q11.2 population.

Conclusions.—We report a 14% incidence of ACF in patients with a 22q11.2 deletion, significantly higher than in the general population. We suggest, therefore, that newborns with ACF be referred for further screening for the 22q11.2 deletion syndrome (Fig 1, Table 1 and Table 2).

▶ Asymmetric crying facies (ACF), also known as hypoplastic or absent depressor anguli oris muscle (DAOM), is a benign newborn physical examination finding that is noted in 0.3% to 0.6% of infants.[1] Normally, the DOAM pulls the corner of the mouth downward during crying or frowning (Fig 1); however, if the DOAM is hypoplastic or absent, the affected side will not turn downward while the infant is crying and appear "crooked." The prognosis is good, because the condition does not affect infant feeding. In addition, the lesion becomes less noticeable with age as the child cries less frequently and eventually, the ipsilateral risorius muscle can help compensate.

In this study, Pasick et al review of medical records on 836 patients with a confirmed 22q11.2 deletion. They report that 117 (14%) had a documented absent DOAM in their medical record. In addition, 91 of the 117 patients

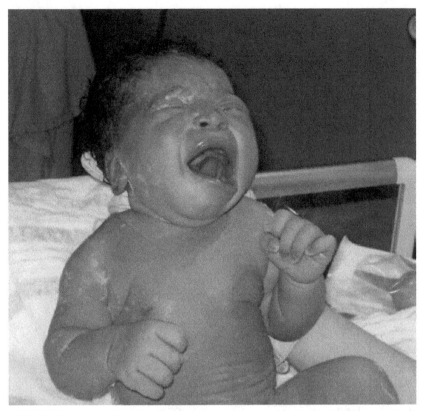

FIGURE 1.—Asymmetric crying facies apparent at the time of birth. (Reprinted from Pasick C, McDonald-McGinn DM, Simbolon C, et al. Asymmetric crying facies in the 22q11.2 deletion syndrome: implications for future screening. *Clin Pediatr.* 2013;52:1144-1148, Copyright 2013, by Clinical Pediatrics. Reprinted by permission of SAGE Publications.)

had a cardiovascular anomaly (Table 1). Because this percentage (14%) is significantly higher than the occurrence of absent DAOM in the general population (0.6%), they recommend that newborns with absent DOAM be referred for further screening for the 22q11.2 deletion syndrome. Although the 14% reported by Pasick et al is interesting, this study is far from conclusive in demonstrating the need to screen for a 22q11.2 deletion syndrome.

The etiology of absent DAOM has not been established. This article on the association between absent DAOM and 22q11.2 deletion syndrome is similar to previous studies examining absent DAOM and cardiac conditions. Since Cayler's first description in 1969,[2] there has been a long history of studies examining the association between this condition and congenital cardiac anomalies (eg, atrial septal defects, ventricular septal defects, patent ductus arteriosus).[3] Several retrospective studies have noted a high percentage of children with cardiac anomalies who also have absent DAOM (Table 2).[2,4,5] As a result, many of these same studies have suggested aggressive testing for cardiac anomalies if absent DAOM is detected.

TABLE 1.—The Prevalence of Coexisting Major Congenital Anomalies in the Patient Population With Both the 22q11.2 Deletion and Asymmetric Crying Facies (N = 117)

Major Congenital Anomaly	Number of Patients (Percentage of Population)
Cardiovascular anomaly	91 (78%)
Palatal/velopharyngeal anomaly	90 (77%)
Cleft palate	6 (5%)
Submucosal cleft palate	28 (24%)
High arched palate	17 (15%)
Velopharyngeal insufficiency	37 (32%)

(Reprinted from Pasick C, McDonald-McGinn DM, Simbolon C, et al. Asymmetric crying facies in the 22q11.2 deletion syndrome: implications for future screening. Clin Pediatr. 2013;52:1144-1148, Copyright 2013, by Clinical Pediatrics. Reprinted by permission of SAGE Publications.)

TABLE 2.—Associations between Absent DOAM and Cardiac Anomalies

Author (Year)	# DAOM Cases	# Cardiac Anomalies	% of DOAM Cases with Cardiac Issues	Study Design	Sample Size
Cayler (1969)	14	14	100%	Retrospective	NA
Pape (1972)	44	22	50%	Retrospective	NA
Levin (1982)	23	12	52%	Retrospective	NA
Dar-Shong (1997)	50	22	44%	Retrospective	NA
Perlman (1973)	41	1	2%	Prospective	6360
Alexiou (1976)	44	3	7%	Prospective	6487
Lahat (2000)	17	1	6%	Prospective	5532

NA indicates not applicable; Adapted from Lahat E, et al. Asymmetric crying facies and associated congenital anomalies. *J Child Neurol.* 2000; 15: 808-810.

The problem with this approach is that many of these associations between absent DAOM and cardiac anomalies are only noted in retrospective studies. A retrospective study design leads to 2 issues. First, absent DAOM is a benign condition that may or may not be documented in the neonatal period. For those infants who are noted to have a cardiac anomaly, there is much more exposure time with the health care system for follow-up visits, including repeat examinations with increased scrutiny for the presence of other potential anomalies. This increased exposure and scrutiny for anomalies (such as absent DAOM) leads to an increased likelihood for detecting this DAOM lesion, and thus, a bias, which may artificially inflate the association of cardiac anomalies and absent DAOM.

Second, if A is found in a high percentage of patients with B, it is not necessarily true that B will be found in a high percentage of patients with A. Just because many patients with a specific cardiac anomaly have absent DAOM, it is not necessarily true that a baby with absent DAOM will have a cardiac issue. For the pediatrician in the nursery who detects an infant with an absent DAOM and is wondering about the possibility of a cardiac issue, the retrospective studies are not applicable. What this pediatrician needs are prospective studies in which an absent DOAM is systematically assessed in a newborn nursery and a standard follow-up for cardiac anomalies is conducted.

Fortunately, these types of studies have been conducted and published[6-8] (Table 2, Rows 4—6). When large cohorts of infants (eg, > 5000 infants) are systematically assessed for absent DAOM and then evaluated for cardiac anomalies, the typical percentage of patients with absent DAOM who later have cardiac issues is 2% to 7%. Furthermore, the risk of any newborn having a minor or major cardiac issue noted in the nursery is approximately 6.5%.[9] As a result, the presence of DAOM is an increased risk factor for a cardiac issue. A good history and a careful cardiac examination is probably sufficient.

In summary, although the percentage of patients with confirmed 22q11.2 deletion who also had absent DAOM was 14%, it is no guarantee that a large percentage of patients with absent DAOM will have 22q11.2 deletion syndrome. A prospective study that first establishes absent DAOM in the nursery and estimates the likelihood of 22q11.2 deletion syndrome is needed first, before regular follow-up 22q11.2 deletion syndrome should be routinely recommended.

M. D. Cabana, MD, MPH

References

1. Rioja-Mazza D, Lieber E, Kamath V, Kalpatthi R. Asymmetric crying facies: a possible marker for congenital malformations. *J Matern Fetal Neonatal Med.* 2005; 18:275-277.
2. Cayler GG. Cardiofacial syndrome. Congenital heart disease and facial weakness, a hitherto unrecognized association. *Arch Dis Child.* 1969;44:69-75.
3. Lin DS, Huang FY, Lin SP, et al. Frequency of associated anomalies in congenital hypoplasia of depressor anguli oris muscle: a study of 50 patients. *Am J Med Genet..* 1997;71:215-218.
4. Levin SE, Silverman NH, Milner S. Hypoplasia or absence of the depressor anguli oris muscle and congenital abnormalities, with special reference to the cardiofacial syndrome. *S Afr Med J.* 1982;61:227-231.
5. Pape KE, Pickering D. Asymmetric crying facies: an index of other congenital anomalies. *J Pediatr.* 1972;81:21-30.
6. Lahat E, Heyman E, Barkay A, Goldberg M. Asymmetric crying facies and associated congenital anomalies. *J Child Neurol.* 2000;15:808-810.
7. Perlman M, Reisner SH. Asymmetric crying facies and congenital anomalies. *Arch Dis Child.* 1973;48:627-629.
8. Alexiou D, Manolidis C, Papaevangellou G, Nicolopoulos D, Papadatos C. Frequency of other malformations in congenital hypoplasia of depressor anguli oris muscle syndrome. *Arch Dis Child.* 1976;51:891-893.
9. Hoffman JI, Kaplan S. The incidence of congenital heart disease. *J Am Coll Cardiol.* 2002;39:1890-1900.

10 Infectious Diseases and Immunology

Intussusception Risk after Rotavirus Vaccination in U.S. Infants
Yih WK, Lieu TA, Kulldorff M, et al (Harvard Med School and Harvard Pilgrim Health Care Inst, Boston, MA; et al)
N Engl J Med 370:503-512, 2014

Background.—International postlicensure studies have identified an increased risk of intussusception after vaccination with the second-generation rotavirus vaccines RotaTeq (RV5, a pentavalent vaccine) and Rotarix (RV1, a monovalent vaccine). We studied this association among infants in the United States.

Methods.—The study included data from infants 5.0 to 36.9 weeks of age who were enrolled in three U.S. health plans that participate in the Mini-Sentinel program sponsored by the Food and Drug Administration. Potential cases of intussusception and vaccine exposures from 2004 through mid-2011 were identified through procedural and diagnostic codes. Medical records were reviewed to confirm the occurrence of intussusception and the status with respect to rotavirus vaccination. The primary analysis used a self-controlled risk-interval design that included only vaccinated children. The secondary analysis used a cohort design that included exposed and unexposed person-time.

Results.—The analyses included 507,874 first doses and 1,277,556 total doses of RV5 and 53,638 first doses and 103,098 total doses of RV1. The statistical power for the analysis of RV1 was lower than that for the analysis of RV5. The number of excess cases of intussusception per 100,000 recipients of the first dose of RV5 was significantly elevated, both in the primary analysis (attributable risk, 1.1 [95% confidence interval, 0.3 to 2.7] for the 7-day risk window and 1.5 [95% CI, 0.2 to 3.2] for the 21-day risk window) and in the secondary analysis (attributable risk, 1.2 [95% CI, 0.2 to 3.2] for the 21-day risk window). No significant increase in risk was seen after dose 2 or 3. The results with respect to the primary analysis of RV1 were not significant, but the secondary analysis showed a significant risk after dose 2.

Conclusions.—RV5 was associated with approximately 1.5 (95% CI, 0.2 to 3.2) excess cases of intussusception per 100,000 recipients of the first dose. The secondary analysis of RV1 suggested a potential risk, although the study of RV1 was underpowered. These risks must be considered in light of the demonstrated benefits of rotavirus vaccination. (Funded by the Food and Drug Administration.)

▶ Although still not well recognized by many in the community, most pediatricians are aware that rotavirus infection is the leading cause of gastroenteritis worldwide. It is estimated to lead to 200 000 deaths and 10 million episodes of severe diarrhea annually. Deaths are uncommon in developed countries, but the burden of disease associated with hospitalization of severe cases is high in the absence of vaccination. However, the development and uptake of vaccines for rotavirus disease suffered a major setback in 1999 when the first licensed vaccine (RotaShield) was withdrawn from the market after it was linked with a substantially elevated risk of intussusception, a rare acute bowel obstruction that can have fatal consequences if not treated promptly and appropriately.

This new study and a companion study examined intussusception risk associated with the 2 second-generation vaccines (the pentavalent Rotateq, RV5, and the monovalent Rotarix, RV1) that have been widely licensed and introduced to many national immunization programs since the mid-2000s. Introduction of these vaccines followed large-scale clinical trials that recruited infants in sufficiently large numbers to rule out adverse event risks of similar magnitude to those found with the first vaccine. However, a series of postmarketing surveillance studies from Brazil, Mexico, and Australia that first appeared in 2011 identified elevated risks of intussusception associated with varying strengths and levels of uncertainty with each of the new vaccines. The new studies report the first clear confirmation of these risks in US data.

Yih et al examined data on infants who received either RV5 or RV1 within 3 managed health plans between 2004 and 2011 and identified cases of intussusception from administrative databases using relevant International Classification of Diseases (Ninth Revision) codes supplemented by case-notes review. A total of 124 confirmed cases were identified, and 2 methods of analysis (discussed subsequently) produced broadly similar findings: about 1.5 additional cases of intussusception could be expected for every 100 000 recipients of the (first dose of) RV5 vaccine. No clear evidence of increased risk in the week after second and third doses could be seen. Numbers of cases receiving RV1 vaccine were too small to enable statistical analysis.

It is interesting to compare these results with a larger study (306 cases) on the same question that we published a year earlier using nationwide data from Australia.[1] The overall pattern of results is remarkably similar except that with larger numbers, the Australian study was able to identify more clearly the risks associated with both vaccines (at similar levels) and with dose 2 as well as dose 1. The report of the Australian study focused attention primarily on relative risk estimates, which were 7- to 9-fold in days 1 to 7 after dose 1, with 95% confidence intervals indicating uncertainty out to around 3 times higher or lower relative risks. Against a higher background incidence of intussusception in Australia and allowing for risk after dose 2 as well as dose 1, these relative risks translated to around 6 additional cases per 100 000 vaccinated.

Yih et al focused on reporting absolute risk estimates, which (as they admit) are less likely to be transportable between settings with different base rates. The estimated attributable risk of 1.5 additional cases per 100 000 almost immediately reassures the reader (correctly) that the risk associated with this vaccine is quite clearly outweighed by the benefits that have been documented not only in randomized trials but also in extensive postmarketing surveillance. Even with what appears to be a higher attributable risk in Australia, our calculations showed a clear net benefit of an estimated 6500 cases of severe gastroenteritis prevented per annum at the cost of 14 additional intussusceptions (within a national population of 22 million).

The challenge of assessing the relative costs and benefits of vaccines has increased with the rapidly rising number of vaccines coming onto the market, some of which address diseases such as rotavirus that are not as life threatening as the historic main targets of vaccination. In this context, careful and comprehensive surveillance is important so that even rare side effects such as intussusception may be studied with reasonable precision after a vaccine has been licensed. This is easier in systems in which vaccines are nationally funded and systematically provided, such as Australia.

It is also important to note that adverse side effects of vaccination can be validly studied using "case-only" methods, provided that the ascertainment of cases is comprehensive and not associated in any way with the determination of vaccination history. Although somewhat challenging to present (because of its slightly "abstruse" logic[2]), this method has advantages over more traditional cohort and case-control epidemiological designs, not only because comparison children not suffering the adverse event are not required but also because the method automatically controls for confounding factors that are fixed for each child (such as socioeconomic position). Because of their small number of cases, Yih et al adopted a somewhat nonstandard approach to the case-only analysis, relying on external information to control for the important confounding effect of age on the risk of intussusception. With a larger number of cases, internal control of age effects using the self-controlled case series method is possible and may be more reliable.

The logic of the case-only method emphasizes that the statistical information in adverse-effect studies is driven by the number of cases, not by the total number of children or of vaccine doses that might be available for study. In this regard, these US studies of rotavirus vaccine risk give the impression that they have recruited just enough cases to provide "statistically significant" signals of risk. An underrecognized side effect of placing undue emphasis on the arbitrary threshold of "$P < .05$" is that although "significant" findings may be conventionally interpreted to rule out the null hypothesis, they will often fail to rule out a number of other possibilities, such as large relative risks. Only by the accumulation of many sets of results from a range of settings, using methods and measures that are as standardized as possible, can we hope to learn with adequate precision about the actual magnitude of rare vaccine-associated effects. In this regard it might have been appropriate for a leading "journal of record" such as the *New England Journal of Medicine* to request that more emphasis be given to reviewing all the available data on this important topic.

J. Carlin, PhD

References

1. Carlin JB, Macartney KK, Lee KJ, et al. Intussusception Risk and Disease Prevention Associated With Rotavirus Vaccines in Australia's National Immunization Program. *Clin Infect Dis.* 2013;57:1427-1434.
2. Weldeselassie YG, Whitaker HJ, Farrington CP. Use of the self-controlled case-series method in vaccine safety studies: review and recommendations for best practice. *Epidemiology & Infection.* 2011;139:1805-1817.

Vaccine for Prevention of Mild and Moderate-to-Severe Influenza in Children

Jain VK, Rivera L, Zaman K, et al (GlaxoSmithKline Vaccines, King of Prussia, PA; Hospital Maternidad Nuestra Señora de la Altagracia, Santo Domingo, Dominican Republic; International Ctr for Diarrheal Disease Res, Dhaka, Bangladesh; et al)
N Engl J Med 369:2481-2491, 2013

Background.—Commonly used trivalent vaccines contain one influenza B virus lineage and may be ineffective against viruses of the other B lineage. We evaluated the efficacy of a candidate inactivated quadrivalent influenza vaccine (QIV) containing both B lineages.

Methods.—In this multinational, phase 3, observer-blinded study, we randomly assigned children 3 to 8 years of age, in a 1:1 ratio, to receive the QIV or a hepatitis A vaccine (control). The primary end point was influenza A or B confirmed by real-time polymerase chain reaction (rt-PCR). Secondary end points were rt-PCR—confirmed, moderate-to-severe influenza and rt-PCR—positive, culture-confirmed influenza. The vaccine efficacy and the effect of vaccination on daily activities and utilization of health care resources were assessed in the total vaccinated cohort (2584 children in each group) and the per-protocol cohort (2379 children in the QIV group and 2398 in the control group).

Results.—In the total vaccinated cohort, 62 children in the QIV group (2.40%) and 148 in the control group (5.73%) had rt-PCR—confirmed influenza, representing a QIV efficacy of 59.3% (95% confidence interval [CI], 45.2 to 69.7), with efficacy against culture-confirmed influenza of 59.1% (97.5% CI, 41.2 to 71.5). For moderate-to-severe rt-PCR—confirmed influenza, the attack rate was 0.62% (16 cases) in the QIV group and 2.36% (61 cases) in the control group, representing a QIV efficacy of 74.2% (97.5% CI, 51.5 to 86.2). In the per-protocol cohort, the QIV efficacy was 55.4% (95% CI, 39.1 to 67.3), and the efficacy against culture-confirmed influenza 55.9% (97.5% CI, 35.4 to 69.9); the efficacy among children with moderate-to-severe influenza was 73.1% (97.5% CI, 47.1 to 86.3). The QIV was associated with reduced risks of a body temperature above 39°C and lower respiratory tract illness, as compared with the control vaccine, in the per-protocol cohort (relative risk, 0.29 [95% CI, 0.16 to 0.56] and 0.20 [95% CI, 0.04 to 0.92], respectively). The QIV was immunogenic against all four strains. Serious adverse events occurred in

36 children in the QIV group (1.4%) and in 24 children in the control group (0.9%).

Conclusions.—The QIV was efficacious in preventing influenza in children. (Funded by GlaxoSmithKline Biologicals; ClinicalTrials.gov number, NCT01218308.)

▶ Last influenza season marked the first season that 2 influenza B strains were included in the standard seasonal influenza vaccine formulation, making the new quadrivalent vaccine a mixture of 2 influenza A and 2 influenza B strains. This change was informed by surveillance data indicating that having only 1 lineage of the influenza B strain each year missed the circulating influenza B strain about half of the time. Effectiveness data also demonstrated that the trivalent vaccine was less effective at preventing disease due to the mismatched B strain compared with the matched B strain.

In this clinical trial, the investigators compared the safety and effectiveness of 1 of the approved quadrivalent inactivated influenza vaccines with a hepatitis A vaccine serving as the control for the prevention of symptomatic laboratory-confirmed influenza. The study enrolled more than 5000 children between the ages of 3 to 8 years and was extremely well executed with comprehensive surveillance for influenza disease using modern molecular detection methods.

Overall, the vaccine efficacy for the prevention of all laboratory-confirmed influenza was nearly 60% and was nearly 75% for the prevention of moderate to severe disease—efficacy values comparable to other previous reports. Vaccine efficacy against all laboratory-confirmed disease in children 3 to 4 years of age was lower than in children 5 to 8 years of age, similar to other reports of inactivated influenza vaccine. The point estimates of efficacy against moderate-to-severe disease were higher and more similar between age groups, being 67.5 for 3- to 4-year-olds and 76.2 for 5- to 8-year-olds. Only 1 influenza B strain circulated during the influenza season making it impossible to determine whether the new quadrivalent vaccine was actually effective in preventing infection with both influenza B strains.

What was not studied in this report was a comparison of the live and the inactivated quadrivalent vaccines. Earlier efficacy studies comparing trivalent live influenza vaccines and the inactivated influenza vaccines had clearly shown that in children between the ages of 2 to 5 years, the live attenuated vaccine was significantly more effective.

So what is the bottom line? First, quadrivalent vaccines are preferred over trivalent preparations, despite the inability of this study to compare the 2. Second, in normal healthy children, at least between the ages of 2 to 5 years, it is highly likely that live attenuated quadrivalent vaccine will be more efficacious than the inactivated vaccine.

K. M. Edwards, MD

Duration of Protection After First Dose of Acellular Pertussis Vaccine in Infants

Quinn HE, Snelling TL, Macartney KK, et al (Univ of Sydney, New South Wales, Australia; The Univ of Western Australia, West Perth, Australia)
Pediatrics 133:e513-e519, 2014

Objective.—Data on the effectiveness of the diphtheria–tetanus–acellular pertussis (DTaP) vaccine in the first 4 years of life are sparse. We evaluated the vaccine effectiveness (VE) of 1 and 2 doses of DTaP before 6 months of age and of 3 doses from 6 months of age in Australia, where, since 2003, a fourth dose is not given until 4 years.

Methods.—We matched reported pertussis cases aged 2 to 47 months between January 2005 and December 2009 to controls from a population-based immunization register by date of birth and region of residence. VE by number of doses and age group was calculated as (1 − odds ratio) × 100%.

Results.—VE against hospitalization increased from 55.3% (95% confidence interval [CI], 42.7%−65.1%) for 1 dose before 4 months of age to 83.0% (95% CI, 70.2%−90.3%) for 2 doses before 6 months. The VE of 3 doses of DTaP against all reported pertussis was 83.5% (95% CI, 79.1%−87.8%) between 6 and 11 months, declining to 70.7% (95% CI, 64.5%−75.8%) between 2 and 3 years of age and 59.2% (95% CI, 51.0%−66.0%) between 3 and 4 years of age.

Conclusions.—DTaP provided good protection against pertussis in the first year of life from the first dose. Without a booster dose, the effectiveness of 3 doses waned more rapidly from 2 to 4 years of age than previously documented for children >6 years of age who had received 5 doses.

▶ Pertussis infection remains a potential public health threat, despite the availability of a pertussis vaccine and high vaccination rates. The current incidence of pertussis is between 10 000 to 40 000 cases annually. Furthermore, there are appropriately 10 to 20 deaths due to pertussis reported annually.[1]

One reason for the persistence of pertussis is the issue of "waning" immunity. Even with completion of the recommended childhood acellular pertussis vaccination series, there is an increasing risk of pertussis infection for the patient with each passing year since the receipt of the most recent dose of diphtheria–tetanus–acellular pertussis (DTaP). It is estimated that protective immunity after the completion of the DTaP vaccination series declines after 4 to 12 years.[2] Based on data from the 2010 pertussis outbreak in California, it is estimated the DTaP is 42% less effective each year.[3] As a result, the Centers for Disease Control and Prevention (CDC) has recommended 2 strategies to prevent pertussis spread. These include vaccination of pregnant women with tetanus toxoid, reduced diphtheria toxoid, and acellular pertussis (Tdap) during each pregnancy and immunization of all infant contacts, including parents, grandparents, siblings, and caretakers.

Quinn and colleagues study the phenomenon of waning immunity but focus instead on the initial doses of DTaP among children less than 4 years of age. The study is a case-control design that takes advantage of difference in vaccination schedules in Australia and data collected during a recent pertussis epidemic from 2008—2011 in the same country. Since 2003, the fourth DTaP dose is not given until 4 years of age in Australia. As a result, the authors were able to estimate DTaP vaccine effectiveness (VE) after the first and second doses, based on a comparison of rates of immunization in the cases and controls. The results noted that for infants less than 1 year old who received 3 doses of DTaP, the VE was 84%; however, at 3 years of age, the VE was only 59%. These results are graphically modeled in Fig 3.

Overall, the results suggest that there is excellent protection for infants after 1 or 2 doses of DTaP. This finding is reassuring for clinicians and public health officials because it helps support the practice that the first dose of DTaP be administered as early as 6 weeks of age. In addition, the drop in immunity between 2 to 3 years of age supports the idea for a booster dose in the second year of life. The authors note that "this an important consideration in the context of maternal Tdap immunization, because there may be a reduced immune response after the primary series of DTaP in infants born to mothers who have received Tdap in the third trimester of pregnancy." In 2011, the Advisory Committee on Immunization Practices updated the recommendations for use of Tdap in pregnant women.[4]

This study by Quinn and colleagues is an important public health and pediatric study that examines the effect of the effectiveness of the initial doses of DTaP among children less than 4 years of age. The results help public health practitioners understand how to best structure DTaP vaccine schedules for infants and young children. Overall, these results support the current dosing schedule for DTaP; however, as pediatricians, we should not forget the CDC's second strategy for the use of Tdap in pregnant women and infant contacts.[4] We need

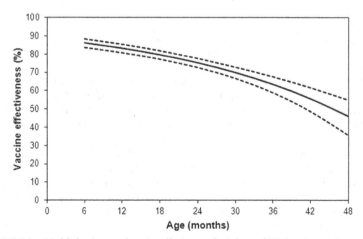

FIGURE 3.—Modeled estimates of vaccine effectiveness for 3 doses of DTaP (versus no doses) against pertussis notification by age. *Note*: Effectiveness (solid line) and pointwise 95% confidence intervals (dotted lines) were estimated from the best fitting fractional polynomial transformation of the age*vaccine interaction, being a first degree cubic polynomial. (Reprinted from Quinn HE, Snelling TL, Macartney KK, et al. Duration of protection after first dose of acellular pertussis vaccine in infants. *Pediatrics*. 2014;133:e513-e519, with permission from the American Academy of Pediatrics.)

to work collaboratively with our colleagues in obstetrics and family medicine to make sure our messages about the importance of Tdap are consistent to families and pregnant women. Pediatricians can iterate these recommendations to pregnant women during their prenatal visits, as well as encounters with older siblings. In the end, public health promotion and disease prevention is a cross-disciplinary, team sport.

M. D. Cabana, MD, MPH

References

1. Centers for Disease Control and Prevention. Pertussis (Whooping Cough) http://www.cdc.gov/pertussis/about/faqs.html. Accessed March 18, 2014.
2. Wendelboe AM, Van Rie A, Salmaso S, Englund JA. Duration of immunity against pertussis after natural infection or vaccination. *Pediatr Infect Dis J.* 2005;24:s54-s61.
3. Klein NP, Bartlett J, Rowhani-Rahbar A, Fireman B, Baxter R. Waning Protection after Fifth Dose of Acellular Pertussis Vaccine in Children. *N Engl J Med.* 2012; 367:1012-1019.
4. Centers for Disease Control and Prevention (CDC). Updated recommendations for use of tetanus toxoid, reduced diphtheria toxoid and acellular pertussis vaccine (Tdap) in pregnant women and persons who have or anticipate having close contact with an infant aged ,12 months—Advisory Committee on Immunization Practices (ACIP), 2011. *MMWR.* 2011;60:1424-1426.

A Randomized Trial to Increase Acceptance of Childhood Vaccines by Vaccine-Hesitant Parents: A Pilot Study
Williams SE, Rothman RL, Offit PA, et al (Vanderbilt Univ School of Medicine, Nashville, TN; Children's Hosp of Philadelphia, PA)
Acad Pediatr 13:475-480, 2013

Objective.—A cluster randomized trial was performed to evaluate an educational intervention to improve parental attitudes and vaccine uptake in vaccine-hesitant parents.

Methods.—Two primary care sites were randomized to provide families with either usual care or an intervention (video and written information) for vaccine-hesitant parents. Eligible parents included those presenting for their child's 2-week well-child visit with performance on the Parent Attitudes about Childhood Vaccines (PACV) survey suggesting vaccine hesitancy (score ≥ 25). Enrollees completed PACV surveys at the 2-month well-child visit and vaccination status at 12 weeks of age was assessed. The primary outcome was the difference in PACV scores obtained at enrollment and 2 months between the 2 groups. The proportion of on-time vaccination was also compared at 12 weeks.

Results.—A total of 454 parents were approached, and 369 (81.3%) participated; 132 had PACV scores of ≥ 25 and were enrolled, 67 in the control group (mean PACV score 37) and 55 in the intervention group (mean PACV score 40). Two month PACV surveys were completed by 108 ($\sim 90\%$) of enrollees. Parents in the intervention group had a significant decrease in PACV score at 2 months compared to control (median difference 6.7, $P = .049$); this remained significant after adjustment for baseline PACV score, race/ethnicity, and income ($P = .044$). There was no difference in the on-time receipt of vaccines between groups at 12 weeks.

Conclusions.—A brief educational intervention for vaccine-hesitant parents was associated with a modest but significant increase in measured parental attitudes toward vaccines.

▶ Vaccine hesitancy—a general term primarily used in the pediatric setting to describe parents' reluctance to accept childhood vaccines in sum, in part, or on time—has become an issue of considerable public health significance in the past 15 years. Parental refusal or delay of vaccines is an important contributor to underimmunization and increases the risk of children developing and transmitting vaccine-preventable disease.[1] It also appears that it is on the rise: the proportion of US parents who claimed a nonmedical exemption for their child from required school-entry vaccines essentially doubled between 2006 and 2011.[2]

Much work has been done to understand the origins of and factors inherent to vaccine hesitancy. Common themes include parental perceptions of vaccine safety and efficacy, parental beliefs about disease and immunization, and the influence of social and mass media on parental vaccine decision making. However, there have been comparatively few well-designed and rigorously evaluated interventions to reduce parental vaccine hesitancy or refusal. This study is one of those few.

Even so, the study has limitations. Foremost, the extent to which the authors' results are clinically meaningful is somewhat muddled by their use of parental vaccine attitudes and beliefs, rather than actual parent behavior (ie, vaccine uptake), as the primary outcome. For instance, it remains unclear whether the significantly greater reduction in parental hesitant attitudes and beliefs that the authors observed among intervention parents compared with control parents is correlated with any increase in vaccine uptake in the short- or long-term.

Despite these limitations, this pilot study offers promise. The demonstration of a significant and positive effect on parental vaccine attitudes through the use of a short patient-centered intervention integrated into clinical care with minimal provider effort is encouraging. In the end, no one intervention will be the cure-all for vaccine hesitancy. This study starts us on the path to having an adequate supply of effective interventions from which to choose.

D. J. Opel, MD, MPH

References

1. Glanz JM, McClure DL, Magid DJ, et al. Parental refusal of pertussis vaccination is associated with an increased risk of pertussis infection in children. *Pediatrics.* 2009;123(6):1446-1451.
2. Omer SB, Richards JL, Ward M, Bednarczyk RA. Vaccination policies and rates of exemption from immunization, 2005-2011. *The New England Journal of Medicine.* 2012;367(12):1170-1171.

Multistate Outbreak of Listeriosis Associated with Cantaloupe

McCollum JT, Cronquist AB, Silk BJ, et al (Ctrs for Disease Control and Prevention, Atlanta, GA; Colorado Dept of Public Health and Environment, Denver; et al)
N Engl J Med 369:944-953, 2013

Background.—Although new pathogen–vehicle combinations are increasingly being identified in produce-related disease outbreaks, fresh produce is a rarely recognized vehicle for listeriosis. We investigated a nationwide listeriosis outbreak that occurred in the United States during 2011.

Methods.—We defined an outbreak-related case as a laboratory-confirmed infection with any of five outbreak-related subtypes of *Listeria monocytogenes* isolated during the period from August 1 through October 31, 2011. Multistate epidemiologic, trace-back, and environmental investigations were conducted, and outbreak-related cases were compared with sporadic cases reported previously to the Listeria Initiative, an enhanced surveillance system that routinely collects detailed information about U.S. cases of listeriosis.

Results.—We identified 147 outbreak-related cases in 28 states. The majority of patients (127 of 147, 86%) were 60 years of age or older. Seven infections among pregnant women and newborns and one related miscarriage were reported. Of 145 patients for whom information about hospitalization was available, 143 (99%) were hospitalized. Thirty-three of the 147 patients (22%) died. Patients with outbreak-related illness were significantly more likely to have eaten cantaloupe than were patients 60 years of age or older with sporadic illness (odds ratio, 8.5; 95% confidence interval, 1.3 to ∞). Cantaloupe and environmental samples collected during the investigation yielded isolates matching all five outbreak-related subtypes, confirming that whole cantaloupe produced by a single Colorado farm was the outbreak source. Unsanitary conditions identified in the processing facility operated by the farm probably resulted in contamination of cantaloupes with *L. monocytogenes*.

Conclusions.—Raw produce, including cantaloupe, can serve as a vehicle for listeriosis. This outbreak highlights the importance of preventing produce contamination within farm and processing environments.

▶ In 1988, Linnan et al described an outbreak of human listeriosis associated with Mexican soft cheese in the *New England Journal of Medicine*. The investigation of this outbreak led to the realization that the bacterial pathogen *Listeria monocytogenes*, the etiologic agent of listeriosis, is transmitted to humans via ingestion of contaminated food.[1] Many physicians remember the association of listeriosis with soft cheeses, but *L monocytogenes* is ubiquitous in the environment and has been found to contaminate many food products including dairy, meat, seafood, raw produce, and, more recently, whole cantaloupes. Yet, listeriosis is a rare disease: the Centers for Disease Control and Prevention reported only 1651 cases in the United States during 2009–2011. Why is the incidence so low if *L monocytogenes* is so widespread?

One plausible explanation is the very high infectious dose, which is estimated to be at least 1 billion bacteria. Food that is preprocessed with contaminated equipment and stored for relatively long periods of time at refrigerator temperatures is usually the culprit because *L monocytogenes*, unlike other bacterial pathogens, can replicate at 4 °C. In addition, listeriosis occurs almost exclusively in individuals with a predisposing condition. Pregnant women and neonates, older adults, and persons with immunocompromising conditions are at higher risk than others for invasive infection with *L monocytogenes*. The incidence of pregnancy-associated cases varies among case series, but overall approximately 14% of all cases are pregnancy associated. Although the mother typically has a mild, influenza-like syndrome, fetal and neonatal infection can be severe with neonatal case-fatality rates ranging from 22% to 45%. Listeriosis in immunocompromised nonpregnant individuals has a high mortality as well. Indeed, among the group of foodborne, gastrointestinal diseases, listeriosis has the highest case-fatality rate. Therefore, susceptible patients who present with signs and symptoms consistent with listeriosis have to be treated empirically until bacteremia or meningitis with *L monocytogenes* are ruled out. This includes febrile newborns, pregnant mothers, and nonpregnant immunocompromised individuals.

As pediatricians, we are particularly interested in the well-being and outcome of newborns. In contrast to the other high-risk groups, newborns are typically infected in utero via the hematogenous route. *L monocytogenes* colonizes the placenta via the maternal bloodstream and subsequently spreads to the fetus. Depending on the gestational age, this leads to spontaneous abortion, preterm labor, or neonatal disease. Combined data from the most recent and largest series of pregnancy-associated listeriosis in the United States include the reported illness and outcomes of approximately 350 mother and newborn pairs.[2,3] The most common clinical manifestations in the mother are fever, chills, flulike illness, preterm labor, abdominal pain, and decreased fetal movement. The average duration of maternal symptoms before diagnosis is 1 week, although incubation times up to 70 days have been reported. The most common clinical manifestations in live newborns are bacteremia and meningitis. Diagnosis can be made by positive culture from neonatal or maternal blood, neonatal cerebrospinal fluid, or placenta.

Treatment of listeriosis consists of intravenous antibiotics, most often ampicillin with or without gentamicin. Reports demonstrate that pregnancy-associated listeriosis can be effectively treated with intravenous (IV) antibiotics administered to the mother resulting in the birth of healthy newborns. During the third trimester the recommended duration of IV antibiotics is 14 days. Earlier in gestation, antibiotic therapy may have to be longer, although because of the lack of randomized case-control studies, the optimal duration of IV antibiotics is unknown. Among 14 case reports of women who developed listeriosis during the first or second trimester, 9 were treated with IV ampicillin or penicillin with or without gentamicin for 9 days to 4 weeks. In all instances, both mother and neonate survived without sequelae. Neonates with bacteremia and meningitis have to be treated with IV ampicillin for 14 and 21 days, respectively.

Listeriosis can occur either sporadically or as a foodborne disease outbreak. McCollum et al reports a large US listeriosis outbreak in 28 states associated with whole cantaloupes that lead to 147 cases (Fig 1 in the original article); 99% of patients were hospitalized, and the mortality rate was 22%. The majority of patients were 60 years of age or older, and 88% had 1 or more potentially immunosuppressive conditions. Four pregnant women and 3 neonates were infected, a relatively low number compared with previously reported outbreaks. Inadequate facility and equipment design of a cantaloupe farm in Colorado, which precluded effective cleaning and sanitization of cantaloupe-contact surfaces, was identified as the source of this outbreak. Overall, the affected patient population, clinical manifestations, and outcomes were relatively typical in comparison to other outbreaks of listeriosis. However, it is relatively unusual for whole fruits as opposed to precut cantaloupes to be the source of this outbreak.

The bottom line is that any food product that is not thoroughly reheated before consumption can be a vehicle for *L monocytogenes* transmission. At-risk patients need to be evaluated and empirically treated for listeriosis because of the high mortality associated with this disease.

A. Bakardjiev, MD

References

1. Linnan MJ, Mascola L, Lou XD, et al. Epidemic listeriosis associated with Mexican-style cheese. *N Engl J Med.* 1988;319:823-828.
2. Mylonakis E, Paliou M, Hohmann EL, Calderwood SB, Wing EJ. Listeriosis during pregnancy: a case series and review of 222 cases. *Medicine.* 2002;81:260-269.
3. Jackson KA, Iwamoto M, Swerdlow D. Pregnancy-associated listeriosis. *Epidemiol Infect.* 2010;138:1503-1509.

Elimination of Endemic Measles, Rubella, and Congenital Rubella Syndrome From the Western Hemisphere: The US Experience
Papania MJ, Wallace GS, Rota PA, et al (Ctrs for Disease Control and Prevention, Atlanta, GA; et al)
JAMA Pediatr 168:148-155, 2014

Importance.—To verify the elimination of endemic measles, rubella, and congenital rubella syndrome (CRS) from the Western hemisphere, the Pan American Health Organization requested each member country to compile a national elimination report. The United States documented the elimination of endemic measles in 2000 and of endemic rubella and CRS in 2004. In December 2011, the Centers for Disease Control and Prevention convened an external expert panel to review the evidence and determine whether elimination of endemic measles, rubella, and CRS had been sustained.

Objective.—To review the evidence for sustained elimination of endemic measles, rubella, and CRS from the United States through 2011.

Design, Setting, and Participants.—Review of data for measles from 2001 to 2011 and for rubella and CRS from 2004 to 2011 covering the US resident population and international visitors, including disease epidemiology, importation status of cases, molecular epidemiology, adequacy of surveillance, and population immunity as estimated by national vaccination coverage and serologic surveys.

Main Outcomes and Measures.—Annual numbers of measles, rubella, and CRS cases, by importation status, outbreak size, and distribution; proportions of US population seropositive for measles and rubella; and measles-mumps-rubella vaccination coverage levels.

Results.—Since 2001, US reported measles incidence has remained below 1 case per 1 000 000 population. Since 2004, rubella incidence has been below 1 case per 10 000 000 population, and CRS incidence has been below 1 case per 5 000 000 births. Eighty-eight percent of measles cases and 54% of rubella cases were internationally imported or epidemiologically or virologically linked to importation. The few cases not linked to importation were insufficient to represent endemic transmission. Molecular epidemiology indicated no endemic genotypes. The US surveillance system is adequate to detect endemic measles or rubella. Seroprevalence and vaccination coverage data indicate high levels of population immunity to measles and rubella.

Conclusions and Relevance.—The external expert panel concluded that the elimination of endemic measles, rubella, and CRS from the United States was sustained through 2011. However, international importation continues, and health care providers should suspect measles or rubella in patients with febrile rash illness, especially when associated with international travel or international visitors, and should report suspected cases to the local health department.

▶ The introduction of measles vaccine in 1963 and rubella vaccine in 1969 ushered in an era of unprecedented progress in the control of these diseases. The gradual introduction of school immunization requirements beginning in the late 1970s has led to a largely immune population in the United States and, despite some setbacks, the very real possibility of eradicating measles and rubella (Fig 1 in the original article). In 2000, the United States eliminated measles and rubella and congenital rubella syndrome in 2004.[1,2] As part of its efforts to eliminate these diseases from North and South America, the Pan American Health Organization in 2011 requested that each member country review its national data to verify elimination.[3] To assess whether elimination has been sustained in the United States, the Centers for Disease Control and Prevention (CDC) convened an expert panel in December 2011 to review data on measles, rubella, and congenital rubella syndrome epidemiology, molecular epidemiology, surveillance adequacy, and population immunity. This report describes the US experience with measles, rubella, and congenital rubella syndrome elimination and confirms their elimination.

There are 3 levels of public health control of disease transmission. Eradication refers to the reduction of the incidence of a disease to zero worldwide; this has only been achieved for smallpox; efforts for eradication of poliomyelitis and dracunculiasis are ongoing. Elimination is the absence of endemic disease transmission in a defined geographic area[4]; endemic transmission is usually defined as chains for transmission lasting ≥12 months. Control refers to reduction of incidence to disease to an acceptable (nonzero) level. It is important to note that elimination does not imply complete absence of cases because cases can be imported and lead to limited local transmission.

The incidence of measles in the United States has remained below 1 case per million since 2001. Of the 911 cases that occurred between 2001 and 2011, 372 (41%) were imported either by US citizens who acquired infection abroad or by foreign nationals visiting the United States. Fifty-two percent of measles cases were associated with outbreaks, primarily involving unvaccinated individuals. The longest outbreak lasted 11 weeks. Using molecular epidemiology techniques, there was no evidence of sustained transmission beyond 10 weeks of measles virus genotypes not stemming from importations. Additionally serological data from the 1999–2004 National Health and Nutrition Examination Survey (NHANES) among 6- to 29-year-old participants found measles antibody seroprevalence of 95.9%.

The incidence of reported rubella cases is even lower. Seventy-seven cases of rubella were reported in that United States between 2004 and 2011; 60% occurred in adults 20 to 49 years of age, and 33 cases (58% for whom country of birth was known) cases were in people born outside the United States. Forty-two cases were either imported or transmitted from an imported case. There were 4 cases of congenital rubella syndrome during this period; 3 were in women exposed overseas, and 1 was in an American woman who had been previously immunized. NHANES data indicate rubella antibody seroprevalence was 91.3% in 2004.

Immunization against both measles and rubella is high in the United States. States estimate that 85.1% to 97.8% of 19- to 35-month-old children had received measles, mumps, rubella vaccine (MMR) in 2010 and that 94.8% of kindergarten entrants had received 2 doses of MMR in 2010. The proportion of students who claim exemptions from immunization varies by state from 0.1% in Minnesota to 6.2% in Washington, and students whose families elect to exempt them from school immunization requirements for nonmedical reasons tend to cluster together, which can lead to situations in which sustained transmission occurs.

The report concludes that measles, rubella, and congenital rubella syndrome continue to occur at only very low levels in the United States, consistent with elimination. Pediatricians in practice can contribute to the national and international effort to eliminate measles by immunizing their patients and discouraging personal belief exemptions to immunization, by diagnosing and rapidly reporting suspected cases to local health departments, and by cooperating with health department investigations. Patients with febrile nonvesicular rash illnesses returning from international travel should trigger a high index of suspicion.

G. W. Rutherford, MD, AM

References

1. Flebelkorn AP, Redd SB, Gallagher K, et al. Measles in the United States during the postelimination era. *J Infect Dis.* 2010;202:1520-1528.
2. Meissner HC, Reef SE, Cochi S. Elimination of rubella from the United States: a milestone on the road to global elimination. *Pediatrics.* 2006;117:933-935.
3. World Health Organization. Progress towards measles elimination, Western hemisphere, 2002-2003. *Wkly Epidemiol Rec.* 2004;79:149-151.
4. World Health Organization. Monitoring progress towards measles elimination. *Wkly Epidemiol Rec.* 2010;85:490-494.

Epidemiology of Tuberculosis in Young Children in the United States

Pang J, Teeter LD, Katz DJ, et al (Univ of Washington, Seattle; Houston Methodist Res Inst, TX; Ctrs for Disease Control and Prevention, Atlanta, GA; et al)
Pediatrics 133:e494-e504, 2014

Objectives.—To estimate tuberculosis (TB) rates among young children in the United States by children's and parents' birth origins and describe the epidemiology of TB among young children who are foreign-born or have at least 1 foreign-born parent.

Methods.—Study subjects were children <5 years old diagnosed with TB in 20 US jurisdictions during 2005–2006. TB rates were calculated from jurisdictions' TB case counts and American Community Survey population estimates. An observational study collected demographics, immigration and travel histories, and clinical and source case details from parental interviews and health department and TB surveillance records.

Results.—Compared with TB rates among US-born children with US-born parents, rates were 32 times higher in foreign-born children and 6 times higher in US-born children with foreign-born parents. Most TB cases (53%) were among the 29% of children who were US born with foreign-born parents. In the observational study, US-born children with foreign-born parents were more likely than foreign-born children to be infants (30% vs 7%), Hispanic (73% vs 37%), diagnosed through contact tracing (40% vs 7%), and have an identified source case (61% vs 19%); two-thirds of children were exposed in the United States.

Conclusions.—Young children who are US born of foreign-born parents have relatively high rates of TB and account for most cases in this age group. Prompt diagnosis and treatment of adult source cases, effective contact investigations prioritizing young contacts, and targeted testing and treatment of latent TB infection are necessary to reduce TB morbidity in this population.

▶ Current estimates of childhood (0–14 years of age) tuberculosis (TB) are probably inaccurate, and this is particularly true for children less than 5 years of age. This is because of the underreporting of childhood TB, but mainly because of the difficulty confirming TB in children who usually have paucibacillary TB and from whom it is difficult to obtain suitable specimens for bacteriologic confirmation of TB.

Childhood TB was for decades a neglected disease; children were not regarded as of epidemiologic importance because they are rarely infectious. However, young children (aged < 5 years) are markers of recent transmission of *Mycobacterium tuberculosis*, and the very young develop the most serious forms of disease with high morbidity and mortality. Older children and young adolescents may contribute to continuous spread of *M tuberculosis* because they will more frequently suffer from infectious adult-type pulmonary TB. Furthermore, infected children are a future source of TB disease (adult reactivation disease), and in developing communities children will constitute a significant proportion of the TB disease burden.

World Health Organization (WHO) notification data report only children with TB < 15 years despite recommendations in 2006 for disaggregation by ages 0 to 4 and 5 to 14 years. WHO estimates for children with TB are very low—5 30 000 children in 2012 (6% of total TB burden),[1] compared with a recent meta-analysis based on published cases that estimated almost 1 million cases in 2010.[2] The natural history of TB disease after infection predicts higher rates in young children (< 5 years) compared with older children. This often does not reflect in studies, such as a recent household contact study from Karachi, Pakistan, in which 73% of the identified TB cases < 15 years of age were children between 11 to 14 years of age, most likely missing the young children, as bacteriologic confirmation is easier in older children who can effectively cough and expectorate sputum.[3]

The diagnosis of TB in young children often requires a high index of suspicion and the acceptance of a diagnosis on grounds of a constellation of history of contact with a TB source case, symptoms, signs, and chest radiographic findings without bacteriologic confirmation. Even when such cases are diagnosed, they are often not reported, leading to a low estimate in especially the 0- to 4- year-old age group.

Finding ways to improve detection of TB in young children is important. One such method is identifying high-risk groups, such as foreign-born children in developed countries and, as shown by Pang et al,[4] even children born in developed countries to foreign-born parents (Table 2in the original article).

Although their data are most likely correct, there is the risk of selection bias because health workers may have included TB in the differential diagnosis of foreign-born families, while they may not have included it in US-born families' differential diagnosis. The fact that 64% (44 of 69 in whom cultures were done) US-born children had culture-confirmed TB compared with only 7% (1 of 14) foreign-born children may indicate later presentation or late consideration of TB in US-born children, given that, on the other hand, contact with a source case was known in only 19% of foreign-born children compared with 61% in US-born children.[4]

Estimates of childhood TB as well as disease spectrum and severity vary widely in different countries. In low-TB-burden countries, population pyramids have a narrow base of young children, compared with developing countries with high TB burden where the population pyramid's base of young children as well as young adults is often wide. This distribution of age within populations partially explains the higher proportion of young children contributing to TB notifications (up to 20%) in high-burden countries compared with developed countries with low TB burden (5% young children).

The low burden of TB disease and better resources make it possible for low-burden TB countries not to rely only on passive (symptomatic) screening for TB but active screening of high-risk groups including systematic contact investigation of identified TB cases. This allows for improved and earlier diagnosis, resulting in a lower frequency of severe disease, as well as improved recording and reporting of cases. It is thus interesting to note that only 56% of reported cases in the study had bacteriologic results available or done and that more than half of those with cultures for *M tuberculosis* done, had a positive result—an indication of possible underreporting or underdiagnosis.

In high-TB-burden countries both underdiagnosis and underreporting of TB in children is well known. Screening of child contacts of infectious TB cases is rarely done, and passive case finding in children presenting with symptoms relies heavily on the individual health worker's index of suspicion of TB and available diagnostic resources. Even if the diagnosis is made, reporting of cases remains poor. A recent study from Cape Town, South Africa, showed that only approximately 60% of culture-confirmed hospital-diagnosed cases were recorded in an electronic TB register, with the most serious cases (death and TB meningitis) the least likely to be reported.[5] In another study from Indonesia only 1.6% of hospital-diagnosed TB cases in children was notified to the National TB Program in Java.[6]

Since 2006 WHO requested reporting of TB in children disaggregated according to ages 0 to 4 and 5 to 14 years. This stratification is to assist in assessing the accuracy of child TB notification data from different countries, but unfortunately this is still incompletely done. Some high-burden countries only report sputum smear-positive for acid-fast bacilli cases, which presents in 5% to 10% of young children with TB, if specimens are obtained.

Suspicion is the key to the diagnosis of childhood TB, and the experience of Pang et al[4] emphasizes again the great importance of history when considering the diagnosis of TB in children in a low-incidence setting. Recent, or distant immigration from high-TB-burden countries must constitute a risk factor for childhood TB. Cough for any length of time in a household contact, or in the child, should lead to a consideration of possible TB and appropriate investigation.

H. S. Schaaf, MBChB

P. R. Donald, MBChB

References

1. World Health Organization. *Global Tuberculosis Report.* Geneva, Switzerland: WHO; 2013. WHO/HTM/TB/2013.11.
2. Jenkins HE, Tolman AW, Yuen CM, et al. Incidence of multidrug-resistant tuberculosis disease in children: systematic review and global estimates. *Lancet.* 2014;383:1572-1579, http://www.ncbi.nlm.nih.gov/pubmed/?term=jenkins+he%2C+becerra+m.
3. Batra S, Ayaz A, Murtaza A, Ahmad S, Hasan R, Pfau R. Childhood tuberculosis in household contacts of newly diagnosed TB patients. *PLoS One.* 2012;7:e40880.

4. Pang J, Teeter LD, Katz DJ, et al. Tuberculosis epidemiologic studies consortium. Epidemiology of tuberculosis in young children in the United States. *Pediatrics.* 2014;133:e494-e504, http://www.ncbi.nlm.nih.gov/pubmed/24515517.
5. Du Preez K, Schaaf HS, Dunbar R, et al. Incomplete registration and reporting of culture-confirmed childhood tuberculosis diagnosed in hospital. *Public Health Action.* 2011;1:19-24, http://www.ingentaconnect.com/content/iuatld/pha.
6. Lestari T, Probandari A, Hurtig AK, Utarini A. High caseload of childhood tuberculosis in hospitals on Java Island, Indonesia: a cross sectional study. *BMC Public Health.* 2011;11:784, http://www.ncbi.nlm.nih.gov/pubmed/21985569.

Absence of Detectable HIV-1 Viremia after Treatment Cessation in an Infant

Persaud D, Gay H, Ziemniak C, et al (Johns Hopkins Univ School of Medicine, Baltimore, MD; Univ of Mississippi Med Ctr, Jackson; et al)

N Engl J Med 369:1828-1835, 2013

An infant born to a woman with human immunodeficiency virus type 1 (HIV-1) infection began receiving antiretroviral therapy (ART) 30 hours after birth owing to high-risk exposure. ART was continued when detection of HIV-1 DNA and RNA on repeat testing met the standard diagnostic criteria for infection. After therapy was discontinued (when the child was 18 months of age), levels of plasma HIV-1 RNA, proviral DNA in peripheral-blood mononuclear cells, and HIV-1 antibodies, as assessed by means of clinical assays, remained undetectable in the child through 30 months of age. This case suggests that very early ART in infants may alter the establishment and long-term persistence of HIV-1 infection.

▶ It has been more than 30 years since the first descriptions of what would come to be known as AIDS were published in the *Morbidity and Mortality Weekly Report.*[1] In that time, tremendous progress has been made in the prevention and treatment of human immunodeficiency virus (HIV) worldwide. The uniqueness of this virus lies with the cell types in which it establishes infection; the relative lack of adaptation between host and pathogen, leading to prolonged and progressive infection; and the fact that it is a sexually transmitted infection that relentlessly destroys the host immune system, leading to opportunistic infections and death.

Before the roll out of antiretroviral therapy worldwide, life expectancy in the countries with the greatest burden of HIV had plummeted by as much as 20 years. Although advances in our understanding of this disease have been accumulating, they have done so in a Hegelian fashion with occasional major scientific/clinical advances in an otherwise steady accumulation of knowledge. These breakthroughs have usually led to unanticipated outcomes.

For example, although the introduction of zidovudine monotherapy in the late 1980s, the first available antiretroviral, did not lead to sustained suppression of HIV or improved long-term survival in HIV-infected adults, it demonstrated a powerful protective effect against the transmission of HIV from mothers to infants and remains the standard of care for perinatal prophylaxis today. The introduction of protease inhibitors in 1996–1997 has resulted in the prolonged survival of patients with HIV by the use of potent combination therapy. However, protease inhibitor–based therapy allowed researchers ultimately to find the cellular reservoir, central memory T cells, by extrapolating from the kinetics of viral decline on potent combination therapy. This reservoir currently prevents full eradication of HIV from an individual. Large-scale rollout of antiretroviral medications to less resourced areas has resulted in millions of individuals benefiting from potent combination therapy but studies still show that only a minority of individuals achieve an undetectable plasma RNA once the treatment cascade from original testing to initiation of therapy is compiled.

It is with this perspective that the report from Persaud et al in the *New England Journal of Medicine* has been published. The investigators describe the clinical course of a premature infant (35 weeks) delivered to a mother who was unaware of her HIV status and thus did not receive prenatal antiretrovirals (ARVs) or intravenous azidothymidine (AZT) during delivery. The infant was started on triple combination therapy at 31 hours of life after HIV DNA and RNA analyses had been sent from separate specimens. The results subsequently showed the infant to be HIV infected with plasma RNA level greater than the mothers' and a positive DNA polymerase chain reaction (PCR). Therapy was tailored at 1 week of life, and the infant was followed for the first 18 months with a rapid response to treatment and undetectable plasma RNA at the time the child was lost to follow-up.

The child's mother brought her back to care 6 months later and reported that no therapy had been given. Routine laboratory analyses were performed, and to the surprise of the treating physician, there was no evidence of HIV infection using standard tests including Western blot, HIV RNA, and HIV DNA. Several experts in pediatric immunology and the kinetics of the viral reservoir were contacted, and the child underwent more sophisticated testing, which again failed to reveal evidence of ongoing HIV infection. If an assay was positive, it was intermittently so and always at the limit of detection of the study, casting doubt as to whether the result was "real" or spurious. The child has been off therapy for 2 years and continues to have periodic follow-up to determine her HIV status.

Although clearly a benefit to this young individual, this case raises a multitude of questions in the basic and clinical sciences as well as future issues of implementation. When does in utero infection occur? Traditionally, an infant is thought to have been infected in utero if an HIV nucleic acid–based test drawn before 48 hours of life is positive. Historically, the nucleic acid test has been a DNA PCR indicating early integration of viral DNA into the host cell, but current standards also allow for the use of an RNA PCR for diagnosis as well. Although these tests indicate that the infant was infected before delivery, they do not indicate when infection actually occurred. The fetal thymus starts to produce T cells at the end of the first trimester, and recent fetal tissue analyses have indicated that there are abundant CD4+ CCR5+ cells in intestinal tissue, the primary target of acute HIV infection, as early as 22 weeks' gestation.[2] In theory, then, it is possible for a fetus to be infected with HIV at least as early as 22 weeks' gestation and possibly as early as 14 to 15 weeks. Clinical analyses looking at in utero infection compared with the timing of maternal ARV initiation speculate that the majority of infections occur between 28 and 36 weeks' gestation because there appear to be lower in utero infection rates when women are started on antiretroviral therapy at 28 weeks compared with 36 weeks' gestation.[3] Of course, it is not known with any certainty whether a fetus can be infected as early as 15 to 20 weeks' gestation or that, if it were, it could survive to delivery; however, the potential exists. Once an infant is identified as HIV infected in utero, what are the treatment options for immediate therapy?

Current ARV treatment regimens in HIV infected neonates are extremely limited. Our knowledge of neonatal antiretroviral medication pharmacokinetics (PK) provides clinicians with treatment dosing for only a few nucleoside analogues at birth including AZT, lamivudine (3TC), emtricitabine (FTC), and stavudine (d4T) in term infants. Only 2 of these drugs have limited PK supporting preterm infant dosing (AZT and 3TC).[4] There are also data on treatment dosing starting at 2 weeks of age in term neonates for didanosine (DDI), nevirapine, and lopinavir/ritonavir. For all other antiretrovirals, PK and safety data are not sufficient to allow recommendations for doses appropriate for use in HIV-infected neonates. The infant in this case report was initially treated with AZT and 3TC at standard doses for age, and nevirapine 2 mg/kg/dose BID. Simulations from previous studies support an investigational dose of nevirapine of 6 mg/kg/dose BID for the first 4 weeks of life in term neonates (to be used in International Maternal, Pediatric, Adolescent AIDS Clinical Trial [IMPAACT] P1115).

Lopinavir/ritonavir is no longer recommended in infants less than 2 weeks of age and 42 weeks' post conceptional age because there have been serious side effects (bradycardia, complete atrioventricular block, heart failure, renal failure, respiratory failure, metabolic acidosis, hypotonia, and central nervous system depression), especially in preterm infants. The liquid formulation contains ethanol and propylene glycol and the contribution of these compounds in conjunction with lopinavir/ritonavir with these observed toxicities remains unclear. Although there is interest in using integrase inhibitors for both prevention and treatment of HIV in neonates, current PK analysis of maternal dosing with washout studies in neonates has led to highly variable elimination with half-lives of 9 to 88 hours in the first days of life.[5] In addition, integrase inhibitors compete for bilirubin binding sites and could theoretically lead to kernicterus or bilirubin encephalopathy. However, finding an appropriate dose of nevirapine, which can be used as a bridge to the use of alternative agents, appears to be the least insurmountable of the potential problems faced by this strategy.

When should therapy begin? As soon as possible after birth? One week? Two weeks? This remains an important and as yet unanswered question. Studies in adult patients who were identified with acute HIV infection only 1 to 2 weeks after acquisition are underway. Evidence thus far has shown that it is possible to reduce the potential reservoir of HIV if therapy is initiated as soon as infection is identified. Whether remission can be obtained, as in the child described in this study, remains to be documented. There is also circumstantial evidence that neonates have a smaller potential T-cell reservoir because central memory T cells in the peripheral blood of newborns are detected consistently but in small numbers.[6] However, memory T cells can be tissue specific, and as mentioned, there are ample intestinal T cells susceptible to infection and to transformation to memory cells early in gestation. Also, there is a recent in vitro study indicating that maternal exposure to malaria antigens primes the fetus to produce memory cells that are more susceptible to HIV acquisition.[7] In addition, the size of the reservoir is probably also larger than was first described. Recent evidence from the Siliciano laboratory[8] has indicated that the memory reservoir is 60-fold greater than the standard assays have indicated. Whether the reservoir is more established in neonates than previously thought or whether it is primarily established after delivery is a critical question to be answered in any controlled trial because the success or failure of this strategy may depend on this single issue.

Finally, where does this strategy fit into the armamentarium used to prevent perinatal transmission? Clearly, the now well-established protocol of treating HIV-infected women maximally during pregnancy and providing prophylaxis to the infant after delivery reduces perinatal transmission to less than 2%. This is a primary prevention strategy adding clear medical benefit to the mother. Reducing the number of perinatal transmissions worldwide will rest predominantly on identifying pregnant women as early as possible who are HIV-infected and starting them on treatment. The strategy used for the infant in this report represents a failure of identification, maintenance in care, and primary prevention. If it can be replicated, then it has potential in countries with low numbers of HIV-infected neonates to reduce those numbers even further for persons who slip through without notice, but it is probably impractical as a widespread intervention given current data.

HIV has become one of the most studied and intransigent pathogens in human history in only 30 years and remains highly stigmatizing for those it affects. The report by Persaud et al has reinvigorated the field concerning the possibility of remission after established infection and the potential for "cure." It has raised many questions posed here and probably more to come as investigators begin to plot a trajectory for controlled trials. With some luck and persistence, it may lead to one of those Hegelian moments.

Addendum: After completing this commentary, the National Institutes of Health announced that at a routine clinical visit, the child in question had a detectable HIV RNA assay twice within a 3-day period and a decrease in T-cell counts. She is now back on ARV and doing well. Although a disappointment, it is still a remarkable achievement for her to have been off therapy for more than 2 years without evidence of HIV infection. All of the questions raised in this commentary remain valid and will require further study to increase the probability of prolonged remission and the potential for "cure" in the future.

M. D. Foca, MD

References

1. Centers for Disease Control (CDC). Pneumocystis pneumonia—Los Angeles. *MMWR Morb Mortal Wkly Rep.* 1981;30:250-252.
2. Bunders MJ, van der Loos CM, Klarenbeek PL, et al. Memory CD4+ CCR5+ T cells are abundantly present in the gut of newborn infants to facilitate mother-to-child transmission of HIV-1. *Blood.* 2012;120:4383-4390.
3. Lallemant M, Jourdain G, Le Coeur S, et al. A trial of shortened zidovudine regimens to prevent mother-to-child transmission of human immunodeficiency virus

type 1. Perinatal HIV Prevention Trial (Thailand) Investigators. *N Engl J Med.* 2000;343:982-991.

4. Mirochnick M, Nielsen-Saines K, Pilotto JH, et al. Nelfinavir and lamivudine pharmacokinetics during the first two weeks of life. *Pediatr Infect Dis J.* 2011; 30:769-772.

5. Clarke DF, Acosta E, Bryson Y, et al. Raltegravir (RAL) pharmacokinetics (PK) and safety in neonates: washout PK of transplacental RAL (IMPAACT P1097). 13th International Workshop on Clinical Pharmacology of HIV Therapy; March 16-18, 2012; Barcelona, Spain. Oral Abstract O_22.

6. Schatorjé EJ, Gemen EF, Driessen GJA, Leuvenink J, van Hout RW, de Vries E. Paediatric reference values for the peripheral T cell compartment. *Scand J Immunol.* 2012;75:436-444.

7. Steiner KL, Malhotra I, Mungai PL, Muchiri EM, Dent AE, King CL. In utero activation of fetal memory T cells alters host regulatory gene expression and affects HIV susceptibility. *Virology.* 2012;425:23-30.

8. Ho YC, Shan L, Hosmane NN, et al. Replication-competent noninduced proviruses in the latent reservoir increase barrier to HIV-1 cure. *Cell.* 2013;155: 540-551.

Comparative Effectiveness of Empiric Antibiotics for Community-Acquired Pneumonia

Queen MA, Myers AL, Hall M, et al (Univ of Missouri School of Medicine, Kansas City; The Children's Hosp Association, Overland Park, KS; et al)
Pediatrics 133:e23-e29, 2014

Background and Objective.—Narrow-spectrum antibiotics are recommended as the first-line agent for children hospitalized with community-acquired pneumonia (CAP). There is little scientific evidence to support that this consensus-based recommendation is as effective as the more commonly used broad-spectrum antibiotics. The objective was to compare the effectiveness of empiric treatment with narrow-spectrum therapy versus broad-spectrum therapy for children hospitalized with uncomplicated CAP.

Methods.—This multicenter retrospective cohort study using medical records included children aged 2 months to 18 years at 4 children's hospitals in 2010 with a discharge diagnosis of CAP. Patients receiving either narrow-spectrum or broad-spectrum therapy in the first 2 days of hospitalization were eligible. Patients were matched by using propensity scores that determined each patient's likelihood of receiving empiric narrow or broad coverage. A multivariate logistic regression analysis evaluated the relationship between antibiotic and hospital length of stay (LOS), 7-day readmission, standardized daily costs, duration of fever, and duration of supplemental oxygen.

Results.—Among 492 patients, 52% were empirically treated with a narrow-spectrum agent and 48% with a broad-spectrum agent. In the adjusted analysis, the narrow-spectrum group had a 10-hour shorter LOS ($P = .04$). There was no significant difference in duration of oxygen, duration of fever, or readmission. When modeled for LOS, there was no

TABLE 2.—Adjusted Outcomes

	Narrow-Spectrum ($n = 256$)	Broad-Spectrum ($n = 236$)	P
LOS, h	43 (39−46)	52.3 (48−57)	.04
Duration of supplemental oxygen, h	15.6 (12−20)	21.8 (17−29)	.18
Duration of fever, h	6.5 (5−9)	9.1 (7−12)	.23
Standardized cost per day, $	2209 (2088−2338)	2160 (2042−2286)	.62
Standardized pharmacy cost per day, $	170 (153−188)	188 (170−208)	.26
Readmission within 7 days[a]	Reference	5.1 (0.3−83.6)	.25

Data are least-squares means (95% CI) unless otherwise indicated and were adjusted for age, gender, race, government insurance, concurrent diagnosis of asthma or reactive airway disease, previous antibiotic therapy, atypical antibiotic therapy, presence of effusion on chest radiograph, diagnosis of viral lower respiratory tract infection, admission to the ICU, blood culture utilization, presence of a positive blood culture, baseline hospital rates for cephalosporin use, tachypnea, fever, and abnormal WBC.
[a]Data are adjusted odds ratios (95% CI) for broad-spectrum/penicillin therapy.
(Reprinted from Queen MA, Myers AL, Hall M, et al. Comparative Effectiveness of Empiric Antibiotics for Community-Acquired Pneumonia. Pediatrics. 2014;133:e23-e29. Copyright © 2014, by the American Academy of Pediatrics.)

difference in average daily standardized cost ($P = .62$) or average daily standardized pharmacy cost ($P = .26$).

Conclusions.—Compared with broad-spectrum agents, narrow-spectrum antibiotic coverage is associated with similar outcomes. Our findings support national consensus recommendations for the use of narrow-spectrum antibiotics in children hospitalized with CAP (Table 2).

▶ Community-acquired pneumonia (CAP) is common both worldwide and in the United States, where it is diagnosed in more than 150 000 children annually.[1] In US children's hospitals, CAP accounts for more antibiotic days of therapy than any other condition.[2] Therefore, optimizing antibiotic use for pediatric CAP is a high priority. In 2011, the Pediatric Infectious Diseases Society (PIDS) and the Infectious Diseases Society of America (IDSA) addressed this issue with the first publication of clinical practice guidelines for the management of CAP in children.[3] These guidelines recommend narrow-spectrum antibiotics—amoxicillin, ampicillin, or penicillin—for most children with uncomplicated CAP. This decision was based on the epidemiology of pediatric CAP, for which *Streptococcus pneumoniae* is the most common bacterial cause. Importantly, greater than 90% of the *S pneumoniae* currently circulating are susceptible to penicillin for infections where high drug levels can be achieved, including the respiratory tract. The effectiveness of narrow-spectrum therapy for pneumonia has been demonstrated in pediatric studies,[4,5] but multicenter studies using detailed chart review had not yet been performed.

Queen et al have answered this call. These investigators conducted a multi-center retrospective cohort study comparing narrow-spectrum antibiotics with broad-spectrum antibiotics for the treatment of children hospitalized with CAP.[6] Their analysis included 492 children admitted to 1 of 4 freestanding children's hospitals during calendar year 2010. To align with the PIDS/IDSA guidelines, they focused on previously healthy children without severe or complicated disease. The outcomes included hospital length of stay (LOS); readmission within 7 days; surrogates for duration of clinical illness including fever and need for supplemental oxygen; and cost. Children with pneumonia were identified using the Pediatric Health Information System database; however, chart review was performed on each patient to collect supplemental clinical, diagnostic, and therapeutic information.

In the final cohort, roughly half of these children were given narrow-spectrum agents (penicillin, amoxicillin, ampicillin, or amoxicillin-clavulanate), the other half receiving broader-spectrum drugs (second- or third-generation cephalosporins or quinolones). Combination therapy with a macrolide was allowed but occurred in the minority (16%) of patients. To address the threat of confounding by indication—that children given broad-spectrum agents might be sicker than those given narrow-spectrum drugs—the authors used propensity score matching using a variety of clinical and demographic variables. In the final analyses, outcomes were similar between children treated with narrow- or broad-spectrum antibiotics (Table 2).

The strengths of this study included the multicenter cohort design, detailed chart review to both validate the diagnosis and collect important clinical outcome data, extensive use of exclusion to identify children who fit the criteria for narrow-spectrum antibiotic use according to PIDS/IDSA guidelines, and propensity score modeling to address the potential for confounding by indication. Notable limitations included the classification of amoxicillin-clavulanate as a narrow-spectrum drug for CAP and the lack of power calculations for the subcohorts without macrolide use or for each clinical outcome.

Overall, Queen et al should be commended for this important study. These data support PIDS/IDSA recommendations for the use of narrow-spectrum antibiotics for children hospitalized for pneumonia. Because of the known prevalence of this condition coupled with recent studies demonstrating that most hospitalized children receive broad-spectrum drugs,[5,7] the impact of these findings can be substantial. Given the global crisis of antimicrobial resistance, it is critical to find evidence-based approaches to limit the unnecessary use of broad-spectrum antimicrobial agents. Prescribing penicillin or ampicillin for children hospitalized with CAP is an excellent start.

J. S. Gerber, MD, PhD

References

1. Lee GE, Lorch SA, Sheffler-Collins S, Kronman MP, Shah SS. National hospitalization trends for pediatric pneumonia and associated complications. *Pediatrics.* 2010;126:204-213.
2. Gerber JS, Kronman MP, Ross RK, et al. Identifying targets for antimicrobial stewardship in children's hospitals. *Infect Control Hosp Epidemiol.* 2013;34:1252-1258.
3. Bradley JS, Byington CL, Shah SS, et al. The management of community-acquired pneumonia in infants and children older than 3 months of age: clinical practice guidelines by the Pediatric Infectious Diseases Society and the Infectious Diseases Society of America. *Clin Infect Dis.* 2011;53:e25-e76.
4. Neuman MI, Hall M, Hersh AL, et al. Influence of hospital guidelines on management of children hospitalized with pneumonia. *Pediatrics.* 2012;130:e823-e830.
5. Williams DJ, Hall M, Shah SS, et al. Narrow vs broad-spectrum antimicrobial therapy for children hospitalized with pneumonia. *Pediatrics.* 2013;132:e1141-e1148.

6. Queen MA, Myers AL, Hall M, et al. Comparative effectiveness of empiric antibiotics for community-acquired pneumonia. *Pediatrics.* 2014;133:e23-e29.
7. Ross RK, Hersh AL, Kronman MP, et al. Impact of infectious diseases society of america/pediatric infectious diseases society guidelines on treatment of community-acquired pneumonia in hospitalized children. *Clin Infect Dis.* 2014;58: 834-838.

Empiric Combination Therapy for Gram-Negative Bacteremia

Sick AC, Tschudin-Sutter S, Turnbull AE, et al (Univ of Pittsburgh Med Ctr, PA; Univ Hosp Basel, Switzerland; Johns Hopkins Bloomberg School of Public Health, Baltimore, MD; et al)
Pediatrics 133:e1148-e1155, 2014

Background.—Empirical combination antibiotic regimens consisting of a β-lactam and an aminoglycoside are frequently employed in the pediatric population. Data to demonstrate the comparative benefit of empirical β-lactam combination therapy relative to monotherapy for culture-proven Gram-negative bacteremia are lacking in the pediatric population.

Methods.—We conducted a retrospective cohort study of children treated for Gram-negative bacteremia at The Johns Hopkins Hospital from 2004 through 2012. We compared the estimated odds of 10-day mortality and the relative duration of bacteremia for children receiving empirical combination therapy versus empirical monotherapy using 1:1 nearest-neighbor propensity-score matching without replacement, before performing regression analysis.

Results.—We identified 226 matched pairs of patients well balanced on baseline covariates. Ten-day mortality was similar between the groups (odds ratio, 0.84; 95% confidence interval [CI], 0.28 to 1.71). Use of empirical combination therapy was not associated with a decrease in the duration of bacteremia (−0.51 days; 95% CI, −2.22 to 1.48 days). There was no survival benefit when evaluating 10-day mortality for the severely ill (pediatric risk of mortality III score ≥15) or profoundly neutropenic patients (absolute neutrophil count ≤100 cells/mL) receiving combination therapy. However, a survival benefit was observed when empirical combination therapy was prescribed for children growing multidrug-resistant Gram-negative organisms from the bloodstream (odds ratio, 0.70; 95% CI, 0.51 to 0.84).

Conclusions.—Although there appears to be no advantage to the routine addition of an aminoglycoside to a β-lactam as empirical therapy for children who have Gram-negative bacteremia, children who have risk factors for MDRGN organisms appear to benefit from this practice.

▶ Sepsis due to Gram-negative bacteremia occurs in normal hosts but is a more frequent problem for the immune-compromised or neutropenic patient. Delayed treatment or improper antibiotic choice is associated with adverse outcomes, so appropriate empiric antibiotic treatment is crucial. The issue of combination therapy (broad-spectrum β-lactam plus aminoglycoside) versus single agent (broad-spectrum beta lactam) for children with Gram-negative sepsis remains unsettled. Although early trials showed a survival advantage for combination therapy, more recent studies with broader-spectrum β-lactams do not show an all-cause mortality advantage of combination therapy. Furthermore, combination therapy is associated with increased adverse events. That the issue is unsettled is evidenced by the number of Cochrane Database Systematic Reviews on this clinical question analyzing nearly 70 studies involving thousands of children and adults.[1-3]

The authors report data from Johns Hopkins Hospital where they analyzed outcome in patients with Gram-negative bacteremia comparing patients treated with a broad-spectrum β-lactam antibiotic to patients given broad-spectrum β-lactam antibiotic plus an aminoglycoside. The design was retrospective and monotherapy versus combination therapy patient pairs were matched by propensity-score of illness severity. They document that mortality is not significantly improved by the use of combination therapy unless the infection is due to an organism that is resistant to the chosen agent. Because antibiotic susceptibility is not known at the time that therapy is initiated, they advise considering host or local factors that may increase the likelihood of multidrug-resistant Gram-negative bacterial carriage and using that information to guide mono versus combination empiric therapy.

The definitive, prospective, double-blind, randomized controlled trial to address this clinical issue would be challenging because Gram-negative sepsis cannot be easily differentiated from Gram-positive sepsis, and empiric antibiotic regimens to compare would be even more complex. However, these data do provide useful information that can influence practice. Given the benefit in patients with infection due to resistant bacteria, the authors advise that empiric combination treatment should be reserved for those at high risk of this condition. These include patients with known colonization with multidrug-resistant Gram-negative bacteria (MDRGNs), patients treated with broad-spectrum antibiotics within 30 days, patients undergoing prolonged hospitalization, and a high prevalence of MDRGNs in the community. The authors then point out that knowledge of susceptibility data in one's hospital and community will allow rational choices to be made about empirical use of beta lactam.

Finally, their primary finding of equivalent survival with susceptible organisms is also critically important and should have an impact on practice. Patients given monotherapy who had Gram-negative bacteremia from a susceptible organism had comparable survival and cleared their bacteremia as quickly as those given combination treatment. Therefore, even if a high-risk patient is initially given combination therapy, if susceptibility data show bacterial sensitivity to the β-lactam, the aminoglycoside could be stopped to reduce risk of toxicity or other adverse events.

J. Tureen, MD

References

1. Paul M, Soares-Weiser K, Grozinsky S, Leibovici L. Beta-lactam versus beta-lactam-aminoglycoside combination therapy in cancer patients with neutropaenia. *Cochrane Database Syst Rev.* 2003;(3):CD003038.

2. Paul M, Silbiger I, Grozinsky S, Soares-Weiser K, Leibovici L. Beta lactam antibiotic monotherapy versus beta lactam-aminoglycoside antibiotic combination therapy for sepsis. *Cochrane Database Syst Rev.* 2006;(1):CD003344.
3. Paul M, Lador A, Grozinsky-Glasberg S, Leibovici L. Beta lactam antibiotic monotherapy versus beta lactam-aminoglycoside antibiotic combination therapy for sepsis. *Cochrane Database Syst Rev.* 2014;(1):CD003344.

The influence of children's day care on antibiotic seeking: a mixed methods study

Rooshenas L, Wood F, Brookes-Howell L, et al (Univ of Bristol, UK; Cardiff Univ, UK)
Br J Gen Pract 64:e302-e312, 2014

Background.—Preschool-aged children are the highest consumers of antibiotics, but consult mainly for viral infections. Little is known about how day care, which is common in this age group, influences primary care consulting and treatment-seeking behaviours.

Aim.—To investigate daycare providers' approaches to excluding and/or readmitting children with infections, and the consequences for parents' consulting and antibiotic-seeking behaviours.

Design and Setting.—Cross-sectional survey, document analysis, and qualitative interviews of daycare providers and parents in South East Wales, UK.

Method.—A total of 328 daycare providers were asked to complete a survey about infection exclusion practices and to provide a copy of their sickness exclusion policy. Next, 52 semi-structured interviews were conducted with purposively selected questionnaire responders and parents using their services. Questionnaire responses underwent bivariate analysis, policies underwent document analysis, and interviews were thematically analysed using constant comparison methods.

Results.—In total 217 out of 328 (66%) daycare providers responded; 82 out of 199 (41%) reported advising parents that their child may need antibiotics and 199 out of 214 (93%) reported advising general practice consultations. Interviews confirmed that such advice was routine, and beliefs about antibiotic indications often went against clinical guidelines: 24% ($n = 136$) of sickness exclusion policies mentioning infections made at least one non-evidence-based indication for 'treatment' or antibiotics. Parent interviews revealed that negotiating daycare requirements lowered thresholds for consulting and encouraged antibiotic seeking.

Conclusion.—Daycare providers encourage parents to consult general practice and seek antibiotics through non-evidence-based policies and practices. Parents' perceptions of daycare providers' requirements override their own beliefs of when it is appropriate to consult and seek treatment.

▶ As anyone who has had young children in early education and child-care settings knows, the daily decisions regarding how mildly ill children are handled—exclusion and return-to-care policies and practices—are often not evidence based and can cause considerable economic and social stress for families and coworkers. The teacher/caregivers are the "gatekeepers" of the process, yet they have little health education.

The study by Rooshenas et al in the United Kingdom provides some insight as to why this process occurs. It is an important study in that it adds another piece of evidence in a complicated puzzle that crosses several domains—economic, social, and medical—and perhaps explains why it is so difficult to solve. This is not a small problem. In the United States, about two-thirds of children younger than 6 years old require nonparental child care.[1] Children in group child-care settings experience more and longer illnesses than children cared for at home.[2] When children in child care become ill, they sometimes require exclusion. Child illness accounts for 40% of parents' absence from work.[3] However, several studies show a large proportion of exclusions are unnecessary and do not agree with published US national guidelines.[4-6] In an effort to get the child back in care and the parent back to work, child-care exclusions lead to increased health care visits and inappropriate use of urgent care and emergency department resources,[7] as well as inappropriate requests for antibiotics.[8]

As reviewed in this article, the main findings of this study are not novel. However, this study does demonstrate that the problem is not limited to the United States, which is both comforting and disturbing. The uniqueness of this study is in its methodology, which demonstrates through qualitative methods some of the reasons why child-care providers make the decisions they do and offers insight into possible solutions. In Wales, each registered childminder (family child care home provider) and nursery manager (child care center director) is required to develop written exclusion criteria for handling mildly ill children; however, no training or guidance is provided by the Welsh regulatory body for child-care settings. Only 1 of 3 local health departments in the geographic area of study stated that it referred child-care providers to the UK Health Protection Agency guidelines[9] for guidance on exclusion criteria.

Given the lack of health training and written guidance, it is not surprising that the review of written policies showed either a lack of any recommendations or inappropriate recommendations for exclusion and treatment of many common childhood infections. The semistructured interviews validated that the policies were an accurate representation of daily practice and further demonstrated child-care providers' lack of medical knowledge, underlying erroneous health beliefs about efficacy of antibiotics, fears of serious illness, and desire to protect themselves from liability resulted in inappropriate exclusions, requests for doctor visits, and requests for antibiotics before the child returns to care. As one frustrated parent put it, "so you're in a situation where someone who knows nothing about medicine is actually telling you what you should be doing."

The limitations of this study are well outlined by the authors—namely, the possibility of recall and social desirability biases in addition to the researchers own inherent biases in analyzing the qualitative data. Yet use of document review, coupled with semistructured interviews, allows for rich information retrieval, exploration of new hypotheses, and discovery of new determinants of the condition under study that might be missed by a more quantitative approach using vignettes or questionnaire surveys that also reflect investigators preconceived notions. This same approach was used in a study of US Navy and

Baltimore child-care centers[10] and formed the basis for a questionnaire survey demonstrating lack of awareness and knowledge of the national guidelines.[11] The identified themes were very similar.

What can we take away from this study, and how does it apply to the United States? Unfortunately, this study shows that without guidance to help write exclusion criteria, child-care providers will write policies that are not evidence based and reflect lay health beliefs, causing undesirable outcomes such as inappropriate exclusions, excess health care visits, and requests for antibiotics. However, the association between written policy and child-care provider practices, as validated by this study, suggests that if evidence-based policies could be generated at the local level, then perhaps they would be implemented. The United States is not much better than the United Kingdom with respect to this problem. Evidence-based guidelines[12] have existed in the United States for more than 2 decades, yet awareness and knowledge of them by child-care providers, pediatricians, and parents alike is poor.[11] A user-friendly version of the guidelines exists and is in wide circulation among child-care providers; however, the effectiveness has not been studied.[13]

The national guidelines and the user-friendly publication of them have been in use in the US Navy child-care system for more than 5 years and, anecdotally, appear to be well received. Program licensing and regulations occur at the state level; however, few have adopted the national guidelines. The process of changing state child-care licensing regulations is cumbersome and sometimes political (personal experience). Child-care programs are permitted to write their own exclusion criteria as long as, at a minimum, they meet the generally sparse state requirements. This process unfortunately allows lay health beliefs and non—evidence-based recommendations to be added and work their way into practice. In the United States, a solution to this complicated but important problem will involve policy change at the state level coupled with policy, education, and user-friendly materials pushed to the local level. This field of research now clearly needs to move into the evaluation of effective interventions.

T. R. Shope, MD, MPH

References

1. US Census Bureau. Who's minding the kids? Child care arrangements: Spring 2011. http://www.census.gov/prod/2013pubs/p70-135.pdf. Accessed October 31, 2011.
2. Wald ER, Guerra N, Byers C. Upper respiratory tract infections in young children: duration of and frequency of complications. *Pediatrics.* 1991;87:129-133.
3. Bell DM, Gleiber DW, Mercer AA, et al. Illness associated with child day care: a study of incidence and cost. *Am J Public Health.* 1989;79:479-484.
4. Copeland KA, Harris EN, Wang NY, Cheng TL. Compliance with American Academy of Pediatrics and American Public Health Association illness exclusion guidelines for child care centers in Maryland: who follows them and when? *Pediatrics.* 2006;118:e1369-e1380.
5. Hashikawa AN, Juhn YJ, Nimmer M, et al. Unnecessary child care exclusions in a state that endorses national exclusion guidelines. *Pediatrics.* 2010;125:1003-1009.
6. Friedman JF, Lee GM, Kleinman KP, Finkelstein JA. Child care center policies and practices for management of ill children. *Ambul Pediatr.* 2004;4:455-460.

7. Hashikawa AN, Brousseau DC, Singer DC, Gebremariam A, Davis MM. Emergency department and urgent care for children excluded from child care. *Pediatrics*. 2014;134:e120-e127.

8. Skull SA, Ford-Jones EL, Kulin NA, Einarson TR, Wang EE. Child care center staff contribute to physician visits and pressure for antibiotic prescription. *Arch Pediatr Adolesc Med*. 2000;154:180-183.

9. Guidance on infection control in schools and other childcare settings. Health Protection Agency, United Kingdom. http://www.hpa.org.uk/webc/hpawebfile/hpaweb_c/1194947358374. Accessed July 18, 2014.

10. Shope T, Duggan A, Wilson M. Exclusion of mildly ill children from child care centers: focus groups of pediatricians, parents and child care providers. Pediatric research abstracts from Pediatric Academic Society annual meeting. 2000;47:225A.

11. Copeland KA, Duggan AK, Shope TR. Knowledge and beliefs about guidelines for exclusion of ill children from child care. *Ambul Pediatr*. 2005;5:365-371.

12. *Caring for Our Children National Health and Safety Performance Standards for Out-Of-Home Child Care and Early Education Programs*. 2011. 3rd ed. American Academy of Pediatrics; 2011.

13. Aronson SS, Shope TR. *Managing Infectious Diseases in Child Care and Schools: A Quick Reference Guide*. 3rd ed. Elk Grove Village, IL: American Academy of Pediatrics; 2013.

Recent Trends in Outpatient Antibiotic Use in Children

Vaz LE, Kleinman KP, Raebel MA, et al (Boston Children's Hosp, MA; Harvard Med School and Harvard Pilgrim Health Care Inst, Boston, MA; Kaiser Permanente Colorado Inst for Health Res, Denver)
Pediatrics 133:1-11, 2014

Objective.—The goal of this study was to determine changes in antibiotic-dispensing rates among children in 3 health plans located in New England [A], the Mountain West [B], and the Midwest [C] regions of the United States.

Methods.—Pharmacy and outpatient claims from September 2000 to August 2010 were used to calculate rates of antibiotic dispensing per person-year for children aged 3 months to 18 years. Differences in rates by year, diagnosis, and health plan were tested by using Poisson regression. The data were analyzed to determine whether there was a change in the rate of decline over time.

Results.—Antibiotic use in the 3- to <24-month age group varied at baseline according to health plan (A: 2.27, B: 1.40, C: 2.23 antibiotics per person-year; $P < .001$). The downward trend in antibiotic dispensing slowed, stabilized, or reversed during this 10-year period. In the 3- to <24-month age group, we observed 5.0%, 9.3%, and 7.2% annual declines early in the decade in the 3 plans, respectively. These dropped to 2.4%, 2.1%, and 0.5% annual declines by the end of the decade. Third-generation cephalosporin use for otitis media increased 1.6-, 15-, and 5.5-fold in plans A, B, and C in young children. Similar attenuation of decline in antibiotic use and increases in use of broad-spectrum agents were seen in other age groups.

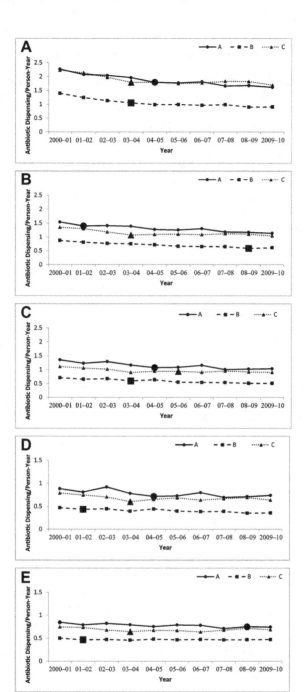

FIGURE 1.—Rates of antibiotic dispensing per person-year of enrollment for children aged as follows: A, 3 to 24 months; B, 2 to <4 years; C, 4 to <6 years; D, 6 to <12 years; and E, 12 to <18 years. Values are for each health plan (A–C) between 2000 and 2010. Note: axes differ for the last 2 age groups. Enhanced marker reflects year of greatest change in decline of antibiotic rate. Although 95% CIs were calculated, the results were too small to be visible on graphs. (Reproduced with permission from Pediatrics. Vaz LE, Kleinman KP, Raebel MA, et al. Recent trends in outpatient antibiotic use in children. *Pediatrics*. 2014;133:1-11, Copyright 2014, with permission from the American Academy of Pediatrics.)

Conclusions.—Antibiotic dispensing for children may have reached a new plateau. Along with identifying best practices in low-prescribing areas, decreasing broad-spectrum use for particular conditions should be a continuing focus of intervention efforts (Fig 1).

▶ Despite well-documented improvements over 2 decades, antibiotic overuse and misuse remain important public health and patient safety problems in the United States. Antibiotic overuse is a major factor underlying the ongoing and alarming rate of rise in antibiotic resistance both in the United States and globally. There is also mounting evidence that antibiotic exposure during infancy—some of which is likely unnecessary—alters the gut microbiome in a way that may increase a child's predisposition for chronic diseases including asthma, allergy, and obesity. Because the vast majority of antibiotic use in pediatrics originates in outpatient settings, it is important to understand physicians' prescribing patterns in this environment. This allows identification of practice patterns that are modifiable and can serve as targets for interventions designed to reduce antibiotic overuse and mitigate its harms.

In a study by Vaz et al, antibiotic prescribing patterns for children were examined within 3 large health plans across the United States. The authors found significant variability in antibiotic prescribing rates between plans (Fig 1). Whether this is merely a reflection of the underlying geographic variations in prescribing culture or if this is more related to influence of the health plans themselves remains somewhat uncertain, but it is intriguing to consider the possibility that the system of care delivery is the root of the variability. This study also highlights one of the major antibiotic misuse issues, which is the overuse of second-line agents, such as macrolides or cephalosporins for common conditions.

One example is use of macrolides for pharyngitis. Most episodes of pharyngitis are caused by viruses rather than bacteria such as *Streptococcus pyogenes* (group A strep), and even if group A strep is the target pathogen, macrolide resistance is well described. Understanding why this occurs and development and implementation of interventions that can promote greater use of first-line agents is imperative.

This study also examined temporal trends in rates of antibiotic prescribing over a decade from 2000 through 2010. During the first part of the decade, prescribing rates declined, but this trend appears to have plateaued or, in some cases, changed direction and increased during the latter part of the past decade (Fig 1). This finding is important because there is evidence that antibiotic overuse remains significant, especially for conditions that are typically of viral origin.

Furthermore, the authors highlight the importance of a single condition, otitis media (OM), to the overall volume of antibiotic prescribing in children. Reductions in the rate of OM diagnosis (which frequently results in an antibiotic prescription), rather than changes in the tendency to prescribe antibiotics for OM, were responsible for much of the early declines in antibiotic use during the study period. This may reflect both physicians' application of more stringent clinical criteria to make the diagnosis of OM and also changes in care-seeking patterns on the part of patients and families. Continued emphasis on the application of evidence-based and stringent clinical criteria for the diagnosis of bacterial upper respiratory tract infections in children (including for sinusitis and pharyngitis in addition to OM) is essential to further reductions in antibiotic overuse.

The major limitation of this study is one of generalizability; the data are derived from 3 large health plans but may not reflect prescribing practices outside of these plans. However, the findings are in line with previously published studies from nationally representative data sources.

Antibiotic prescribing practices are not set in stone. They can and do change over time. Furthermore, and perhaps more important, this study suggests the possibility that factors embedded into the system of care delivery have the potential to substantially affect prescribing practices. It is important to dig deeper and identify which system factors facilitate most judicious antibiotic use. Promising strategies include clinical decision support, greater use of rapid testing for viruses at the point of care and audit and feedback with benchmarking to enable providers to compare their prescribing practices to peer physicians.[1,2]

A. L. Hersh, MD, PhD

References

1. Caliendo AM, Gilbert DN, Ginocchio CC, et al. Infectious Diseases Society of America (IDSA). Better tests, better care: improved diagnostics for infectious diseases. *Clin Infect Dis.* 2013;57:S139-S170.
2. Gerber JS, Prasad PA, Fiks AG, et al. Effect of an outpatient antimicrobial stewardship intervention on broad-spectrum antibiotic prescribing by primary care pediatricians: a randomized trial. *JAMA.* 2013;309:2345-2352.

Accuracy of tympanic and forehead thermometers in private paediatric practice

Teller J, Ragazzi M, Simonetti GD, et al (Private Paediatric Practice, Langnau i.E., Switzerland; Univ of Bern, Switzerland)
Acta Paediatr 103:e80-e83, 2014

Aim.—To compare infrared tympanic and infrared contact forehead thermometer measurements with traditional rectal digital thermometers.

Methods.—A total of 254 children (137 girls) aged one to 24 months (median 7 months) consulting a private paediatric practice because of fever were prospectively recruited. Body temperature was measured using the three different devices.

Results.—The median and interquartile range for rectal, tympanic and forehead thermometers were 37.6 (37.1–38.4)°C, 37.5 (37.0–38.1)°C and 37.5 (37.1–37.9)°C, respectively ($p < 0.01$). The limits of agreement in the Bland-Altman plots were −0.73 to +1.04°C for the tympanic thermometer and −1.18 to +1.64°C for the forehead thermometer. The specificity of both the tympanic and forehead thermometers for detecting fever above 38°C was good, but sensitivity was low. Forehead measurements were susceptible to the use of a radiant warmer.

Conclusion.—Both the tympanic and forehead devices recorded lower temperatures than the rectal thermometers. The limits of agreement were particularly wide for the forehead thermometer and considerable for the tympanic thermometer. In the absence of valid alternatives, because of the ease to use and little degree of discomfort, tympanic thermometers can still be used with some reservations. Forehead thermometers should not be used in paediatric practice.

▶ Fever in children is a frequent source of vexation for parents and providers alike. The term "fever phobia" has been used to describe the concern and anxiety about the adverse effects of fevers. With the increasing number of options available, the choice of a thermometer itself potentially adds to this issue.

Rectal thermometry remains the gold standard for detection of fever in infants and young children. Oral temperatures are generally considered to be acceptable in cooperative, school-age children. Both of these routes have some limitations, which has led to interest in the development and validation of alternative methods. The role for newer thermometers—in particular, tympanic membrane and temporal artery thermometers—continues to evolve as more evidence becomes available about their performance, indications, and limitations. A growing body of literature compares the different thermometers in emergency rooms, inpatient units, and intensive care units. In contrast, a dearth of information exists about thermometer performance in private pediatric practice.

The present article by Teller et al adds to the conversation by way of a head-to-head comparison of modern, commercially available thermometers in a private pediatric practice. The population comprised infants and toddlers presenting to the clinic with a complaint of fever. This study design takes advantage of a natural opportunity for putting different thermometers to the test. For the tympanic membrane thermometer, the sensitivity and specificity for detection of fever were 0.72 and 0.97, respectively. These findings are in line with previous studies comparing tympanic membrane to rectal temperatures in other clinical settings. The temporal artery thermometer, in contrast, had poor sensitivity (0.42) and but still had reasonable specificity (0.96). Importantly, it was more subject to error because of external factors and gave a wider range of values than the tympanic membrane thermometer. Both devices were found to record lower temperatures compared with rectal thermometry. The conclusion from these data is that forehead temperatures should not be routinely used for definitive temperature measurement in the community practice setting. The authors used modern thermometers, which are likely of interest and relevant to the general pediatrician in clinical practice. The limitations of this study include the use of only 1 brand of thermometer, a relatively narrow age range (1–24 months), the potential influence of radiant warmers, and the use of single measurements by a single provider (ie, no information available on reproducibility or interobserver reliability).

Temperature measurement raises a number of practical issues. The convenience, price, and durability of commercially available instruments are important considerations. Widespread use and acceptance of newer devices such as temporal artery and tympanic membrane thermometers is reflected by their inclusion as a recommended means to measure temperature in clinical practice guidelines.[1,2] Products on the market range in price from $5 to $500. The number of options complicates the generalizability of studies that use 1 type or brand of thermometer. Practically speaking, this issue is relevant when deciding what equipment to purchase and training clinical staff in proper use of the instruments. Additionally, continued research is needed to validate the accuracy and reproducibility of results in everyday use for both tympanic and temporal artery thermometry.

Of course, concern for fever should always be contextualized in the overall clinical assessment of the child. The numerical reading on the thermometer is of secondary importance to a good clinical assessment of the patient. However, when precise fever detection explicitly matters, such as the trigger for further workup in a feverish newborn, rectal thermometry is clearly irreplaceable at present. An ideal instrument should be noninvasive, convenient, inexpensive, and, most important, accurate and reliable in measuring core body temperature. This study lends support to the use of tympanic membrane thermometers. As a result, the Holy Grail with all of these characteristics is still elusive.

G. S. Kelly, MD

M. Crocetti, MD, MPH

References

1. Canadian Paediatric Society. *Temperature measurement in paediatrics.* 2013, http://www.cps.ca/documents/position/temperature-measurement. Accessed July 23, 2014.
2. National Institute for Health and Care Excellence. *Feverish illness in children: assessment and initial management in children younger than 5 years.* 2013, http://www.nice.org.uk/CG047. Accessed July 23, 2014.

Management of Febrile Neonates in US Pediatric Emergency Departments
Jain S, Cheng J, Alpern ER, et al (Emory Univ and Children's Healthcare of Atlanta, GA; Lurie Children's Hosp of Chicago, IL; et al)
Pediatrics 133:187-195, 2014

Background.—Blood, urine, and cerebrospinal fluid cultures and admission for antibiotics are considered standard management of febrile neonates (0–28 days). We examined variation in adherence to these recommendations across US pediatric emergency departments (PEDs) and incidence of serious infections (SIs) in febrile neonates.

Methods.—Cross-sectional study of neonates with a diagnosis of fever evaluated in 36 PEDs in the 2010 Pediatric Health Information System database. We analyzed performance of recommended management (laboratory testing, antibiotic use, admission to hospital), 48-hour return visits to PED, and diagnoses of SI.

Results.—Of 2253 neonates meeting study criteria, 369 (16.4%) were evaluated and discharged from the PED; 1884 (83.6%) were admitted. Recommended management occurred in 1497 of 2253 (66.4%; 95% confidence interval, 64.5–68.4) febrile neonates. There was more than twofold variation across the 36 PEDs in adherence to recommended management, recommended testing, and recommended treatment of febrile neonates. There was significant variation in testing and treatment between admitted and discharged neonates ($P < .001$). A total of 269 in 2253 (11.9%) neonates had SI, of whom 223 (82.9%; 95% confidence interval, 77.9–86.9) received recommended management.

Conclusions.—There was wide variation across US PEDs in adherence to recommended management of febrile neonates. One in 6 febrile neonates was discharged from the PED; discharged patients were less likely to receive testing or antibiotic therapy than admitted patients. A majority of neonates with SI received recommended evaluation and management. High rates of SI in admitted patients but low return rates for missed infections in discharged patients suggest a need for additional studies to understand variation from the current recommendations.

▶ The need to address the ever-increasing variation in health care delivery and resource utilization in the United States has been recognized as a top priority by the Agency for Healthcare Research and Quality (AHRQ). In this article, Jain and colleagues explored adherence to and variation from guidelines regarding the management of febrile neonates. According to the authors, "Delineating variation across hospitals is a critical first step for learning the source of variation. Once the source of variation is determined, interventions may be designed to reduce variation and improve adherence to recommended evidence-based guidelines." The authors are suggesting that if variation from guidelines for managing febrile infants exists, then steps should be taken to reduce the variation.

Using data from the PHIS database, they reviewed the management of 2253 febrile neonates by 36 pediatric emergency departments (PED) to determine to what extent management adhered to current guidelines and whether there was variation in management among the various PED. Overall they found that about 73% of the febrile neonates were managed according to the 1993 AHRQ guidelines: full "sepsis workup" (complete blood count, urinalysis, lumbar puncture, cultures of the blood, urine, and cerebral spinal fluid), hospitalization, and initiation of intravenous antibiotics.[1] However they found striking variation among the PED ranging from 38.9% to 90.2% in adherence to diagnostic guidelines and 39% to 100% to guidelines for treatment; 269 (or 12%) had a "serious infection" (SI), of which urinary tract infections accounted for 27%. Although somewhat difficult to determine, it appears that there were 8 cases of bacterial meningitis and 63 cases of sepsis. Only 1 of the cases of SI was among the newborns who were not admitted to the hospital.

This paper picks up the now 50-year-old theme that Dr Sarah Long has referred to as the "bacteremia bandwagon"[2] that began in 1973 with McGowan's publication in the *New England Journal of Medicine*.[3] The recognition that some well-appearing infants and children had serious bacterial infections

(SBI) has led to various approaches such as the Rochester criteria to identify infants at low or not low risk for an SBI.[4] A consistent theme in the literature has been the argument that a clinician cannot reliably exclude the possibility of a SBI by his or her clinical exam, particularly in the first month of life. As a result, guidelines for management call for the use of laboratory tests including a complete blood count, lumbar puncture, urine obtained by catheter or suprapubic aspiration, and intravenous antibiotics even in neonates who are well appearing.

The study by Jain shows substantial variation in adherence to the guidelines for managing febrile neonates (Fig 2 and Table 3 in the original article) but is unable to address the reasons for the variation or provide evidence of an association between differences in outcome for those PED that adhered to the guidelines and those that did not. Among the 369 newborns who were not initially admitted to the hospital, only 1 (0.3%) was subsequently found to have an SBI and, as far as can be determined from the information in the article, had no adverse consequences from a management strategy that differed from the guidelines.

There are probably 2 reasons why guidelines are not followed. First the clinician may be unaware of the guidelines. This seems extremely unlikely given the fact that the guidelines have been around for 20 years and the study took place in PED of academic children's hospitals. The other reason is that clinicians are confident that they can use their clinical assessment of the baby and the reliability of the family to determine which, if any, aspect of the guidelines they will follow.

When not following guidelines can be clearly linked to worse outcomes or increased costs, clinicians can usually be convinced to follow them, but when this link is unclear, it is likely that variation in care processes will continue. Establishing a convincing link between variation in management and variation in outcome for febrile neonates, especially those who are well appearing, is unlikely, given the heterogeneity of the causes of fever and the relatively rare occurrence of SBI. The authors have provided convincing evidence that variation and nonadherence to the guidelines is common, but evidence that increasing adherence to them will be of benefit remains to be established.

P. C. Young, MD

References

1. Baraff LJ, Bass JW, Fleisher GR, et al. Practice guideline for the management of infants and children 0 to 36 months of age with fever without source. Agency for Health Care Policy and Research. *Ann Emerg Med.* 1993;22:1198-1210.
2. Long SS. Antibiotic therapy in febrile children: "best-laid schemes". *J Pediatr.* 1994;124:585-588.
3. McGowan JE Jr, Bratton L, Klein JO, Finland M. Bacteremia in febrile children seen in a walk-in pediatric clinic. *N Engl J Med.* 1973;288:1309-1312.
4. Jaskiewicz JA, McCarthy CA, Richardson AC, et al. Febrile Infant Collaborative Study Group. Febrile infants at low risk for serious bacterial infection—an appraisal of the Rochester criteria and implications for management. *Pediatrics.* 1994;94:390-396.

Immune deficiency in Ataxia-Telangiectasia: a longitudinal study of 44 patients

Chopra C, Davies G, Taylor M, et al (Queen's Med Centre, Nottingham, UK; Great Ormond Street Hosp and Inst of Child Health, London; Univ of Birmingham, UK; et al)

Clin Exp Immunol 176:275-282, 2014

Ataxia-Telangiectasia (A-T) is a genetic condition leading to neurological defects and immune deficiency. The nature of the immune deficiency is highly variable, and in some cases causes significant morbidity and mortality due to recurrent sinopulmonary infections. Although the neurological defects in A-T are progressive, the natural history of the immune deficiency in A-T has not been evaluated formally. In this study we analyse the clinical history and immunological data in 44 patients with A-T who attended the National Ataxia-Telangiectasia clinic in Nottingham between 2001 and 2011. Using patient medical records and Nottingham University Hospitals (NUH) National Health Service Trust medical IT systems, data regarding clinical history, use of immunoglobulin replacement therapy, total immunoglobulin levels, specific antibody levels and lymphocyte subset counts were obtained. T cell receptor spectratyping results in some patients were already available and, where possible, repeat blood samples were collected for analysis. This study shows that subtle quantitative changes in certain immunological parameters such as lymphocyte subset counts may occur in patients with A-T over time. However, in general, for the majority of patients the severity of immune deficiency (both clinically and in terms of immunological blood markers) does not seem to deteriorate significantly with time. This finding serves to inform the long-term management of this cohort of patients because, if recurrent respiratory tract infections present later in life, then other contributory factors (e.g. cough/swallowing difficulties, underlying lung disease) should be investigated aggressively. Our findings also offer some form of reassurance for parents of children with A-T, which is otherwise a progressively severely debilitating condition.

▶ Ataxia-telangiectasia (AT) is a rare, autosomal recessive disorder with multisystem manifestations. Although the most familiar features of AT to clinicians are motor impairments, such as ataxia, secondary to a neurodegenerative process, and oculocutaneous telangiectasia, the disorder is also characterized by chronic sinopulmonary infections, increased risk of lymphoreticular cancer, hypersensitivity to ionizing radiation, and progressive immunodeficiency.[1] The disease is caused by a mutation in the *ATM* (ataxia-telangiectasia mutated) gene on chromosome 11 that encodes the ATM protein, which is associated with cell cycle control and DNA repair, and hence the varied features of the disorder.[2]

It is known that the manifestations of immune deficiency within the population of patients with AT is highly variable. Patients may have poor polysaccharide antibody responses, lymphopenia, low total immunoglobulin levels, and low immunoglobulin G.[2] However, less well known is the natural history of the immune deficiency. AT is a rare disease, with a prevalence estimated to be less than 1 in 100 000.[3] Few cohorts have been established to characterize the natural history of the different features of the disease. A previous analysis of 100 patients from the Johns Hopkins AT Clinic suggested that the immune deficiency is rarely progressive; however, the data was cross-sectional.[4] This study by Chopra et al from the United Kingdom National Ataxia-Telangiectasia Clinic at the Nottingham University Hospitals is a longitudinal analysis of 44 patients with AT who were seen at the clinic from 2001 to 2011.

The study found that, in general, there was no evidence of clinically significant immunological deterioration over time for this group of patients with AT. This analysis is helpful information for clinicians because patients with AT may have frequent respiratory tract infections. These infections are unlikely to be a harbinger of deteriorating immune function but instead point to another manifestation of the disorder—deteriorating swallowing function. Previous studies have suggested that pulmonary infections may be more likely related to oropharyngeal dysphagia and aspiration.[5] Deteriorating swallowing function over time is consistent with the neurodegenerative nature of AT. In addition, these symptoms tend to manifest in the second decade of life and can be mitigated by modifications in feeding routines and food consistency.

Unfortunately, there is no cure for AT at this time; however, these studies help clinicians understand how to better manage this chronic disorder and maximize health outcomes and quality of life for these patients.

M. D. Cabana, MD, MPH

References

1. Woods CG, Taylor AMR. Ataxia telangiectasia in the British Isles: the clinical and laboratory features of 70 affected individuals. *Q J Med.* 1992;82:169-179.
2. McKinnon PJ. ATM and the molecular pathogenesis of ataxia telangiectasia. *Annual Rev Pathol.* 2012;7:301-321.
3. Swift M, Morrell D, Cromartie E, Chamberlin AR, Skolnick MH, Bishop DT. The incidence and gene frequency of ataxia-telangiectasia in the United States. *Am J Hum Genet.* 1986;39:573-583.
4. Nowak-Wegrzyn A, Crawford TO, Winkelstein JA, Carson KA, Lederman HM. Immunodeficiency and infections in ataxia-telangiectasia. *J Pediatr.* 2004;144:505-511.
5. Lefton-Greif MA, Crawford TO, Winkelstein JA, et al. Oropharyngeal dysphagia and aspiration in patients with ataxia-telangiectasia. *J Pediatr.* 2000;136:225-231.

11 Miscellaneous

Frequency and Variety of Inpatient Pediatric Surgical Procedures in the United States
Sømme S, Bronsert M, Morrato E, et al (Children's Hosp Colorado, Aurora; Univ of Colorado Denver, Aurora)
Pediatrics 132:e1466-e1472, 2013

Objective.—Pediatric surgical procedures are being performed in a variety of hospitals with large differences in surgical volume. We examined the frequency and variety of inpatient pediatric surgical procedures in the United States by hospital type and geographic region using a nationally representative sample.

Methods.—The 2009 Kids' Inpatient Database for patients <18 years old was used to calculate surgical frequencies by using International Classification of Diseases, Ninth Revision, Clinical Modification, (ICD-9-CM) codes. We performed stratified analysis by hospital type (free-standing children's hospital, children's unit within an adult hospital, and general hospital) and geographic region (South, West, Midwest, Northeast) to compare frequencies of surgical procedures.

Results.—A total of 216 081 procedures were projected for 2009 with the top 20 procedures accounting for >90% of cases. As many as 40% of all pediatric inpatient surgical procedures are being performed in adult general hospitals. Infrequent complex low-volume neonatal surgical procedures (pullthrough for Hirschsprung disease, surgery for malrotation, esophageal atresia repair, and diaphragmatic hernia repair) were 6.8 to 16 times more likely to occur in a children's hospital. Significant regional variation in procedure frequency rates occurred for appendectomy and cholecystectomy.

Conclusions.—This report is the first to characterize pediatric surgical inpatient volume in the United States. Such data may influence the distribution of pediatric surgeons, number of trainees, and training curricula for pediatric surgeons, pediatricians, general surgeons and other surgical specialists who might operate on children. In addition, it raises the question of whether complex pediatric surgical procedures should preferably be performed at dedicated high volume children's hospitals.

▶ This snapshot of the distribution of pediatric surgical care in the United States reveals that although complex cases are 10 times more likely to be performed in a children's hospital than in a non-children's hospital, there is a significant amount of complex surgery being performed on children in non-children's hospitals. The most likely explanation for this is not that an adult surgeon is actually performing these procedures (it is hard to imagine an adult surgeon taking on a tracheoesophageal fistula repair). Rather, the huge financial incentive to hold onto complex pediatric patients drives non-children's hospitals to hire pediatric surgeons to come there and operate even when there may be a children's hospital within easy transfer distance. There are geographic regions where children's hospitals are scarce, and it is possible that these account for a small proportion of cases being performed in non-children's hospitals, but these areas are so underpopulated compared with the rest of the country that their contribution is likely to be minimal.

In adult surgery, research has shown that individual surgeon volume is highly correlated with superior patient outcomes. There are some data in pediatric surgery supporting better outcomes in higher volume centers, but this has not been shown for individual surgeons as it has in adult endocrine surgery, esophageal surgery, and pancreatic surgery.[1-4] The reality is that many pediatric surgical procedures are incredibly rare even in high-volume centers, so a "high-volume" surgeon may do no more than 1 resection of sacrococcygeal teratoma every couple of years (and there are several other examples of this). Also, high-volume centers often have 20 to 25 pediatric surgeons. So even though the center may be high-volume, the individual surgeons are not necessarily high volume. In pediatric surgery, the center is the appropriate unit of measure rather than the surgeon. It is not necessarily the higher volume but rather the comprehensive resources available in high-volume centers that usually lead to better outcomes.

The current picture that is described in this article by Sømme et al is provocative because it demonstrates the need and sets the stage for a system that will optimize resources for the surgical care of children in this country. To understand shortcomings of the current system and help it evolve toward better outcomes, it is crucial to track outcomes data. This article provides a broad overview about procedures in aggregate, but more granular analysis is required to make meaningful conclusions about how to redesign a system to optimize outcomes. In addition, because the analysis only focused on inpatient surgical procedures, the information provided accounts for only a fraction of the procedures being performed on children in this country. It is likely that adult surgeons are performing an even higher proportion of procedures such as hernia repairs than they are inpatient surgical procedures, but this information is hard to come by, and the potential impact on outcomes is unknown. When considering how to optimize outcomes for children undergoing surgery, it is not just presence or absence of a pediatric surgeon, or the volume of surgery performed at a center, that is important.

Safely and effectively caring for children undergoing complex surgical procedures requires a system and a multidisciplinary care team that can support the complex needs of these patients. Recognition of this fact led to the creation of a document titled "Optimal Resources for Children's Surgical Care in the United States,"[5] which was published this year and has been endorsed by the American Pediatric Surgical Association, the American College of Surgeons, and the Society for Pediatric Anesthesia. The authors recognize a mismatch between individual patient needs and available clinical resources for some infants and children receiving surgical care and argue that this systematically results in suboptimal outcomes. The document describes center classifications as "basic," "advanced," and "comprehensive" and clearly defines the procedures that should be taking place in institutions in each of these categories. Effective allocation of operations to appropriately resourced centers should optimize outcomes and improve the value of services delivered by reducing the risk of a complication.

For the proposed system to go into effect, regulation by an external authority such as the Joint Commission will be necessary. The financial incentive for poorly equipped centers to hold on to complex pediatric patients is too powerful to be overcome by anything other than a strongly enforced system of regionalization. There are existing models of regionalization for surgical care; for example, the American College of Surgeons' trauma verification program has been successful in matching patient needs with adequate resources. It is crucial to define geographic areas where there is a lack of appropriate resources to inform ongoing dialogue about workforce issues in pediatric surgery. The most significant impact of a regionalized system is likely to be seen not in these rural areas but in well-resourced areas where there are well-equipped children's hospitals but financial incentives are interfering with appropriate transfer to higher level care facilities.

If such a system does go into effect, it will be essential to track outcomes and cost to demonstrate that regionalization of care improves the value of services delivered. To determine the true impact of center type on patient outcomes, it is essential that outcomes are captured accurately and appropriate adjustment is made for patient comorbidities. The American College of Surgeons National Surgical Quality Improvement Project-Pediatric (ACS NSQIP-P) reports risk-adjusted 30-day outcomes for about 50 children's hospitals across the country, and the data that it has generated have led to impressive advances in quality improvement.[6] As of right now, however, there is no mechanism to reliably measure risk-adjusted outcomes in non-children's hospitals, so we are missing the other side of the coin. Additionally, NSQIP-P is limited, in that it only tracks outcomes for 30 days postoperatively, and many of the crucial outcomes in pediatrics have to do with long-term neurocognitive development and other issues affecting patient quality of life. Ongoing accrual of data (both short and long term, and across all the center levels) will allow for the system to adapt and continue to match patients and resources appropriately to optimize outcomes without creating the need for unnecessary transfers.

L. Berman, MD

J. Sosa, MD

References

1. Boudourakis LD, Wang TS, Roman SA, Desai R, Sosa JA. Evolution of the surgeon-volume, patient-outcome relationship. *Ann Surg.* 2009;250:159-165.
2. Sosa JA, Bowman HM, Gordon TA, et al. Importance of hospital volume in the overall management of pancreatic cancer. *Ann Surg.* 1998;228:429-438.
3. Sundelof M, Lagergren J, Ye W. Surgical factors influencing outcomes in patients resected for cancer of the esophagus or gastric cardia. *World J Surg.* 2008;32:2357-2365.

4. Kandil E, Noureldine SI, Abbas A, Tufano RP. The impact of surgical volume on patient outcomes following thyroid surgery. *Surgery.* 2013;154:1346-1352.
5. Oldham KT. Optimal resources for children's surgical care. *J Pediatr Surg.* 2014; 49:667-677.
6. Saito JM, Chen LE, Hall BL, et al. Risk-adjusted hospital outcomes for children's surgery. *Pediatrics.* 2013;132:e677-e688.

Pediatric Shopping-Cart-Related Injuries Treated in US Emergency Departments, 1990-2011

Martin KJ, Chounthirath T, Xiang H, et al (The Res Inst at Nationwide Children's Hosp, Columbus, OH)
Clin Pediatr 53:277-285, 2014

This study investigates the effect of the 2004 US shopping cart safety standard on shopping-cart-related injuries among children younger than 15 years of age by retrospectively analyzing data from the National Electronic Injury Surveillance System. An estimated 530 494 children younger than 15 years were treated in US emergency departments for shopping-cart-related injuries from 1990 to 2011, averaging 24 113 children annually. The most commonly injured body region was the head (78.1%). The annual concussion/closed head injury rate per 10 000 children increased significantly ($P < .001$) by 213.3% from 0.64 in 1990 to 2.02 in 2011. Although a shopping cart safety standard was implemented in the United States in 2004, the overall number and rate of injuries associated with shopping carts have not decreased. In fact, the number and rate of concussions/closed head injuries have continued to climb. Increased prevention efforts are needed to address these injuries among children.

▶ Shopping carts are a potential source of injury for young children. In 2005, approximately 24 200 children younger than 15 years were treated in US emergency departments (ED), with the head and neck being the most common body region affected, and 4% required hospital admission. Despite a 2004 voluntary shopping cart safety standard developed by the American Society for Testing and Materials (ASTM), there has been no evaluation comparing injuries before and after.

The authors conducted a retrospective analysis of data from the National Electronic Injury Surveillance System (NEISS), which tracks injuries treated in US hospitals due to sports and recreational activities, as well as consumer products. NEISS diagnoses were categorized as concussion/closed head injury, laceration, soft-tissue injury, fractures, and other.

The results suggest that an estimated 530 494 children younger than age 15 years treated for injuries due to shopping carts during this time period (1990–2011). This suggests that 1 child is injured every 22 minutes. The average patient age was 2.8 years, with a median of 2 years. The average annual rate of injury was 4.07 injuries per 10 000 children, with males having a higher rate of injury. It is not surprising that those children aged 0 to 4 years had a higher rate of 10.38 injuries per 10 000 children versus those 5 to 14 years of 0.94

injuries per 10 000 children. Children aged 0 to 4 years experienced 84.5% of shopping-cart-related injuries, and 3.1% of patients required hospital admission.

Falls from the shopping cart accounted for the majority of injuries (70.4%) followed by running into the cart (7.9%), cart tips over (6.2%), and entrapment of extremities in the cart (6.1%). Patients aged 0 to 4 years were 2.37 time more likely to fall out of the cart than older children, whereas those 5 to 14 years were 1.72 time more likely to be involved in cart tip-overs, 3.95 time more likely to have an entrapment, and 3.19 time more likely to run into a cart.

What is concerning is that there was no change in the annual number or rate of injuries during the study period, but there was a 57.6% increase in children falling out of shopping carts, most due to children aged 0 to 4 years (Fig 2).

The head was injured 78.1% of the time, upper extremities 13.8%, and lower extremities 6.0%. The majority of head injuries occurred in younger children (90.7%), and the majority of admitted children had a head injury (78.5%). Older children sustained more knee and foot injuries. Mechanism of injury included soft tissue injury (41.2%), concussion/closed head injury (29.8%), and laceration (17.4%). Younger children were 2.97 times more likely to have a concussion/closed head injury, and those who fell out of a shopping cart were 4.32 times more likely to be diagnosed with concussion than patients with other injury mechanisms. For all children, the rate of concussions increased by 254% (Fig 3).

Children aged 0 to 4 years are at highest risk for a shopping-cart-related injury, most likely due to a fall and sustaining a head injury. The 2004 American Society for Testing and Materials standard in the United States addressed

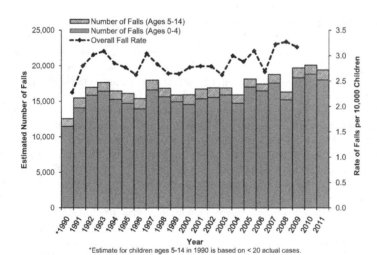

FIGURE 2.—Estimated number and rate of falls among children younger than 15 years of age treated in emergency departments in the United States for injuries associated with shopping carts according to year and age group, 1990-2011. (Reprinted from Martin KJ, Chounthirath T, Xiang H, et al. Pediatric shopping-cart-related injuries treated in US emergency departments, 1990-2011. *Clin Pediatr.* 2014;53:277-285, with permission from The Author(s).)

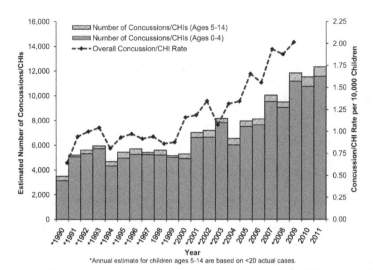

FIGURE 3.—Estimated number and rate of concussions/closed head injuries (CHIs) among children younger than 15 years of age treated in emergency departments in the United States for injuries associated with shopping carts according to year and age group, 1990-2011. (Reprinted from Martin KJ, Chounthirath T, Xiang H, et al. Pediatric shopping-cart-related injuries treated in US emergency departments, 1990-2011. *Clin Pediatr.* 2014;53:277-285, with permission from The Author(s).)

performance and labeling requirements and restraint systems but did not address cart stability, which is part of the European standard. In 2012, the Consumer Product Safety Commission (CPSC) released a safety alert about head injury in young children falling out of shopping carts, but this action still does not address cart stability.

An estimated life span of a shopping cart is 2 to 8 years. As of 2015, the majority of carts should conform to the 2004 standard; however, this study suggests the injury rate overall has not changed. Moreover, the rate of concussions/closed head injuries has skyrocketed since 2004. There is an even greater need for improved shopping cart stability standards, design changes, and store-based and public education.

What are parents to do then they go grocery shopping with a 5-month-old infant, and a 2-year-old child? Shopping carts have warning labels that refer to "children ages 6 months to 48 months AND 15 lbs up to 35 lbs." The warnings add: "Do not allow child to ride in the basket," and "Do not use your own personal infant carrier or car seat." What is the parent's recourse?

Basically, the parent is forced to ignore the warnings, and hope that nothing bad happens. Although there are restraints in the cart seat for a 2-year-old, they only secure at the waist, and as a result, the restraints can be overcome easily by a toddler. The parent is then faced with placing the 5-month-old in a car seat in the basket or carrying the 5 month-old in the store in a soft carrier. Some stores have a carlike cart with a low-to-the-ground toy car (often with 2 seats), attached to a shortened shopping cart with cart seat. These carts provide some help; however, they are often in short supply. Other stores have mini-carts for young children to push alongside the parent, but their use by a child depends on the child's coordination and cooperation.

The bottom line is, until cart stability and better restrains are addressed, when you go shopping, it's better to go without your children. But if you must: plan in advance and be very, very cautious and careful.

S. Fuchs, MD

Impact of the 2010 FIFA (Federation Internationale de Football Association) World Cup on Pediatric Injury and Mortality in Cape Town, South Africa
Zroback C, Levin D, Manlhiot C, et al (Univ of Toronto, Ontario, Canada; The Hosp for Sick Children, Toronto, Ontario, Canada; et al)
J Pediatr 164:327-331, 2014

Objective.—To examine how a mass-gathering event (the Federation Internationale de Football Association World Cup, 2010, South Africa) impacts trauma and mortality in the pediatric (≤ 18 years) population.

Study Design.—We investigated pediatric emergency visits at Cape Town's 3 largest public trauma centers and 3 private hospital groups, as well as deaths investigated by the 3 city mortuaries. We compared the 31 days of World Cup with equivalent periods from 2007-2009, and with the 2 weeks before and after the event. We also looked at the World Cup period in isolation and compared days with and without games in Cape Town.

Results.—There was significantly decreased pediatric trauma volume during the World Cup, approximately 2/100 000 (37%) fewer injuries per day, compared with 2009 and to both pre- and post-World Cup control periods ($P < .001$). This decrease occurred within a majority of injury subtypes, but did not change mortality. There were temporal fluctuations in emergency visits corresponding with local match start time, with fewer all-cause emergency visits during the 5 hours surrounding this time (-16.4%, $P = .01$), followed by a subsequent spike ($+26.2\%$, $P = .02$). There was an increase in trauma 12 hours following matches ($+15.6\%$, $P = .06$).

Conclusions.—In Cape Town, during the 2010 Federation Internationale de Football Association World Cup, there were fewer emergency department visits for traumatic injury. Furthermore, there were fewer all-cause pediatric emergency department visits during hometown matches. These results will assist in planning for future massgathering events.

▶ This study examines the association between a unique sporting event, the 2010 Federation Internationale de Football Association (FIFA) World Cup, and the frequency of pediatric injury and pediatric emergency department (ED) volume.

There have been several studies that have documented the effect of mass-gathering sporting or cultural events on health services utilization. One type of analysis focuses on the effects of a distant mass-gathering event on local health care infrastructure and utilization. For example, there are published analyses on the effect of the 1997–2002 Champions League soccer games, and the 2006–2010 Super Bowls, World Series, and National Basketball Association (NBA) Finals on pediatric ED volume.[1,2] Only the NBA Finals were associated with a decrease in ED attendance 6 to 8 hours postgame.

Another type of analysis focuses on the effects of a local mass-gathering event and the potential strain on local health care infrastructure and utilization. There have been fewer pediatric studies in this area because the majority of studies have focused on adult outcomes and utilization. McQueen documented that children and young adults may have different reasons for seeking medical attention at large gatherings. Children (ages 16 years or less) at a large outdoor music festival were more likely to suffer from being "crushed in a crowd," having syncopal events, or complaining of nausea, compared with young adults (ages 17–25 years) who were seen for alcohol-related illness.[3] However, local events have been documented to have positive effects as well. For example, the 1996 Olympic Games led to a temporary reduction in downtown traffic patterns in Atlanta. These changes were associated with lower ozone rates and lower rates of pediatric asthma events.[4]

It is in this context that Zroback et al analyze the frequency of pediatric injury in Cape Town, the second largest city in South Africa and the site of eight of the 2010 World Cup matches. The authors conducted 2 types of comparisons: annual trends (pediatric injury frequency in 2007, 2008, 2009, and 2010) and hourly trends (pediatric injury frequency each hour in relation to the start of a World Cup match in 2010).

Based on the limited, published work in this area, it is not clear if a large mass-gathering event, such as a World Cup, would be associated with an increase or a decrease in pediatric injury. For example, large projects to improve infrastructure, such as transportation and housing, accompanied the long-term preparation for the World Cup. In addition, the influx of tourism, increased police security, and a temporary boost in employment may have effects on the local economy and subsequent effects on child welfare and health. However, mass events, can also be associated with increased crime, such as "hooliganism" and increased vehicle traffic, which may have negative effects on child health or increase the frequency of injury.

The authors reported a decrease in pediatric trauma volume during the 2010 World Cup period compared with a similar period in 2009, as well as the time periods in the weeks before and after the 2010 World Cup. However, it is not really clear if the period during the 2010 World Cup experienced a decline in pediatric trauma volume. In reviewing the data over a longer time horizon (beyond the 2009 to 2010 comparison), there are other possible interpretations.

For example, it is possible that pediatric injury may have increased in 2009, as national resources normally allotted for child welfare or safety were diverted or distracted in the preparation and buildup to the World Cup. In looking at the multivariable linear regression models in Table 1, there is no difference between the 2010 World Cup period compared with the 2007 period or the 2008 period.

As a result, it is not clear if 2010 represents a difference in admission rates over the previous years or whether 2009 was actually the aberration. Childhood injury and morbidity and injury may have increased in the period immediately before the 2010 World Cup as public resources and attention were focused

TABLE 1.—Factors Associated with Injury-Related Paediatrics Emergency Department Visits in Multivariable Linear Regression Models (Further Adjusted for Population and Day of the Week, Data Not Shown)

Associated Factors	Ratio of Admission Rate with 95% CI	Change in Admission Rate (per 100 000 Children) with 95% CI	P Value
Age category			
0-4 years old	1.587 (1.227; 1.948)	+4.027 (+1.554; +6.500)	.001
5-9 years old	0.919 (0.689; 1.148)	−0.558 (−2.130; +1.014)	.49
10-14 years old	0.834 (0.750; 0.924)	−1.137 (−1.722; −0.552)	<.01
15-18 years old	reference category	reference category	
Sex (male)	1.722 (1.639; 1.806)	+3.954 (+3.498; +4.410)	<.001
Period			
Control 2007	1.001 (0.886; 1.115)	+0.005 (−0.746; +0.755)	.99
Control 2008	1.001 (0.891; 1.111)	+0.006 (−0.713; +0.725)	.99
Control 2009	1.344 (1.237; 1.451)	+2.256 (+1.554; +2.958)	<.001
Control 2010 pre-World Cup	1.315 (1.190; 1.439)	+2.063 (+1.245; +2.881)	<.001
Control 2010 post-World Cup	1.376 (1.249; 1.504)	+2.469 (+1.634; +3.304)	<.001
2010 World Cup	reference category	reference category	
Landmark games	1.026 (0.836; 1.217)	+0.170 (−1.062; +1.402)	.79
Cape Town games	0.905 (0.754; 1.056)	−0.645 (−1.672; +0.381)	.22

Reprinted from Journal Pediatrics. Zroback C, Levin D, Manlhiot C, et al. Impact of the 2010 FIFA (Federation Internationale de Football Association) World Cup on Pediatric Injury and Mortality in Cape Town, South Africa. J Pediatr. 2014;164:327-331, Copyright 2014, with permission from Elsevier.

elsewhere. There are recent examples of this phenomenon. For example, in the buildup to the 2014 World Cup in Brazil, over 25 billion reais (11 billion US dollars) was spent in World Cup related projects and infrastructure improvements, which could have been spent on health care, education, and other public transportation projects.[4]

The bottom line is that child health care and injury prevention are long-term, societal investments. Large cultural and sporting events are also important for society. However, I do not think planners of such events can claim that there will be potential spillover benefits from these events on child health. I would be skeptical of any argument that such spending on a short-term, 1-time event will have long-term, or even short-term, benefits for child health.

Finally, another fascinating aspect of this study is the hour-to-hour analysis of changes in pediatric ED visits in relation to the start of a World Cup game (Fig 1).

Immediately before and after games, there is a notable decrease in pediatric ED visits. However, 12 hours after the start of a game (approximately 9 to 10 hours after a game is completed), there is a spike in ED visits.

It is not clear if the injury or illness actually occurred in the time period immediately after a game, so they may represent a real spike in injuries after a World Cup game. There are other interpretations. In general, for minor illnesses and injuries, children cannot take themselves to an ED because they are dependent on their parents or guardians for transportation. The timing of these ED presentations may instead reflect a delay in presentation and caregiver preferences in the timing of pediatric ED visits. Alternatively, these data may represent the difficulty in traveling to a health care facility immediately after a mass gathering due to crowd control issues. For each of these potential explanations, there are different interventions (eg, policing after World Cup games, parental public

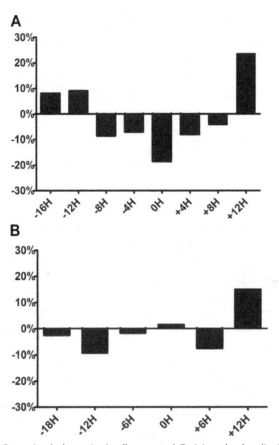

FIGURE 1.—Proportional change in **A**, all-causes and **B**, injuryrelated pediatric admission (vs expected) per hour relative to game start in Cape Town. (Reprinted from Zroback C, Levin D, Manlhiot C, et al. Impact of the 2010 FIFA (Federation Internationale de Football Association) world cup on pediatric injury and mortality in cape town, South Africa. *J Pediatr.* 2014;164:327-331, Mosby Inc.)

health education, improved transportation) that event planners should consider for future mass gatherings. For ED administrators and public health officials, these data can also help with future staffing and planning.

World Cup effects on pediatric ED attendance may or may not be similar to the effects of the Super Bowl; however, for those clinicians who work or moonlight in pediatric ED (especially those colleagues in Phoenix, Arizona), the next Super Bowl for the National Football League will be held on February 1, 2015, in Phoenix. Kick off is at 3:30 p.m. (Pacific Time). Pick and plan your shifts accordingly.

M. D. Cabana, MD, MPH

References

1. Farrell S, Doherty GM, Mccallion WA, Shields MD. Do major televised events affect pediatric emergency department attendances or delay presentation of surgical conditions? *Pediatr Emerg Care.* 2005;21:306-308.

2. Kim TY, Barcega BB, Denmark TK. Pediatric emergency department census during major sporting events. *Pediatr Emerg Care.* 2012;28:1158-1161.
3. Mcqueen CP. Care of children at a large outdoor music festival in the United Kingdom. *Prehosp Disaster Med.* 2010;25(3):223-226.
4. Friedman MS, Powell KE, Hutwagner L, Graham LM, Teague WG. Impact of changes in transportation and commuting behaviors during the 1996 Summer Olympic Games in Atlanta on air quality and childhood asthma. *JAMA.* 2001; 285:897-905.

Variation in Outcomes of Quality Measurement by Data Source

Angier H, Gold R, Gallia C, et al (Oregon Health & Science Univ, Portland; Kaiser Permanente Northwest, Portland, OR; Oregon Health Authority, Salem; et al)
Pediatrics 133:e1676-e1682, 2014

Objective.—To evaluate selected Children's Health Insurance Program Reauthorization Act claims-based quality measures using claims data alone, electronic health record (EHR) data alone, and both data sources combined.

Methods.—Our population included pediatric patients from 46 clinics in the OCHIN network of community health centers, who were continuously enrolled in Oregon's public health insurance program during 2010. Within this population, we calculated selected pediatric care quality measures according to the Children's Health Insurance Program Reauthorization Act technical specifications within administrative claims. We then calculated these measures in the same cohort, by using EHR data, by using the technical specifications plus clinical data previously shown to enhance capture of a given measure. We used the k statistic to determine agreement in measurement when using claims versus EHR data. Finally, we measured quality of care delivered to the study population, when using a combined dataset of linked, patient-level administrative claims and EHR data.

Results.—When using administrative claims data, 1.0% of children (aged 3–17) had a BMI percentile recorded, compared with 71.9% based on the EHR data (κ agreement [k] $\leq$ 0.01), and 72.0% in the combined dataset. Among children turning 2 in 2010, 20.2% received all recommended immunizations according to the administrative claims data, 17.2% according to the EHR data ($k = 0.82$), and 21.4% according to the combined dataset.

Conclusions.—Children's care quality measures may not be accurate when assessed using only administrative claims. Adding EHR data to administrative claims data may yield more complete measurement.

▶ Angier and colleagues describe an important component of quality measurement as they summarize the reliability and contrasts between measures presented based on distinct data sources. This article represents an important link in several chains of thought, ranging from empirical demonstrations of data comparability to sophisticated analyses of the most desirable presentation of impact measurement.

Focusing on data sources in the 20th century, much of what we learned about clinical medicine came from the admittedly imperfect information recorded in the medical record. Although there were occasional efforts to directly observe clinical practice, collect outcomes, or both, studies of quality focused initially on structural aspects of care, and then evolved toward process and occasionally outcomes measurement. With the creation of Medicare in the 1960s and the passage of legislation that created Peer Review Standards Organizations (PRSOs that have evolved into PROs) in the 1970s, audits of quality moved more routinely into the inpatient arena, focusing on information contained in the inpatient medical chart. Lohr and Brook at RAND and Roos in Manitoba, Canada, pioneered the use of electronically available administrative data (generated by routine health care operations, such as billings) as proxies for health care processes. Administrative data carefully used could reduce the burden for quality measurement.

As the National Committee for Quality Assurance developed the Healthcare Employee Data Information Set as the de facto measurement system for managed care, attention turned to the use of administrative data for routine performance measurement. Work done with managed care plans demonstrated that administrative data could have a role, but it was not definitive absent augmentation by chart review. This article builds on that tradition of technical assessments regarding the quality of electronic data.

Today, the modern hope for efficient "low-friction" access to information about the processes of care turns to the electronic health record (EHR). We learn herein that the EHR can augment administrative data: the new technology can enhance performance measurement. Common sense tells us that different data sources will produce different results. Medical science requires that people put in the hard work to demonstrate the extent to which such seemingly obvious truths are borne out by data. In doing this, implicit belief becomes explicit empirical knowledge—or by its refutation the field is forced to reconsider what it believes. Such articles are a cornerstone to advancing our understanding of the practice of medicine. This article specifically demonstrates that the EHR may have an important role for enhancing clinical quality measures.

While appreciating what this article accomplishes, we should recognize what it does not intend to do. For example, the variation in performance that results from the different data sources reminds us that old problems can persist through new technologies. The old adage of "garbage in, garbage out" holds equally well whether the data are generated by claims forms or by checkboxes or other structured fields in the EHR. This article does not try to validate the information in the EHR. Medical records, whether paper or electronic, are prone to error and bias. It remains for others to evaluate the accuracy of the EHR data in the context of clinical quality measurement.

The exercise of measuring quality is imperfect by nature. Potential measures typically serve as proxies for an ethereal ideal of optimal care. A more nuanced appreciation of this article recognizes that measurement is an exercise in distinguishing signal from noise. The value of a quality measure stands in its capacity to identify enough signal compared with the noise to accomplish at least 1 of 2 tasks: to estimate the absolute level of performance for a specified entity or to demonstrate meaningful differences between different entities, even when measurement of the absolute performance level may be biased.

This article shows that the absolute performance score is highly dependent on the data source. It would be useful for future research papers to assess the extent to which this limitation permits or prevents comparison across different entities using identical data sources. Turning to practice, this article reminds us both that reporting data sources is fundamental to good practice and that different data sources may work in different contexts. Researchers can observe that the value of data is always specific to the questions you would like it to address.

This important technical paper on pediatric quality measurement also provides us with an opportunity to highlight the work of the Pediatric Quality Measures Program, which includes 7 Centers of Excellence assembled by the Agency for Healthcare Research and Quality in collaboration with the Centers for Medicare and Medicaid Services, 1 of which is at Seattle Children's Hospital and lead by 1 of the Angier article's authors (RMS). The Centers of Excellence are charged with working with diverse stakeholders to develop and enhance quality measures for public and private purchasers and others. In our Center of Excellence's work at the Icahn School of Medicine at Mount Sinai, we have found limitations to EHR data. For example some fields are populated by internal administrative systems, which may be imprecise, for example, regarding the timing of arrival on a unit. Our measure development work is looking at how to enhance the precision of data to meet the needs for quality measurement.

At the end of the day, it remains for the field of pediatric quality measurement to build off of this work to define optimal methods, create optimal measures, and identify optimal data sources for answering the diversity of specific questions required to assess and/or compare the quality of health care, whether for accountability purposes or for improvement. We also need to define acceptable methods that can serve specific purposes even when they are not perfect. These are distinct but related tasks.

L. C. Kleinman, MD, MPH

E. Shemesh, MD

Rates of Medical Errors and Preventable Adverse Events Among Hospitalized Children Following Implementation of a Resident Handoff Bundle
Starmer AJ, Sectish TC, Simon DW, et al (Boston Children's Hosp, MA; et al)
JAMA 310:2262-2270, 2013

Importance.—Handoff miscommunications are a leading cause of medical errors. Studies comprehensively assessing handoff improvement programs are lacking.

Objective.—To determine whether introduction of a multifaceted handoff program was associated with reduced rates of medical errors and preventable adverse events, fewer omissions of key data in written hand-offs, improved verbal handoffs, and changes in resident-physician workflow.

Design, Setting, and Participants.—Prospective intervention study of 1255 patient admissions (642 before and 613 after the intervention) involving 84 resident physicians (42 before and 42 after the intervention) from July-September 2009 and November 2009-January 2010 on 2 inpatient units at Boston Children's Hospital.

Interventions.—Resident handoff bundle, consisting of standardized communication and handoff training, a verbal mnemonic, and a new team handoff structure. On one unit, a computerized handoff tool linked to the electronic medical record was introduced.

Main Outcomes and Measures.—The primary outcomes were the rates of medical errors and preventable adverse events measured by daily systematic surveillance. The secondary outcomes were omissions in the printed handoff document and resident time-motion activity.

Results.—Medical errors decreased from 33.8 per 100 admissions (95% CI, 27.3-40.3) to 18.3 per 100 admissions (95% CI, 14.7-21.9; $P < .001$), and preventable adverse events decreased from 3.3 per 100 admissions (95% CI, 1.7-4.8) to 1.5 (95% CI, 0.51-2.4) per 100 admissions ($P = .04$) following the intervention. There were fewer omissions of key handoff elements on printed handoff documents, especially on the unit that received the computerized handoff tool (significant reductions of omissions in 11 of 14 categories with computerized tool; significant reductions in 2 of 14 categories without computerized tool). Physicians spent a greater percentage of time in a 24-hour period at the patient bedside after the intervention (8.3%; 95% CI 7.1%-9.8%) vs 10.6% (95% CI, 9.2%-12.2%; $P = .03$). The average duration of verbal handoffs per patient did not change. Verbal handoffs were more likely to occur in a quiet location (33.3%; 95% CI, 14.5%-52.2% vs 67.9%; 95% CI, 50.6%-85.2%; $P = .03$) and private location (50.0%; 95% CI, 30%-70% vs 85.7%; 95% CI, 72.8%-98.7%; $P = .007$) after the intervention.

Conclusions and Relevance.—Implementation of a handoff bundle was associated with a significant reduction in medical errors and preventable adverse events among hospitalized children. Improvements in verbal and written handoff processes occurred, and resident workflow did not change adversely.

▶ Increasing data and research point to communication and handoffs as key factors in both poor quality of health care as well as patient safety events. This being said, the communication and handoff arena is not as well understood or developed, nor is it taught as routinely, as physiology in medical education. In actuality, the effect of communication and handoffs on health care quality has only intensified with the regulation of resident work hours, wide infusion of electronic means of interaction that often replace face-to-face communication, and general pushes toward more reasonable work hours for attending physicians as the Generation X folks and beyond become an increasing majority of the workforce. The article by Starmer and colleagues is an important piece because of its systematic implementation and evaluation of an intervention geared solely to improve communication and handoffs. In particular, this article is unique and robust because of its intentional pre–post design, a priori power calculations, well-designed evaluation schema, and broad menu of key outcomes to be assessed. The investigators report, in summary, that a multipronged communication intervention coupled with chart reviews and time-motion observations for evaluation was associated with a statistically significant decrease in medical errors on 2 units within 1 children's hospital over a 3-month intervention period.

The authors provide a thoughtful discussion of concrete considerations that are study limitations. For readers to digest this work and put it in perspective, 1 additional limitation needs consideration: sustainability. The field of quality improvement research is rife with examples of good ideas and interventions implemented for short but intensely scrutinized time periods. These studies often report impact on the outcomes of interest. What is sorely needed to truly improve care is enduring cultural change—in this case, among the health care providers for handoffs—which ensures these new behaviors persist beyond the period of intense study observation. This dilemma in quality improvement research is analogous to the often discrepant findings of what can be accomplished in a controlled, clinical trial versus what happens in routine, "uncontrolled" clinical care. How do we make the often time-pressed task of handoffs reliably occur using mindful communication as routine as putting on a seatbelt in our cars? How do we ensure providers would feel uncomfortable and actually stop a handoff discussion if they are repeatedly interrupted, so that they can consciously seek out a quiet venue to have this key conversation and exchange in? This is a daunting cultural norm shift before us if we are to achieve it for each provider. The task is no less daunting than eradicating polio seemed decades ago. The investigators here, however, are on to something, it seems, and have essentially done a proof-of-concept prototype with a small-scale, both in provider scope and time, demonstration.

For providers, educators, operational staff, and policy makers, the key implications of this research are many. First, this study highlights need and potential impact of standardizing and broadly applying communication and handoff training across medical school and residency curriculum. This topic is as crucial as knowing how to perform a cardiovascular examination or the standard approach to preventing and treating asthma. Second, trainees are obviously not the only ones involved in handoffs of patients. How do we begin to instill reliable best practices in communication among all practicing physicians? Perhaps the underpinning goals of Maintenance of Certification are a foundation that can be used for this. Third, this study also highlights the potential for tools to facilitate this in the form of computerized handoff tools and automatic import of key information. This adds to the growing list of promises foreseeable due to information technology but still far from being standardized, user-friendly, and broadly available.

The "elevator speech" with regard to this study is that the time is now to systematically research communication and handoffs. The past status quo of assuming providers are adept at communication, despite tiredness and distractions, is put to rest by studies like this that apply the scientific lens to every-day care and show that promising improvements are achievable.

M. R. Miller, MD, MSc

Five-Year Follow-up of Community Pediatrics Training Initiative
Minkovitz CS, on behalf of the Community Pediatrics Training Initiative Workgroup (Johns Hopkins Bloomberg School of Public Health, Baltimore, MD; et al)
Pediatrics 134:83-90, 2014

Objective.—To compare community involvement of pediatricians exposed to enhanced residency training as part of the Dyson Community Pediatrics Training Initiative (CPTI) with involvement reported by a national sample of pediatricians.

Methods.—A cross-sectional analyses compared 2008–2010 mailed surveys of CPTI graduates 5 years after residency graduation with comparably aged respondents in a 2010 mailed national American Academy of Pediatrics survey of US pediatricians (CPTI: $n = 234$, response $= 56.0\%$; national sample: $n = 243$; response $= 59.9\%$). Respondents reported demographic characteristics, practice characteristics (setting, time spent in general pediatrics), involvement in community child health activities in past 12 months, use of ≥ 1 strategies to influence community child health (eg, educate legislators), and being moderately/very versus not at all/minimally skilled in 6 such activities (eg, identify community needs). χ^2 statistics assessed differences between groups; logistic regression modeled the independent association of CPTI with community involvement adjusting for personal and practice characteristics and perspectives regarding involvement.

Results.—Compared with the national sample, more CPTI graduates reported involvement in community pediatrics (43.6% vs 31.1%, $P < .01$) and being moderately/very skilled in 4 of 6 community activities ($P < .05$). Comparable percentages used ≥ 1 strategies (52.2% vs 47.3%, $P > .05$). Differences in involvement remained in adjusted analyses with greater involvement by CPTI graduates (adjusted odds ratio 2.4, 95% confidence interval 1.5–3.7).

Conclusions.—Five years after residency, compared with their peers, more CPTI graduates report having skills and greater community pediatrics involvement. Enhanced residency training in community pediatrics may lead to a more engaged pediatrician workforce.

▶ One of our favorite quotes as medical educators is from Plutarch who said, "The mind is not a vessel to be filled, but a fire to be kindled." This article addresses the important question of whether residency programs funded by the Dyson Community Pediatrics Training Initiative (CPTI) successfully kindled such a flame and had an impact on trainees beyond their time in residency.

The last decade has seen tremendous changes in the US health care system. The battle around health care reform highlights the need for physician advocates and community-level advocacy as changes are implemented. Venerable organizations such as the Institute of Medicine and the Robert Wood Johnson Foundation have called attention to the critical need for physicians who have the capacity to transform not just the health of individuals but of communities. Thus, the culture of medicine is shifting to require that all practicing pediatricians, regardless of specialty area, have foundational skills in community pediatrics. CPTI responded to this call to action by funding 10 pediatric programs across the country to incorporate the principles of community pediatrics into their curricula. We applaud the authors for developing a study to answer the question important to many educators—whether their intervention affects knowledge, skills, and behaviors beyond the training period. In addition, we feel that an important outcome of this study is to highlight what practicing pediatricians are doing in the area of community pediatrics and advocacy and where the training gaps remain.

This study includes a control group of pediatricians not in a CPTI program who took the American Academy of Pediatrics general survey. Some of these pediatricians who trained at non-CPTI sites had some form of community pediatrics curricula; however, if anything, their inclusion in this comparison would underestimate the effects of the CPTI curriculum.

Those pediatricians who had not graduated from a CPTI program reported a greater sense of responsibility for community child health yet they also reported lower skill levels compared with the levels reported by graduates of CPTI sponsored programs. This dichotomy does not surprise us. Those trained in the CPTI programs might better understand that they do not bear the sole "responsibility" of community health but would value their role as a partner with the community in creating positive change and would know the steps to engage and serve as a resource.

Although CPTI respondents reported higher level of skills, it is encouraging that in both groups, about half of respondents had used at least 1 community health "strategy," such as participating on a board or educating a legislator. In contrast, use of "skills" such as speaking publicly and researching population data, was low in both groups (Table 4 in the original article). Perhaps it was easier for respondents to recall participating in concrete activities rather than demonstrating broad and somewhat abstract "skills" such as identifying community needs.

Somewhat surprising and concerning is that approximately one-quarter of both groups reported not being able to identify community resources for individual patients. Perhaps respondents were not interpreting this question as broadly as we do. We hesitate to think that any practicing pediatrician would not know how to connect a family with a food bank or a library. These respondents were not asked about the availability of such community resources in their area, but presumably even the most underserved of areas would have at least a few resources.

This article shines light on an area about which we have little data: what are practicing pediatricians doing with regard to community pediatrics and advocacy? The answers are encouraging but also underscore the continuing need for CPTI and similar curricula in other programs. The new pediatric residency requirement of a "minimum of 2 ambulatory educational units that include elements of community pediatrics and child advocacy" allows flexibility but can be broadly interpreted without including key skills like identifying community resources and needs.[1] In addition, new program requirements allow for longitudinal experiences and enhanced individualized curricula.

At our institution, we took advantage of this new flexibility by revamping our mandatory Physician in Community curriculum from a 1-month Post Graduate Year (PGY)-2 rotation to a structured and integrated curriculum that spans the PGY-1 and 2 years and moves from community skills to systems and advocacy skills over time. This format emerged via feedback from our trainees, who, regardless of professional interest, reported that they wanted more community pediatrics skills earlier in their training and valued learning how to be effective advocates. In addition, we greatly appreciate the authors' conclusion about the increasing importance of developing physician leaders in the community.

We launched the Pediatric Leadership for the Underserved residency program in 2004, incorporating explicit leadership skills and development and underserved medicine into the core of standard clinical training.[2] It has become clear to us that the everyday structure of clinical medicine and our clinical learning environments provide the perfect opportunity for our trainees to gain insight into and develop their leadership skills.

Community health and advocacy are areas in which pediatrics is truly a leader among medical specialties. We must continue to kindle the fire by developing and incorporating innovative curricula across the educational spectrum to prepare physicians to use their unique position to meet the health needs of our communities.

A. K. Kuo, MD
A. Whittle, MD

References

1. Accreditation Council on Graduate Medical Education. ACGME Program Requirements for Graduate Medical Education in Pediatrics. https://www.acgme.org/acgmeweb/Portals/0/PFAssets/2013-PR-FAQ-PIF/320_pediatrics_07012013.pdf. Accessed July 27, 2014.
2. Kuo AK, Thyne SM, Chen HC, West DC, Kamei RK. An innovative residency program designed to develop leaders to improve the health of children. *Acad Med.* 2010;85:1603-1608.

The 2011 ACGME Standards: Impact Reported by Graduating Residents on the Working and Learning Environment
Schumacher DJ, Frintner MP, Jain A, et al (Boston Med Ctr, MA; American Academy of Pediatrics, Elk Grove Village, IL)
Acad Pediatr 14:149-154, 2014

Objective.—Changes in Accreditation Council for Graduate Medical Education (ACGME) requirements, including duty hours, were implemented in July 2011. This study examines graduating pediatrics residents' perception of the impact of these standards.

Methods.—A national, random sample survey of 1000 graduating pediatrics residents was performed in 2012; a total of 634 responded. Residents were asked whether 9 areas of their working and learning environments had changed with the 2011 standards. Three combined change scores were created for: 1) patient care, 2) senior residents, and 3) program effects, with scores ranging from −1 (worse) to 1 (improved). Respondents were also asked about hours slept and perceived change in hours slept.

Results.—Most respondents felt that several areas had worsened, including continuity of care and senior resident workload, or not changed, including supervision and sleep. Mean change scores that included all study variables except those related to sleep all showed worsening: patient care (mean −0.37); senior residents (mean −0.36), and program effects (mean −0.06) ($P < .01$). Respondents reported a mean of 6.7 hours of sleep in a 24-hour period, with the majority (71%) reporting this amount of sleep has not changed with the 2011 standards.

Conclusions.—In the year after implementation of the 2011 ACGME standards, graduating pediatrics residents report no changes or a worsening in multiple components of their working and learning environments, as well as no changes in the amount of sleep they receive each day.

▶ Schumacher et al report the dissatisfaction of senior pediatric residents 1 year after the implementation of greater work-hour restrictions on postgraduate level (PL)-1s in 2011. The senior residents expressed the opinion that continuity of care had worsened and their workload had increased without an improvement in hours of sleep or change in supervision. Notably, similar dissatisfaction to the 2011 Accreditation Council for Graduate Medical Education (ACGME) standards was also expressed by residents in other specialties[1] and pediatric program directors.[2] However, dissatisfaction was voiced after the 2003 ACGME duty-hour restrictions were implemented, and the sky did not fall—but neither did the hoped-for benefits appear to accrue for patients or residents.[3] Following the implementation of the 2011 regulations, the 2003 requirements seem like the new "good old days." So what should we make of this?

Residents may resist change only to have the resistance fade after a 3-year "generation" of residents turns over and the change is accepted by successors as "normal"; an example is the introduction of hospitalists.[4] The important question, then, is whether the "new normal" does, in fact, adversely affect clinical care and education.

Continuity of care clearly is affected by shorter resident "shifts," as well as an increased number of transitions and individuals responsible for care. Continuity is also considered a righteous virtue by those of us from a previous era, epitomized in action by such icons as Marcus Welby, MD. But times have changed; shifts and handovers are here to stay. More has been written about handovers in the past several years than in the previous quarter century. This attention has been prompted by restrictions to work hours, but the need to improve handovers is not so much generated by work hour restrictions as revealed by them. Increasing the number of handovers has magnified a problem that existed before work hours were restricted. Structure and supervision can and need to improve handovers and, in the process, improve both clinical care and education. Whether the number of handovers, rather than the quality of handovers, will remain a problem remains to be seen.

The workload of PL-3s likely has increased as PL-1 work hours were restricted and PL-3 work hours were not. But is this a bad thing? Traditionally, PL-1s worked longer and harder than PL-3s, who had "earned" the right to less night call and fewer hours. Yet perhaps this tradition should be questioned. To prepare for independent practice, PL-3s need opportunities to make decisions. Although residents tend to view increased workload as affecting education adversely,[5] the nature of the work as well as the quantity needs to be considered. The distribution of workload needs to reflect the educational needs of PL-3s to assume more responsibility and develop skills in supervision and clinical decision making, rather than being simply a convenient administrative alternative to compensate for the reduced work hours of PL-1s. In many programs, the distribution of workload may well need to be addressed, but the goal is for the responsibility and workload of PL-3s to be appropriate for their level, not for it to be low.

So we come back to the question: What should we make of the dissatisfaction of senior residents (and program directors) 1 year after the implementation of the 2011 regulations? Should we take a "this too shall pass" attitude" or wring our hands? Or recognize the need for better data about the relationship between work hours, patient safety, and education?[6] Thomas Nasca, the chief executive officer of the ACGME, has recognized the need to "remedy the information gap" by providing waivers to groups in internal medicine and surgery to conduct large, multicenter trials to "answer fundamental questions related to the impact of duty hour standards on patient safety and resident education in the real world setting of health care delivery."[7] We look forward with great anticipation to the results of these studies.

K. B. Roberts, MD

References

1. Drolet BC, Christopher DA, Fischer SA. Residents' response to duty-hour regulations—a follow-up national survey. *N Engl J Med.* 2012;e35:31-34.
2. Drolet BC, Whittle SB, Khokhar MT, Fischer SA, Pallant A. Approval and perceived impact of duty hour regulations: survey of pediatric program directors. *Pediatrics.* 2013;132:819-824.
3. Philibert I, Chang B, Flynn T, et al; for the 2001–2002 Accreditation Council for Graduate Medical Education Work Group on Resident Duty Hours and the Learning Environment. The 2003 common duty hour limits: process, outcome, and lessons learned. *J Grad Med Educ.* 2009;1:334-337.
4. Landrigan CP, Muret-Wagstaff S, Chiang VW, Nigrin DJ, Goldmann DA, Finkelstein JA. Senior resident autonomy in a pediatric hospitalist system. *Arch Pediatr Adolesc Med.* 2003;157:206-207.
5. Haferbecker D, Fakeye O, Medina SP, Fieldston ES. Perceptions of educational experience and inpatient workload among pediatric residents. *Hosp Pediatr.* 2013;3:276-284.
6. Roberts KB. Patient safety, work hour regulations, and resident education. *Pediatrics.* 2013;132:919-920.
7. Nasca TJ. Letter to members of the graduate medical education community. Accreditation Council for Graduate Medical Education. March 13, 2014.

Well-Child Care Clinical Practice Redesign for Serving Low-Income Children

Coker TR, Moreno C, Shekelle PG, et al (Mattel Children's Hosp, Los Angeles, CA; Univ of Illinois College of Medicine, Chicago; RAND, Santa Monica, CA; et al)
Pediatrics 134:e229-e239, 2014

Our objective was to conduct a rigorous, structured process to create a new model of well-child care (WCC) in collaboration with a multisite community health center and 2 small, independent practices serving predominantly Medicaid-insured children. Working groups of clinicians, staff, and parents (called "Community Advisory Boards" [CABs]) used (1) perspectives of WCC stakeholders and (2) a literature review of WCC practice redesign to create 4 comprehensive WCC models for children ages 0 to 3 years. An expert panel, following a modified version of the Rand/UCLA Appropriateness Method, rated each model for potential effectiveness on 4 domains: (1) receipt of recommended services, (2) family-centeredness, (3) timely and appropriate follow-up, and (4) feasibility and efficiency. Results were provided to the CABs for selection of a final model to implement. The newly developed models rely heavily on a health educator for anticipatory guidance and developmental, behavioral, and psychosocial surveillance and screening. Each model allots a small amount of time with the pediatrician to perform a brief physical examination and to address parents' physical health concerns. A secure Web-based tool customizes the visit to parents' needs and facilitates previsit screening. Scheduled, non-face-to-face methods (text, phone) for parent communication with the health care team are also critical to these new models of care. A structured process that engages small community practices and community health centers in clinical practice redesign can produce comprehensive, site-specific, and innovative models for delivery of WCC. This process, as well as the models developed, may be applicable to other small practices and clinics interested in practice redesign.

▶ Most pediatricians perform well-child-care (WCC) visits in manner that would be familiar to the founders of the American Academy of Pediatrics in 1930—1 clinician and 1 child—parent dyad at a time in a face-to-face communication. This time-honored format works for most but not all families. Although the standards for WCC visits are set high,[1] many recommended developmental and preventive services are not carried out, and parents report that their major concerns are not addressed.[2]

The study by Coker and her colleagues asks, "Can the design of WCC visits in the first 3 years of life be modified to improve the quality of anticipatory guidance and to more effectively address the concerns of parents in low-income families?" This is an important question considering the many potential and underutilized ideas about the content and process of WCC visits that have been reported in pediatric journals. Consider these:

- Electronic communication for screening, accessing parent concerns, and parent education[3,4]
- Group WCC visits (references listed in text)
- Health educator or developmental specialist as part of the office team[5]
- Selected WCC visits by e-mail correspondence only[6]
- Increased attention to the physical and mental health of parents[7]
- Family/child risk stratification to plan for different time allotments for visits
- Motivational learning[8]
- The Reach Out and Read early literacy program[9]
- Colocating with other professionals in pediatric practice (eg, mental health therapist)
- WCC visits in places other than the pediatric office (eg, day-care centers, preschools)
- Parent groups in an office practice to discuss normal development and behavior
- Parent groups to teach behavior modification in families with oppositional children[10]

Some of these proposed changes are supported by randomized controlled trials, but few have been integrated into WCC visits in most pediatric offices and clinics.

The study by Coker et al used a qualitative research process. Clinicians, staff, and parents from a multisite community clinic and private practices in low-income communities met to develop alternative models for WCC visits that considered feasibility, acceptability to parents and clinicians, and cost. An expert panel then rated each model for provision of recommended services, family-centered perspective, feasibility, and efficiency. Results of the expert panel and a literature review were analyzed by the 2 clinical groups for selection of a final model. The 2 models of care that emerged from this process shared many attributes:

- A health educator for anticipatory guidance and developmental, behavioral, and psychosocial screening
- Abbreviated amount of time with a pediatrician (for physical examinations and addressing physical health concerns)
- Standardized questionnaires and eliciting parent concerns assessed electronically either at home before the visit or at the clinic
- Scheduled non—face-to-face (text, phone) communications with the health care team

The group WCC model proposed by the community clinic group comprised 6 parent—child dyads (same-age children) meeting with a health educator at each WCC visit over a 2-hour period. Reviewing results of screening tools, addressing parent concerns, and standard anticipatory guidance would be accomplished through a group discussion. The model proposed by the private practice group shares components of WCC with a health educator, pediatrician, and medial assistant. Forty minutes is allotted to each patient. In both models, the pediatrician is available for physical examinations a limited amount of time, leaving added time for the pediatrician's regular appointments.

The engagement of parents, staff, and pediatricians is a significant strength of this study. How often are parents or staff in a pediatric practice asked to reflect and comment on the content and style of office visits? Experts were involved as a resource to those who provide and receive care. The central role of the health educator in both models is a departure from traditional WCC visits. It reflects recognition that 1 clinician cannot accomplish everything with current time and financial restraints. Both models of care provide additional time (compared with most current WCC visits) for conversations with parents to assess their understanding of early child care, to instruct, and to provide an opportunity to express concerns. These models of care bring a balance to the contemporary overreliance on standardized questionnaires to detect developmental delays and behavioral conditions.[11] With increased time for conversation between a parent and health care provider, both models of WCC have the potential for strengthening the promotion of healthy development and for not being limited to screen only for developmental and behavioral pathology. Furthermore, these models of WCC visits provide opportunities to teach residents effective clinical communication skills.

A moment of disclosure: 50 years ago, I developed a group WCC model in my primary care practice and in resident teaching clinics.[12] Subjectively, the results were spectacular for the parents and for me as an effective method to teach parents and provide care for babies. Children were seen for health supervision visits in the first 2 years of life in small groups of parents and infants. Beginning with the first well-child visit after birth, a group of 5 or 6 infants and parents met (usually 45 minutes) to discuss recommended WCC topics. Parent concerns guided the discussion. In this model, the pediatrician is in the role of both an educator and facilitator while making use of shared parent concerns with children of similar developmental age. Parents learned from each other as well as from the clinician-facilitator. After the group discussion, a physical and developmental examination took place in either the group setting or individually. I was most impressed with the added value of group WCC in creating a supporting group of parents who shared their parenting experience while observing a range of normal patterns of development and behavior among the children in the group.

Randomized controlled studies of group WCC are limited by different group models, frequency of visits, and small samples. These studies show improved attendance at group WCC visits, fewer calls between visits, more time for personal issues, more open-ended questions, and more discussion of recommended WCC topics compared with traditional WCC.[13,14] No difference could be documented in maternal knowledge or provision of social support.[15] Group WCC in high-risk families did not result in better outcomes in child development status, maternal–child interactions, home environment, or provider time; in this study, attendance at group WCC visits was lower than for traditional care.[16]

In a recent study, pediatricians agreed that building trust between a parent and pediatrician is the most effective tool to ensure successful WCC visits and that trust develops over time with repeated visits.[17] Parents believed that a trusting relationship with the pediatrician was necessary to effectively address their concerns.[18] Can a therapeutic relationship built on trust develop in WCC when a health educator plays a central role? I suspect that trust would be a result of the collective work of the office staff, not always focused on 1 individual. That said, the increased time for education in both models and the opportunity for a shared discussion among parents in the group model may trump the 1-to-1 trust bond of traditional practice. Both models will benefit from randomized controlled trials. The study by Coker et al informs us that the time is right for rethinking WCC visits.[19]

M. T. Stein, MD

References

1. Hagan JF, Shaw JS, Duncan PM, eds. Bright Futures: Guidelines for Health Supervision of Infants, Children, and Adolescents. 3rd ed. Elk Grove Villiage, IL: American Academy of Pediatrics; 2008.
2. Kogan MD, Schuster MA, Yu SM, et al. Routine assessment of family and community health risks: parent views and what they receive. *Pediatrics*. 2004;113: 1934-1943.
3. Carroll AE, Bauer NS, Dugan TM, Anand V, Saha C, Downs SM. Use of computerized decision aid for developmental surveillance and screening. *JAMA Pediatr.* 2014;168:815-821.
4. Sterner R, Howard B. CHADIS. http://www.childhealthcare.org. Accessed August 13, 2014.
5. Zuckerman B, Parker S, Kaplan-Sanoff M, Augustyn M, Barth MC. Healthy steps: a case study of innovation in pediatric practice. *Pediatrics*. 2004;114: 820-826.
6. Bergman DA, Beck A, Rahm AK. The use of internet-based technology to tailor well-child care encounters. *Pediatrics*. 2009;124:e37-e43.
7. Schor EL, American Academy of Pediatrics Task Force on the Family. Family pediatrics: report of the task force on the family. *Pediatrics*. 2003;111: 1541-1571.
8. Schwartz RP. Motivational interviewing (patient-centered counseling) to address childhood obesity. *Pediatr Ann.* 2010;39:154-158.
9. Needlman R, Toker KH, Dreyer BP, Klass P, Mendelsohn AL. Effectiveness of a primary care intervention to support reading aloud: a multi-center evaluation. *Ambul Pediatr.* 2005;5:209-215.
10. Stein MT. Group-based parenting-skill training in primary care offices: are we ready for the challenge? *JAMA Pediatr.* 2014;168:7-9.
11. Stein MT. Strategies to enhance developmental and behavioral services in primary care. In: Wolraich ML, Drotar DD, Dworkin PH, Perrin EC, eds. *Developmental-Behavioral Pediatrics: Evidence and Practice*. Philadelphia: Mosby Elevier; 2008.
12. Stein MT. The providing of well baby care within parent-infant groups. "Pediatricians are encouraged to explore the parent-infant group model in their practices". *Clin Pediatr.* 1977;16:825-828.
13. Osborn LM, Woolley FR. Use of groups in well child care. *Pediatrics*. 1981;67: 701-706.
14. Dodds M, Nicholson L, Muse B, Osborn LM. Group health supervision visits more effective than individual visits in delivering health care information. *Pediatrics*. 1993;91:668-670.
15. Rice RL, Miles CE, Slater CJ. An analysis of group versus individual health supervision visits. *Amer J Dis Children.* 1992;146:488.
16. Taylor JA, Davis RL, Kemper KJ. A randomized controlled trial of group versus individual well child care for high-risk children: maternal-child interaction and developmental outcomes. *Pediatrics*. 1997;99:e9.

17. Tanner JL, Stein MT, Olson LM, Frintner MP, Redecki L. Reflections on well-child care: a national study of pediatric clinicians. *Pediatrics*. 2009;124:849-857.
18. Radecki L, Olson LM, Frintner MP, Tanner JL, Stein MT. What do families want from well-child care? Including parents in the rethinking discussion. *Pediatrics*. 2009;124:858-865.
19. Schor EL. Rethinking well-child visits. *Pediatrics*. 2004;41:210-216.

Group Well-Child Care: An Analysis of Cost

Yoshida H, Fenick AM, Rosenthal MS (Univ of Washington, Seattle; Yale Univ, New Haven, CT)
Clin Pediatr 53:387-394, 2014

Objective.—To determine if group well-child visits (WCV) can be cost neutral compared with individual WCV by varying health care providers, group size, and physician salary.

Method.—We created 6 economic models to evaluate the costs of WCV: 3 for individual WCV delivered by (1) advanced practice registered nurse (APRN), (2) resident, and (3) attending and 3 for group WCV delivered by (4) APRN with a nurse and social worker; (5) resident with an attending, nurse, and child life specialist; and (6) attending with a nurse. For group WCV, we performed sensitivity analyses on group size and duration of provider participation.

Results.—We achieved cost-neutrality at 4 families in the APRN group WCV model; at 3, 4, 5, and 6 families in the resident model with 30, 45, 60, and 90 minutes of attending supervision, respectively; and at 4 and 5 families in the low and high attending salary model, respectively.

Conclusion.—Group WCV can be delivered in a cost-neutral manner by optimizing group size and provider participation.

▶ Considering the huge effort that pediatricians put into well-child care (WCC)—probably about one-third of all primary care pediatric visits—the lack of research on the economics of WCC is surprising. One culprit might be the difficulty of specifying outputs. Some are easy and minimalist: immunizations, assessments of growth and development, perhaps. Bright Futures has clarified basic standards, but there is much beyond those that can and, arguably should, be approached. One study found, for example, "192 discrete health advice directives that pediatricians are expected to deliver to patients/guardians" simply from AAP policy statements."[1] Many others have suggested the importance of teaching parenting skills, observing the irony that driving a car requires proof of knowledge and skill, whereas child rearing is entrusted to anyone who can manage to become pregnant.

Imparting knowledge is not the only output of the WCC visit. Many experienced practitioners think that perhaps the most important result of WCC visits may be to establish and nurture a "therapeutic alliance," a relationship of mutual trust and even emotional closeness between family and clinician, which allows parents to confide their fears and trepidations and secures the future of excellent care for both well and sick situations.

Clearly, then, the outputs of WCC are numerous, variable, and hard to measure, especially in the long term, which is so important to pediatrics. With so many variables, although the traditional 1-on-1 WCC visit has much to satisfy both patients and clinicians, it is not surprising that many alternatives to that model have been suggested. Some practices use technical advances to better collect information from families (eg, online questionnaires) or convey information to them (eg, handouts and online videos). Others substitute an advance practice registered nurse for a pediatrician. Still others try to assemble groups of patients to receive WCC together. Most of these innovations aim at better delivery of information, and the group model promotes social ties among patients as well. Although the article overestimates the deficiencies of current WCC efforts—the citations of ineffectiveness are unconvincing, and strong distinctions need to be made for different settings and populations to properly assess needs and deficits—there is no question that a lot could be done better.

Yoshida et al address themselves to a small but important component to the group care alternative: if you were head of a clinic and wanted to have group visits, what would the production function of alternative personnel inputs be, keeping cost constant? This narrow question avoids assessing various outputs as well as alternative technologies. The narrowness of the question provides some practical guidance to a clinic that has decided to try group WCC visits.

The general conclusion of their economic analysis without an output discriminator is predictable—using lower paid personnel can enable longer visits, as can including more families in the group. The limits of size are set at from 3 to 6 families.

Although the article's general economic approach is admirable, the specifics of their calculations could be questioned. Overhead is not dealt with adequately, especially for the difficult logistical task of arranging group visits. They posit nurses rather than medical assistants rooming patients, which probably doubles the cost of that function. The salaries of pediatricians in New Haven will not reflect that in other parts of the country. And crucially, in fee-for-service situations, they do not consider the possibility of insurance paying for the group visits or the level of such payments.

WCC certainly could use more research. I would suggest staying away from cost-benefit studies because the variable outputs and especially the long-term effects would be so difficult to assess. Instead, cost-effectiveness studies that compared specific outputs under variable input conditions would be better. Most likely, there is no one superior approach to WCC, but rather many alternatives depending on circumstances. Choosing which outputs to emphasize will vary with the specific practitioner, the practice setting, and the patient population.

For future work, the most important variable could be the composition of the research teams. There is a yawning gulf between an academic clinic with residents and a clinic population as opposed to a private practice with experienced pediatricians and middle-class families. Research collaboration between academic researchers and private practitioners might lead to particularly rich and fruitful results, difficult as it is to bridge these 2 disparate worlds. In such collaboration, William Bruce Cameron's observation could be apposite: "Not everything that counts can be counted, and not everything that can be counted counts."

B. N. Shenkin, MD, MAPA

Parents' Experiences With Pediatric Care at Retail Clinics
Garbutt JM, Mandrell KM, Allen M, et al (Washington Univ School of Medicine, St Louis, MO)
JAMA Pediatr 167:845-850, 2013

Importance.—Little is known about the use of retail clinics (RCs) for pediatric care.

Objective.—To describe the rationale and experiences of families with a pediatrician who also use RCs for pediatric care.

Design and Setting.—Cross-sectional study with 19 pediatric practices in a Midwestern practice-based research network.

Participants.—Parents attending the pediatrician's office.

Main Outcomes and Measures.—Parents' experience with RC care for their children.

Results.—In total, 1484 parents (91.9% response rate) completed the self-administered paper survey. Parents (23.2%) who used the RC for pediatric care were more likely to report RC care for themselves (odds ratio, 7.79; 95% CI, 5.13-11.84), have more than 1 child (2.16; 1.55-3.02), and be older (1.05; 1.03-1.08). Seventy-four percent first considered going to the pediatrician but reported choosing the RC because the RC had more convenient hours (36.6%), no office appointment was available (25.2%), they did not want to bother the pediatrician after hours (15.4%), or they thought the problem was not serious enough (13.0%). Forty-seven percent of RC visits occurred between 8 AM and 4 PM on weekdays or 8 AM and noon on the weekend. Most commonly, visits were reportedly for acute upper respiratory tract illnesses (sore throat, 34.3%; ear infection, 26.2%; and colds or flu, 19.2%) and for physicals (13.1%). While 7.3% recalled the RC indicating it would inform the pediatrician of the visit, only 41.8% informed the pediatrician themselves.

Conclusions and Relevance.—Parents with established relationships with a pediatrician most often took their children to RCs for care because access was convenient. Almost half the visits occurred when the pediatricians' offices were likely open.

▶ Ready access to acute care (particularly for adults) especially during evenings and weekends, has long been neglected by our health care system. Large drugstore chains and retailers with pharmacies have taken advantage of their access to capital and their high visibility in communities to establish retail-based clinics (RBCs) on their premises to fill that access gap. Although they appear to have become financially successful, serious questions surround RBCs. Do they further fragment an already-fragmented system? Do they provide high-quality care? Do they succumb to the temptation to drive further profits by prescribing too many medicines to be bought at the parent company's store where they are located?

This simple but wonderfully direct study looks at some of these questions by simply asking parents—all of whom they found in the waiting rooms of a private practice primary care research network in the St Louis area—about their use of and experience with RBC visits for their children. The study finds that an amazing percentage of patients have been seen in RBCs—25%. They find that parents use RBCs because of "convenience." Parents felt RBCs were preferable to seeing their primary care physician (PCP) even though almost half the RBC visits were at times the PCP offices were open (Table 4 in the original article). Almost half of RBC visits (with chief complaints described in Table 5) involved a 30-minute wait, and 11% involved more than an hour wait. In addition, many parents had no or only partial insurance for the RBC visit.

When these data are reviewed objectively, it is difficult to believe that RBC care is indeed more convenient for patients and families; however, something about "convenience" must draw them there. What is it about the way these private offices are run that deflects patients to RBCs? Whatever it is, given that all the study subjects already had a pediatrician, it is unlikely that simply increasing insurance coverage or designating some physician as the PCP will not be sufficient to address these parents' perceived needs of acute care for their children.

Although RBCs seem to be adding something that parents value, there are deficits to the choice that they are making. Continuity of provider is obviously violated. Moreover, the lack of communication between RBC and their home practice shows lack of medical continuity as well.[1] Most dismaying, however, is the finding of how many antibiotics were prescribed in clearly inappropriate clinical situations, if the parents' accounts can be believed: 67.7% of patients with colds or "flu" were treated with antibiotics, and 28.6% of patients with a negative rapid strep test were treated with antibiotics. This is clearly not a definitive study, but anecdotal reports nationwide support this finding and make these

TABLE 5.—Reasons Parents Reported for Seeking Pediatric Care at a Retail Clinic

Reason	No. (%)[a]
Sore throat	118 (34.3)
Ear infection	90 (26.2)
Colds or flu	66 (19.2)
Physical	45 (13.1)
Flu shot	30 (8.7)
Rash	14 (4.1)
Allergies	8 (2.3)
Asthma care	8 (2.3)
Cut or wound	8 (2.3)
Pink eye	6 (1.7)
Other immunizations	4 (1.2)
Sprain/strain	2 (0.6)
Bladder or urinary tract infection	1 (0.3)
Burn	0

[a]N = 344. Percentages sum to more than 100% because parents could select more than 1 reason.

Reprinted from Garbutt JM, Mandrell KM, Allen M, et al. Parents' Experiences With Pediatric Care at Retail Clinics. JAMA Pediatr. 2013;167:845-850, Copyright 2013.

results not unexpected but are nonetheless disturbing. This prima facie evidence of poor quality is shocking, alarming, and deserving of urgent further study.

How, then, should pediatricians respond to the rise in RBCs? One clear finding is that a significant percentage of parents, even those with an established relationship with a pediatrician, want better access, but most still strongly prefer their PCP. Almost all patients in the study knew about RBCs, but most did not use them. As a result, it would seem that pediatricians, whom the authors report are currently ignoring RBCs almost entirely, should develop an explicit strategy to provide the benefits to patients that RBCs seem to provide. Many practices already offer extended hours and walk-in times. Many practices band together to offer weekend and evening care that no individual practice could provide alone. They could also provide more explicit information to patients about expected waiting times and take measures within their offices to minimize these times. If they intend to serve the public, they need to serve the public.

It is unlikely that RBCs will be part of any long-term solution for pediatrics. Mixed adult and pediatric facilities such as emergency departments rarely serve children well. Acute pediatrics might seem "easy," but that is true only for the most experienced practitioners, who are unlikely to gravitate to RBCs. For the public to be served properly, the profession must find ways to make care as easy to access as possible.

From a policy point of view, it is actually a positive for the American system that innovations such as RBCs do arise; in more socialized systems, such innovation would be much more difficult. The challenge, however, is to ensure that good medicine is not driven out simply by profitable exploitation of lack of consumer knowledge of medical quality that they themselves cannot validate. This is a role that is best assumed by professional societies, which should be guardians of quality, and governmental agencies who should support such guardianship.

B. N. Shenkin, MD, MAPA
R. A. Dudley, MD, MBA

Reference

1. Reid RO, Ashwood JS, Friedberg MW, Weber ES, Setodji CM, Mehrotra A. Retail clinic visits and receipt of primary care. *J Gen Intern Med*. 2013;28:504-512.

Vaccine Financing From the Perspective of Primary Care Physicians
O'Leary ST, Allison MA, Lindley MC, et al (Children's Hosp Colorado, Aurora; Ctrs for Disease Control and Prevention, Atlanta, GA; et al)
Pediatrics 133:367-374, 2014

Objectives.—Because of high purchase costs of newer vaccines, financial risk to private vaccination providers has increased. We assessed among pediatricians and family physicians satisfaction with insurance payment for vaccine purchase and administration by payer type, the proportion who have considered discontinuing provision of all childhood vaccines for financial reasons, and strategies used for handling uncertainty about insurance coverage when new vaccines first become available.

Methods.—A national survey among private pediatricians and family physicians April to September 2011.

Results.—Response rates were 69% (190/277) for pediatricians and 70% (181/260) for family physicians. Level of dissatisfaction varied significantly by payer type for payment for vaccine administration (Medicaid, 63%; Children's Health Insurance Program, 56%; managed care organizations, 48%; preferred provider organizations, 38%; fee for service, 37%; $P < .001$), but not for payment for vaccine purchase (health maintenance organization or managed care organization, 52%; Child Health Insurance Program, 47%; preferred provider organization, 45%; fee for service, 41%; $P = .11$). Ten percent of physicians had seriously considered discontinuing providing all childhood vaccines to privately insured patients because of cost issues. The most commonly used strategy for handling uncertainty about insurance coverage for new vaccines was to inform parents that they may be billed for the vaccine; 67% of physicians reported using 3 or more strategies to handle this uncertainty.

Conclusions.—Many primary care physicians are dissatisfied with payment for vaccine purchase and administration from third-party payers, particularly public insurance for vaccine administration. Physicians report a variety of strategies for dealing with the uncertainty of insurance coverage for new vaccines.

▶ Few physicians would argue with the dramatic impact that newer immunizations have had on morbidity and mortality in pediatric practice. But at what cost comes this success? At last, we are able to discuss both the financial impact on the primary care physician and the future uncertainty of being able to continue this success story with newer vaccines that provide protection.

This study examines the financial reality of the business aspect of new vaccines that require multiple doses of product, often costing in excess of $100 per dose. The primary care physician must purchase these vaccines in advance, without knowledge of whether the new vaccine is a covered benefit and whether it will be reimbursed at a level that will achieve a modest profit or produce a substantial loss.

This situation clearly creates a dangerous gamble for a physician whose mantra has not included price discussions with the parents and contract negotiations with each insurance carrier, who then may deny this new vaccine or set an arbitrary payment for the product. Who would have thought that this financial risk would force primary care providers to charge separately "up front" for the provision of new immunizations? Other equally unsatisfying strategies are described in the article (Table 2). Regardless of what strategy is applied, parents are troubled by the approach of carving out a new vaccine. They want protection for their children as soon as they hear about the new immunization that is being advertised by a vaccine manufacturer.

We have seen the impact of expensive new pharmacological agents in adult medicine in the treatment of hepatitis C with expensive medications that are too

TABLE 2.—Physicians' Reported Use of Payment Strategies When Vaccines are First Available

Strategy	HPV Peds	HPV FM	MCV4 Peds	MCV4 FM	Tdap Peds	Tdap FM	Rotavirus Peds	Rotavirus FM
Inform patients that their health plan may not cover it, and therefore they may be billed for it	76%	80%	62%	67%	48%*	59%	50%	55%
Ask patients to determine whether their health plan will cover the vaccine before administering the vaccine	49%*	63%	33%*	47%	23%*	36%	23%*	37%
Delay offering the vaccine to any patients until most health plans are covering it	64%*	47%	50%*	34%	35%*	16%	49%*	33%
Ask patients to sign a statement indicating that they will pay for the vaccine if their health plan denies coverage	41%*	55%	32%*	44%	27%	41%	25%*	39%
Check whether each patient's health plan will cover the vaccine before offering the vaccine to the patient	41%	43%	36%	32%	30%	33%	32%	29%

FM, family medicine physicians; Peds, pediatricians.
*Significantly different from FM; $P \leq .05$ using Mantel–Haenszel χ^2 test for comparison between specialties.
Reproduced with permission from Pediatrics. O'Leary ST, Allison MA, Lindley MC, et al. Vaccine Financing From the Perspective of Primary Care Physicians. Pediatrics. 2014;133:367-374, Copyright © 2014, by the American Academy of Pediatrics.

new to be a covered benefit, but whose efficacy is not in question. Who is to pay the price?

The article mentions, but does not document, the magnitude of vaccine purchase for a pediatrician in a mid-sized private practice. Informal studies place that value at $90 000 per physician per year, and this cost often exceeds personnel costs as the largest overhead item for practice expenses.

This study cites but does not detail the recommendations of the American Academy of Pediatrics (AAP) Private Sector Advocacy Advisory Committee in both "The Business Case for Pricing Vaccines" and "The Business Case for Pricing Immunization Administration." Legal constraints have likely prevented the AAP from endorsing a simple principle to pay physicians 118% to 128% of acquisition cost for vaccine purchase and at least resource-based relative value scale payment for vaccine administration, rather than "cherry picking" this fee and paying physicians as little as $2 to $5 per vaccine administered.

There is mention of a complex marketplace and variation across states. Payment by private payers in Colorado may be vastly different from that received by practices in California. Much like chemotherapy costs, vaccine provision will continue to grow as an important part of the insurance policy. However, why should the reimbursement for this critical piece of medical care be reimbursed differently in Massachusetts than in Texas?

The benefits of future, newer vaccine will be great, but the costs are a moving target. A significant percentage of primary care physicians are contemplating not providing immunizations because the economic risks are too great to stay in this business. It behooves us to consider a consistent national policy for payment—a policy that would reward physicians by encouraging them not to miss an opportunity to prevent disease and not to be worried about the economic consequences. All of us would welcome the opportunity to save children without the threat of ever considering the denial of service. But, as mentioned by the AAP's Section on Administration and Practice Management: "No margin, no mission."

R. L. Oken, MD

Changes in Language Services Use by US Pediatricians

DeCamp LR, Kuo DZ, Flores G, et al (Johns Hopkins Univ School of Medicine, Baltimore, MD; Univ of Arkansas for Med Sciences, Little Rock; Univ of Texas-Southwestern and Children's Med Ctr, Dallas; et al)
Pediatrics 132:e396-e406, 2013

Background and Objectives.—Access to appropriate language services is critical for ensuring patient safety and reducing the impact of language barriers. This study compared language services use by US pediatricians in 2004 and 2010 and examined variation in use in 2010 by pediatrician, practice, and state characteristics.

Methods.—We used data from 2 national surveys of pediatricians (2004: $n = 698$; 2010: $n = 683$). Analysis was limited to postresidency pediatricians with patients with limited English proficiency (LEP). Pediatricians reported use of ≥ 1 communication methods with LEP patients: bilingual family member, staff, physician, formal interpreter (professional, telephone), and primary-language written materials. Bivariate analyses examined 2004 to 2010 changes in methods used, and 2010 use by characteristics of pediatricians (age, sex, ethnicity), practices (type, location, patient demographics), and states (LEP population, Latino population growth, Medicaid/Children's Health Insurance Program language services reimbursement). Multivariate logistic regression was performed to determine adjusted odds of use of each method.

Results.—Most pediatricians reported using family members to communicate with LEP patients and families, but there was a decrease from 2004 to 2010 (69.6%, 57.1%, $P < .01$). A higher percentage of pediatricians reported formal interpreter use (professional and/or telephone) in 2010 (55.8%) than in 2004 (49.7%, $P < .05$); the increase was primarily attributable to increased telephone interpreter use (28.2%, 37.8%, $P < .01$). Pediatricians in states with reimbursement had twice the odds of formal interpreter use versus those in nonreimbursing states (odds ratio 2.34; 95% confidence interval 1.24–4.40).

Conclusions.—US pediatricians' use of appropriate language services has only modestly improved since 2004. Expanding language services reimbursement may increase formal interpreter use.

▶ The changing demographic profile of the American population is old news in pediatrics.[1] We stand at the leading edge of demographic trends and recognized the impact of these trends several decades ago. Our daily interactions with patients and families highlight the need for effective communication, but it is not clear how to best address these challenges. We need effective communication strategies that can be adapted to a variety of settings and that do not interrupt the flow of the provider—patient interaction. DeCamp et al document changes in how pediatricians communicate with patients of low English proficiency (LEP) from 2004 to 2010 (Table 2 in the original article).

The authors highlight the need for objective standards to assess providers' proficiency in a second language and the challenge of developing individual approaches versus systems approaches. I'm encouraged by the fact that policies (Medicaid/CHIP coverage of interpreter services) have a measurable, and positive, impact on providers' behavior (Table 4 in the original article, Rows 9 and 10); however, states vary in their coverage of interpreter services, and providers in some settings still rely on family members as interpreters.

This study, which analyzed national data based on individual pediatricians' experiences, is an important step forward in defining the issues we need to address through research as well as policy development. I look forward to additional studies that will leverage our collective experiences and define new strategies to optimize communication with our patients.

E. Fuentes-Afflick, MD, MPH

Reference

1. Flores G. Culture and the patient-physician-relationship: achieving cultural competency in health care. *J Pediatr.* 2000;136:14-23.

Minority Faculty Development Programs and Underrepresented Minority Faculty Representation at US Medical Schools
Guevara JP, Adanga E, Avakame E, et al (The Children's Hosp of Philadelphia, PA; Rutgers Univ, New Brunswick, NJ; et al)
JAMA 310:2297-2304, 2013

Importance.—Diversity initiatives have increased at US medical schools to address underrepresentation of minority faculty.

Objective.—To assess associations between minority faculty development programs at US medical schools and underrepresented minority faculty representation, recruitment, and promotion.

Design.—Secondary analysis of the Association of American Medical Colleges Faculty Roster, a database of US medical school faculty.

Participants.—Full-time faculty at schools located in the 50 US states or District of Columbia and reporting data from 2000-2010.

Exposure.—Availability of school-wide programs targeted to underrepresented minority faculty in 2010.

Main Outcomes and Measures.—Percentage of underrepresented minority faculty, defined as self-reported black, Hispanic, Native American, Alaskan Native, Native Hawaiian, or Pacific Islander faculty. Percentage of underrepresented minority faculty was computed by school and year for all faculty, newly appointed faculty, and newly promoted faculty. Panel-level analyses that accounted for faculty clustering within schools were conducted and adjusted for faculty- and school-level variables.

Results.—Across all schools, the percentage of underrepresented minority faculty increased from 6.8% (95% CI, 6.7%-7.0%) in 2000 to 8.0% (95% CI, 7.8%-8.2%) in 2010. Of 124 eligible schools, 36 (29%) were identified with a minority faculty development program in 2010. Minority faculty development programs were heterogeneous in composition, number of components, and duration. Schools with minority faculty development programs had a similar increase in percentage of underrepresented minority faculty as schools without minority faculty development programs (6.5%-7.4% vs 7.0%-8.3%; odds ratio [OR], 0.91 [95% CI, 0.72-1.13]). After adjustment for faculty and school characteristics, minority faculty development programs were not associated with greater representation of minority faculty (adjusted OR, 0.99 [95% CI, 0.81-1.22]), recruitment (adjusted OR, 0.97 [95% CI, 0.83-1.15]), or promotion (adjusted OR, 1.08 [95% CI, 0.91-1.30]). In subgroup analyses, schools with programs of greater intensity (present for ≥ 5 years and with more components) were associated with greater increases in underrepresented minority representation than schools with minority faculty development programs of less intensity.

Conclusions and Relevance.—The percentage of underrepresented minority faculty increased modestly from 2000 to 2010 at US medical schools. The presence of a minority faculty development program targeted to underrepresented minority faculty was not associated with greater underrepresented minority faculty representation, recruitment, or promotion. Minority faculty development programs that were of greater intensity were associated with greater increases in underrepresented minority faculty representation.

▶ A diverse workforce in academic medicine is broadly recognized as a core value to an institution based on numerous examples of the strengths of diverse teams in the workplace. Medical school minority faculty development programs are one approach to recruiting, promoting, and retaining underrepresented minority (URM) faculty. Individual program evaluations and characteristics of successful programs based on individual faculty member outcomes are available, but this article supplements a rich database of the Association of American Medical Colleges to perform a national program-level evaluation. We should not be surprised or disappointed at the lack of differences in the growth of minority faculty representation at schools with programs versus schools without formal programs. The authors acknowledge that the heterogeneity of the programs and the multiple sources of supplemental information presented analytic challenges.

In addition, the program-level versus individual faculty member analysis does not account for the impact of department-level faculty development programming, and I would also add professional organization or other national programs. However, a key message should be underscored with the finding that schools that did make a difference had been in business longer (≥ 5 years) and had more components to their programs. The change we want to come will be the result of a marathon, not a sprint, to success.

Although the article does not specifically refer to pediatric faculty, the findings and the challenge of promoting diversity has relevance across the basic science and clinical faculties. Walker and Stapleton[1] call attention to the need to increase pediatric faculty diversity, recognizing that the problem starts early in the pipeline with a limited 1.4% increase in URM entering medical students from 2007 to 2012. The proportion of URM graduates of pediatric residency programs increased from 9% to 15% from 2003 to 2009, but this increase was not statistically significant $(P = .09)$.[2] This limited growth occurred at a time when nonwhite babies made up a majority of the children born in 2011.

Pediatricians are on the front line of addressing the multicultural health issues and challenges for this new pediatric population. There is evidence of positive movement from most of the pediatric organizations with the bottom line being the need for a universal call to promote and support diversity and inclusion from the recruitment of medical students to professorial promotion and academic leadership. An overwhelming number of medical students beginning matriculation, both majority and URM, report the intention to pursue a career in clinical practice in contrast to a full-time academic faculty career. Those of us in academic medicine have to seize this observation as an opportunity to model enthusiasm for the enriching career of an academician, in education, research, service, leadership, and advocacy. Let's make that a priority for all of our students and embrace our URM students for the multicultural perspectives they bring to the table.

R. R. Jenkins, MD

References

1. Walker LR, Stapleton FB. Pediatric Faculty Diversity: A New Landscape for Academic Pediatrics in the 21st Century. *JAMA Pediatrics.* 2013;167(11):989-990.
2. Jenkins RR. Diversity and Inclusion: Strategies to Improve Pediatrics and Pediatric Health Care Delivery. *Pediatrics.* 2014;133(2):327-330.

Commercialism in US Elementary and Secondary School Nutrition Environments: Trends From 2007 to 2012

Terry-McElrath YM, Turner L, Sandoval A, et al (Univ of Michigan, Ann Arbor; Univ of Illinois at Chicago)
JAMA Pediatr 168:234-242, 2014

Importance.—Schools present highly desirable marketing environments for food and beverage companies. However, most marketed items are nutritionally poor.

Objective.—To examine national trends in student exposure to selected school-based commercialism measures from 2007 through 2012.

Design, Setting, and Participants.—Annual nationally representative cross-sectional studies were evaluated in US public elementary, middle, and high schools with use of a survey of school administrators.

Exposures.—School-based commercialism, including exclusive beverage contracts and associated incentives, profits, and advertising; corporate food vending and associated incentives and profits; posters/advertisements for soft drinks, fast food, or candy; use of food coupons as incentives; event sponsorships; and fast food available to students.

Main Outcomes and Measures.—Changes over time in school-based commercialism as well as differences by student body racial/ethnic distribution and socioeconomic status.

Results.—Although some commercialism measures—especially those related to beverage vending—have shown significant decreases over time, most students at all academic levels continued to attend schools with one or more types of school-based commercialism in 2012. Overall, exposure to school-based commercialism increased significantly with grade level. For 63.7% of elementary school students, the most frequent type of commercialism was food coupons used as incentives. For secondary students, the type of commercialism most prevalent in schools was exclusive beverage contracts, which were in place in schools attended by 49.5% of middle school students and 69.8% of high school students. Exposure to elementary school coupons, as well as middle and high school exclusive beverage contracts, was significantly more likely for students attending schools with mid or low (vs high) student body socioeconomic status.

Conclusions and Relevance.—Most US elementary, middle, and high school students attend schools where they are exposed to commercial efforts aimed at obtaining food or beverage sales or developing brand recognition and loyalty for future sales. Although there have been significant decreases over time in many of the measures examined, the continuing high prevalence of school-based commercialism calls for, at minimum, clear and enforceable standards on the nutritional content of all foods and beverages marketed to youth in school settings.

▶ Food marketing influences children's food choices—both immediately and over time as they become loyal customers.[1-3] This is why corporations market to children, and also why it is essential for anyone concerned about children's health to understand how and where children are exposed to marketing. Terry-McElrath et al's nationally representative study of trends in the marketing of food in schools provides important data about children's exposure to marketing in this environment where they are a captive and impressionable target population.[4]

The findings of this study are consistent with our own 2006 national survey of schools[5] and with other local studies that found high prevalence of in-school marketing and modest, if any, financial returns to participating schools.[6-8] Given their large data set and repeat measures over time, Terry-McElrath et al are able to examine additional questions, such as the following: Has the volume of food and beverage marketing in schools changed over time? and Are there observed differences in school marketing based on the age, ethnicity, or socioeconomic status of the children?

The particular time span of the current data, 2007 through 2012, covers the time period during which self-regulation measures announced by the food and beverage industries were put in place.[9-11] The Alliance School Beverage Guidelines, in particular, were intended to limit portion sizes and reduce the number of beverage calories shipped to schools; and industry-sponsored research has reported a significant reduction in the number of beverage calories shipped to schools between 2004 and 2010.[12] This is generally consistent with Terry-McElrath et al's finding that between 2007 and 2012, the percentage of students attending a school with an exclusive beverage contract (EBC) decreased (from 10.2% to 2.9% for elementary schools, from 67.4% to 49.5% for middle schools, and from 74.5% to 69.8% for high schools).

More impressive than the reduction in beverage calories available to students during the school day, however, is the number of students still exposed to food marketing at school. Terry-McElrath et al found that in 2012, 71.5% of elementary school students, 72.7% of middle school students, and 89.7% of high school students in the United States were exposed to some form of food marketing in school (Table 3 in the original article). Even with the self-regulation of the "Alliance School Beverage Guidelines" in place, nearly 70% of high school students nationally were in 2012 exposed to the relentless (ie, daily, in multiple locations in their school) marketing associated with EBCs. Fewer calories are sold in schools as part of these contracts, but the sale of reduced-calorie versions of products serves also to advertise full-calorie primary products, likely influencing children's purchase preferences outside of school.[13]

It is also troubling that despite food industry self-regulation that eschews the use of food coupons in elementary schools,[14] 63.7% of elementary school students attended schools in 2012 where food coupons were distributed. The available data do not shed light on the contrast between the self-regulation commitment of the Children's Food and Beverage Advertising Initiative and the facts on the ground; it may be that companies not participating in the initiative are providing coupons, some participating companies are not complying, or both.

Although marketing is often justified by schools' need to raise funds, the available evidence shows unequivocally that, overall, schools receive minimal funds as a result of participating in marketing initiatives. Terry-McElrath et al report that in 2012, the annual per-pupil profit of schools that received any profits from EBCs was $1.75 for elementary schools, $1.54 for middle schools, and $4.18 for high schools. Moreover, coupons, the most prevalent form of food marketing in elementary schools, are not associated with funding at all.

In our research, we found that in the 2003–2004 school year, 67.2% of US district public schools had some form of advertising by corporations that sell foods of minimal nutritional value or foods high in fat and sugar.[5] Terry-McElrath et al found that in 2012, more than 70% of elementary and middle school students and nearly 90% of high school students are exposed to food marketing at school. Although the studies are not exactly parallel, it is clear that the situation has not improved since 2004—and arguably is worse. This suggests that industry self-regulation has not reduced marketing of foods of little or no nutritional value in schools. By focusing solely on the number of calories for sale at schools, policy makers have allowed the door to food marketing at school to remain open and for children to be persuaded at school to want, buy, and eat foods that are unhealthy for them when eaten to excess.[15]

Given the limited amount of time they have with patients, pediatricians are hard-pressed to influence the food choices essential to their patients' health. The food industry, in contrast, works to influence children's preferences and choices daily by marketing to them wherever they are—at home watching television, on their computers, and in their schools.[15,16] Schools, as a public space, are subject to legislative and regulatory actions that can limit food marketing.[17,18] Terry-McElrath et al's findings should help pediatricians both to understand the extent to which children are marketed to at school and the need to press for laws and policies to protect them from it.

A. Molnar, PhD

F. Boninger, PhD

References

1. Hastings G, McDermott L, Angus K, Stead M, Thomson S. The Extent, Nature and Effects of Food Promotion to Children: A Review of the Evidence Geneva: World Health Organization: July 2006. http://www.who.int/dietphysicalactivity/publications/Hastings_paper_marketing.pdf. Accessed July 14, 2014.
2. Harris JL, Bargh JA, Brownell KD. Priming effects of television food advertising on eating behavior. *Health Psychol.* 2009;28:404-413.
3. Committee on Communications. Children, adolescents, and advertising. *Pediatrics..* 2006;118:2563-2569.
4. Terry-McElrath YM, Turner L, Sandoval A, Johnson LD, Chaloupka FJ. Commercialism in US elementary and secondary school nutrition environments: Trends from 2007-2012. *JAMA-Pediatr.* 2014;168:234-242.
5. Molnar A, Garcia DR, Boninger F, Merrill B. *A National Survey of the Types and Extent of the Marketing of Foods of Minimal Nutritional Value in Schools.* Tempe, AZ: Commercialism in Education Research Unit. http://nepc.colorado.edu/publication/national-survey-types-and-extent-marketing-foods-minimal-nutritional-value-schools. Accessed July 14, 2014.
6. Brent BO, Lunden S. Much ado about very little: the benefits and costs of school-based commercial activities. *Leadersh Policy Sch.* 2009;8:307-336.
7. Polascek M, O'Roarke K, O'Brien L, Blum JW, Donahue S. Examining compliance with a statewide law banning junk food and beverage marketing in Maine schools. *Public Health Rep.* 2012;127:216-223.
8. Nestle M. Soft drink "pouring rights": marketing empty calories. *Public Health Rep.* 2000;115:308-319.
9. Kolish ED, Enright M. *The Children's Food and Beverage Advertising Initiative: A Report on Compliance and Progress During 2012.* Arlington, VA: Council of Better Business Bureaus, Inc. http://www.bbb.org/Global/Council_113/CFBAIReportonComplianceandProgressDuring2012.pdf. Accessed July 14, 2014.
10. Memorandum of Understanding. Washington, DC: American Beverage Association; 2006. http://www.ameribev.org/files/336_MOUFinal28signed29.pdf. Accessed July 14, 2014.
11. American Beverage Association. *Alliance School Beverage Guidelines Final Progress Report.* Washington, DC: American Beverage Association. http://www.ameribev.org/files/240_SchoolBeverageGuidelinesFinalProgressReport.pdf. Accessed July 14, 2014.
12. Wescott RF, Fitzpatrick BM, Phillips E. Industry self-regulation to improve student health. *Am J Public Health.* 2012;102:1928-1936.

13. Moss M. *Salt Fat Sugar: How the Food Giants Hooked US*. New York: Random House; 2013.
14. Kolish ED. *Letter to Margo Wootan (CSPI) Explicating CFBAI Elementary Schools Principles*. Arlington, VA: Council of Better Business Bureaus, Inc; December 14, 2009. http://www.bbb.org/us/storage/0/SharedDocuments/CSPIresponse12-14-09.pdf. Accessed July 14, 2014.
15. Molnar A, Boninger F, Harris MD, Libby KM, Fogarty J. *Promoting Consumption at School: Health Threats Associated with Schoolhouse Commercialism—The Fifteenth Annual Report on Schoolhouse Commercializing Trends: 2011-2012*. Boulder, CO: National Education Policy Center. http://nepc.colorado.edu/publication/schoolhouse-commercialism-2012. Accessed July 14, 2014.
16. Montgomery KC, Chester J. Interactive food and beverage marketing: targeting adolescents in the digital age. *J Adolesc Health*. 2009;45:S18-S29.
17. ChangeLab Solutions. *Model Statute Limiting Food Marketing at Schools*. Oakland, CA: ChangeLab Solutions November 2013. http://changelabsolutions.org/publications/food-marketing-schools. Accessed July 14, 2014.
18. Harris JL, Graff SK. Protecting children from harmful food marketing: options for local government to make a difference. *Prev Chronic Dis*. 2011;8:A92.

Association Between Casino Opening or Expansion and Risk of Childhood Overweight and Obesity

Jones-Smith JC, Dow WH, Chichlowska K (Johns Hopkins Bloomberg School of Public Health, Baltimore, MD; Univ of California, Berkeley; Independent Consultant, Sacramento, CA)
JAMA 311:929-936, 2014

Importance.—Economic resources have been inversely associated with risk of childhood overweight/obesity. Few studies have evaluated whether this association is a direct effect of economic resources or is attributable to unmeasured confounding or reverse causation. American Indian-owned casinos have resulted in increased economic resources for some tribes and provide an opportunity to test whether these resources are associated with overweight/obesity.

Objective.—To assess whether openings or expansions of American Indian–owned casinos were associated with childhood overweight/obesity risk.

Design, Setting, and Participants.—We used repeated cross-sectional anthropometric measurements from fitness testing of American Indian children (aged 7-18 years) from 117 school districts that encompassed tribal lands in California between 2001 and 2012. Children in school districts encompassing American Indian tribal lands that either gained or expanded a casino were compared with children in districts with tribal lands that did not gain or expand a casino.

Main Outcomes and Measures.—Per capita annual income, median annual household income, percentage of population in poverty, total population, child overweight/obesity (body mass index [BMI] ≥85th age- and sex-specific percentile) and BMI z score.

Results.—Of the 117 school districts, 57 gained or expanded a casino, 24 had a preexisting casino but did not expand, and 36 never had a casino. The mean slots per capita was 7 (SD, 12) and the median was 3 (interquartile range [IQR], 0.3-8). Among districts where a casino opened or expanded, the mean change in slots per capita was 13 (SD, 19) and the median was 3 (IQR, 1-11). Forty-eight percent of the anthropometric measurements were classified as overweight/obese (11 048/22 863). Every casino slot machine per capita gained was associated with an increase in per capita annual income ($\beta = \$541$; 95% CI, \$245-\$836) and a decrease in percentage in poverty ($\beta = -0.6\%$; 95% CI, -1.1% to -0.20%) among American Indians living on tribal lands. Among American Indian children, every slot machine per capita gained was associated with a decreased probability of overweight/obesity by 0.19 percentage points (95% CI, -0.26 to -0.11 percentage points) and a decrease in BMI z score ($\beta = -0.003$; 95% CI, -0.005 to -0.0002).

Conclusions and Relevance.—In this study, opening or expanding a casino was associated with increased economic resources and decreased risk of childhood overweight/obesity. Given the limitations of an ecological study, further research is needed to better understand the mechanisms behind this association.

▶ Native American children and youth are disproportionately both poor and overweight compared with non-Hispanic whites, and these differences are most pronounced for those living on tribal lands.[1,2] Poverty is a disease, a social determinant of obesity and a potential epigenetic influence on trans-generational health. This well designed ecological study by Jones-Smith and colleagues comes at a time when understanding the effects of a positive economic "shock" on rates of obesity in California's tribal communities has profound significance. There is a striking paucity of truly unbiased research on the individual and community-wide effects of casinos in the scientific literature, and the small number of investigations provide mixed evidence of health benefits compared with the predictable associations of increased substance abuse, crime, and bankruptcy.

This study sheds light on the cost and benefits of casino ownership in Indian Country and comes on the heels of a 2010 study by Costello et al showing that casino-related profit sharing among all members of the Eastern Band of Cherokee Indians was associated with significant reductions in rates of mental health and behavioral disorders among youth while improving educational outcomes.[3] A 2012 study by Wolfe et al also demonstrated that an exogenous increase in income may improve both health status and well-being through policies that improve economic development.[4]

The researchers evaluated the effect of increased economic resources on the risk for obesity in 117 school districts that encompassed tribal lands between 2001 and 2012. They found a small but significant dose response between increased family income and a decreased risk for overweight/obesity in children and youth. By our account, the effect, although small, is stunning. If the modest increase in per capita income can be shown to have such a salutary effect on overweight/obesity in other communities of poverty, we may have ammunition to attempt replication of the poverty reduction model seen in the United Kingdom between 1999 and 2010. As documented by Jane Waldfogel in Britain's War on Poverty, the Blair government prioritized the reduction in childhood poverty in 1999. Through a combination of programs designed to raise income in families (increase in the minimum wage, paid maternity and paternity leave and tax credits) and an increase in services including universal preschool, the rate of childhood poverty declined from 26.1% to 10.6% over the 11-year period.[5]

This study has some obvious limitations, many of which the authors acknowledged in their discussion. For one, they did not examine differences between individual- and community-level changes with regard to access to healthy foods, the built environment or proximity to communities with higher average incomes. From the point of view of potential generalizability to other tribal lands, it is vital that we understand the complex array of social and economic changes that may have contributed to the reduction in overweight/obesity. What distinguished the communities that had no casino? Which tribal communities engaged in profit sharing, and which invested in community infrastructure? If the long-term health implications of poverty are truly greatest when experienced early in life, how long will it take to recognize the long-term effects of these interventions on children under age 5? What about the health and weight status of women of childbearing age? What might be short- and long-term effects of casinos on cultural well-being, and what are the health costs of those changes?

The authors were careful to note that their conclusions could not be generalized to tribal lands with greater than 80% poverty because they did not observe that level of poverty, yet they compared the casino effect to the Pathways Study. The Pathways Study was an ambitious multicenter study to test the effect of a school-based behavioral intervention on rates of overweight/obesity in Native American children. The study included communities where poverty rates approached 80%. Although ineffective at producing unbiased results within a 3-year study period, the investigators recognized that there is not likely any such thing as a one-size-fits-all approach to obesity prevention or reduction.[6] The same is undoubtedly true of poverty. It is critical that we use research to inform and guide our advocacy and public policy toward the reduction of poverty. Studies such as this one show that small steps in poverty reduction can improve the health of individuals and the community. What remains is the need for ongoing research on the best ways to achieve poverty reduction and the political will to act on it.

Casinos are the elephant in the room for many American tribal communities. They are a means to economic self-sufficiency for some tribes but for others are unprofitable or incomprehensible. For the US government to begin to address the failure of the reservation system, there needs to be a systemic reexamination of economic development efforts on tribal lands. One step in the right direction was President Obama's designation of the Choctaw Nation as 1 of 5 Promise Zones in his 2014 State of the Union address.[7] One small step...

J. A. Oski, MD, MPH

N. Branco, MD, MPH

References

1. United States Census Bureau. Facts for Features. http://www.census.gov/newsroom/releases/archives/facts_for_features_special_editions/cb12-ff22.html. Accessed June 12, 2014.
2. Wang Y. Disparities in pediatric obesity in the United States. *Adv Nutr.* 2011;2: 23-31.
3. Costello EJ, Erklani A, Copeland W, Angold A. Association of Family Income Supplements in Adolescence with Development of Psychiatric and Substance Abuse Disorders in Adulthood Among an American Indian Population. *JAMA.* 2010; 303(19):1954-1960.
4. Wolfe B, Jakubowski J, Haveman R, Courey M. The Income and Health Effects of Tribal Casino Gaming on American Indians. *Demography.* 2012;49:499-524.
5. Waldfogel J. Britain's War on Poverty. Russell Sage Foundation. 2010.
6. Gittelsohn J, Davis SM, Steckler A, et al. Pathways: Lessons Learned and Future Directions for School-based Interventions Among American Indians. *Prev Med.* 2003;37:S107-S112.
7. The White House. State of The Union. http://www.whitehouse.gov/sotu. Accessed on June 12, 2014.

Sleep Timing Moderates the Concurrent Sleep Duration–Body Mass Index Association in Low-Income Preschool-Age Children

Miller AL, Kaciroti N, LeBourgeois MK, et al (Univ of Michigan, Ann Arbor; Univ of Colorado, Boulder)
Acad Pediatr 14:207-213, 2014

Objective.—To test the independent main and moderating effects of sleep timing on body mass index (BMI) in low-income preschool-age children (M = 4.11 years, SD = 0.54).

Methods.—Parents reported demographics and children's sleep concurrently, and a subset of children was followed longitudinally. Child height and weight were measured and BMI z score (BMIz) calculated. Regression analysis evaluated main effects of sleep timing (bedtime, weekday-to-weekend schedule shifting, napping) on concurrent BMIz and future rate of change, and their moderating effects on the sleep duration–BMIz association.

Results.—Of 366 children (longitudinal subsample = 273), 50% were boys, 57% white, and 37% overweight or obese. Nocturnal sleep duration predicted concurrent BMIz, but not rate of change in BMIz over time. Bedtime was a moderator; the sleep duration–BMIz association was present only among children with bedtimes after 9 PM ($\beta = -0.44$; 95% confidence interval $-0.69, -0.18$). Schedule shifting was a moderator; the association between greater nocturnal sleep duration and lesser rate of future BMIz increase was present only among children with the most consistent sleep schedules (<45-minute delay in weekend bedtime: $\beta = -0.12$; 95% confidence interval $-0.23, -0.01$). Daytime napping did not moderate the nocturnal sleep duration–BMIz association. Covariates (sleep-disordered breathing, soda consumption, home chaos) did not explain these associations.

TABLE 2.—Unadjusted Parameter Estimates and 95% Confidence Intervals From Final Cross-Sectional Models Predicting Child Concurrent BMI z Score (n = 366)

Parameter	B (SE) for:			
	Model A: Nocturnal Sleep Duration	Model B: Nocturnal Sleep + Bedtime	Model C: Nocturnal Sleep + Shifting	Model D: Nocturnal Sleep + Napping
Nocturnal sleep duration	−0.15 (0.07)*	−0.23 (0.10)*	−0.15 (0.08)*	−0.15 (0.08)†
Bedtime		−0.18 (0.10)*		
Shifting			−0.02 (0.07)	
Napping				0.05 (0.08)
Nocturnal sleep duration × bedtime		−0.18 (0.08)*		
SDB	0.43 (0.40)	0.37 (0.40)	0.45 (0.41)	0.43 (0.40)
Caffeine	0.10 (0.10)	0.08 (0.10)	0.10 (0.10)	0.10 (0.10)
CHAOS	0.01 (0.02)	−0.002 (0.02)	0.01 (0.02)	0.01 (0.02)

BMI = body mass index; SDB = sleep-disordered breathing; CHAOS = Confusion, Hubbub, and Order Scale.
*$P < .05$.
†$P < .10$.
Reprinted from Miller AL, Kaciroti N, LeBourgeois MK, et al. Sleep Timing Moderates the Concurrent Sleep Duration-Body Mass Index Association in Low-Income Preschool-Age Children. Acad Pediatr. 2014;14:207-213, with permission from Acta Paediatrica and John Wiley and sons, www.interscience.wiley.com.

Conclusions.—Among low-income preschoolers, sleep timing moderated the nocturnal sleep duration—BMIz association. Understanding how sleep timing and sleep duration relate to childhood obesity is important for prevention efforts.

► Sleep duration has decreased among people of all ages. In addition, this decline parallels the rise in the prevalence of obesity. The mechanisms through which sleep duration are thought to affect obesity include changes in metabolic pathways, such as appetite hormone dysregulation (ie, leptin and ghrelin).[1] Cross-sectional study findings support the relationship between short sleep duration and obesity in different age groups.

The effect of short sleep duration on obesity risk is a particularly important issue for preschool-age children. The National Sleep Foundation recommends 11 to 13 hours of sleep for this age group.[2] However, these children are documented to have a notably late bedtime (after 9 PM), as well as short average sleep duration time.[3] Longitudinal evidence in this population has been limited.

In this respect, Miller and colleagues present an important and timely study of sleep duration and obesity risk in a large sample of low-income preschool-age children. They tested the association of nighttime sleep duration with body mass index (BMI) z-score (BMIz) and the association between nighttime sleep duration with BMIz rate of change over 1 year, while accounting for sleep timing as a moderator of these relationships. Findings showed that longer sleep duration and later bedtime were associated with decreased BMIz (Table 2). Three sleep timing variables were examined as moderators: "usual bedtime" on weekdays, weekday to weekend sleep shifting, and daytime napping. Only bedtime significantly interacted with sleep duration ($P < .02$).

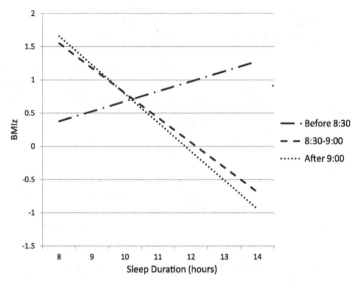

FIGURE 1.—Association between nocturnal sleep duration and concurrent body mass index z score (BMIz) by tertile of bedtime (cross-sectional sample). (Reprinted from Miller AL, Kaciroti N, Lebourgeois MK, et al. Sleep timing moderates the concurrent sleep duration—body mass index association in low-income preschool-age children. *Acad Pediatr.* 2014;14:207-213, with permission from Academic Pediatric Association.)

To examine interactions, bedtime was split into tertiles: before 8:30 PM, 8:30 to 9:00 PM, and after 9 PM. Cross-sectional results showed that children who went to bed at or after 8:30 PM and slept less had higher BMIz (Fig 1), but with increasing sleep duration, BMIz decreased. Among those who went to bed early (before 8:30 PM), sleep duration was positively, but not significantly, related to BMIz. Longitudinal findings showed that longer sleep duration was significantly and inversely related to 1-year BMIz rate of change, among those who had less than a 45-minute shift in their bedtime from weekday to weekend (Fig 2). The authors concluded that sleep timing played a moderating role in how short sleep contributes to obesity.

In addition, to the findings noted by authors, there are other findings worth mentioning. Fig 1 shows that children who slept about 10.5 hours had a healthy BMIz, regardless of the child's bedtime. Furthermore, children with a bedtime at or after 8:30 PM and who slept the recommended amount (11—13 hours) had a significantly lower BMIz. In addition, sleep shifting > 45 minutes showed a similar trend with decreasing BMIz with longer sleep duration. A limitation of the study is that authors did not provide sample sizes that corresponded to the various regression lines in Figs 1 and 2.

Authors conclude that pediatric providers should emphasize earlier bedtimes in addition to adequate sleep duration to prevent obesity. Based on these findings, however, a bedtime at or after 8:30 PM may have been a protective risk factor. Further investigation is needed to understand how bedtime plays a role in the sleep-obesity relationship. Indeed, preschool-age children in this study who slept at least 10.5 hours, regardless of bedtime, had a healthy weight

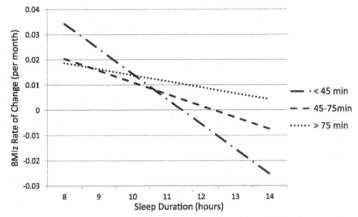

FIGURE 2.—Association between nocturnal sleep duration and rate of body mass index z score (BMIz) change by tertile of weekday to weekend bedtime shift (longitudinal sample). (Reprinted from Miller AL, Kaciroti N, Lebourgeois MK, et al. Sleep timing moderates the concurrent sleep duration—body mass index association in low-income preschool-age children. *Acad Pediatr.* 2014;14:207-213, with permission from Academic Pediatric Association.)

status. Therefore, an alternative conclusion to draw from these findings is simple: preschool-age children should obtain an adequate amount of sleep.

As for providers and public health educators, there are several take-home messages. Children should sleep the recommended amount to ensure that their bodies are rested and metabolically recovered. An early bedtime may not necessarily be required.

S. M. Martinez, PhD, MS

References

1. Spiegel K, Tasali E, Penev P, Van Cauter E. Brief communication: sleep curtailment in healthy young men is associated with decreased leptin levels, elevated ghrelin levels, and increased hunger and appetite. *Ann Intern Med.* 2004;141:846-850.
2. National Sleep Foundation. http://www.sleepfoundation.org/article/sleep-topics/children-and-sleep. Accessed September 28, 2012.
3. Owens JA, Jones C. Parental knowledge of healthy sleep in young children: results of a primary care clinic survey. *J Dev Behav Pediatr.* 2011;32:447-453.

Parent Perspectives on the Design of a Personal Online Pediatric Immunization Record

Kitayama K, Stockwell MS, Vawdrey DK, et al (Columbia Univ, NY; New York-Presbyterian Hosp)
Clin Pediatr 53:238-242, 2014

Objective.—To examine desired characteristics of an online immunization record for parents from a predominantly Latino, low-income population.

Methods.—Four focus groups were conducted with parents (n = 29) from an urban, primarily Latino, low-income population in New York. The data were collected and analyzed during winter 2008-2009.

Results.—Participants expressed interest in using an online immunization record that has the ability to show a child's immunization status and to access consumer health information related to vaccinations. Participants suggested that the online record be translated into multiple languages and provide user-friendly interfaces. Participants were enthusiastic about the benefits offered by the online immunization record, highlighting having an electronic copy of their child's immunization record available. Concerns over disclosing personal information were raised, and safeguards to protect confidentiality were requested.

Conclusions.—If concerns about privacy are adequately addressed, parents of low-income, urban children are likely to use and benefit from an online immunization record.

▶ This article written by Kitayama and colleagues is particularly relevant for the 2015 edition of the YEAR BOOK OF PEDIATRICS because we are entering the formative years of the digital patient-engagement revolution. Many clinical, consumer-driven, policy, and financial factors are coalescing to create an environment in which patient engagement with empowering digital tools will be "the blockbuster drugs of this century."[1,2]

Providers across the country are now deploying electronic tools and communication standards that enable their patients to "review, download, and transmit" their own health data to meet the federal Meaningful Use Program Stage 2 requirements.[3] Furthermore, in 2014 through the effects of the Affordable Care Act, value-based reimbursement incentives are percolating throughout the health care system. These incentives are beginning to encourage providers to partner with their patients to keep them healthy, free from chronic disease exacerbations, and out of the hospital. Meanwhile, US consumers, who have been mightily empowered by the Internet in industries such as banking and travel, are now looking to use connected communication tools to empower themselves in health care.[4]

At this crucial moment, Kitayama and colleagues remind us that as we engage patients with electronic-communication tools such as a personal health record, we need to include those patients who are at risk of being marginalized—the poor, the less educated, and immigrant families who have specific cultural, language, and documentation-status needs.

We should focus on empowering historically underserved patients with engagement tools not only because it is the compassionate thing to do but also because data are accumulating to suggest that it is also the most cost-effective thing to do. Rask and colleagues, for example, showed that indigent public-hospital diabetes patients who were more activated, as measured by a standard patient-activation scale, were more likely to get foot checks and eye exams compared with their less activated counterparts in the same social circumstances.[5] Quantifying the cost of this effect, Hibbard and colleagues found that patients with the lowest activation scores cost the system between 8% to 21% more than patients who are the most activated.[6]

The authors stated the limitations of this study well, prompting the need for continued rigorous evaluation of patient-facing digital health engagement tools—including quantitative outcomes-based evaluation. Nevertheless, insights that we should apply to digital patient-empowerment tools for traditionally underserved populations include the need to translate information from the provider-facing health record and patient education into many languages and the desire for this study population to receive more than just data but actual information. For example, the study participants asked: "Is my child up-to-date on his or her vaccinations? The request from this population is for applicable knowledge to be synthesized from the personal health record data. For example, study participants requested knowing "What diseases can my children get and not get, given all vaccines they've received?"

Finally, although we often think of the discerning, wealthy health care consumer demanding convenience and privacy, the authors of this article remind us that these factors are even more important for mothers with limited resources and for families with varying immigration documentation.

S. Bokser, MD, MPH

References

1. Kish L. The Blockbuster Drug of the Century: An Engaged Patient? [HL7 Standards Blog]. http://www.hl7standards.com/blog/2012/08/28/drug-of-the-century/. Accessed May 19, 2014.
2. Chase D. Patient Engagement is the Blockbuster Drug of the Century. Forbes. http://www.forbes.com/sites/davechase/2012/09/09/patient-engagement-is-the-blockbuster-drug-of-the-century/. Accessed May 19, 2014.
3. Centers for Medicare & Medicaid Services. https://www.cms.gov/Regulations-and-Guidance/Legislation/EHRIncentivePrograms/Downloads/stage1vsStage2Comp TablesforEP.pdf. Accessed May 19, 2014.
4. Pew Research Center/CHCF Health Survey: August 7-September 6, 2012. http://www.pewinternet.org/2013/02/12/the-internet-and-health/. Accessed May 30, 2014.
5. Rask KJ, Ziemer DC, Kohler SA, Hawley JN, Arinde FJ, Barnes CS. Patient activation is associated with healthy behaviors and ease in managing diabetes in an indigent population. *Diabetes Educ.* 2009;35(4):622-630.
6. Hibbard JH, Greene J, Overton V. Patients with lower activation associated with higher costs; delivery systems should know their patients' 'scores'. *Health Aff.* 2013;32(2):216-222.

Twelve tips for using social media as a medical educator
Kind T, Patel PD, Lie D, et al (George Washington Univ, DC; Univ of Louisville School of Medicine, KY; Keck School of Medicine of Univ of Southern California, Los Angeles, CA)
Med Teach 36:284-290, 2014

Background.—We now live, learn, teach and practice medicine in the digital era. Social networking sites are used by at least half of all adults.

TABLE.—Twelve Tips for Using Social Media as a Medical Educator

1. Identify and then reflect upon your digital identity and goals for using social media
2. Select a tool based upon goals and the strength of platforms available to support educational activities
3. Observe and establish comfort first. Think, then contribute
4. Make some initial connections and tap into the power of a community
5. Know and apply existing social media guidelines for the responsible use of social media
6. Develop individual guiding principles with which you are comfortable
7. Keep all patient information private
8. Handling "friend" requests from trainees: Know your options and their consequences
9. Share credible information: disseminate evidence-based health information, enhancing public health
10. Engage, learn, reflect, and teach
11. Research: Advance your academic productivity by expanding your professional network
12. Mentor and be mentored: demonstrate responsible social media use

Adapted from Kind T, Patel PD, Lie D, et al. Twelve tips for using social media as a medical educator. Med Teach. 2014;36:284-290, Copyright 2014.

Engagement with social media can be personal, professional, or both, for health-related and educational purposes. Use is often public. Lapses in professionalism can have devastating consequences, but when used well social media can enhance the lives of and learning by health professionals and trainees, ultimately for public good. Both risks and opportunities abound for individuals who participate, and health professionals need tips to enhance use and avoid pitfalls in their use of social media and to uphold their professional values.

Aims and Methods.—This article draws upon current evidence, policies, and the authors' experiences to present best practice tips for health professions educators, trainees, and students to build a framework for navigating the digital world in a way that maintains and promotes professionalism.

Results and Conclusions.—These practical tips help the newcomer to social media get started by identifying goals, establishing comfort, and connecting. Furthermore, users can ultimately successfully contribute, engage, learn, and teach, and model professional behaviors while navigating social media (Table).

▶ We are living in a digital world today with social media being the latest tools we health care providers have to use in our daily work with patients, learners, and colleagues and also in own personal lives for connecting and engaging with family, friends, and our communities. This article provides practical information for health care providers considering using social media or who are relatively new to it, and also for experienced users who may be looking for ideas to enhance their use.

For those starting out, social media can seem overwhelming. However, the authors break down the task of using social media into 12 key concepts or tips (Table). Each tip has important questions to consider and presents practical examples and ideas of how your answers to the questions could be applied to your own particular situation. These tips help to sort out the questions you should be asking before starting to use these tools and develop your online persona.

For the seasoned user, the tips can serve to reaffirm your appropriate use of social media, as a reminder of potential pitfalls of inappropriate use, and to help reaffirm your online persona. Even an experienced user may not have come across all of these concepts, and this is a good article to review them. One example is how to handle "friending" trainees.

As with any new tool or technology, there are pros and cons to their use, and the best use balances these elements. The key issue of how best to use these tools in our professional and personal lives is explored, pointing out the how social media tools can be overwhelming or easy to use, a time-sink or time-saver, and very distracting or rewarding to use.

The writing style is conversant and sounds like one is discussing the issues with a friend or expert. For a new user, the "conversations in your head" should help build confidence to begin using these tools. For a seasoned user, a particular question should resonate with your experience and make your reflect more on it. The questions should help you to reaffirm your use, possibly abandon some practices and wish to explore other tools.

The key tips for me are the following: to think about your goals for social medial use and what you hope to do when using these tools (Tip 1); to develop social media use principles that are true to your offline self and online persona (Tip 6); being willing to try using these tools to engage, learn, reflect, and teach (Tip 10); and to balance the competing issues to use social media in a responsible way that you are proud of (Tips 1—12). Even in this short list, the most important ones are to know your purpose for using these tools and to balance the issues. If your purpose is clear, then the necessary balance becomes easier to accomplish successfully.

Although relatively new, social media tools have been in existence long enough for some behavioral norming standards to occur. As these tools develop with more time and use, as well as the availability of different, future technology, behavioral norming will need to continue to change. This article organizes key concepts so that the ideas and questions should remain relevant and applicable to developing standards and new tools in the future.

D. M. D'Alessandro, MD

Educational and Vocational Outcomes of Adults With Childhood- and Adult-Onset Systemic Lupus Erythematosus: Nine Years of Followup
Lawson EF, Hersh AO, Trupin L, et al (Univ of California, San Francisco; Univ of Utah, Salt Lake City)
Arthritis Care Res 66:717-724, 2014

Objective.—To compare educational and vocational outcomes among adults with childhood-onset systemic lupus erythematosus (SLE) and adult-onset SLE.

Methods.—We used data derived from the 2002—2010 cycles of the Lupus Outcomes Study, a longitudinal cohort of 1,204 adult subjects with SLE. Subjects ages 18—60 years living in the US (n = 929) were included in the analysis and were classified as childhood-onset SLE if age at diagnosis was <18 years (n = 115). Logistic regression was used to assess the unadjusted and adjusted effect of childhood-onset SLE, sex, race/ethnicity, baseline age, urban or rural location, and US region on the likelihood of completing a bachelor's degree. Generalized estimating equations were used to assess the effect of childhood-onset SLE, demographics, education, and disease-related factors on the odds of employment, accounting for multiple observations over the study period.

Results.—Subjects with childhood-onset SLE were on average younger (mean ± SD 29 ± 10 years versus 44 ± 9 years), with longer disease duration (mean ± SD 15 ± 10 years versus 11 ± 8 years). Subjects with adult-onset SLE and childhood-onset SLE subjects were equally likely to complete a bachelor's degree. However, subjects with childhood-onset SLE were significantly less likely to be employed, independent of demographic and disease characteristics (odds ratio 0.62, 95% confidence interval 0.42−0.91).

Conclusion.—While subjects with SLE are just as likely as those with adult-onset SLE to complete college education, childhood-onset SLE significantly increases the risk of not working in adulthood, even when controlling for disease and demographic factors. Exploring reasons for low rates of employment and providing vocational support may be important to maximize long-term functional outcomes in patients with childhood-onset SLE.

▶ This report highlights some of the social and vocational challenges that children with chronic disorders, such as systemic lupus erythematosus (SLE), confront as they grow into adulthood. This issue has relevance for all medical providers who care for children. SLE is sometimes disabling and, especially if renal disease is present, progressive; it also has many comorbidities, many of which have an impact during the working years. Young adults who have onset chronic illness in childhood are liable to confront lower educational and then occupational outcomes regardless of the specific diagnosis. Adults with childhood-onset chronic illness have been shown to fare worse than adults without such illnesses on educational, vocational, and income outcomes and have about 50% of college graduation, being currently employed, and have significantly lower mean incomes.[1]

Factors such as gender; socioeconomic status of child's family, especially based on highest level of graduation of either parent, educational attainment, and current employment; as well as current school attendance are all variables that should be controlled in assessing impacts of the illness on the child's vocational outcomes. Various complex mechanisms, such as absenteeism from school or work, that can affect occupational readiness and educational attainment must also be considered when reviewing data on different outcomes in adults who had childhood-onset chronic impairments. More adults with adult-onset chronic illness start college than those whose illness was diagnosed during preadult years. Also important, although most adults who had childhood-onset chronic illness complete high school and are employed, they are likely to have poorer educational and occupational outcomes than adults without a chronic illness.

Other chronic disorders are more static, are less progressive, and have less likelihood of neurologic impairments. A child with juvenile idiopathic arthritis, for example, is more similar to unaffected peers on educational and other outcomes during transition from adolescence to adulthood than those with active SLE with central nervous system involvement.[2]

Other variables have been examined and interventions to ameliorate dysfunctions based on, for example, family dysfunctions and parental functioning have been fruitful.[3,4]

Multiple studies demonstrate that caregiver burden and health risks may be accentuated in the case of adults caring for children with a serious health condition or disability and that intervention focused on the caregiver has a positive impact on long-term social, educational, and vocational outcomes for the child.[5,6]

Advances in clinical medicine are extending the life spans of youngsters with illnesses that formerly had life-threatening consequences. Medical providers are in a unique position to identify some of the avoidable barriers to a successful educational, social, and vocational outcome for their patients with childhood-onset chronic disorders and to assist families in identifying resources to overcome them. Family disarray, parental dysfunctions, overly restrictive expectations for social, educational, and vocational outcomes are among those that, if unaddressed, can further burden and increase the impairment of the child or adolescent with a chronic illness. There is a growing and urgent need for good data on the impact of newer medical interventions on social, educational, or occupational outcomes. The use of new biologic agents, gene therapies, and other advances has yet to be evaluated in terms of those outcomes.

E. M. Sills, MD

References

1. Maslow GR, Haydon A, McRee AL, Ford CA, Halpern CT. Growing up with a chronic illness: social success, educational/vocational distress. *J Adolesc Health.* 2011;49:206-212.
2. Gerhardt CA, McKordon KD, Vannatta K, et al. Educational and occupational outcomes among young adults with juvenile idiopathic arthritis. *Arthritis Rheum.* 2008;59:1385-1391.
3. Ireys HT, Sillis EM, Kolodner KB, Walsh BB. A social support intervention for parents of children with juvenile rheumatoid arthritis: results of a randomized clinical trial. *J Pediatr Psychol.* 1996;21:633-641.
4. Lustig JL, Ireys HT, Sillis EM, Walsh BB. Mental health of mothers of children with juvenile rheumatoid arthritis: appraisal as a mediator. *J Pediatr Psychol.* 1996;21:719-733.
5. Silver EJ, Ireys HT, Bauman LJ, Stein REK. Psychological outcomes of a support intervention in mothers of children with ongoing health conditions: the parent-to-parent network. *J Community Psychol.* 1997;25:249-264.
6. Ireys HT, Salkever DS, Kolodner KB, Bijur PE. Schooling, employment, and idleness in young adults with serious physical health conditions: effects of age, disability status, and parental education. *J Adolesc Health.* 1996;19:25-33.

12 Musculoskeletal

Shoulder Injuries Among US High School Athletes, 2005/2006–2011/2012
Robinson TW, Corlette J, Collins CL, et al (Nationwide Children's Hosp, Columbus, OH; et al)
Pediatrics 133:272-279, 2014

Objectives.—The objective of this study was to describe shoulder injuries in a nationally representative sample of high school athletes playing 9 sports. A national estimate of shoulder injuries among high school athletes was subsequently calculated.

Methods.—Injury data were collected in 9 sports (boys' football, soccer, basketball, wrestling, and baseball; girls' soccer, volleyball, basketball, and softball) during the 2005–2006 through 2011–2012 academic years from a nationally representative sample of high schools via High School Reporting Information Online.

Results.—During the 2005–2006 through 2011–2012 academic years, high school athletes in this study sustained 2798 shoulder injuries during 13 002 321 athlete exposures, for an injury rate of 2.15 per 10 000 athlete exposures. This corresponds to a nationally estimated 820 691 injuries during this time period. Rates of injury were higher in competition as compared with practice (rate ratio = 3.17 [95% confidence interval: 2.94–3.41]). The highest rate of injury was in football (4.86) and the lowest in girls' soccer (0.42). The most common types of injury were strain/sprain (37.9%) and dislocation/separation (29.2%). Boys were more likely than girls to sustain their injuries after contact with another person or with the playing surface. Surgical repair was required for 7.9% of the injuries. Time loss from athletic participation varied among sports, with 40.7% of athletes returning within 1 week, whereas 8.2% were medically disqualified for their season/career.

Conclusions.—High school shoulder injury rates and patterns varied by sport and gender. Prospective epidemiologic surveillance is warranted to discern trends and patterns to develop evidence-based interventions to prevent shoulder injuries.

▶ Athletes get shoulder injuries. This is not new news. What makes this study unique is the large sample size and robust data collection methods; these allow for identification of important sport and gender differences in injury patterns, which have implications for injury prevention strategies.

Data were collected using the National High School Sports-Related Injury Surveillance System, High School Reporting Online (RIO), an Internet-based sports injury surveillance system. Athletic trainers from a nationally representative sample of high schools collect data in a prospective manner, by submitting weekly reports online to describe the details of any injury that (1) occurred as a result of participation in an organized practice or competition, (2) required medical attention by an athletic trainer or physician, and (3) resulted in restriction of athlete's participation for at least 1 day. Injury rates are reported per athlete exposure, which is a much more accurate way of estimating injury risk than percentage of athletes injured because it takes into account exposure time. An athlete exposure is defined as 1 athlete participating in 1 practice or competition, which is the most common way of reporting exposure time in sports injury surveillance studies.

That shoulder injury patterns were found to differ by gender and sport may not be that surprising. For males, particularly in football and wrestling, about 90% of the time shoulder, injuries resulted from contact with another player, the playing surface, or equipment, and only 10% were noncontact injuries (due to overuse). Contrast this with the pattern seen among female athletes, among whom 43% of the shoulder injuries were noncontact in nature (Table 2 in the original article).

These results have significant implications for future research, specifically that one size may not fit all when it comes to developing prevention strategies for shoulder injuries. For male athletes, the data suggest an approach that focuses on improvements in the protective equipment, emphasis on proper tackling and wrestling techniques, and stricter officiating. Conversely, for female athletes, prevention strategies most likely to be successful may include limits on practice time or number of serves and overhead motions in volleyball practices, and better preseason conditioning and upper body strengthening. Numerous studies have shown reduction in lower extremity injuries among female athletes who participate in neuromuscular training—a combination of strengthening exercises for the core and lower extremities and plyometrics (repetitive jumping exercises) coupled with instructor feedback to the athletes regarding proper form.[1] This study suggests the next horizon for neuromuscular training programs may be in adapting them to the upper extremity and investigating their effect on shoulder injury rates in female athletes.

C. R. LaBella, MD

Reference

1. Myer GD, Sugimoto D, Thomas S, Hewett TE. The influence of age on the effectiveness of neuromuscular training to reduce anterior cruciate ligament injury in female athletes: a meta-analysis. *Am J Sports Med.* 2013;41:203-215.

Effects of Bracing in Adolescents with Idiopathic Scoliosis
Weinstein SL, Dolan LA, Wright JG, et al (Univ of Iowa; Hosp for Sick Children, Toronto, Ontario, Canada; et al)
N Engl J Med 369:1512-1521, 2013

Background.—The role of bracing in patients with adolescent idiopathic scoliosis who are at risk for curve progression and eventual surgery is controversial.

Methods.—We conducted a multicenter study that included patients with typical indications for bracing due to their age, skeletal immaturity, and degree of scoliosis. Both a randomized cohort and a preference cohort were enrolled. Of 242 patients included in the analysis, 116 were randomly assigned to bracing or observation, and 126 chose between bracing and observation. Patients in the bracing group were instructed to wear the brace at least 18 hours per day. The primary outcomes were curve progression to 50 degrees or more (treatment failure) and skeletal maturity without this degree of curve progression (treatment success).

Results.—The trial was stopped early owing to the efficacy of bracing. In an analysis that included both the randomized and preference cohorts, the rate of treatment success was 72% after bracing, as compared with 48% after observation (propensity-score—adjusted odds ratio for treatment success, 1.93; 95% confidence interval [CI], 1.08 to 3.46). In the intention-to-treat analysis, the rate of treatment success was 75% among patients randomly assigned to bracing, as compared with 42% among those randomly assigned to observation (odds ratio, 4.11; 95% CI, 1.85 to 9.16). There was a significant positive association between hours of brace wear and rate of treatment success ($P < 0.001$).

Conclusions.—Bracing significantly decreased the progression of high-risk curves to the threshold for surgery in patients with adolescent idiopathic scoliosis. The benefit increased with longer hours of brace wear. (Funded by the National Institute of Arthritis and Musculoskeletal and Skin Diseases and others; BRAIST ClinicalTrials.gov number, NCT00448448.)

▶ There are nearly 4000 surgical procedures for adolescent idiopathic scoliosis per annum in the United States. Unfortunately, to date, there has been no evidence-based validation of noninvasive options. Even apart from surgical risks, this is important because of the psychological and physical consequences of major surgery at this important point in adolescent development.

We cannot yet predict whether an individual with scoliosis has a curve that will progress to the surgical range, so every clinical presentation merits consideration for preventative treatment with postural bracing. Bracing itself can be an emotional issue during adolescence, particularly with the challenges of body image and peer acceptance in this age group.

This high-quality study by Weinstein and colleagues helps define and the success of the technique, enabling us to inform and educate patients and parents of their choices. This information will help them participate in shared decision making about the treatment with the best evidence available to them.

This work by a multicenter, international group attempts to address inadequacies in previous studies evaluating bracing for scoliosis. Strong efforts were made to optimize the study design and to overcome inherent challenges by performing a randomized, controlled trial, by defining and measuring success as skeletal maturity without progression to surgery, failure as progression to a surgical range, and accurate real-time measurement of patient adherence to therapy. Because a bracing study cannot be double-blinded, the results were interpreted by blinded personnel, further enhancing and validating the results.

Ultimately the authors were unable to accrue and retain patients sufficiently with only 15% recruitment, hence a compromise preference arm was opened, which, it is acknowledged, decreases the level of evidence. However, the preference and randomized wings had similar results, lending strength to the conclusions (Table 2 in the original article).

For the bracing group, the rate of treatment success was 72%, and for the observation group, the rate of treatment success was 48% (propensity-score-adjusted odds ratio for treatment success, 1.93; 95% confidence interval, 1.08–3.46).

Weinstein et al have shown that bracing of adolescents with idiopathic adolescent scoliosis can prevent progression to the surgical range. In addition, their finding that 12.9 hours of brace wear was associated with 90% to 93% success rate in preventing curve progression to the surgical range may allow us to prescribe this treatment to our patients in more socially acceptable hours of the day (Fig 2 in the original article).

Interestingly, the quality of life (PedsQL scores) in both the bracing and observation group were similar, suggesting bracing does not worsen teenage angst more than just answering study questionnaires! They also showed that the current criteria for bracing overtreats many curves, the natural history of which would not be to progress, even without intervention. Hopefully future evaluation of data will help us narrow the treatment indications.

Besides all the important and applicable clinical results and statistical findings, this work demonstrates that it is feasible to undertake rigorous, methodologically sound studies in children's orthopedics where high-level studies are rare. The investigators have not yet analyzed their data relative to maturity, curve pattern or magnitude, or patient sex. Hopefully, their future analysis will allow us to identify specific subsets of patients who can avoid surgery with appropriate bracing, thus allowing us to achieve more patient-specific treatments for those with adolescent idiopathic scoliosis.

N. T. O'Malley, MD
J. O. Sanders, MD

Botulinum Toxin A for Nonambulatory Children with Cerebral Palsy: A Double Blind Randomized Controlled Trial

Copeland L, Edwards P, Thorley M, et al (Royal Children's Hosp, Parkville, Victoria, Australia; et al)
J Pediatr 165:140-146, 2014

Objectives.—To examine the efficacy and safety of intramuscular botulinum toxin A (BoNT-A) to reduce spasticity and improve comfort and ease of care in nonambulant children with cerebral palsy (CP).

Study Design.—Nonambulant children with CP (n = 41; Gross Motor Function Classification System level IV = 3, level V = 38; mean age 7.1 years, range 2.3-16 years, 66% male) were randomly allocated to receive either intramuscular BoNT-A injections (n = 23) or sham procedure (n = 18) combined with therapy. The analysis used generalized estimating equations with primary outcome the Canadian Occupational Performance Measure (COPM) at 4 weeks postintervention and retention of effects at 16 weeks. Adverse events (AE) were collected at 2, 4, and 16 weeks by a physician masked to group allocation.

Results.—There were significant between group differences favoring the BoNT-A-treated group on COPM performance at 4 weeks (estimated mean difference 2.2, 95% CI 0.8, 3.5; $P = .002$) and for COPM satisfaction (estimated mean difference 2.2, 95% CI 0.5, 3.9; $P = .01$). These effects were retained at 16 weeks for COPM satisfaction (estimated mean difference 1.8, 95% CI 0.1, 3.5; $P = .04$). There were more mild AE at 4 weeks for the BoNT-A group ($P = .002$), however, there were no significant between-group differences in the reporting of moderate and serious AE.

Conclusions.—In a double-blind randomized sham-controlled trial, intramuscular BoNT-A and therapy were effective for improving ease of care and comfort for nonambulant children with CP. There was no increase in moderate and severe AE in the children who had BoNT-A injections compared with the sham group.

▶ The dilemma that faces the rehabilitation team when treating children with cerebral palsy is the inability to compare a given intervention with its absence. The authors of this article take on this challenge by using a "sham" protocol for mimicking intramuscular injections with botulinum toxin A (BTA). Subjects in the treatment and sham groups received topical EMLA at injection sites. The treatment group received intranasal fentanyl before injection. Sham subjects received intranasal saline and blunt needle pressure to the injection sites. A total of 31.6% of the subjects correctly identified the intervention grouping immediately after the procedure, leaving 68.4% who did not know. Because the main outcome of the study was based on parent report, it was important that the sham procedure was effective in ensuring that the parents were blinded to the child's group assignment. These authors appropriately provide information examining the fidelity of the sham procedure and a discussion of the problems associated with masking an invasive intervention.

Unfortunately, the difficulty with assessing the benefits of BTA does not end with successful blinding. Patient selection and randomization is critical because children with cerebral palsy who share similar mobility skills as classified by the Gross Motor Function Classification System (GMFCS) may not respond to BTA in the same way. Only 3 subjects were evaluated in the less severely affected GMFCS IV category (3 in the BTA group and 0 in the sham group), compared with 38 patients in the GMFCS V category. Limiting this report to include just GMFCS V patients would increase confidence in the results.

Clearly defining treatment goals is the most important part of any therapeutic program that includes BTA. There is a tendency to make the BTA injection the focus of the therapy plan. These authors rightly emphasize that the injections are an adjunct and not the therapy itself. Unless this is explained to families in advance, expectations for the benefits from BTA injections may be more than what is possible, and the results may be disappointing. In this study, the primary outcome was defined as comfort and ease of care as measured by the Canadian Occupational Performance Measure (COPM), which was based on parent report.

On average, the effects of BTA injections last 3 months with a wide range in duration. The therapist in conjunction with the family and treating physician must decide whether the effect of a single treatment warrants continued injections. Investigations looking at the effects of BTA after the second or third injection cycle are hard to find. Often the best response reported by families is after the first time BTA is given with diminishing returns afterward. As mentioned in this article, the high rate of comorbidities in nonambulatory patients with cerebral palsy requires caution when BTA injections are repeated on a 3- to 4-month schedule. The decision boils down to whether the benefits are enough to justify discomfort to the child and the risk of adverse effects.

This investigation is an important contribution because it tackles difficult issues that have plagued clinical research to determine the effects of BTA injections and the broader question of assessment of therapies for children with cerebral palsy. The scientific literature is populated with many anecdotal reports, case series, and inadequately designed and underpowered studies. There are only a few reports of investigations that use an effective double-blind procedure. Almost all of the studies suffer from inadequate sample size, clearly pointing to the need for multicenter collaboration. In this study, intramuscular BTA combined with therapy appear to be effective for improving parent perception of ease of care and comfort for nonambulatory children with CP (primarily GMFCS V).

I am looking forward to future studies by this group and others to corroborate and expand these findings. In the final analysis, treating cerebral palsy requires years of consistent and thoughtful hard work by dedicated families and therapists with a clear eye on appropriate and achievable goals.

F. S. Pidcock, MD

Utility of Head Computed Tomography in Children with a Single Extremity Fracture

Wilson PM, Chua M, Care M, et al (Cincinnati Children's Hosp Med Ctr, OH)
J Pediatr 164:1274-1279, 2014

Objectives.—To determine the clinical and forensic utility of head computed tomography (CT) in children younger than 2 years of age with an acute isolated extremity fracture and an otherwise-negative skeletal survey.

Study Design.—Retrospective chart review of children younger than 2 years of age who obtained a skeletal survey in the Cincinnati Children's Hospital Medical Center Emergency Department during the 159-month study period. Clinically important head injury was determined based on previously defined Pediatric Emergency Care Applied Research Network criteria. Forensically significant head injury was defined as that which increased the concern for inflicted injury. The rate of head CT relative to patient age and location of fracture (proximal vs distal extremity, upper vs lower extremity) was determined via χ^2 tests.

Results.—Of the 320 children evaluated, 37% received neuroimaging, 95.7% of which had no signs of skull fracture or intracranial trauma. Five children (4.3%) with head imaging had traumatic findings but no children in the study had clinically significant head injury. Three of these children had previous concerns for nonaccidental trauma and findings on head CT that were forensically significant. There was a greater rate of head imaging in children in the younger age groups and those with proximal extremity fractures ($P < .05$).

Conclusions.—In young children who present with an isolated extremity fracture, clinicians should consider obtaining head CT in those who are younger than 12 months of age, have proximal extremity fractures, or who have previous evaluations for nonaccidental trauma. Evaluation with head CT in children without these risk factors may be low yield.

▶ In clinical practice, missing a case of child abuse puts vulnerable children at risk for serious—sometimes life threatening—future injury, a reality that is well documented in the pediatric medical literature.[1-3] In an effort to identify victims of abuse before catastrophic injury, physicians are often reminded to consider abuse in the differential diagnosis of injury in young children, evaluate all suspicious injuries thoroughly, and report reasonable suspicions to child protective services. This is easier said than done. Pediatricians often struggle to meet these recommendations, wanting to limit unnecessary testing, accusations, and reporting while meeting their obligations to protect children. In these high-stakes diagnoses, balancing benefit and risk can be difficult when deciding on how much testing is enough.

Wilson and colleagues provide data to help hone the evaluation process, suggesting that computed tomography (CT) scan of the head can often be omitted in the evaluation of a child with a single fracture when a skeletal survey is otherwise negative. There are caveats, however. Age, developmental ability, and social history matter—in this study and in practice. The risk that a fracture is due to child abuse is highest in infancy, as is the risk of occult head injury in abuse victims.[4] Head imaging remains necessary in the youngest children and is recommended by the American Academy of Pediatrics for infants with suspicious fractures.[5] Finally, imaging modality also matters, and in the near future, the use of fast-sequence magnetic resonance imaging[6] will hopefully replace radiating CT scans as the study of choice for brain imaging in neurologically asymptomatic infants.

C. W. Christian, MD

References

1. Sheets LK, Leach ME, Koszewski IJ, Lessmeier AM, Nugent M, Simpson P. Sentinel injuries in infants evaluated for child physical abuse. *Pediatrics*. 2013;131:701-707.
2. Jenny C, Hymel KP, Ritzen A, Reinert SE, Hay TC. Analysis of missed cases of abusive head trauma. *JAMA*. 1999;281:621-626.
3. Ravichandiran N, Schuh S, Bejuk M, et al. Delayed Identification of Pediatric Abuse-Related Fractures. *Pediatrics*. 2010;125:60-66.
4. Rubin DM, Christian CW, Bilaniuk LT, Zazyczny KA, Durbin DR. Occult head injury in high-risk abused children. *Pediatrics*. 2003;111:1382-1386.
5. Flaherty EG, Perez-Rossello JM, Levine MA, Hennrikus WL. Evaluating children with fractures for child physical abuse. *Pediatrics*. 2014;133:e477-e489.
6. Patel DM, Tubbs RS, Pate G, Johnston JM Jr, Blount JP. Fast-sequence MRI studies for surveillance imaging in pediatric hydrocephalus. *J Neurosurg Pediatr*. 2014;13:440-447.

13 Neurology Psychiatry

Effects of Hypothermia for Perinatal Asphyxia on Childhood Outcomes
Azzopardi D, for the TOBY Study Group (King's College London, UK; et al)
N Engl J Med 371:140-149, 2014

Background.—In the Total Body Hypothermia for Neonatal Encephalopathy Trial (TOBY), newborns with asphyxial encephalopathy who received hypothermic therapy had improved neurologic outcomes at 18 months of age, but it is uncertain whether such therapy results in longer-term neurocognitive benefits.

Methods.—We randomly assigned 325 newborns with asphyxial encephalopathy who were born at a gestational age of 36 weeks or more to receive standard care alone (control) or standard care with hypothermia to a rectal temperature of 33 to 34°C for 72 hours within 6 hours after birth. We evaluated the neurocognitive function of these children at 6 to 7 years of age. The primary outcome of this analysis was the frequency of survival with an IQ score of 85 or higher.

Results.—A total of 75 of 145 children (52%) in the hypothermia group versus 52 of 132 (39%) in the control group survived with an IQ score of 85 or more (relative risk, 1.31; $P = 0.04$). The proportions of children who died were similar in the hypothermia group and the control group (29% and 30%, respectively). More children in the hypothermia group than in the control group survived without neurologic abnormalities (65 of 145 [45%] vs. 37 of 132 [28%]; relative risk, 1.60; 95% confidence interval, 1.15 to 2.22). Among survivors, children in the hypothermia group, as compared with those in the control group, had significant reductions in the risk of cerebral palsy (21% vs. 36%, $P = 0.03$) and the risk of moderate or severe disability (22% vs. 37%, $P = 0.03$); they also had significantly better motor-function scores. There was no significant between-group difference in parental assessments of children's health status and in results on 10 of 11 psychometric tests.

Conclusions.—Moderate hypothermia after perinatal asphyxia resulted in improved neurocognitive outcomes in middle childhood. (Funded by the United Kingdom Medical Research Council and others; TOBY Clinical-Trials.gov number, NCT01092637.)

▶ Therapeutic hypothermia is now standard of care throughout the developed world. From meta-analyses of the major randomized clinical trials, it is apparent that improved neurologic outcome at 18 months favors treatment, with a number needed to treat of 7 (95% confidence interval 5–10) to prevent 1 child from suffering death or major developmental impairment.[1] However, it is still uncertain whether these outcome improvements are sustainable. There is concern that those that infants who appeared normal or with mild impairments at 18 to 22 months of age may develop more significant cognitive or motor impairments by school age.

In a follow-up study of the Cool-Cap trial, examination findings seen at 18 months were sustained at 6 years as determined by parental interview with WeeFIM (Functional Independence Measures for Children).[2] Because of significant loss to follow-up, a direct association between treatment with hypothermia and outcome at 7 to 8 years of age could not be determined. However, the results were reassuring in that children who were doing well at 18 months of age were also likely to be doing well at school age. In the Eunice Kennedy Shriver National Institute of Child Health and Human Development (NICHD) network trial,[3] although significant differences existed for mortality in the groups, there was only a trend toward a difference in the primary outcome of death or an IQ < 70 (47% vs 62%, $P = .06$) at school age, but fewer children suffered death or severe disability in the treated group. Overall treatment with hypothermia resulted in a lower death rate and did not result in an increase in the rate of severe disability.

The TOBY trial now reports improved neurodevelopmental outcomes at 6 to 7 years of age for those newborns treated with therapeutic hypothermia. The primary outcome was survival with an IQ score > 85, which is only 1 SD from the mean of 100 and differs by a full standard deviation from the NICHD cutoff point of IQ < 70. Just over half (52%) of the treated children in the TOBY trial survived with an IQ > 85 compared with only 39% ($P = .04$) in the control group, with a number needed to treat of 8 (95% CI 4–145) for any 1 child to survive with a good outcome at 6 to 7 years of age. There was a loss to follow-up rate of 15%, and these children tended to have poorer outcomes at 18 months of age. In addition, 41 of the 184 who survived could not complete testing, presumably because of motor, cognitive, or behavioral impairments.

To evaluate the impact of the loss to follow-up and those who could not fully be tested, they performed sensitivity analyses by imputing the scores from the 18-month outcomes for those who were lost and also by assigning those who could not complete testing to the group with an IQ < 85. They also found that rates of death did not differ between the 2 groups at 29% versus 30% and that more children in the hypothermia treatment group survived without neurologic impairments (45% vs 28%), had lower rates of cerebral palsy (CP; 21% vs 36%) and fewer suffered moderate-severe disability (22% vs 37%). Another interesting finding was that fewer children in the treated group required special education resources (8.2% vs 26.9%, $P = .01$), which highlights the substantial impact that hypothermia therapy has on the use of financial and educational resources.

The choice of the primary outcome (survival with IQ > 85) and the higher follow-up rates compared with the publications from the NICHD Network and the Cool-Cap Study resulted in the authors being able to conclude that treatment with hypothermia after perinatal asphyxia in the newborn period results in improved outcomes at 6 to 7 years of age. The high follow-up rate and frequency of the outcome of survival with IQ > 85 provided the power needed to detect a difference between the treatment groups. This result was substantiated by the sensitivity analyses as well as the secondary outcomes, such as less severe disability and less CP in the treated group. This study, together with the results of the Cool-Cap study and the NICHD Network study, demonstrate that hypothermia therapy does provide sustained benefit in terms of both mortality and morbidity at school age. We eagerly await the school-age outcomes of the other large trials as well as a meta-analysis of all the trials at school age.

S. L. Bonifacio, MD

D. M. Ferriero, MD

References

1. Jacobs SE, Berg M, Hunt R, Tarnow-Mordi WO, Inder TE, Davis PG. Cooling for newborns with hypoxic ischaemic encephalopathy. *Cochrane Database Syst Rev.* 2013;1:CD003311.
2. Guillet R, Edwards AD, Thoresen M, et al. Seven- to eight-year follow-up of the CoolCap trial of head cooling for neonatal encephalopathy. *Pediatr Res.* 2012; 71(2):205-209.
3. Shankaran S, Pappas A, McDonald SA, et al. Childhood outcomes after hypothermia for neonatal encephalopathy. *N Engl J Med.* 2012;366(22):2085-2092. PMCID: 3459579.

Prevalence of Prader—Willi Syndrome among Infants with Hypotonia
Tuysuz B, Kartal N, Erener-Ercan T, et al (Istanbul Univ, Turkey; et al)
J Pediatr 164:1064-1067, 2014

Objective.—To investigate the prevalence of Prader—Willi syndrome (PWS) in infants with hypotonia between the ages of 0 and 2 years.

Study Design.—Karyotyping studies were performed in all infants with hypotonia. The study group was composed of infants with hypotonia for whom the karyotyping was found to be normal. Fluorescence in situ hybridization and methylation analysis were performed simultaneously in the study group. Molecular studies for uniparental disomy were undertaken in the patients without deletions with an abnormal methylation pattern.

Results.—Sixty-five infants with hypotonia with a mean age of 8 months were enrolled. A deletion was detected in 6 patients by fluorescence in situ hybridization analysis. Only 1 patient had no deletion but had an abnormal methylation pattern. A maternal uniparental disomy was observed in this patient. PWS was diagnosed in 10.7 % (7/65) of the infants with hypotonia.

Conclusion.—The prevalence of PWS syndrome is high among infants with hypotonia. PWS should be considered by pediatricians and neonatologists in the differential diagnosis of all newborns with hypotonia. Early diagnosis of PWS is important for the management of these patients.

▶ The article by Tuysuz et al summarizes the experience in infants with hypotonia by undergoing systematic evaluation to identify the cause by using standard cytogenetic studies with fluorescent in situ hybridization (FISH) followed by syndrome-specific methylation analysis for the chromosome 15q11-q13 region disturbed in Prader-Willi syndrome (PWS). PWS is due to errors in genomic imprinting with loss of paternally expressed genes in this chromosome region generally as a de novo 15q11-q13 deletion. The identification of PWS via these genetic testing methods was found in 10% of their enrolled infant cohort, which emphasizes the importance of developing and systematically pursuing a differential diagnosis after clinical evaluation and examination. Ordering syndrome-specific genetic testing was required because standard chromosome studies alone did not identify or confirm the diagnosis.

The diagnosis of PWS was not assisted by the use of the clinical consensus diagnostic criteria reported by Holm et al[1] because hypotonia was the only major diagnostic criteria identifiable in their infant cohort. The Holm et al diagnostic criteria are more useful in older patients, but recent advances in genetic technology have significantly augmented the criteria. These advances include syndrome-specific genetic testing such as DNA methylation and chromosomal microarray analysis. Microarrays are many-fold, more powerful than standard cytogenetic testing. The Holm et al article was published before discovery of advanced genetic testing methods including FISH analysis for identifying the chromosome 15q11-q13 deletion in PWS.

The diagnostic challenges in infancy identified in the report by Tuysuz et al are enhanced by features shared in common with other syndromic and nonsyndromic disorders due to multiple causes such as metabolic, mitochondrial, sepsis, muscle disease, fetal insults, and congenital defects. Other cardinal features seen in PWS are not readily evident during the neonatal period. Hyperphagia and obesity; growth hormone deficiency with short stature and small hands and feet; craniofacial features represented by a narrow forehead, almond-shaped eyes and a small chin; and oral pathology with enamel hypoplasia and sticky, dry saliva are more evident at later ages. Hence, important diagnostic signs or symptoms for PWS are not present during infancy to alert the primary care physician or neonatologist (most often encountering this patient population at the earliest age) to suspect PWS as the most likely cause and to order syndrome-specific genetic tests required for laboratory diagnosis.

The report by Tuysuz et al further illustrates the importance of chromosomal microarrays to be performed early during laboratory assessments but requires a longer period of time to complete compared with standard chromosome testing and FISH. The chromosome 15q11-q13 deletion is seen in approximately 70% of cases consisting of 2 types (a larger type I deletion or smaller type II deletion) when using microarray analysis, and the remaining patients will require syndrome-specific methylation analysis for both PWS or the sister syndrome, Angelman syndrome (AS), both of which are due to errors in genomic imprinting on chromosome 15. AS is an entirely different clinical disorder and most commonly due to the same chromosome 15q11-q13 deletion but of maternal origin. AS also shares in common with PWS the clinical presentation of hypotonia but without the same severity and level of feeding problems seen in PWS infants; it should nonetheless be considered when chromosomal testing identifies a 15q11-q13 deletion but without identifying the parent of origin by genotyping or syndrome-specific methylation to distinguish between these 2 rare genomic imprinting disorders.

Clinicians need to be vigilant in considering the causation of congenital hypotonia and specifically genetic disorders including PWS. Most clinicians are not trained in clinical genetics or dysmorphology and may be unaware of pertinent genetic testing options and priorities, often syndrome-specific, when processing the growing list of causes (both common and rare) in developing a differential diagnosis. In addition, PWS generally does not recur, and families present with a negative family history for this disorder which lowers the likelihood that the nonclinical geneticist will pursue timely and appropriate syndrome-specific genetic testing options initially, and possibly avoid invasive procedures such as gastrostomy tube placement and muscle biopsies or other diagnostic tests. Better awareness of rare genetic conditions such as PWS and AS is needed by the medical community and recognized advances in genetic testing and options applicable to the patient and their findings. A clinical genetics consult would be advisable to assist in identifying potential causes and to prioritize and select the most appropriate diagnostic tests to lower the costs and obtain results in a timely fashion needed for diagnosis and treatment.

Diagnostic testing for infants with severe congenital hypotonia should initially include standard chromosomal testing and syndrome-specific methylation analysis for PWS/AS in view of a normal family history and often followed by structural chromosomal microarrays to rule out or establish the diagnosis more quickly and accurately to address the clinical course and treatment. More accurate information about the diagnosis and prognosis will then be shared with the family along with genetic counseling. This process will be both cost-effective for families and time-saving for doctors and health care providers for infants and hopefully lead to better outcomes.

M. G. Butler, MD, PhD

Reference

1. Holm VA, Cassidy SB, Butler MG, et al. Prader-Willi syndrome: consensus diagnostic criteria. *Pediatrics.* 1993;91:398-402.

Stroke and nonstroke brain attacks in children

Mackay MT, Chua ZK, Lee M, et al (Royal Children's Hosp Melbourne, Parkville, Australia; et al)
Neurology 82:1-7, 2014

Objectives.—To determine symptoms, signs, and etiology of brain attacks in children presenting to the emergency department (ED) as a first step for developing a pediatric brain attack pathway.

Methods.—Prospective observational study of children aged 1 month to 18 years with brain attacks (defined as apparently abrupt-onset focal brain dysfunction) and ongoing symptoms or signs on arrival to the ED. Exclusion criteria included epilepsy, hydrocephalus, head trauma, and isolated

TABLE 2.—Presenting Symptoms and Signs of Pediatric Brain Attacks

	No. (%)	95% CI, %
Symptom		
Headache	169/301 (56)	50–62
Vomiting	109/301 (36)	31–42
Focal weakness	103/297 (35)	29–40
Focal numbness	74/295 (24)	20–30
Visual disturbance	67/297 (23)	18–28
Febrile or afebrile seizures	62/301 (21)	16–26
Altered mental status	60/299 (21)	16–25
Dizziness	60/297 (20)	16–25
Speech disturbance	50/298 (17)	13–22
Ataxia	42/297 (14)	10–19
Loss of consciousness	34/299 (11)	8–16
Faint	33/297 (11)	8–15
Vertigo	10/295 (3)	16–61
Other symptoms	61/300 (20)	16–25
Sign		
Focal weakness	93/301 (31)	26–36
Focal sensory disturbance	40/301 (13)	10–18
Speech disturbance	24/301 (8)	5–12
Leg weakness	45/297 (15)	11–20
Facial weakness	44/297 (15)	11–19
Arm weakness	43/297 (14)	11–19
Hand weakness	35/297 (12)	8–16
Ataxia	31/297 (10)	7–14
Inability to walk	29/293 (10)	7–14
Eye movement abnormality	26/295 (9)	6–13
Arm sensory disturbance	26/293 (9)	6–13
Leg sensory disturbance	20/292 (7)	4–10
Visual defects	21/295 (7)	4–11
Dysarthria	18/296 (6)	4–9
Facial sensory disturbance	11/291 (4)	2–7
GCS abnormal, <15	83/292 (28)	23–33
GCS score <9	12/292 (4)	2–7
Pupillary abnormality	7/280 (3)	1–5
Hand sensory disturbance	9/277 (3)	1–6
Dysphasia	9/301 (3)	1–6
Paralysis	2/297 (0.7)	0.8–2
Sensory neglect	1/296 (0.3)	0.8–2
Other neurologic signs	24/300 (8)	5–12
No neurologic signs	102/298 (34)	29–40

Abbreviations: CI = confidence interval; GCS = Glasgow Coma Scale.
Mackay MT, Chua ZK, Lee M, et al. Stroke and nonstroke brain attacks in children. J Neurology. 2014;82:1-7, Copyright 2014.

headache. Etiology was determined after review of clinical data, neuroimaging, and other investigations. A random-effects meta-analysis of similar adult studies was compared with the current study.

Results.—There were 287 children (46% male) with 301 presentations over 17 months. Thirty-five percent arrived by ambulance. Median symptom duration before arrival was 6 hours (interquartile range 2–28 hours). Median time from triage to medical assessment was 22 minutes (interquartile range 6–55 minutes). Common symptoms included headache (56%), vomiting (36%), focal weakness (35%), numbness (24%), visual disturbance (23%), seizures (21%), and altered consciousness (21%). Common

TABLE 5.—Random-Effects Meta-Analysis: Comparison of 1,117 Combined Adult Brain Attacks From 3 Studies[6,8,9] with 301 Pediatric Brain Attacks From Current Study

Diagnoses	Children %	Children 95% CI	Adult Meta-analysis %	Adult Meta-analysis 95% CI
Conditions encountered in both groups				
Stroke	7	4.4–10.5	73.1	64.7–81.5
Migraine[a]	27.9	22.9–33.3	2.4	0–5.7
Seizures/epilepsy	15.2	11.4–20	4.3	2.3–6.2
Psychiatric	6	3.6–9.3	1.5	0.4–3.2
Syncope	4.7	2.6–7.7	1.7	0.7–2.8
Encephalopathy[a]	3	1.6–6	1	0–2.7
CNS demyelination[b] (n = 411)	2	0.7–4.3	0.2	0.01–1.3
PNS/mononeuritis[a]	1.7	0.5–3.8	2.1	0.9–3.1
CNS infection[b] (n = 411)	1.3	0.4–3.4	0.5	0.01–1.7
CNS tumors	1	0.2–2.9	2.1	0.5–3.6
Cord lesion[b] (n = 350)	0.7	0.1–2.4	0.9	0.2–2.5
Other neurologic[a]	6	3.6–9.3	0.6	0.1–1.2
Other non-neurologic[a]	6	3.6–9.3	2	0–4.4
Conditions not encountered in children				
Systemic infection	0	0–1.2	3.4	2.3–4.4
Toxic metabolic	0	0–1.2	2.3	1.4–3.3
Vestibular	0	0–1.2	1.7	0.9–2.4
Trauma[b] (n = 411)	0	0–1.2	1	0.3–2.5
Cardiac[b] (n = 411)	0	0–1.2	0.97	0.3–2.4
Joint/musculoskeletal[b] (n = 356)	0	0–1.2	0.8	0.2–2.4
Dementia/delirium	0	0–1.2	0.8	0.3–1.3
Subdural[a]	0	0–1.2	0.5	0–1
TGA[a]	0	0–1.2	0.5	0–1
Conditions not described in adult studies				
Bell palsy[c]	9.6	6.5–13.5	NA	NA
Headache NOS[c]	4	2–7	NA	NA
Cerebellitis[c]	2.3	0.9–4.7	NA	NA
Drug intoxication[c]	1.3	0.4–9.3	NA	NA

Abbreviations: CI = confidence interval; NA = not applicable; NOS = not otherwise specified; PNS = peripheral nervous system; TGA = transient global amnesia.
Editor's Note: Please refer to original journal article for full references.
[a]Data available for 2 studies.
[b]One study, therefore random meta-analysis was not performed and 95% CIs are presented for the individual study.
[c]Not stated as diagnoses in adult studies and therefore removed from meta-analysis.
Mackay MT, Chua ZK, Lee M, et al. Stroke and nonstroke brain attacks in children. J Neurology. 2014;82:1-7, Copyright 2014.

signs included focal weakness (31%), numbness (13%), ataxia (10%), or speech disturbance (8%). Neuroimaging included CT imaging (30%), which was abnormal in 27%, and MRI (31%), which was abnormal in 62%. The most common diagnoses included migraine (28%), seizures (15%), Bell palsy (10%), stroke (7%), and conversion disorders (6%). Relative proportions of conditions in children significantly differed from adults for stroke, migraine, seizures, and conversion disorders.

Conclusions.—Brain attack etiologies differ from adults, with stroke being the fourth most common diagnosis. These findings will inform development of ED clinical pathways for pediatric brain attacks.

▶ Although uncommon in childhood, stroke affects approximately 5000 children in the United States per year. Pediatricians and emergency medicine physicians are often the first to evaluate these children and need to be prepared to recognize the signs of a stroke and make the diagnosis. Advances in neurocritical care have led to strategies to help minimize the extent of the stroke and prevent additional brain injury due secondary effects (often related to brain swelling) or recurrent stroke. Hence, early recognition of the stroke is critical.

As in adults, strokes present with a "brain attack"—sudden onset focal brain dysfunction. The particular manifestations depend on the part of the brain affected (Table 2). These can include a focal deficit—most commonly weakness on one side of the face and body—changes in speech, double vision, or gait ataxia.

A first-time seizure can also be the initial manifestation of stroke, as can a sudden-onset, severe headache. In the study by Mackay et al, a single emergency department evaluated 287 children with 301 presentations of brain attacks over the span of 17 months—about 4 children per week (Table 5). A stroke was the culprit in a nontrivial proportion: 7%. Stroke mimics include migraine, which can cause dramatic focal deficits that cannot be clinically distinguished from a stroke. Although seizures can result from an acute stroke, a focal seizure from any other cause (such as an underlying brain malformation) can lead to hemiparesis or aphasia if motor or language cortex was involved. It can be impossible to clinically distinguish a postictal Todd paresis from an acute stroke.

Fortunately, standard magnetic resonance imaging can easily confirm, or rule out, a stroke. Sequences such as diffusion-weighted imaging (DWI) can detect infarcted brain within minutes of an ischemic stroke, and iron-sensitive sequences can detect a hemorrhagic stroke. (CT scans are highly sensitive for blood but will not detect an acute infarction less than 6 to 12 hours old and are particularly insensitive for small infarcts and those in the posterior fossa.) Urgent brain imaging should be considered in any child with a first brain attack.

H. J. Fullerton, MD, MAS

A Randomized Controlled Trial of Clinician-Led Tactile Stimulation to Reduce Pain During Vaccination in Infants

Taddio A, Ho T, Vyas C, et al (Univ of Toronto, Ontario, Canada; Dr Tommy Ho Paediatric Clinic, Toronto, Ontario, Canada; et al)
Clin Pediatr 53:639-644, 2014

Background.—Clinician-led tactile stimulation (rubbing the skin adjacent to the injection site or applying pressure) has been demonstrated to reduce pain in children and adults undergoing vaccination.

Objective.—To evaluate the analgesic effectiveness of clinician-led tactile stimulation in infants undergoing vaccination.

Methods.—This was a partially blinded randomized controlled trial that included infants undergoing vaccination in a private clinic in Toronto. Infants were randomly allocated to tactile stimulation or no tactile stimulation immediately prior to, during, and after vaccination. The primary outcome was infant pain, assessed using a validated observational measure, the Modified Behavioral Pain Scale (MBPS; range = 0-10).

Results.—Altogether, 121 infants participated (n = 62 tactile stimulation; n = 59 control); demographics did not differ (P > .05) between groups. MBPS scores did not differ between groups: mean = 7.2 (standard deviation = 2.4) versus 7.6 (1.9); P = .245.

Conclusion.—Tactile stimulation cannot be recommended as a strategy to reduce vaccination pain in infants because of insufficient evidence of a benefit.

▶ Repeated painful procedures have long-term negative physical and psychological consequences in children.[1] The impact of pain and distress from medical procedures as simple as immunizations injections and venipuncture ranges from negative memories to avoidance behaviors to hypersensitivity and anxiety related to subsequent procedures as a child and even later as adults. Among children, infants are the most vulnerable not only because of repeated exposures to painful immunizations but also because of the immaturity of their pain pathways, which leads them to experience pain with greater intensity.[2,3] The most frequent cause of medical procedural pain for infants and children are immunizations. This significant iatrogenic pain burden may result in delay and even noncompliance in receiving immunizations.

Given the importance of vaccinations for global public health, identifying an effective method for reducing the pain burden of immunizations on infants and children is therefore paramount.

In its most recent study, Taddio et al conducted a randomized controlled trial of clinician-led tactile stimulation to reduce pain during vaccination in infants. Several methods for reducing pain from immunization injections have been investigated, including topical anesthetics, cognitive behavioral methods, and a number of techniques based on the gate control theory of pain transmission.

Gate control theory hypothesizes that pain signal transmission from afferent pain fibers can be inhibited by nonnoxious physical stimuli (eg, rubbing, massaging) in proximity to the painful stimuli. Because of their simplicity and easy availability, techniques based on the gate control theory to reduce pain from immunizations have received a significant amount of attention. In fact, tactile stimulation has gathered enough evidence in children and adults to be included in evidence-based clinical practice guidelines for reducing pain from childhood vaccinations in Canada.[4] However, the lack of studies involving infants does not support a recommendation at this time. The only other study of tactile stimulation on infants' immunization pain was conducted by Taddio as well and did not show any benefit.[5]

It is within this context that the present study by Taddio et al is important. First, it is trying to clarify the mixed picture of tactile stimulation efficacy, particularly in infants. Additionally, in the present study, Taddio et al tried to address some of the limitations of previous studies. In particular, the consistency of tactile stimulation was ensured by using the same clinician throughout the study (instead of the parent in the previous study). Infants received different vaccines, but the study intervention involved only 1 injection. In addition, the same injection and stimulation site was used. Not surprisingly, the study findings in terms of pain scores before and after the injection and cry duration are consistent with other studies using the same pain assessment tool, providing some further credibility to the results of the present study.

Although this study has a number of limitations inherent to its design, some of them warrant highlighting. The effect of tactile stimulation was measured in a context in which other known methods to reduce pain from immunizations were used (sucrose administration and rapid intramuscular injection without aspiration) and so it is conceivable, especially for infants, that the added benefit of tactile stimulation in this context is minimal but may be greater if other methods for pain reduction are not used. The method to apply tactile stimulation was not standardized with possible variability in the amount of pressure applied. Combined with the fact that the clinician delivering the tactile stimulation and the vaccinations was aware of the study hypothesis, it is conceivable that a greater amount of pressure was applied in response to the pain and distress of the infant as perceived by the clinician during the injection, possibly resulting in discomfort from the pressure itself and resulting in biased data. Additionally, there were no indications if the infants had been breastfed just before the immunization. We know that breastfeeding can reduce pain and distress from immunizations.[4] There was also no mention of the position of the infant (supine vs erect). Previous studies have shown that position has an impact on pain scores from immunizations.[4] More important, there was no data collection of the pain history of some of the infants in the study. Some of them may have been presensitized to painful stimuli because of previous significant medical procedures, surgeries, prematurity, and prolonged hospitalizations.

We have 2 well-designed studies of tactile stimulation for immunization pain reduction in infants that are negative, whereas it has been found to be effective in children and adults in multiple studies. It does beg the question, is there something more fundamental explaining these findings? The pain reduction properties of tactile stimulation are based on gate control theory. This theory requires mature descending pain pathways to work. We know that newborns have immature descending pain pathways, and although it is unclear exactly when these mature, it is likely that there is variability of how quickly these pathways mature during the first year of life.[3] Without mature descending pathways, it is therefore not surprising that tactile stimulation, either from parents or clinicians, does not deliver any significant change in response to pain in infants. In addition, we know that because of these immature descending pathways, infants are likely to have stronger response to the same painful stimuli as other children. This consideration would explain why studies of tactile stimulation and transcutaneous electrical nerve stimulation units have shown positive results in older children and adults but not in infants.[6]

Tactile stimulation for infants does not appear to be effective in reducing the pain burden from immunizations. The search for simple and readily available methods to reduce pain from vaccinations in infants needs to continue. Interestingly a recent study of lidocaine 2.5% and prilocaine 2.5% cream (EMLA), conducted mostly on infants and using the same pain assessment method as the present study, showed positive results and no increase in wait times.[7]

With additional positive studies, topical anesthetics could become the standard of care for preventing vaccination pain in infants. In the meantime, continuing to educate parents and clinicians on the importance of minimizing distress and pain from vaccination needs to remain a priority, and other methods that have been validated such as sucrose, breastfeeding, proper positioning, and injection technique need to be better disseminated.

P. Scemama de Gailluly, MD, MBA

References

1. Kennedy RM, Luhmann J, Zempsky WT. Clinical implications of unmanaged needle-insertion pain and distress in children. *Pediatrics.* 2008;122:S130-S133.
2. Fitzgerald M, Walker SM. Infant pain management: a developmental neurobiological approach. *Nat Clin Pract Neurol.* 2009;5:35-50.
3. Pattinson D, Fitzgerald M. The neurobiology of infant pain: development of excitatory and inhibitory neurotransmission in the spinal dorsal horn. *Reg Anesth Pain Med.* 2004;29:36-44.
4. Taddio A, Appleton M, Bortolussi R, et al. Reducing the pain of childhood vaccination: an evidence-based clinical practice guideline. *CMAJ.* 2010;182: E843-E855.
5. Hogan ME, Probst J, Wong K, Riddell RP, Katz J, Taddio A. A randomized-controlled trial of parent-led tactile stimulation to reduce pain during infant immunization injections. *Clin J Pain.* 2014;30:259-265.
6. Lander J, Fowler-Kerry S. Tens for children's procedural pain. *Pain.* 1993;52: 209-216.
7. Abuelkheir M, Alsourani D, Al-Eyadhy A, Temsah MH, Meo SA, Alzamil F. Emla(R) cream: a pain-relieving strategy for childhood vaccination. *J Int Med Res.* 2014;42:329-336.

Lorazepam vs Diazepam for Pediatric Status Epilepticus: A Randomized Clinical Trial

Chamberlain JM, for the Pediatric Emergency Care Applied Research Network (PECARN) (Children's Natl Med Ctr, Washington, DC; et al)
JAMA 311:1652-1660, 2014

Importance.—Benzodiazepines are considered first-line therapy for pediatric status epilepticus. Some studies suggest that lorazepam may be more effective or safer than diazepam, but lorazepam is not Food and Drug Administration approved for this indication.

Objective.—To test the hypothesis that lorazepam has better efficacy and safety than diazepam for treating pediatric status epilepticus.

Design, Setting, and Participants.—This double-blind, randomized clinical trial was conducted from March 1, 2008, to March 14, 2012. Patients aged 3 months to younger than 18 years with convulsive status epilepticus presenting to 1 of 11 US academic pediatric emergency departments were eligible. There were 273 patients; 140 randomized to diazepam and 133 to lorazepam.

Interventions.—Patients received either 0.2 mg/kg of diazepam or 0.1 mg/kg of lorazepam intravenously, with half this dose repeated at 5 minutes if necessary. If status epilepticus continued at 12 minutes, fosphenytoin was administered.

TABLE 3.—Primary and Secondary Efficacy and Safety Outcomes[a]

| Outcome | Age 3 mo to <3 y | | Age 3 to <13 y | | Age ≥13 y | | Overall | |
	No./Total No. (%)							
	Diazepam	Lorazepam	Diazepam	Lorazepam	Diazepam	Lorazepam	Diazepam	Lorazepam
Primary Outcomes								
Efficacy	48/72 (66.7)	38/62 (61.3)	44/55 (80.0)	49/60 (81.7)	9/13 (69.2)	10/11 (90.9)	101/140 (72.1)	97/133 (72.9)
Efficacy (per-protocol population)	35/48 (72.9)	32/48 (66.7)	36/43 (83.7)	44/50 (88.0)	7/11 (63.6)	9/9 (100.0)	78/102 (76.5)	85/107 (79.4)
Need for assisted ventilation (all randomized patients)	11/77 (14.3)	16/71 (22.5)	12/68 (17.6)	10/63 (15.9)	3/17 (17.6)	0/14	26/162 (16.0)	26/148 (17.6)
Secondary Outcomes								
Patients requiring only a single dose of study medication	41/72 (56.9)	34/62 (54.8)	37/55 (67.3)	38/60 (63.3)	9/13 (69.2)	8/11 (72.7)	87/140 (62.1)	80/133 (60.2)
Patients requiring a second dose of study medication	27/72 (37.5)	25/62 (40.3)	14/55 (25.5)	17/60 (28.3)	1/13 (7.7)	2/11 (18.2)	42/140 (30.0)	44/133 (33.1)
Patients requiring study medication plus additional anticonvulsant medication(s)	15/72 (20.8)	15/62 (24.2)	4/55 (7.3)	6/60 (10.0)	2/13 (15.4)	0/11	21/140 (15.0)	21/133 (15.8)
Patients responding to fosphenytoin or phenytoin within 10 min	6/15 (40.0)	2/15 (13.3)	0/4	1/6 (16.7)	0/2	NA	6/21 (28.6)	3/21 (14.3)
Recurrence within 1 h	6/48 (12.5)	3/38 (7.9)	5/44 (11.4)	6/49 (12.2)	0/9	1/10 (10.0)	11/101 (10.9)	10/97 (10.3)
Recurrence within 4 h	23/48 (47.9)	25/38 (65.8)	11/44 (25.0)	12/49 (24.5)	5/9 (55.6)	1/10 (10.0)	39/101 (38.6)	38/97 (39.2)
Any respiratory depression (all severities)	38/77 (49.4)	32/71 (45.1)	33/68 (48.5)	21/63 (33.3)	3/17 (17.6)	1/14 (7.1)	74/162 (45.7)	54/148 (36.5)
Sedation (Riker score <3)	35/77 (45.5)	44/71 (62.0)[b]	38/68 (55.9)	47/63 (74.6)[b]	8/17 (47.1)	8/14 (57.1)	81/162 (50.0)	99/148 (66.9)[b]
Aspiration pneumonia	0/77	1/71 (1.4)	1/68 (1.5)	1/63 (1.6)	1/17 (5.9)	0/14	2/162 (1.2)	2/148 (1.4)
Secondary Time Outcomes, Median (IQR), min								
No. of noncensored patients	51	42	46	53	11	11	108	106
Time to status epilepticus cessation	3.0 (1.0-9.0)	4.0 (1.0-10.0)	2.0 (1.0-7.0)	2.0 (1.0-6.5)	3.0 (1.0-5.0)	1.0 (0.0-2.0)	2.5 (1.0-12.5)	2.0 (1.0-11.0)
Time to recovery from sedation	114.0 (60.0-121.0)	60.0 (49.0-176.0)	120.0 (55.0-174.0)	136.0 (111.5-180.0)	10.5 (4.5-25.0)	5.0 (1.0-35.0)	104.5 (60.0-125.0)	120.0 (53.0-174.5)

Abbreviations: IQR, interquartile range; NA, not applicable.
[a] Efficacy analysis includes all patients who received study medication and were experiencing generalized convulsive SE. Patients who were enrolled more than once were only included for the first visit. The per-protocol analysis excludes patients with significant protocol deviations (see Methods section).
[b] $P < .05$.

Main Outcomes and Measures.—The primary efficacy outcome was cessation of status epilepticus by 10 minutes without recurrence within 30 minutes. The primary safety outcome was the performance of assisted ventilation. Secondary outcomes included rates of seizure recurrence and sedation and times to cessation of status epilepticus and return to baseline mental status. Outcomes were measured 4 hours after study medication administration.

Results.—Cessation of status epilepticus for 10 minutes without recurrence within 30 minutes occurred in 101 of 140 (72.1%) in the diazepam group and 97 of 133 (72.9%) in the lorazepam group, with an absolute efficacy difference of 0.8% (95% CI, −11.4% to 9.8%). Twenty-six patients in each group required assisted ventilation (16.0% given diazepam and 17.6% given lorazepam; absolute risk difference, 1.6%; 95% CI, −9.9% to 6.8%). There were no statistically significant differences in secondary outcomes except that lorazepam patients were more likely to be sedated (66.9% vs 50%, respectively; absolute risk difference, 16.9%; 95% CI, 6.1% to 27.7%).

Conclusions and Relevance.—Among pediatric patients with convulsive status epilepticus, treatment with lorazepam did not result in improved efficacy or safety compared with diazepam. These findings do not support the preferential use of lorazepam for this condition.

Trial Registration.—clinicaltrials.gov Identifier: NCT00621478 (Table 3).

▶ Convulsive status epilepticus is one of the most frequent neurologic emergencies in the pediatric population with an estimated incidence of 17 to 23 in 100 000.[1-3] The vast majority of pediatricians will encounter at least a few cases of children with active status epilepticus in their professional and even personal lives, and their initial management will significantly determine prognosis. Mortality in pediatric status epilepticus continues to be high at approximately 1% to 3%[2,4-7] and severe clinical complications and cognitive impairment after status epilepticus are common.[5] Several clinical studies have shown that earlier administration of appropriate treatment improves the prognosis of pediatric convulsive status epilepticus.[8-10] All pediatricians should be familiar with the optimal initial management for status epilepticus.

The study by Chamberlain et al is unique for several reasons. First, it addresses one of the most clinically relevant questions in pediatric status epilepticus: what is the optimal initial treatment? In addition, the study population is very large ($N = 273$) and comes from 11 academic pediatric emergency departments in the United States. These features allow a more confident generalization of results to the population of interest: all children with convulsive status epilepticus. Third, this study is focused on patients 3 months to 18 years of age. Status epilepticus in children aged less than 3 months and in adults have different etiologies, clinical characteristics, treatments, and outcomes. The characteristics of pediatric convulsive status epilepticus are usually diluted in series with neonatal and adult cases. The present study addresses the specific treatment for children with convulsive status epilepticus. Finally, the outcomes were objectively defined and data collection was standardized yielding high-quality data.

Evidence to support the best first-line treatment in pediatric convulsive status epilepticus is limited. The Veterans Affairs cooperative trial randomized patients to 4 first-line treatments for status epilepticus: intravenous diazepam followed by intravenous phenytoin, intravenous lorazepam, intravenous phenobarbital, and intravenous phenytoin.[11] In that study, lorazepam was superior to phenytoin, but not to diazepam followed by phenytoin.[11] Further, in an intention-to-treat analysis, there were no differences among the 4 treatment groups.[11] Since then, lorazepam has become widely used as the first-line treatment for pediatric convulsive status epilepticus, although there were no children in the VA study. For children, the preference of lorazepam as first-line therapy is essentially based on the large North London series of 182 pediatric patients (1 month to 16 years of age) with convulsive status epilepticus, in which treatment with intravenous lorazepam was associated with a 3.7 (95% confidence interval 1.7–7.9) times greater likelihood of seizure cessation than was treatment with rectal diazepam.[9]

However, several studies show that there is no clear benefit of one benzodiazepine over the others for convulsive status epilepticus.[12] Lorazepam disadvantages include the following: (1) the need for an intravenous line to administer it decreases its practical usefulness in convulsive status epilepticus, a situation in which getting a line may be particularly challenging. (2) It requires a specific temperature and expires after a relatively short period making it more difficult to store and distribute. For this reason, other first-line treatments are being increasingly considered. A recent double-blind, randomized, noninferiority trial in 893 patients compared the efficacy of intramuscular midazolam with that of intravenous lorazepam for children and adults in status epilepticus treated before arrival at the hospital.[13] Intramuscular midazolam was found to be at least as safe and effective as intravenous lorazepam for prehospital seizure cessation.[13] In this study, the time saved by using the intramuscular route appears to at least offset the delay in the drug onset of action (intramuscular vs intravenous).[13]

In a classic prospective study, 44 children (ages 6 months to 5 years) were treated with rectal diazepam during 59 generalized seizures with a rate of seizure resolution of 80%.[14] In 10% diazepam failed, whereas intravenous diazepam was effective, and in 10%, diazepam failed after rectal and intravenous administration.[14] These rates are similar if not superior to those of intravenous lorazepam. In addition, the therapeutic effect in that study was significantly correlated with the duration of convulsions before treatment: early treatment (convulsions ≤15 minutes) had effect in 96% and late treatment (convulsions >15 minutes) was effective in 57% of the cases.[14] No respiratory depression or serious side effects were observed.[14] In a different comparison, diazepam and lorazepam showed no difference in efficacy in a series of 48 children with status epilepticus treated in the emergency department.[15]

The present study by Chamberlain and colleagues adds to the literature by showing that intravenous lorazepam did not result in improved efficacy or safety compared with intravenous diazepam (Table 3). The study shows lack of superiority of any drug when comparing intravenous lorazepam and intravenous diazepam. Although the study design is a randomized controlled trial, the level of evidence of the findings is that of an observational study because the randomized clinical trial was not designed to test noninferiority. To definitively demonstrate noninferiority, studies with a noninferiority design may be required in the future. From a clinical practice point of view, this study significantly adds to the growing body of literature that suggests that there are limited differences in efficacy and safety among different benzodiazepines as first-line treatment for pediatric status epilepticus. In short, when faced with a child with convulsive status epilepticus, always ensure proper airway patency. Protect the patient from trauma and avoid any movement restraints. Importantly, rapid administration of the first benzodiazepine is more important than choosing the ideal one because there is currently limited evidence to support the superiority of lorazepam versus midazolam or diazepam. Lastly, swift workup and treatment of etiologies is crucial. As more evidence on status treatment becomes available, time to treatment emerges as a much more important variable than any specific agent.

I. Sánchez Fernández, MD

T. Loddenkemper, MD

References

1. Chin RF, Neville BG, Peckham C, Bedford H, Wade A, Scott RC. Incidence, cause, and short-term outcome of convulsive status epilepticus in childhood: prospective population-based study. *Lancet.* 2006;368:222-229.
2. Coeytaux A, Jallon P, Galobardes B, Morabia A. Incidence of status epilepticus in French-speaking Switzerland: (EPISTAR). *Neurology.* 2000;55:693-697.
3. DeLorenzo RJ, Hauser WA, Towne AR, et al. A prospective, population-based epidemiologic study of status epilepticus in Richmond, Virginia. *Neurology.* 1996;46:1029-1035.
4. Loddenkemper T, Syed TU, Ramgopal S, et al. Risk factors associated with death in in-hospital pediatric convulsive status epilepticus. *PloS One.* 2012;7:e47474.
5. Raspall-Chaure M, Chin RF, Neville BG, Scott RC. Outcome of paediatric convulsive status epilepticus: a systematic review. *Lancet Neurol.* 2006;5:769-779.
6. Singh RK, Stephens S, Berl MM, et al. Prospective study of new-onset seizures presenting as status epilepticus in childhood. *Neurology.* 2010;74:636-642.
7. Wu YW, Shek DW, Garcia PA, Zhao S, Johnston SC. Incidence and mortality of generalized convulsive status epilepticus in California. *Neurology.* 2002;58:1070-1076.
8. Alldredge BK, Wall DB, Ferriero DM. Effect of prehospital treatment on the outcome of status epilepticus in children. *Pediatr Neurol.* 1995;12:213-216.
9. Chin RF, Neville BG, Peckham C, Wade A, Bedford H, Scott RC. Treatment of community-onset, childhood convulsive status epilepticus: a prospective, population-based study. *Lancet Neurol.* 2008;7:696-703.
10. Eriksson K, Metsäranta P, Huhtala H, Auvinen A, Kuusela AL, Koivikko M. Treatment delay and the risk of prolonged status epilepticus. *Neurology.* 2005; 65:1316-1318.
11. Treiman DM, Meyers PD, Walton NY, et al. A comparison of four treatments for generalized convulsive status epilepticus. Veterans Affairs Status Epilepticus Cooperative Study Group. *N Engl J Med.* 1998;339:792-798.
12. Glauser TA. Designing practical evidence-based treatment plans for children with prolonged seizures and status epilepticus. *J Child Neurol.* 2007;22:38S-46S.
13. Silbergleit R, Durkalski V, Lowenstein D, et al. Intramuscular versus intravenous therapy for prehospital status epilepticus. *N Engl J Med.* 2012;366:591-600.
14. Knudsen FU. Rectal administration of diazepam in solution in the acute treatment of convulsions in infants and children. *Arch Dis Child.* 1979;54:855-857.
15. Qureshi A, Wassmer E, Davies P, Berry K, Whitehouse WP. Comparative audit of intravenous lorazepam and diazepam in the emergency treatment of convulsive status epilepticus in children. *Seizure.* 2002;11:141-144.

Injury Among Children and Young Adults With Epilepsy

Prasad V, Kendrick D, Sayal K, et al (Univ of Nottingham, England; et al)
Pediatrics 133:827-835, 2014

Objective.—To investigate whether children and young adults with epilepsy are at a greater risk of fracture, thermal injury, or poisoning than those without.

Methods.—A cohort study was conducted by using the Clinical Practice Research Datalink (1987–2009), a longitudinal database containing primary care records. A total of 11 934 people with epilepsy and 46 598 without, aged between 1 and 24 years at diagnosis, were followed for a median (interquartile range) of 2.6 (0.8–5.9) years. The risk of fractures (including long bone fractures), thermal injuries, and poisonings (including medicinal and nonmedicinal poisonings) was estimated.

Results.—Adjusting for age, gender, Strategic Health Authority region, deprivation, and calendar year at study entry (and, for medicinal poisonings, behavior disorder), people with epilepsy had an 18% increase in risk of fracture (hazard ratio [HR] = 1.18; 95% confidence interval [CI], 1.09–1.27), a 23% increase in risk of long bone fracture (HR = 1.23; 95% CI, 1.10–1.38), a 49% increase in risk of thermal injury (HR = 1.49; 95% CI, 1.27–1.75), and more than twice the risk of poisoning (HR = 2.47; 95% CI, 2.15–2.84), which was limited to poisoning from medicinal products (medicinal HR = 2.54; 95% CI, 2.16–2.99; nonmedicinal HR = 0.96; 95% CI, 0.61–1.52).

Conclusions.—Children and young adults with epilepsy are at a greater risk of fracture, thermal injury, and poisoning than those without. The greatest risk is from medicinal poisonings. Doctors and other health care professionals should provide injury and poison prevention advice at diagnosis and epilepsy reviews (Table 2).

▶ In general, the higher risk of lifetime injuries associated with epilepsy has been well documented. This association may be due to seizure-related trauma or the adverse effects of chronic antiepileptic medications. However, most of these data are from adults with epilepsy.[1,2] As a result, this study by Prasad et al fills in an important gap in our understanding of the risk for injury in children and young adults with epilepsy.

Using a multivariate analysis approach, Prasad et al demonstrate that children with epilepsy had an increased risk of fracture, thermal injury, any poisoning, and poisoning from medicinal products (Table 2).

Although the increased risk of fractures and thermal injuries are most likely related to seizures, the reason for the increased risk of poisoning is not clear. Furthermore, it is difficult to determine whether the cases of poisoning were intentional or unintentional in this data set. A Danish case-control study reported a higher relative risk of suicide for persons with epilepsy compared with persons without epilepsy.[3] This study features an age group in which patients take increasing responsibility for their medical management, eventually assuming primary or sole responsibility for their chronic medications.[4] The increased risk for poisoning

TABLE 2.—Risk of Fractures, Thermal Injuries, and Poisonings in Children and Young Adults With Epilepsy Compared With Those Without

Injury Category	Epilepsy or No Epilepsy	Events, n	Person-years at Risk	Rate per 1000 (95% CI)	HR (95% CI)	Adjusted HR[a] (95% CI)
Any fractures	No epilepsy	2066	143 336	14.4 (13.8–15.0)	1	1
	Epilepsy	948	56 310	16.8 (15.8–17.9)	1.15 (1.07–1.24)	1.18 (1.09–1.27)
Thermal injuries	No epilepsy	415	164 247	2.5 (2.3–2.8)	1	1
	Epilepsy	253	67 231	3.8 (3.3–4.3)	1.51 (1.29–1.77)	1.49 (1.27–1.75)
Any poisonings	No epilepsy	417	165 376	2.5 (2.3–2.8)	1	1
	Epilepsy	408	66 021	6.2 (5.6–6.8)	2.57 (2.24–2.95)	2.47 (2.15–2.84)
Injury subgroups						
Long bone fractures	No epilepsy	931	155 637	6.0 (5.6–6.4)	1	1
	Epilepsy	438	63 454	6.9 (6.3–7.6)	1.17 (1.04–1.31)	1.23 (1.10–1.38)
Medicinal poisonings	No epilepsy	293	164 946	1.8 (1.6–2.0)	1	1
	Epilepsy	341	65 786	5.2 (4.7–5.8)	3.06 (2.62–3.59)	2.54[b] (2.16–2.99)
Nonmedicinal poisonings	No epilepsy	72	164 121	0.4 (1.9–0.6)	1	1
	Epilepsy	26	64 760	0.4 (1.9–0.6)	0.92 (0.59–1.45)	0.96 (0.61–1.52)

[a]All HRs were adjusted for age, gender, SHA region, deprivation, and calendar year at study entry.
[b]HR additionally adjusted for behavior disorder.
Reprinted from Prasad V, Kendrick D, Sayal K, et al. Injury Among Children and Young Adults With Epilepsy. Pediatrics. 2014;133:827–835. Copyright © 2014, by the American Academy of Pediatrics.

may be due to poor medication self-management. Children and young adults need to develop proper medication habits of double-checking the medication name on the bottle, keeping medications in their appropriate container, and developing a system to avoid "doubling up" or forgetting to take a medication.

This cohort study provides more interesting questions than answers, because further work is needed to understand the nature of the poisonings. In addition, it would be helpful to analyze factors that might be associated with later injury (eg, setting of injury, type of seizure disorder). Did the injury occur due to a fall from a height? Or was it associated with a specific sport or activity? Were specific mediations associated with an increased risk of poisoning? It may be possible to screen and provide increased counseling based on these preidentified risk factors. For clinicians, this study offers information about the risk of injuries for children with epilepsy and also reminds us of the importance of anticipatory guidance regarding medication safety.

M. D. Cabana, MD, MPH

References

1. Persson HB, Alberts KA, Farahmand BY, Tomson T. Risk of extremity fractures in adult outpatients with epilepsy. *Epilepsia.* 2002;43:768-772.
2. Neufeld MY, Vishne T, Chistik V, Korczyn AD. Life-long history of injuries related to seizures. *Epilepsy Res.* 1999;34:123-127.
3. Christensen J, Vestergaard M, Mortensen PB, Sidenius P, Agerbo E. Epilepsy and risk of suicide: a population-based case–control study. *Lancet Neurol.* 2007;6: 693-698.
4. Orrell-Valente JK, Jarlsberg LG, Hill LG, Cabana MD. At what age do children start taking daily asthma medicines on their own? *Pediatrics.* 2008;122: e1186-e1192.

Duration and Course of Post-Concussive Symptoms
Eisenberg MA, Meehan WP III, Mannix R (Boston Children's Hosp, MA)
Pediatrics 133:999-1006, 2014

Objectives.—To examine the incidence, duration, and clinical course of individual post-concussive symptoms in patients presenting to a pediatric emergency department (ED) with a concussion.

Methods.—We conducted secondary analysis of a prospective cohort study of patients 11 to 22 years old presenting to the ED of a children's hospital with an acute concussion. The main outcome measure was duration of symptoms, assessed by the Rivermead Post-Concussion Symptoms Questionnaire (RPSQ). Patients initially completed a questionnaire describing mechanism of injury, associated symptoms, past medical history, and the RPSQ, then were serially administered the RPSQ for 3 months after the concussion or until all symptoms resolved.

Results.—Headache, fatigue, dizziness, and taking longer to think were the most common symptoms encountered at presentation, whereas sleep disturbance, frustration, forgetfulness, and fatigue were the symptoms most likely to develop during the follow-up period that had not initially

TABLE 2.—Time to Resolution of Individual Post-Concussive Symptoms

	% Reporting Symptom at Presentation	% Developing Symptom After Initial Assessment	% With Symptoms on Day 7 (N = 234)[a]	% With Symptoms on Day 28 (N = 218)[a]	% With Symptoms on Day 90 (N = 207)[a]	Median Days of Symptom (95% CI)
All symptoms	n/a	n/a	77	32	15	13 (11–15)
Physical symptoms						
Blurry vision	32	5.4	31.6	6	1.4	11 (9–13)
Dizziness	61.3	6.8	53	14.2	3.9	10 (8–12)
Double vision	13.2	2.1	12.8	1.8	0.5	10 (9–11)
Fatigue	64.2	15.4	59.8	21.6	3.4	13 (11–15)
Headache	85.1	3.8	69.2	24.8	5.2	12 (10–14)
Light sensitivity	42.5	10.7	44	13.8	1.9	13 (10–16)
Nausea	41.6	3.9	37.2	8.7	2.4	9 (8–10)
Noise sensitivity	40.4	14	43.2	12.4	1.9	11 (10–12)
Sleep disturbance	11.6	21.6	24.8	10.1	1	16 (10–22)
Cognitive symptoms						
Forgetfulness	42.1	15.8	44	14.	1.9	11 (8–14)
Poor concentration	52.4	13.1	56.8	17	3.4	14 (12–16)
Taking longer to think	57.8	11.1	54.3	18.3	4.3	13 (10–16)
Emotional symptoms						
Depression	22.9	8.6	25.6	8.3	1.4	9 (7–11)
Frustration	27.7	17.4	37.6	14.7	1.4	14 (8–20)
Irritability	25.5	14.5	30.3	14.2	1.9	16 (9–23)
Restlessness	24.6	14.1	31.6	10.6	1.4	12 (9–15)

[a]Number of patients in the study minus patients censored before given time interval.
CI, 95% confidence interval; n/a, not applicable.

Reprinted from Eisenberg MA, Meehan WP III, Mannix R. Duration and Course of Post-Concussive Symptoms. Pediatrics. 2014;133:999-1006. Copyright © 2014, by the American Academy of Pediatrics.

been present. Median duration of symptoms was the longest for irritability (16 days), sleep disturbance (16 days), frustration (14 days), and poor concentration (14 days), whereas nausea, depression, dizziness, and double-vision abated most quickly. One month after injury, nearly a quarter of children still complained of headache, >20% suffered from fatigue, and nearly 20% reported taking longer to think.

Conclusions.—Among patients presenting to a pediatric ED after a concussion, physical symptoms such as headache predominate immediately after the injury, emotional symptoms tend to develop later in the recovery period, and cognitive symptoms may be present throughout (Table 2).

▶ With the increasing media and medical attention on concussions, the wide array of symptomology associated with concussions has generally been well classified. Concussion symptoms tend to cluster in 4 groups, and some people have more or fewer symptoms in different areas. These include physical symptoms (headache, balance problems, light and sound sensitivity, dizziness, nausea/vomiting, numbness/tingling), sleep difficulties (sleeping more/less than usual, trouble falling asleep), cognitive symptoms (feeling foggy or slow, trouble remembering, trouble concentrating), and emotional symptoms (feeling sad, anxious, irritable). Most management approaches for concussions revolve around these 4 domains and include classifying symptoms in each cluster and developing a plan including medical management, behavioral modifications, and guidance for Return to Play and Return to Learn.[1]

Eisenberg et al performed a prospective cohort study that provides a better linear understanding of the duration of individual concussion symptoms over a 12-week period of patients presenting to a tertiary care pediatric emergency department (ED). This provides unique insight into the evolution of these symptom clusters, in particular, over time. It represents the first study to better define the time element of concussion symptoms by following patient symptoms with the Rivermead Post-Concussion Symptoms Questionnaire at 1, 2, 4, 6, 8, and 12 weeks after their ED visit or until they met criteria for symptom resolution. In general terms, the study showed that physical symptoms such as headache and dizziness predominated at initial presentation, emotional symptoms such as frustration and depression often evolved during follow-up and often lasted the longest, and cognitive symptoms such as poor concentration and slow thinking were burdensome throughout the time period followed and often lasted long into the recovery period (Table 2).

Understanding the evolution of these symptoms can be beneficial to a wide breadth of individuals. For patients and their families, it can help normalize the often difficult and stressful process of recovering from a concussion. For school personnel and families, it can provide further reinforcement on the very real and often predominant cognitive symptoms that need to be accommodated in the process of returning to learn. For athletic personnel, it provides another piece of evidence of the sometimes long course of concussion recovery. This study can hopefully provide further validation on the importance of some of our guiding principles in concussion management—"When in doubt, sit it out" as well as gradual guided Return to Play activities accounting for the potential regression in symptoms.

While providing good general data on the timeline of concussion symptoms, I believe there are several limitations to the study. The authors do mention some of these basic limitations. First, there was no control group to account for other variables contributing to self-reported symptoms. Second, the study is limited to self-reported symptoms from the Rivermead Post-concussion Symptoms Questionnaire as would be expected. Third, many of the patients were enrolled after their ED visits, which could reflect initial symptoms hours to days after the injury. Fourth, there were some substantial differences in the patients enrolled who were studied and those lost to follow-up including race/ethnicity and presence of attention-deficit/hyperactivity disorder. Fifth, the authors note the limitations of including patients referred to a tertiary-care pediatric ED as possibly reflecting a more severe subset.

In addition, there are several other limitations on the data and study design that preclude it from helping refine concussion management protocols. First, the study does not provide any individual data on management strategies for patients throughout the follow-up period. There was inclusion of a basic follow-up questionnaire in which patients reported the amount of cognitive and athletic activity on a 5-point scale from full rest to full participation, and for patients to also compare their current school and athletic performance to their preinjury performance. Fifty-seven percent of patients reported at least moderately limiting cognitive activity, 18% reported worse school performance, and only 8.2% of patients reported returning to full athletic activity. Because this questionnaire is also self-reported, there may be wide variations in understanding and accounting of activity levels as well as subjective accounting of school and athletic performance.

The details of medical management may have affected symptom evolution; however, no data describing clinical management are presented. Some patients may be followed at specialty concussion centers including medical management of symptoms such as headaches and sleep problems, whereas others may not seek any health care professional guidance. Some patients may be followed closely and provided detailed counseling on cognitive and physical rest and gradual introduction of Return to Play and Return to Learn instructions, whereas others may be guiding this process on their own. Concussion management can be highly variable based on practitioner preferences, family preferences, and numerous other environmental considerations. As practitioners who manage concussions regularly, we know that careful management of symptoms, regular counseling, and gradual guided introduction of cognitive and physical activity drastically affects the evolution and course of symptoms.

Second, the study does not attempt to qualify the severity of concussions. By excluding patients with Glasgow Coma Score < 13, a coexisting fracture of the skull or long bone, or a coexisting injury to intra-abdominal or intrathoracic organ or spinal cord, the study has effectively excluded more moderate or severe traumatic brain injuries. However, a hot topic in current concussion research is trying to identify early markers that may help us categorize the more severe concussions and guide a different approach to those patients who may be at risk for a more prolonged symptom course. Areas of research include various high-resolution imaging modalities, various biomarkers, and neuropsychologic testing. Although this study provides information about the general timeline of concussion symptoms, future work is needed to help understand why certain patients may have a more pronounced and/or prolonged course as well as how we can identify these patients early. This information will allow us to better tailor our approach and management to optimize care and aid in quicker recovery after diagnosed concussions.

M. Kapadia, MD, MSc

Reference

1. McCrory P, Meeuwisse WH, Aubry M, et al. Consensus statement on concussion in sport: the 4th International Conference on Concussion in Sport held in Zurich. November 2012. *British Journal of Sports Medicine*. 2013;47:250-258.

Use of Selective Serotonin Reuptake Inhibitors during Pregnancy and Risk of Autism

Hviid A, Melbye M, Pasternak B (Statens Serum Institut, Copenhagen, Denmark)
N Engl J Med 369:2406-2415, 2013

Background.—Studies have raised concern about an association between the use of selective serotonin reuptake inhibitors (SSRIs) during pregnancy and an increased risk of autism spectrum disorders in the offspring.

Methods.—We conducted a cohort study of all singleton live births in Denmark from 1996 through 2005 (626,875 births), with follow-up through 2009. Using Danish population registries, we linked information on maternal use of SSRIs before and during pregnancy, autism spectrum disorders diagnosed in the offspring, and a range of potential confounders. We used a survival analysis of the time to diagnosis in the offspring with Poisson regression to estimate rate ratios of autism spectrum disorders according to maternal use of SSRIs.

Results.—During 5,057,282 person-years of follow-up, we identified 3892 cases of autism spectrum disorder (incidence rate, 77.0 per 100,000 person-years). A total of 52 cases during 42,400 person-years of follow-up involved offspring of women who were exposed to SSRIs during their pregnancy (incidence rate, 122.6 per 100,000 person-years). As compared with no use of SSRIs both before and during pregnancy, use during pregnancy was not associated with a significantly increased risk of autism spectrum disorders (fully adjusted rate ratio, 1.20; 95% confidence interval [CI], 0.90 to 1.61). Among women who received SSRIs before pregnancy but not during pregnancy, the corresponding fully adjusted rate ratio was 1.46 (95% CI, 1.17 to 1.81).

Conclusions.—We did not detect a significant association between maternal use of SSRIs during pregnancy and autism spectrum disorder in the offspring. On the basis of the upper boundary of the confidence interval, our study could not rule out a relative risk up to 1.61, and therefore the association warrants further study. (Funded by the Danish Health and Medicines Authority.)

▶ The dramatic increase in diagnosis of autism spectrum disorders (ASD) over the past few decades is one of the issues of greatest attention in the area of child mental health and child development. Although much of the increase is accounted for by better awareness and identification, as well as changing diagnostic criteria, there remains concern about possible environmental or other factors leading to more affected children. The Centers for Disease Control and Prevention currently report the rate of ASD in the United States as 1 of 88 children. Of all the environmental factors proposed as possible culprits, childhood vaccines as a cause has gained the most attention and created the most impact (as seen in parents refusing vaccinations for children), although there is no demonstrated evidence of a link. Yet because of the real possibility of other environmental factors contributing to the incidence of autism, the search continues, especially focusing on environmental exposures that themselves have risen along the same timeline as the rise in ASD diagnoses.

Because several studies have shown that autism is a neurodevelopmental disorder with brain alterations beginning in utero, prenatal environmental exposures are a primary focus of investigation. Autism is associated with alterations in the brain's serotonin pathways, and thus several groups have now looked at the possible impact of maternal prenatal use of medications that affect serotonin systems, especially the commonly used selective-serotonin reuptake inhibitor (SSRI) antidepressants. SSRI medications first came into use in the United States in 1987 and have seen rising rates of prescription across the past few decades, including in pregnant women. Although some time-limited neonatal withdrawal effects have been seen with maternal use of SSRIs, studies of general outcomes of exposed children have not demonstrated any significant long-term adverse effects. These reassuring data, combined with data demonstrating that prenatal maternal depression itself has adverse effects on the developing fetus, has led maternal health care providers to recommend that SSRI antidepressants be considered during pregnancy when the risk of impairing depression is significant.

However, the safety of prenatal SSRI exposure has been called into question by recent case control studies finding an association between exposure and ASD diagnosis.[1-3] This study by Hviid A et al, in contrast, which is a large prospective cohort study, did not find elevated risk (Table 3 in the original article). This study makes use of the comprehensive Danish health registries, allowing for complete, prospectively collected data on all live births in Denmark over a 10-year period.

One of the most obvious potential confounds in these studies is the indication for the medication itself, which needs to be controlled for because maternal depression and other mental health problems are associated with elevated risk of ASD in offspring. All the referenced studies attempt to control for this confound but may not be able to do so completely. In this study, the risk of an association may be overestimated because of a limitation in how maternal mental health history data was collected. On the other hand, the method of ascertaining prenatal SSRI exposure is based on prescription records, which may exaggerate the actual incidence of exposure because not all filled prescriptions are actually consumed; this could bias the results toward underestimation of risk. One other major limitation of this study is the potential lack of generalizability; the prevalence of SSRI use during pregnancy was 1% in this sample, whereas in the United States during the same time frame, SSRI use during pregnancy is reported to be more than 5%.

The bottom line for the moment seems to be that there is a potential modest risk to the fetus from exposure to SSRI antidepressant medication, which must be weighed against the risks to the mother and fetus from inadequately treated mental health conditions. In women for whom the risk of depression during pregnancy without medications is high, SSRI medications should not be ruled out. Notably, even if there is a true association between prenatal antidepressant exposure and autism, this particular environmental exposure would not contribute significantly to an explanation for the rising incidence of ASD because the relative risk found in the positive studies would account for only 0.5% to 3.0% of total ASD cases.

R. Marquardt, MD

R. L. Hendren, DO

References

1. Harrington RA, Lee LC, Crum RM, Zimmerman AW, Hertz-Picciotto I. Prenatal SSRI use and offspring with autism spectrum disorder or developmental delay. *Pediatrics.* 2014 [Epub ahead of print].
2. Rai D, Lee BK, Dalman C, Golding J, Lewis G, Magnusson C. Parental depression, maternal antidepressant use during pregnancy, and risk of autism spectrum disorders: population based case-control study. *BMJ.* 2013;346:f2059.
3. Croen LA, Grether JK, Yoshida CK, Odouli R, Hendrick V. Antidepressant use during pregnancy and childhood autism spectrum disorders. *Arch Gen Psychiatry.* 2011;68:1104-1112.

Accuracy of Brief Screening Tools for Identifying Postpartum Depression Among Adolescent Mothers

Venkatesh KK, Zlotnick C, Triche EW, et al (Massachusetts General Hosp and Brigham and Women's Hosp, Boston; Warren Alpert Med School of Brown Univ, Providence, RI; Brown Univ, Providence, RI; et al)
Pediatrics 133:e45-e53, 2014

Objective.—To evaluate the accuracy of the Edinburgh Postnatal Depression Scale (EPDS) and 3 subscales for identifying postpartum depression among primiparous adolescent mothers.

Methods.—Mothers enrolled in a randomized controlled trial to prevent postpartum depression completed a psychiatric diagnostic interview and the 10-item EPDS at 6 weeks, 3 months, and 6 months postpartum. Three subscales of the EPDS were assessed as brief screening tools: 3-item anxiety subscale (EPDS-3), 7-item depressive symptoms subscale (EPDS-7), and 2-item subscale (EPDS-2) that resemble the Patient Health Questionnaire-2. Receiver operating characteristic curves and the areas under the curves for each tool were compared to assess accuracy. The sensitivities and specificities of each screening tool were calculated in comparison with diagnostic criteria for a major depressive disorder. Repeated-measures longitudinal analytical techniques were used.

Results.—A total of 106 women contributed 289 postpartum visits; 18% of the women met criteria for incident postpartum depression by psychiatric diagnostic interview. When used as continuous measures, the full EPDS, EPDS-7, and EPDS-2 performed equally well (area under the curve >0.9). Optimal cutoff scores for a positive depression screen for the EPDS and EPDS-7 were lower (≥9 and ≥7, respectively) than currently recommended cutoff scores (≥10). At optimal cutoff scores, the EPDS and EPDS-7 both had sensitivities of 90% and specificities of >85%.

Conclusions.—The EPDS, EPDS-7, and EPDS-2 are highly accurate at identifying postpartum depression among adolescent mothers. In primary care pediatric settings, the EPDS and its shorter subscales have potential for use as effective depression screening tools.

▶ Screening for postpartum depression has become more accepted and routine in pediatric offices over the past decade. Now that screening has been established as important and helpful, it is time to refine our understanding of screening to include the choice, length, and validity of screening in diverse populations. The article by Venkatesh et al is a critical contribution to the literature because it begins to address these important questions among a high-risk and underresearched population—a diverse group of adolescent mothers. It not only supports that the Edinburgh Postnatal Depression Scale (EPDS) is an accurate tool in this population by comparing it to a semistructured interview, it seeks to explore whether shorter subscales are accurate and potentially useful in the clinical setting.

While seeking to improve the acceptability for patients and providers by shortening questionnaires, accuracy cannot be forfeited for brevity. The study helps to underscore the importance of validating subscales. The investigators found that the 3-item subscale, which focuses on anxiety, did not perform as well as in identifying postpartum depression as the full EPDS, the 7-item, or the 2-item subscales that targeted depression questions. Therefore, the specific questions and not the length are critical to ensuring accurate identification of postpartum depression.

Furthermore, the study findings reinforce the need to consider standard cut points as guideposts and not strict determinations of "depressed or not depressed." Cut points may need to be adapted based on the population. Understanding these subtleties of screening are crucial to how clinicians use screening tools effectively because they are the ones who must determine what the next steps are for guiding mothers to seek help. The generalizability of the study findings is limited by the fact that the population was derived from a randomized controlled trial aimed at prevention of postpartum depression. However, the study expands our knowledge of a population about whom we know little, and it extends the critical dialogue about postpartum depression screening.

L. H. Chaudron, MD, MS

Adverse Childhood Experiences of Low-Income Urban Youth
Wade R Jr, Shea JA, Rubin D, et al (Children's Hosp of Philadelphia, PA; Univ of Pennsylvania, Philadelphia)
Pediatrics 134:e13-e20, 2014

Background and Objective.—Current assessments of adverse childhood experiences (ACEs) may not adequately encompass the breadth of adversity to which low-income urban children are exposed. The purpose of this study was to identify and characterize the range of adverse childhood experiences faced by young adults who grew up in a low-income urban area.

Methods.—Focus groups were conducted with young adults who grew up in low-income Philadelphia neighborhoods. Using the nominal group technique, participants generated a list of adverse childhood experiences and then identified the 5 most stressful experiences on the group list. The most stressful experiences identified by participants were grouped into a ranked list of domains and subdomains.

Results.—Participants identified a range of experiences, grouped into 10 domains: family relationships, community stressors, personal victimization, economic hardship, peer relationships, discrimination, school, health, child welfare/juvenile justice, and media/technology. Included in these domains were many but not all of the experiences from the initial ACEs studies; parental divorce/separation and mental illness were absent. Additional experiences not included in the initial ACEs but endorsed by our participants included single-parent homes; exposure to violence, adult themes, and criminal behavior; personal victimization; bullying; economic hardship; and discrimination.

Conclusions.—Gathering youth perspectives on childhood adversity broadens our understanding of the experience of stress and trauma in childhood. Future work is needed to determine the significance of this broader set of adverse experiences in predisposing children to poor health outcomes as adults.

▶ Since Felitti et al's landmark series of articles on adverse childhood experiences (ACEs),[1] it has become increasingly clear that ACEs have profound lifelong effects on health, social outcomes, and disparities. The original ACEs papers, however, were based on a largely white, middle-class Kaiser Permanente health maintenance organization population. As such, the generalizability of their findings (and of the ACEs questionnaire itself) to other populations has been less clear. More recent studies have begun adding additional elements to the original list of stressors, reflecting our growing understanding of ACEs and an increasing appreciation for the unique experiences of different populations.[2,3]

The new study by Wade et al addresses an important gap by exploring what youth (18–26 years old) who grew up in low-income Philadelphia neighborhoods perceive to be ACEs in both their own lives and the lives of people they know. In addition to confirming many of the family relationship and personal victimization ACEs examined in previous studies (Table 2 in the original article), these youth identified additional ACEs, especially in the domains of economic hardship and community stressors (eg, neighborhood crime/violence). This work is a valuable contribution to the literature, identifying at least 2 additional major domains that will likely need to be fully incorporated into future ACEs studies. Together, these 4 domains—family relationships, community stressors, personal victimization, and economic hardship—may provide a more complete conceptualization of ACEs than was possible in the original studies. Moreover, the perspectives of the youth in this study align with increasing scientific attention being paid to the powerful effects of neighborhood environments and poverty on health.[4,5]

It is worth noting that focusing specifically on youths' voices has both potential strengths and potential weaknesses. On one hand, youth provide a firsthand, on-the-ground perspective that differs from the perspectives of adult observers. In many respects, youth may know themselves (and their thoughts and experiences) better than anybody else does. The relative immediacy of youth perspectives, for instance, might eventually prove to correlate better with real-time stress-related biological changes that may predispose them to later health problems. On the other hand, what do youth not know that they don't know? What are the limits of their perspective? To what degree, for instance, does these youths' endorsement of single-parent homes as a childhood stressor but not of parental divorce/separation (included in the original ACEs studies) reflect a particular set of experiences among these youth rather than a more generally applicable understanding of societal trends? Similarly, to what degree does the relatively low importance given to poor-quality schools reflect a limited awareness of the impact of school quality on later adult earnings and other key health-related outcomes? And to what degree does the surprisingly infrequent nomination of rape reflect a lack of understanding among youth regarding rape (or, given that focus groups were performed, a social inhibition against even acknowledging the issue)?

Overall, however, the youth participants in the study have given us a valuable platform on which to build. As the field moves forward, this study of low-income, Philadelphia youth reinforces an interesting and important point—that ACEs will likely be different in different populations. Age, gender, race/ethnicity, poverty, and other factors may not only predispose specific populations to certain ACEs but also affect these populations' subjective and biological experiences of them. The key will be identifying, respecting, and leveraging both the universal and population-specific aspects of ACEs in ways that can lead to effective community-based interventions and national policies. In addition, the field will need to merge with other active areas of research and policy to better incorporate positive, resilience-building counterparts to ACEs, placing adverse events in the context of individual, family, and community assets and strengths.

In summary, perhaps the most important take-home messages of this study are that youths' voices matter, that neighborhood environments and poverty must be incorporated into any model of ACEs, and that ACEs are likely to be context-specific, dynamic forces in the human experience. There can be little doubt at this point that ACEs belong on a surprisingly short list of major childhood determinants of adult health. Most of the truly essential child health services occur outside traditional clinical environments, in the social fabric of vulnerable communities made up of vulnerable families with vulnerable children. How effectively child health care providers learn to address core health issues such as economic hardship and community stressors will in large part determine the continued relevance of this profession in the coming years.

P. J. Chung, MD, MS

E. S. Barnert, MD, MPH, MS

References

1. Felitti VJ, Anda RF, Nordenberg D, et al. Relationship of childhood abuse and household dysfunction to many of the leading causes of death in adults. The Adverse Childhood Experiences (ACE) Study. *Am J Prev Med.* 1998;14:245-258.
2. Shonkoff JP, Garner AS, Committee on Psychosocial Aspects of Child and Family Health; Committee on Early Childhood, Adoption, and Dependent Care, Section on Developmental and Behavioral Pediatrics. The lifelong effects of early childhood adversity and toxic stress. *Pediatrics.* 2012;129:e232-e246, http://www. pediatrics.org/cgi/content/full/129/1/e232. Accessed August 13, 2014.
3. Finkelhor D, Shattuck A, Turner H, Hamby S. Improving the adverse childhood experiences study scale. *JAMA Pediatr.* 2013;167:70-75.
4. Brooks-Gunn J, Duncan GJ. The effects of poverty on children. *Future Child.* 1997;7:55-71.
5. Leventhal T, Brooks-Gunn J. The neighborhoods they live in: the effects of neighborhood residence on child and adolescent outcomes. *Psychol Bull.* 2000;126: 309-337.

The Effects of Poverty on Childhood Brain Development: The Mediating Effect of Caregiving and Stressful Life Events

Luby J, Belden A, Botteron K, et al (Washington Univ School of Medicine in St Louis, MO; et al)
JAMA Pediatr 167:1135-1142, 2013

Importance.—The study provides novel data to inform the mechanisms by which poverty negatively impacts childhood brain development.

Objective.—To investigate whether the income-to-needs ratio experienced in early childhood impacts brain development at school age and to explore the mediators of this effect.

Design, Setting, and Participants.—This study was conducted at an academic research unit at the Washington University School of Medicine in St Louis. Data from a prospective longitudinal study of emotion development in preschool children who participated in neuroimaging at school age were used to investigate the effects of poverty on brain development. Children were assessed annually for 3 to 6 years prior to the time of a magnetic resonance imaging scan, during which they were evaluated on psychosocial, behavioral, and other developmental dimensions. Preschoolers included in the study were 3 to 6 years of age and were recruited from primary care and day care sites in the St Louis metropolitan area; they were annually assessed behaviorally for 5 to 10 years. Healthy preschoolers and those with clinical symptoms of depression participated in neuroimaging at school age/early adolescence.

Exposure.—Household poverty as measured by the income-to-needs ratio.

Main Outcomes and Measures.—Brain volumes of children's white matter and cortical gray matter, as well as hippocampus and amygdala volumes, obtained using magnetic resonance imaging. Mediators of interest were caregiver support/hostility measured observationally during the preschool period and stressful life events measured prospectively.

Results.—Poverty was associated with smaller white and cortical gray matter and hippocampal and amygdala volumes. The effects of poverty on hippocampal volume were mediated by caregiving support/hostility on the left and right, as well as stressful life events on the left.

Conclusions and Relevance.—The finding that exposure to poverty in early childhood materially impacts brain development at school age further underscores the importance of attention to the well-established deleterious effects of poverty on child development. Findings that these effects on the hippocampus are mediated by caregiving and stressful life events suggest that attempts to enhance early caregiving should be a focused public health target for prevention and early intervention. Findings substantiate the behavioral literature on the negative effects of poverty on child development and provide new data confirming that effects extend to brain development. Mechanisms for these effects on the hippocampus are suggested to inform intervention.

▶ Children under 18 years of age represent 23% of the US population but comprise 34% of all people in poverty. More than 1 in 5 children in the United States live in poverty, representing more than 16 million children. Poverty places children at risk for a host of problems pertaining to cognitive development and academic achievement, including lower IQs, reduced literacy, and decreased rates of high school graduation and gainful employment in adulthood. Disparities in cognitive development and academic achievement tend to emerge early in childhood and then widen throughout the early elementary school years.

Numerous factors contribute to these socioeconomic gaps in cognitive development: nutrition, environmental toxins, the home learning environment, early schooling, and, as is the focus in this article, caregiving style and differential exposure to early life stressors. Unfortunately, these different pathways are often highly correlated in that disadvantaged families are more likely to be exposed to multiple risk factors than are advantaged families. As such, researchers find it daunting to tease out the mechanisms behind the socioeconomic gap in cognitive development and, in turn, to design effective interventions.

One approach to attempting to disentangle these links is to focus on disparities in specific brain structures or functions, as the authors in this study did

(Fig 1). Although academic achievement is clearly influenced by brain development, until recently the study of socioeconomic disparities in child development operated with virtually no input from neuroscience. Classic work tells us broadly about associations between income and achievement, but neuroscience teaches us that "achievement" is the complex output of multiple cognitive systems supported by different brain regions and networks.

Luby et al found that, relative to their more advantaged peers, children from lower income families had reductions in overall gray and white matter, as well as reductions in the size of the hippocampus and amygdala. These latter brain regions are critical for learning, memory, and emotion development. Previous research has (1) reported links between family socioeconomic background and the structure and function of these structures, and (2) shown that exposure to early life stress and hostile parenting have direct effects on the development of these structures. Importantly, however, this is the first study to "connect the dots," showing that the links between income and hippocampal/amygdala volume are mediated by caregiving support/hostility and exposure to stressful life events (Fig 2).

One limitation in these findings is that children were recruited from a larger study on childhood depression, such that children with depression were oversampled. This limits the generalizability of the study somewhat because it is possible that, for example, the effects of family stress could be more pronounced among children with depression, that childhood depression itself affects parenting style and family stress, or that depression affects these brain structures in ways unrelated to the present study.

Nonetheless, this study has important implications for the design of interventional approaches. Young children spend the vast majority of their time with their parents and other caretakers, and so interventions that lead to more sensitive, responsive parenting may well lead to large gains for children's cognitive, socioemotional, and brain development. Thought-provokingly, policies that target poverty reduction itself may well "get at the source" of socioeconomic disparities in child development. Such policies are likely to reduce parental stress, fatigue,

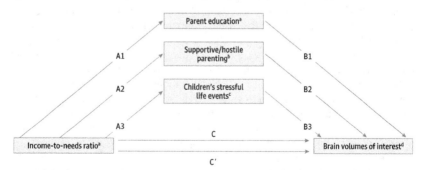

FIGURE 1.—Conceptual model testing multiple mediators of the hypothesized association between income-to-needs ratio and variation in brain volume. [a] Measured at baseline. [b] Measured after baseline but before scan. [c] Between baseline and time of scan. [d] Time of scan. (Reprinted from Luby J, Belden A, Botteron K, et al. The effects of poverty on childhood brain development: the mediating effect of caregiving and stressful life events. *JAMA Pediatr.* 2013;167:1135-1142, with permission from American Medical Association.)

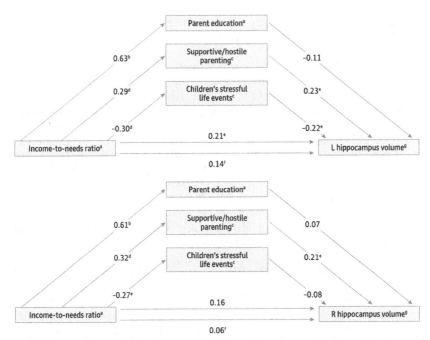

FIGURE 2.—Caregivers' Education, Supportive/Hostile Parenting, and Children's Experiences of Stressful Life Events as Mediators of the Relation Between Income-to-Needs Ratio and Hippocampus Volumes. Values shown are standardized regression coefficients. The top model is for the left (L) hippocampus volume, while the model at the bottom represents the right (R) hippocampus volume. Both models include whole-brain volume and sex as covariates. [a] Measured at baseline. [b] $P < .001$. [c] Measured after baseline but before scan. [d] $P < .01$. [e] $P < .05$. [f] After adding parents' education, supportive/hostile parenting, and children's stressful life events to the model. [g] Time of scan. (Reprinted from Luby J, Belden A, Botteron K, et al. The effects of poverty on childhood brain development: the mediating effect of caregiving and stressful life events. *JAMA Pediatr.* 2013;167:1135-1142, with permission from American Medical Association.)

depression, and chaos in the home, improving the likelihood that parents will have the emotional bandwidth to provide the kind of sensitive and responsive caregiving that children need to thrive.

K. G. Noble, MD, PhD

Sports Participation and Parent-Reported Health-Related Quality of Life in Children: Longitudinal Associations

Vella SA, Cliff DP, Magee CA, et al (Univ of Wollongong, Australia)
J Pediatr 164:1469-1474, 2014

Objective.—To investigate the longitudinal association between sports participation and parent-reported health-related quality of life (HRQOL) in children.

Study Design.—Cohort study that used data drawn from the Longitudinal Study of Australian Children in waves 3 (2008) and 4 (2010).

Participants were a nationally representative sample of 4042 Australian children ages 8.25 (SD = 0.44) years at baseline and followed-up 24 months later.

Results.—After we adjusted for multiple covariates, children who continued to participate in sports between the ages of 8 and 10 years had greater parent-reported HRQOL at age 10 (Eta^2 = .02) compared with children who did not participate in sports ($P \leq .001$), children who commenced participation after 8 years of age ($P = .004$), and children who dropped out of sports before reaching 10 years of age ($P = .04$). Children who participated in both team and individual sports ($P = .02$) or team sports alone ($P = .04$) had greater HRQOL compared with children who participated in individual sports alone (Eta^2 = .01). The benefits of sports participation were strongest for girls ($P < .05$; Eta^2 = .003).

Conclusions.—Children's participation in developmentally appropriate team sports helps to protect HRQOL and should be encouraged at an early age and maintained for as long as possible.

▶ Health-related quality of life (HRQoL) takes into account physical, social, and psychological health domains, which are important for overall health. Recently, research has suggested that sport participation for children and adolescents may have benefits to HRQoL above and beyond those associated with other individual forms of physical activity. Sport has been identified as a leisure-time physical activity specifically that could contribute to greater social and psychological health compared with individual forms of physical activity because of its social nature of participation.

This article is unique in that it investigates the role of participation in sport, contributing to HRQoL longitudinally. Most research to date investigating sport as a leisure-time physical activity specifically has been limited in establishing causality due to its cross-sectional nature of investigation. Participation in team and individual sports contributes to greater HRQoL across domains, compared with nonparticipants or individual sport participation alone, and in particular to social functioning (Table 2).

In practical terms, the definition of an "individual" sport versus a "team" sport is not as clear as what is described in this study. There is not a clear distinction in the literature between individual activities in a group setting versus team sport. Most studies do not distinguish between the 2 and often do not clearly define "team" sport. A traditionally "individual" sport can occur in a "team" setting. For example, a child can swim individually and also as part of a larger swim team. In the end, the social nature of individual athletes on the same team together for some traditionally individual activities such as gymnastics, fencing, or swimming is likely to benefit HRQoL above and beyond children going for a run by themselves. Children especially appreciate physical activity with their friends, which can make it more enjoyable for them. In addition, children may gain other skills through team sports because of the "team" nature of the activity.[1]

Another unique finding is that it is important for people to stay active because once they drop out, their HRQoL lowers to rates similar to nonparticipants. This study is, however, limited by a short duration longitudinal duration (2 years),

TABLE 2.—Adjusted mean PedsQL Total and Subscale Scores at Baseline (Age 8 Years) Stratified by Type of Sports Participation

	Mean* PedsQL Score (95% CI)					
	Total	Physical	Psychosocial	Social	Emotional	School
Participation group						
Participants	79.7 (79.1-80.2)	84.6 (84.0-85.3)	77.0 (76.4-77.6)	80.5 (79.7-81.3)	73.2 (72.5-73.9)	77.4 (76.7-78.1)
Nonparticipants	76.2 (74.9-77.4)	81.1 (79.7-82.5)	73.5 (72.2-74.9)	74.7 (73.0-76.5)	73.2 (71.6-74.8)	72.6 (71.0-74.3)
Dropouts	76.7 (75.3-78.0)	81.1 (80.3-83.3)	73.9 (72.4-75.4)	76.7 (74.9-78.6)	71.8 (70.1-73.5)	73.2 (71.4-74.9)
Commencers	76.3 (75.0-77.6)	81.4 (79.9-82.9)	73.5 (72.1-75.0)	75.7 (73.9-77.5)	71.4 (69.7-73.0)	73.9 (72.2-75.7)
Sports type						
Team and individual	80.9 (79.9-81.8)	85.9 (84.8-86.9)	78.2 (77.1-79.3)	81.8 (80.4-83.1)	73.8 (72.5-75.0)	79.1 (77.8-80.4)
Team sport only	81.2 (80.1-82.3)	86.0 (84.8-87.2)	78.6 (77.4-79.9)	82.6 (81.0-84.2)	75.0 (73.5-76.5)	78.3 (76.8-79.8)
Individual sport only	77.0 (75.6-78.5)	81.3 (79.7-82.9)	74.7 (73.1-76.4)	77.7 (75.6-79.8)	71.1 (69.1-73.0)	75.6 (73.6-77.5)

*Marginal means were estimated using general linear models and were adjusted for sex, neighborhood SEP, household income, parental education, BMI, and pubertal status, and were weighted by population weights.

Reprinted from Journal Pediatrics. Vella SA, Cliff DP, Magee CA, et al. Sports Participation and Parent-Reported Health-Related Quality of Life in Children: Longitudinal Associations. J Pediatr. 2014;164:1469-1474, Copyright 2014, with permission from Elsevier.

and for children aged 8 to 10 years only. In addition, HRQoL is based on parental report.

The implications for practice are to recommend physical activity for health for children and adolescents to tackle the obesity epidemic. More specifically, it is recommended that children and adolescents participate in developmentally appropriate team sports to potentially increase overall physical, social, and psychological health.

R. M. Eime, PhD

Reference

1. Eime RM, et al. A systematic review of the psychological and social benefits of participation in sport for children and adolescents: informing development of a conceptual model of health through sport. *International Journal of Behavioral Nutrition and Physical Activity.* 2013;10:98.

The prognosis of common mental disorders in adolescents: a 14-year prospective cohort study

Patton GC, Coffey C, Romaniuk H, et al (Univ of Melbourne, Parkville, Victoria, Australia; Royal Children's Hosp, Parkville, Victoria, Australia; et al)
Lancet 383:1404-1411, 2014

Background.—Most adults with common mental disorders report their first symptoms before 24 years of age. Although adolescent anxiety and depression are frequent, little clarity exists about which syndromes persist into adulthood or resolve before then. In this report, we aim to describe the patterns and predictors of persistence into adulthood.

Methods.—We recruited a stratified, random sample of 1943 adolescents from 44 secondary schools across the state of Victoria, Australia. Between August, 1992, and January, 2008, we assessed common mental disorder at five points in adolescence and three in young adulthood, commencing at a mean age of $15 \cdot 5$ years and ending at a mean age of $29 \cdot 1$ years. Adolescent disorders were defined on the Revised Clinical Interview Schedule (CIS-R) at five adolescent measurement points, with a primary cutoff score of 12 or higher representing a level at which a family doctor would be concerned. Secondary analyses addressed more severe disorders at a cutoff of 18 or higher.

Findings.—236 of 821 (29%; 95% CI 25−32) male participants and 498 of 929 (54%; 51−57) female participants reported high symptoms on the CIS-R (≥ 12) at least once during adolescence. Almost 60% (434/734) went on to report a further episode as a young adult. However, for adolescents with one episode of less than 6 months duration, just over half had no further common mental health disorder as a young adult. Longer duration of mental health disorders in adolescence was the strongest predictor of clear-cut young adult disorder (odds ratio [OR] for persistent young adult disorder *vs* none $3 \cdot 16$, 95% CI $1 \cdot 86−5 \cdot 37$). Girls ($2 \cdot 12$, $1 \cdot 29−3 \cdot 48$) and adolescents with a background of parental separation

TABLE 2.—Prevalence and Continuity of Common Mental Disorders at 15–29 Years of Age

	Index	Male Participants (n = 821)		Female Participants (n = 929)	
		n	% (95% CI)	n	% (95% CI)
Adolescent phase (waves 2–6)					
Mental disorder by wave (CIS-R ≥12)					
Wave 2 (mean age 15.5 years)	CIS-R	137	17% (14–19)	312	34% (30–37)
Wave 3 (mean age 15.9 years)	CIS-R	103	13% (10–15)	289	31% (28–34)
Wave 4 (mean age 16.4 years)	CIS-R	90	11% (9–13)	247	27% (24–30)
Wave 5 (mean age 16.8 years)	CIS-R	73	9% (7–11)	219	24% (21–26)
Wave 6 (mean age 17.4 years)	CIS-R	59	7% (5–9)	217	23% (20–26)
Persistence of disorder (CIS-R ≥12)					
Never	..	585	71% (68–75)	431	46% (43–50)
1 wave	..	117	14% (12–17)	156	17% (14–19)
≥2 waves	..	119	14% (12–17)	342	37% (34–40)
Young adult phase (waves 7–9)					
Mental disorder by wave					
Wave 7 (mean age 20.7 years)	CIS-R	80	10% (8–12)	201	22% (19–24)
Wave 8 (mean age 24.1 years)	GHQ	122	15% (12–18)	246	27% (24–29)
Wave 9 (mean age 29.1 years)	GHQ	80	10% (8–12)	162	17% (15–20)
Wave 9 (mean age 29.1 years)	CIDI MDD	47	6% (4–7)	128	14% (11–16)
Wave 9 (mean age 29.1 years)	CIDI AD	60	7% (5–9)	140	15% (13–18)
Persistence of disorder					
Never	..	563	69% (65–72)	446	48% (44–52)
1 wave	..	188	23% (20–26)	287	31% (27–34)
≥2 waves	..	70	9% (6–11)	196	21% (18–24)
Continuity and discontinuity from adolescence (waves 2–6) to young adulthood (waves 7–9)*					
No waves in adolescence					
No waves in young adulthood	..	438	75% (71–79)	271	63% (58–68)
1 wave in young adulthood	..	119	20% (17–24)	118	27% (22–32)
≥2 waves in young adulthood	..	28	5% (3–7)	42	10% (7–13)
1 wave in adolescence					
No waves in young adulthood	..	72	61% (50–73)	72	46% (37–55)
1 wave in young adulthood	..	29	25% (15–35)	59	38% (29–47)
≥2 waves in young adulthood	..	16	14% (6–22)	25	16% (9–23)
≥2 waves in adolescence					
No waves in young adulthood	..	53	45% (35–56)	103	30% (25–36)
1 wave in young adulthood	..	39	33% (23–44)	110	32% (26–38)
≥2 waves in young adulthood	..	25	22% (13–30)	129	38% (32–43)

CIS-R = Revised Clinical Interview Schedule. GHQ = General Health Questionnaire. CIDI MDD = Composite International Diagnostic Interview major depressive disorder. CIDI AD = Composite International Diagnostic Interview anxiety disorder.

*Percentages relate to the six strata defined by three levels of adolescent caseness (no waves, one wave, and ≥two waves) and sex.

Reprinted from The Lancet. Patton GC, Coffey C, Romaniuk H, et al. The prognosis of common mental disorders in adolescents: a 14-year prospective cohort study. Lancet. 2014;383:1404-1411, Copyright 2014, with permission from Elsevier.

or divorce (1·62, 1·03–2·53) also had a greater likelihood of having ongoing disorder into young adulthood than did those without such a background. Rates of adolescent onset disorder dropped sharply by the late 20s (0·57, 0·45–0·73), suggesting a further resolution for many patients whose symptoms had persisted into the early 20s.

Interpretation.—Episodes of adolescent mental disorder often precede mental disorders in young adults. However, many such disorders, especially when brief in duration, are limited to the teenage years, with further symptom remission common in the late 20s. The resolution of many adolescent disorders gives reason for optimism that interventions that shorten the duration of episodes could prevent much morbidity later in life.

▶ This Australian longitudinal study is important because it underscores the presence of a modern epidemic. It contains both good and bad news. The study is likely to be representative of contemporary adolescent and young adult populations in many well-developed industrial countries and therefore raises many issues for clinicians and public health officials.

First, the bad news: the rates of adolescent mental health problems are high with a third of boys and a half of girls being defined as a case at least once in adolescence (Table 2; Row 6). This issue requires broad education, prevention, and intervention strategies to be put in place if the epidemic is to be stemmed. A similar package of issues equally applies to young adulthood with its array of complex stressors from tertiary education, finding a future in a competitive job market, as well as late family formation.[1] The good news is that if adolescent depressive conditions can be shortened, the prospects for recurrence in adulthood are lower. The study notes that "for those with a single adolescent episode of less than 6 months' duration, persistence into young adulthood was substantially lower than in those with longer lasting or recurrent episodes."

But why are young women in our modern culture so vulnerable? This study only highlights the issue and does not explore causal mechanisms. So what do we know about the challenges they are facing? Girls are commencing menstruation earlier, a known predisposing factor to adolescent mental health problems.[2] Equally, schools appear to have become more stressful with pressures on young people to complete high school and compete for jobs in the high-skilled service industries.[3,4] Girls face complex choices around identity development, future family formation, and career advancement. In addition, our Western media culture broadcasts body image stereotypes of women, adding further pressure.[5,6]

Where the young person is experiencing mild to moderate depressive features, cognitive behavior therapy is appropriate. However more severe presentations may require a course of antidepressants as well as close follow-up. Other components include consistent screening for suicidality and comorbidity, especially alcohol and marijuana use.[7]

A recent Australian systematic literature review of depression in adolescents and young adults has led to a series of best practice guidelines based on available evidence.[8,9] Examples of online information and early intervention services are MoodGYM[10] or e-Couch.[11] Clinicians ranging from school counselors, to pediatricians, to psychiatrists need to be up to date with a 21st-century tool kit of online education and intervention programs, an understanding of psychotherapeutic treatment approaches, and an understanding of the place for antidepressant or antianxiety medication.

W. Bor, MBBS, DPM, FRANZCP

References

1. Arnett JJ. Emerging adulthood: A theory of development from the late teens through the twenties. *Am Psychol.* 2000;55:469-480.
2. Crockett LJ, Carlo G, Wolff JM, Hope MO. The role of pubertal timing and temperamental vulnerability in adolescents' internalizing symptoms. *Dev Psychopathol.* 2013;25:377-389.
3. Lindsey B. *Human Capitalism: How Economic Growth Has Made Us Smarter—and More Unequal.* Princeton University Press; 2013.
4. Wiklund M, Malmgren-Olsson EB, Ohman A, Bergström E, Fjellman-Wiklund A. Subjective health complaints in older adolescents are related to perceived stress, anxiety and gender - a cross-sectional school study in Northern Sweden. *BMC Public Health.* 2012;12:993.
5. Stromback M, Wiklund M, Salander Renberg E, et al. Complex symptomatology among young women who present with stress-related problems. *Scand J Caring Sci.* 2014 [Epub ahead of print].
6. West P, Sweeting H. Fifteen, female and stressed: changing patterns of psychological distress over time. *J Child Psychol Psychiatry.* 2003;44:399-411.
7. Teesson M, Slade T, Mills K. Comorbidity in Australia: findings of the 2007 National Survey of Mental Health and Wellbeing. *Aust N Z J Psychiatry.* 2009;43:606-614.
8. Beyond Blue. Adolescent and Young Adult Guidelines. http://www.beyondblue.org.au/resources/health-professionals/clinical-practice-guidelines/adolescents-and-young-adults-guidelines. Accessed August 4, 2014.
9. McDermott B, Baigent M, Chanen A, et al. Clinical practice guidelines: Depression in adolescents and young adults. Melbourne, Australia: Beyondblue Expert Working Committee. 2010.
10. The Mood Gym Training Program. https://moodgym.anu.edu.au/welcome. Accessed August 4, 2014.
11. E-couch. https://ecouch.anu.edu.au/welcome. Accessed August 4, 2014.

Cognitive Behavioral Therapy Plus Amitriptyline for Chronic Migraine in Children and Adolescents: A Randomized Clinical Trial

Powers SW, Kashikar-Zuck SM, Allen JR, et al (Cincinnati Children's Hosp Med Ctr, OH)

JAMA 310:2622-2630, 2013

Importance.—Early, safe, effective, and durable evidence-based interventions for children and adolescents with chronic migraine do not exist.

Objective.—To determine the benefits of cognitive behavioral therapy (CBT) when combined with amitriptyline vs headache education plus amitriptyline.

Design, Setting, and Participants.—A randomized clinical trial of 135 youth (79% female) aged 10 to 17 years diagnosed with chronic migraine (≥15 days with headache/month) and a Pediatric Migraine Disability Assessment Score (PedMIDAS) greater than 20 points were assigned to the CBT plus amitriptyline group (n = 64) or the headache education plus amitriptyline group (n = 71). The study was conducted in the Headache Center at Cincinnati Children's Hospital between October 2006 and September 2012; 129 completed 20-week follow-up and 124 completed 12-month follow-up.

Interventions.—Ten CBT vs 10 headache education sessions involving equivalent time and therapist attention. Each group received 1 mg/kg/d of amitriptyline and a 20-week end point visit. In addition, follow-up visits were conducted at 3, 6, 9, and 12 months.

Main Outcomes and Measures.—The primary end point was days with headache and the secondary end point was PedMIDAS (disability score range: 0-240 points; 0-10 for little to none, 11-30 for mild, 31-50 for moderate, >50 for severe); both end points were determined at 20 weeks. Durability was examined over the 12-month follow-up period. Clinical significance was measured by a 50% or greater reduction in days with headache and a disability score in the mild to none range (<20 points).

Results.—At baseline, there were a mean (SD) of 21 (5) days with headache per 28 days and the mean (SD) PedMIDAS was 68 (32) points. At the 20-week end point, days with headache were reduced by 11.5 for the CBT plus amitriptyline group vs 6.8 for the headache education plus amitriptyline group (difference, 4.7 [95% CI, 1.7-7.7] days; $P = .002$). The PedMIDAS decreased by 52.7 points for the CBT group vs 38.6 points for the headache education group (difference, 14.1 [95% CI, 3.3-24.9] points; $P = .01$). In the CBT group, 66% had a 50% or greater reduction in headache days vs 36% in the headache education group (odds ratio, 3.5 [95% CI, 1.7-7.2]; $P < .001$). At 12-month follow-up, 86% of the CBT group had a 50% or greater reduction in headache days vs 69% of the headache education group; 88% of the CBT group had a PedMIDAS of less than 20 points vs 76% of the headache education group. Measured treatment credibility and integrity was high for both groups.

Conclusions and Relevance.—Among young persons with chronic migraine, the use of CBT plus amitriptyline resulted in greater reductions in days with headache and migraine-related disability compared with use of headache education plus amitriptyline. These findings support the efficacy of CBT in the treatment of chronic migraine in children and adolescents.

Trial Registration.—clinicaltrials.gov Identifier: NCT00389038.

▶ Headaches have a significant impact on children. Structured interviews and reviews of academic records have shown that increased severity of headache is associated with poor quality of life and decreased academic performance within the pediatric population.[1] Migraine prevalence in this age group is approximately 8%, and surveys have estimated that chronic migraine has a prevalence of up to 1.75% of the adolescent population within the United States.[2,3] Given the high prevalence of migraine and the negative impact of headache on academic and social development, it is important to identify effective treatments for pediatric headache.

Unfortunately, clinical trials in pediatric headache are fewer in number compared with the adult population, and there is currently no US Food and Drug Administration—approved preventative medication for migraine in the pediatric population. Practitioners need effective, pharmacologic, and nonpharmacologic treatment for the pediatric population.

The clinical trial by Powers et al shows that cognitive behavioral therapy (CBT) is an effective treatment for adolescent patients diagnosed with chronic migraine using International Classification of Headache Disorders—II criteria.[4] The investigators randomized patients into an experimental group of CBT plus amitriptyline and a control group that received educational sessions on headache topics plus amitriptyline therapy. CBT was modified to include a biofeedback component that included thermal and electromyographic monitoring of the relaxation response.

Results from the study showed statistically significant benefit in the CBT group compared with the headache education group in predefined outcome measures. The number of days with headache was reduced by 11.5 days in the CBT plus amitriptyline group versus 6.8 days in the headache education plus amitriptyline group ($P = .002$). Disability measured by Pediatric Migraine Disability Assessment Score was also reduced by 52.7 points in the CBT plus amitriptyline group versus 38.6 in the control group at the 20-week end point ($P = .01$; Table 3 in the original article).

All patients received amitriptyline, which is not FDA-approved for migraine. Behavioral therapies are particularly relevant to treatment of the pediatric population given desires to avoid or supplement pharmacotherapy and the negative impact of that inadequately treated headache has on pediatric patients. It is important that effective nonpharmacologic treatments are identified as such because patient access to such therapies is often limited by lack of insurance coverage and associated financial burden. Well-designed clinical trials showing benefit of a given therapy are crucial to justify increased utilization and improve patient access.

This trial shows strong evidence of efficacy of CBT (modified to include a biofeedback) in combination with amitriptyline in the adolescent population with chronic migraine and thus provides physicians an important tool to advocate for inclusion of nonpharmacologic interventions in their patients' treatment plans. We await the comparison of drug to nondrug treatment. Could biofeedback, which is effective in headache treatment, be as good as CBT modified to include biofeedback?

S. D. Silberstein, MD

J. L. Pomeroy, MD, MPH

References

1. Rocha-Filho PAS, Santos PV. Headaches, quality of life, and academic performance in schoolchildren and adolescents. *Headache: The Journal of Head and Face Pain.* 2014;54:1194-1202.

2. Abu-Arafeh I, Razak S, Sivaraman B, Graham C. Prevalence of headache and migraine in children and adolescents: a systematic review of population-based studies. *Developmental Medicine & Child Neurology.* 2010;52:1088-1097.

3. Lipton RB, Manack A, Ricci JA, Chee E, Turkel CC, Winner P. Prevalence and burden of chronic migraine in adolescents: results of the Chronic Daily Headache in Adolescents Study (C-dAS). *Headache: The Journal of Head and Face Pain.* 2011; 51:693-706.

4. Headache Classification Subcommittee of the International Headache Society. The International Classification of Headache Disorders: 2nd edition. *Cephalalgia.* 2004;24 (suppl 1):9-160.

Health Care Provider-Delivered Adherence Promotion Interventions: A Meta-Analysis

Wu YP, Pai ALH (Univ of Utah, Salt Lake City; Cincinnati Children's Hosp Med Ctr, OH)
Pediatrics 133:e1698-e1707, 2014

Background and Objective.—Improving medical regimen adherence is essential for maximizing the therapeutic potential of treatments for pediatric chronic illness. Health care providers are uniquely positioned to deliver adherence promotion interventions. However, no studies have summarized the effectiveness of health care provider-delivered adherence interventions. The objective of this study was to describe the effectiveness of health care provider-delivered adherence promotion interventions in improving adherence among children who have chronic illness. Data sources include PubMed, PsycINFO, CINAHL, and Scopus. Studies were included if they were randomized-controlled trials of pediatric interventions aiming to increase adherence to the primary regimen for a chronic illness and at least 1 health care provider delivered the intervention.

Results.—A total of 35 randomized-controlled studies including 4616 children were included. Greater improvements in adherence were observed immediately after health care provider-delivered interventions (d = 0.49; 95% confidence interval, 0.32 to 0.66) than at longer-term follow-up (d = 0.32; 95% confidence interval, 0.10 to 0.54). Treatment effect sizes differed across the adherence behaviors measured. There was significant heterogeneity in treatment effects; however, no moderators of treatment effectiveness were identified. This meta-analysis focused on the published literature. In addition, the majority of studies involved children who had asthma and younger children.

Conclusions.—Health care provider-delivered interventions for children who have chronic illness can be effective in improving adherence. Gains in adherence are highest immediately after intervention. Future interventions and studies should include multiple methods of assessing adherence, include active comparators, and address long-term maintenance of adherence gains.

▶ Chronic diseases require lifetime management with a therapeutic regimen to keep the disease under control. Therapeutic advances allow individuals, especially children, to live full and active lives. However, one of the biggest challenges of getting proven, efficacious therapies to improve health status is by supporting individual's efforts with adherence. Adherence to therapeutic regimens for chronic disease management is influenced by a host of factors and is widely studied. Support systems such as those available through family, social networks, and health care providers can be instrumental in facilitating adherence to therapeutic regimens over the long-term. For children and adolescents, support systems are especially important in promoting adherence given cognitive and developmental considerations to facilitate independent disease management.

Health care providers play a unique role, especially in the patient-centered medical home model, in championing adherence efforts for families. This is in part because of the long-term relationship and trust that they are able to establish with families, which is especially enhanced when effective communication and collaboration is evident. Findings from the synthesis of evidence by Wu and colleagues provide important information that validate the unique conditions under which adherence can best be facilitated for families of children with chronic illness and provides an agenda for future research. Family-centered approaches were increasingly emphasized in existing interventions. Given that 1 in 2 adults now manages chronic disease, it is likely that managing multiple disease management regimens are evident within families, and multiple family members benefit from interventions focused on adherence.

One of the most striking findings from this evidence review was the limited effect of adherence promotion for factors unrelated to medication regimens such as diet and physical activity. Although medicines are central for the disease control of major childhood chronic conditions such as asthma and diabetes, diet and physical activity play an instrumental role for the long-term health of a developing child.

The analysis does not provide specific details of interventions but highlights general approaches that are successful in promoting adherence. In terms of encouraging adherence in a busy office setting, a team approach may be more efficient. Wu and colleagues highlight the need for interventions that address comprehensive approaches to adherence for disease management by potentially utilizing ancillary care providers to facilitate adherence efforts beyond medicines. Content should also include behavioral strategies that promote patient skills (eg, tips to remember when to take medicines, how to recognize symptoms). In addition, Wu and colleagues found that treatment effects are strongest immediately after intervention. As a result, the review recognizes the importance of follow-up education.

For health systems and behavioral interventionists, this meta-analysis provides a nice calibration for what is working when it comes to health care provider interventions that promote adherence, and why investment in this area is worthwhile. In addition, this analysis highlights where further work in the field is needed. Given the rapidly evolving health care landscape, the increasing demands on primary care, and a greater push toward care coordination, new approaches are needed in thinking about the health care system role in promoting adherence for children with chronic care needs. The increasing use of health information technology (IT) to increase and triangulate communication and collaboration between health care providers, families, and the developing child living with a chronic condition shows promise in this area. Health IT has significant potential for tailored approaches, efficiencies in adherence promotion, and increasing frequency of intervention over the long-term at low-cost. Future interventions aimed at promoting adherence with chronic disease treatment regimens may consider greater efforts that leverage the common uses of health IT as an intervention medium.

M. R. Patel, PhD, MPH

M. D. Cabana, MD, MPH

14 Newborn

Impact of ART on pregnancies in California: an analysis of maternity outcomes and insights into the added burden of neonatal intensive care
Merritt TA, Goldstein M, Philips R, et al (Loma Linda Univ School of Medicine, CA; et al)
J Perinatol 34:345-350, 2014

Objective.—We reviewed the occurrence of prematurity, low birth weight, multiple gestations, frequency of stillbirths and maternity care-associated variables including hospital stay and hospital charges of women conceiving using assisted reproductive technology (ART) or artificial insemination (AI) compared with women with a history of infertility who conceived naturally, and all other naturally conceived pregnancies in California at non-federal hospitals between 2009 and 2011. At a single center, infants born after ART/AI were compared with infants provided care in the normal nursery.

Study Design.—Publically available inpatient data sets from the California Office of Statewide Health Planning and Development for years 2009–2011 using data from all California non-federal hospitals were used to determine the impact of ART on a variety of pregnancy-related outcomes and infant characteristics. Infant data from a single center was used to determine hospital charges for infants delivered over an 18-month period to compare the hospital and physician charges indexed to similar charges for infants admitted to the 'normal' newborn nursery.

Result.—Among ART/AI pregnancies, there was a 4–5-fold increase in stillbirths, compared with a 2–3-fold increase among women with infertility compared with other naturally conceiving women. ART/AI pregnancies underwent more cesarean sections (fourfold), and a near fourfold increase in the rate of preterm deliveries. Multiple gestations were increased 24–27-fold compared with naturally conceived pregnancies. Maternal hospital stay and hospital charges were increased among those undergoing ART/AI. Infant charges were increased multi-fold for singletons, twins and triplets delivered after ART/AI compared with naturally conceived infants.

Conclusion.—Multiple births, preterm births and a higher overall rate of fetal anomalies were found in California after ART/AI for 2009–2011. Cesarean section rates, longer length of maternal stay and hospital charges among women receiving ART/AI could be lowered if emphasis on elective single embryo transfers was a higher priority among providers. Charges for the care of infants delivered after ART/AI are substantially higher than among naturally conceived infants born late preterm or at term. Families seeking ART/AI need to be informed of the impact of these adverse pregnancy outcomes, including neonatal outcomes and charges for medical care for their infant(s), when considering ART/AI.

▶ Since its inception in 1978, approximately 5 million infants worldwide have been born after in vitro fertilization (IVF). Although assisted reproductive techniques (ART) are a successful treatment for infertility with pregnancy rates generally in the 40% per cycle range, they have also led to an increase in twins and higher order multiple gestations. These multiple gestations, in turn, are associated with a host of pregnancy complications including preterm birth, preeclampsia, gestational diabetes, as well as the neonatal consequences of these complications.

To provide an updated examination of how ART is affecting birth outcomes, Merritt et al conducted a study of the use of ART in California. Using a combination of public and private data from the state and their local institution, they were able to cleverly examine the use and the outcomes related to ART. In California in 2009, ART accounted for 5710 deliveries, of which 30.1% were multiple gestations, and made up 1.4% of the births that year. This number is similar to the national estimate of 1.4%.

Not surprisingly to anyone practicing obstetrics, ART was associated with increased length of stay, as well as greater rates of preterm labor, preterm birth, stillbirths, and fetal anomalies than natural conception, much of this was due to the higher rates of multiple gestations (Figs 1-4). These outcomes, in turn, led to longer lengths of stay for both mothers and babies and increased median charges. The findings in these analyses were not particularly surprising; however, there is a need for updated information, and, as ART use has risen, it appears that the impact on perinatal morbidity and mortality continues to be negative. Because California accounts for 12.8% of the nation's births and

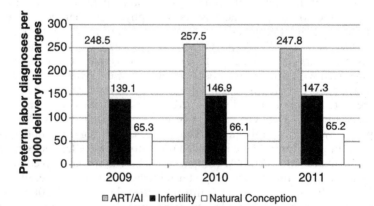

FIGURE 1.—Preterm labor diagnoses among ART/AI, infertility and natural conception delivery discharges, California, 2009—2011. Source: California Office of Statewide Health Planning and Development, Patient Discharge Data, Public Files, 2009—2011. (Reprinted from Merritt TA, Goldstein M, Philips R, et al. Impact of ART on pregnancies in California: an analysis of maternity outcomes and insights into the added burden of neonatal intensive care. *J Perinatol.* 2014;34:345-350, with permission from Nature America, Inc.)

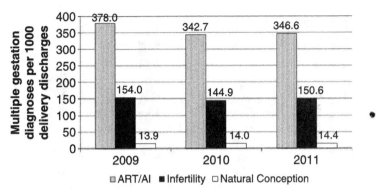

FIGURE 2.—Multiple gestation diagnoses among ART/AI, infertility and natural conception delivery discharges, California, 2009–2011. Source: California Office of Statewide Health Planning and Development, Patient Discharge Data, Public Files, 2009–2011. (Reprinted from Merritt TA, Goldstein M, Philips R, et al. Impact of ART on pregnancies in California: an analysis of maternity outcomes and insights into the added burden of neonatal intensive care. *J Perinatol.* 2014;34:345-350, with permission from Nature America, Inc.)

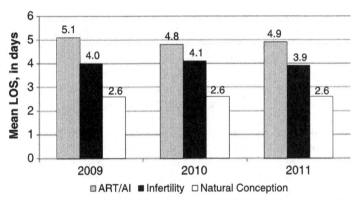

FIGURE 3.—Mean length of stay (LOS) in days among ART/AI, infertility and natural conception delivery discharges, California, 2009–2011. Source: California Office of Statewide Health Planning and Development, Patient Discharge Data, Public Files, 2009–2011. (Reprinted from Merritt TA, Goldstein M, Philips R, et al. Impact of ART on pregnancies in California: an analysis of maternity outcomes and insights into the added burden of neonatal intensive care. *J Perinatol.* 2014;34:345-350, with permission from Nature America, Inc.)

has a particularly diverse population, and given the similar overall rates of ART, the study may be reflective of the nation as a whole. In the end, the authors conclude that the negative impact of ART may be mitigated by increased use of single embryo transfer (SET). In practice, SET involves creating multiple embryos but only putting back 1 in the first IVF cycle (the fresh cycle) and freezing the rest to be used in subsequent IVF cycles (frozen cycles).

I agree with the authors' point on this issue of SET. First, although there may be specific causal impacts on embryonic and fetal development from ART, most studies that find an association between ART and neonatal or childhood outcomes, the effect either disappears or is greatly reduced when controlling for

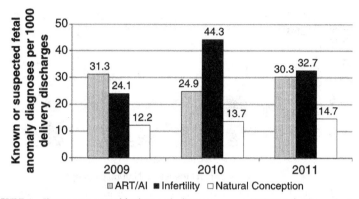

FIGURE 4.—Known or suspected fetal anomaly diagnoses among ART/AI, infertility and natural conception delivery discharges, California, 2009–2011. Source: California Office of Statewide Health Planning and Development, Patient Discharge Data, Public Files, 2009–2011. (Reprinted from Merritt TA, Goldstein M, Philips R, et al. Impact of ART on pregnancies in California: an analysis of maternity outcomes and insights into the added burden of neonatal intensive care. *J Perinatol*. 2014;34:345-350, with permission from Nature America, Inc.)

multiple gestations and the associated preterm births. For example, in a recent article that examined the association between IVF and autism or mental retardation, it was particularly interesting that when the modest increase in mental retardation that was seen in unadjusted analyses was examined in just the preterm, term, or singleton gestations, any difference that existed disappeared. Thus, it does appear from these and many other studies, that the majority of the negative impact from ART results from the approximately 30% multiple gestation rate.

Merritt et al's focus on pushing for specific policies toward SET is refreshing. One feature of most IVF that has an impact on the possibility of routine SET is that the majority of patients pay out of pocket for the ART; however, they have insurance for the costs of the birth. Because the costs per cycle are commonly between $10 000 to $20 000, minimizing the number of cycles has a strong economic incentive for the payors, who are the patients in this case. In a study that examined the payor perspective for the costs of the combination of infertility care plus the pregnancy care, when examined from the insurance perspective, the study indicated that overall costs would be lower from SET, because fewer patients would deliver preterm. However, from the patient perspective, who only bear the costs of IVF, 2 or more embryos was generally cheaper because it would minimize the number of cycles needed to achieve pregnancy. Overall, from a societal perspective, SET was cost-beneficial because the costs of providing ART pale in comparison to the costs of care for multiple gestation pregnancies.

These economic trade-offs underscore the primary problem with IVF. In addition to the economic impact, many couples undergoing IVF believe that achieving twins is not just as good, but even better than singletons. In light of these issues, a study of SET versus double embryo transfer (DET) would be enlightening. Luckily, one has been recently completed. The BEST trial randomized women to receiving either standard DET versus SET with embryos that had undergone genetic testing for aneuploidy. The thinking was that such tested embryos would lead to higher pregnancy rates, perhaps overcoming the pregnancy benefit of transferring 2 embryos. When a single SET cycle was compared with a single DET cycle, this did not bear out. However, a follow-up study compared a single fresh SET cycle plus a single frozen cycle versus DET. In this study, the differences were quite interesting. Although there was no difference in eventual pregnancy and delivery rates, the DET approach lead to higher rates of twinning, preterm birth, neonatal intensive care unit admissions, and low birth weight (as seen in the Merritt study). From a societal perspective, the genetically tested SET approach is superior to DET. However, from a patient perspective, it is still likely to cheaper in the short run to go with DET.

Thus, I believe that it is time for IVF care to be included in all routine insurance products. Such IVF care may be limited to SET or even the genetically tested SET. In doing so, patients would lose the economic incentive toward DET, or more embryos being transferred, and both long-term outcomes would be improved as well as, potentially, the long-term costs. Many European countries have adopted routine SET as the standard, which has led to a reduction in multiple gestations. Such a transition in the United States would likely lead to a far lower rate of multiple gestations and their accompanying neonatal morbidity and mortality. However, to accomplish this will require the cooperation of payors, regulators, and clinicians.

A. B. Caughey, MD, PhD

Obstetric and Neonatal Care Practices for Infants 501 to 1500 g From 2000 to 2009
Soll RF, Edwards EM, Badger GJ, et al (Univ of Vermont, Burlington; Vermont Oxford Network, Burlington)
Pediatrics 132:222-228, 2013

Objective.—To identify changes in clinical practices for infants with birth weights of 501 to 1500 g born from 2000 to 2009.

Methods.—We used prospectively collected registry data for 355 806 infants born from 2000 to 2009 and cared for at 669 North American hospitals in the Vermont Oxford Network. Main outcome measures included obstetric and neonatal practices, including cesarean delivery, antenatal steroids, delivery room interventions, respiratory practices, neuroimaging, retinal exams, and feeding at discharge.

Results.—Significant changes in many obstetric, delivery room, and neonatal practices occurred from 2000 to 2009. Use of surfactant treatment in the delivery room increased overall (adjusted difference [AD] 17.0%; 95% confidence interval [CI] 16.4% to 17.6%), as did less-invasive methods of respiratory support, such as nasal continuous positive airway pressure (AD 9.9%; 95% CI 9.1% to 10.6%). Use of any ventilation (AD −7.5%; 95% CI −8.0% to −6.9%) and steroids for chronic lung disease (AD −15.3%;

95% CI −15.8% to −14.8%) decreased significantly overall. Most of the changes in respiratory care were observed within each of 4 birth weight strata (501–750 g, 751–1000 g, 1001–1250 g, 1251–1500 g).

Conclusions.—Many obstetric and neonatal care practices used in the management of infants 501 to 1500 g changed between 2000 and 2009. In particular, less-invasive approaches to respiratory support increased.

▶ What a long way neonatology has come since 1963, the year Patrick Bouvier Kennedy, a 36-week preemie, born to John and Jacqueline Kennedy, died at 3 days of age from respiratory distress syndrome (RDS).[1] In that era, virtually no babies born at less than 28 weeks' gestation survived. Fast-forward to 2013, the year this article was published. Since that pivotal event in neonatology's history, the gestational age at which babies can survive (with intensive care) dropped by 1 week per decade. So, from 28 weeks in 1963, that "limit of viability" has become 23 weeks, and now, the majority of infants born at 28 weeks' gestation survive. Changes in obstetric and neonatal care practices, most of which are evidence-based, have helped to make this happen.

Soll et al report on changes in neonatal and obstetrical care practices over the past decade. Data were gleaned from their large Vermont-Oxford Network (VON), which includes 355 000 babies cared for at 669 neonatal intensive care units (NICUs) across the United States. The article provides important validation of our practice improvement efforts, demonstrating that when we strive to implement evidence-based practices, we can succeed—although it takes time. Of course, the authors can't prove that increased use of antenatal steroids and less invasive neonatal respiratory support led directly to improved survival and short-term outcomes for these babies, but it's certainly likely. That's what the evidence shows and what we hope for.

It's interesting to note that Soll et al chose to focus on care practices designed to prevent or ameliorate RDS, the very disease that led to Patrick Bouvier Kennedy's death. We've been discussing some of these practice changes for years, but the article nicely demonstrates that we neonatologists really are using fewer steroids for chronic lung disease as well as more noninvasive respiratory support (even for the tiniest babies). Furthermore, the obstetricians are doing more caesarean sections and administering antenatal steroids to just about anyone anticipating preterm birth. These neonatal and perinatal practice changes have undoubtedly led to significant improvements in both mortality and morbidity from RDS.

But what about the brain? The only brain-related care practice examined by Soll et al was the percentage of babies receiving neuroimaging—and that's the only care practice that did not change. The article ends with a sobering conclusion: "How these changes in practice affected patient outcomes is uncertain." Indeed, the VON previously reported morbidity and mortality of the same very low birth weight (VLBW) babies, noting that in 2009, 49% of all VLBW babies and 89% of those with birth weight 501 to 750 grams either died or survived with major neonatal morbidity. We must do better!

Let's hope that the next decade's report from VON includes changes in neuroprotective, neurodevelopmental care practices—both perinatal and neonatal. Numerous clinical trials are ongoing in this domain. Once we have evidence to support their efficacy, we should swiftly implement these practices into our NICUs and perinatal services. Although we continue to strive for more survivors, we must redouble our efforts to ensure that more of those survivors grow up without major neurodevelopmental handicaps.

And while we're working hard to institute practice changes that improve the outcomes of preterm pregnancy, let's not forget our greatest challenge: to figure out how to prevent preterm birth. Wouldn't it be nice if the 2010—2019 VON report contained far fewer premature babies, despite adding more NICUs to the registry? And if the 2020—2029 report didn't exist at all because prematurity just wasn't a significant problem anymore?

C. A. Gleason, MD

Reference

1. Altman L. "A Kennedy Baby's Life and Death." *New York Times.* 2013.

Oral Paracetamol versus Oral Ibuprofen in the Management of Patent Ductus Arteriosus in Preterm Infants: A Randomized Controlled Trial
Oncel MY, Yurttutan S, Erdeve O, et al (Zekai Tahir Burak Maternity Teaching Hosp, Ankara, Turkey; Ankara Univ School of Medicine, Turkey; et al)
J Pediatr 164:510-514, 2014

Objective.—To compare the efficacy and safety of oral paracetamol and oral ibuprofen for the pharmacological closure of patent ductus arteriosus (PDA) in preterm infants.

Study Design.—This prospective, randomized, controlled study enrolled 90 preterm infants with gestational age ≤30 weeks, birthweight ≤1250 g, and postnatal age 48 to 96 hours who had echocardiographically confirmed significant PDA. Each enrolled patient received either oral paracetamol (15 mg/kg every 6 hours for 3 days) or oral ibuprofen (initial dose of 10 mg/kg, followed by 5 mg/kg at 24 and 48 hours).

Results.—Spontaneous closure rate for the entire study group was 54%. After the first course of treatment, the PDA closed in 31 (77.5%) of the patients assigned to the oral ibuprofen group vs 29 (72.5%) of those enrolled in the oral paracetamol group ($P = .6$). The reopening rate was higher in the paracetamol group than in the ibuprofen group, but the reopening rates were not statistically different (24.1% [7 of 29] vs 16.1% [5 of 31]; $P = .43$). The cumulative closure rates after the second course of drugs were high in both groups. Only 2 patient (2.5%) in the paracetamol group and 3 patients (5%) in the ibuprofen group required surgical ligation.

Conclusion.—This randomized, controlled clinical study compared oral paracetamol with ibuprofen in preterm infants and demonstrated that paracetamol may be a medical alternative in the management of PDA.

▶ Over the past decade, the neonatal literature has undergone such dynamic swings vis-à-vis the clinical approach to patent ductus arteriosus (PDA) therapeutics that it is often difficult to define what is best for our patients with a patent ductus. The pendulum has swung from aggressive treatment of nearly all PDAs in preterm neonates to a "kinder, gentler" approach, encouraging a permissive tolerance of ductal shunting and withholding therapy in all except the most hemodynamically significant cases. This latter approach has been advocated in recent years based on the lack of convincing evidence supporting the once common practice of early aggressive pharmacologic closure coupled with the potential side effects of cyclooxygenase (COX) inhibitors, commonly used for therapeutic closure. Although mostly reversible, these side effects can occasionally be clinically challenging and, in some cases, even life-threatening.

However, lack of evidence is not the same as evidence of a lack of effect. Data are again beginning to emerge suggesting possible increased long-term morbidities associated with or exacerbated by not treating a PDA. As such, we are beginning to wonder whether permissive tolerance may have actually evolved into benign neglect. Is it possible that closing the patent ductus is still hemodynamically beneficial for many babies and that an alternative treatment with fewer potential side effects might be helpful in resolving some of these therapeutic dilemmas?

It is in this context that we must evaluate recent studies of paracetamol, the latest addition to the therapeutic arsenal against the persistently patent ductus arteriosus. We published the first series of case reports[1] documenting the efficacy of paracetamol in mediating ductal closure in five premature neonates in 2011. Since 2011, 14 additional observational series have been published, collectively treating a total of 115 infants who either failed standard therapy or who had contraindications to therapy with a COX inhibitor. Overall, these studies show a ductal closure rate above 76%, a degree of therapeutic efficacy similar to that achieved by standard therapy with COX inhibitors.

Although the multitude of case reports has been encouraging, the scientific community was clearly in need of prospective, randomized controlled trials. This study by Oncel et al comparing the efficacy of oral paracetamol with that of oral ibuprofen in mediating ductal closure, offers one of the first such studies, a critically important contribution to the PDA literature. The study, which included 80 preterm neonates less than 30 weeks' gestational age, was powered to detect a 25% difference in ductal closure rate between the 2 drugs, which they did not find. As a result, they concluded that paracetamol, used as a first-line drug, has an efficacy similar to that of ibuprofen in mediating ductal closure. It might be argued that they should have designed and powered the study as a noninferiority trial, thus requiring a substantially greater sample size. However, if we accept that there are significant differences in toxicity, it could reasonably be argued that a less toxic drug, such as paracetamol, which is 80% as effective as ibuprofen, still deserves a respectable place in our therapeutic arsenal.

Are we justified, however, in claiming that the toxicity of paracetamol in neo-nates is low? Available observational data seem to support this. First of all, none of the side effects attributed to the COX inhibitors, including altered platelet function, decreased cerebral, mesenteric, and renal blood flow and spontaneous gastrointestinal perforation, are seen with paracetamol. What may be of theoretical concern with paracetamol is its potential for hepatotoxicity. Of all the patients described to date in the various paracetamol PDA case reports, there were only 3 infants with transiently elevated liver transaminases. Reported clinical experiences of paracetamol overdosages in infants not related to PDA studies also reinforce the concept of lower toxicity in neonates. Of 10 reported cases of neonates exposed to potentially toxic amounts of paracetamol that our search of the literature revealed, long-term outcomes were universally favorable despite transient elevations in liver enzymes reported in half of the cases. To the best of our knowledge, there are no cases in the literature describing permanent liver damage secondary to paracetamol poisoning in a newborn resulting from direct administration of the drug. These assumptions make sense on a theoretical level as well. Hepatotoxicity results from accumulation of a toxic metabolite of paracetamol, N-acetyl-p-benzoquinone imine [NAPQI]. NAPQI production is mediated by the mixed-function cytochrome P-450 oxidase CYP2E1, and, in turn, it can be detoxified by glutathione and eliminated in urine or bile. However, when NAPQI accumulates either as a result of excessive paracetamol intake or of insufficient glutathione reserves, liver damage ensues. Neonates are relatively protected by both low levels of CYP2E1 enzyme activity, thereby slowing oxidative metabolism of paracetamol and reducing production of toxic metabolites[2] and by increased glutathione synthesis, rendering detoxification of the NAPQI formed more efficient.

The well-designed study by Oncel et al raises 2 additional issues that, although not significant, we believe are noteworthy. First, the study showed a trend toward improved ductal closure with paracetamol (77% vs 56%) in the lower gestational age subgroups. However, as there were only 16 infants in the subgroup of ibuprofen infants aged less than 26 weeks and 13 in the comparable paracetamol group; because a sample size of 80 would have been needed to reach significance of $P < .05$ given this degree of difference in response rate, it is not surprising that this difference was not significant. Whether this trend will be confirmed by future studies and, if so, whether it reflects a greater effect of paracetamol in the less mature infants or a decreased sensitivity toward ibuprofen in these infants remain subjects for further study.

Second, there was a trend toward a higher incidence of retinopathy of prematurity (ROP) in the ibuprofen-treated infants. Although the literature on COX inhibitors and ROP appears on the surface to be contradictory, we have postulated[3] reinterpreting these data within the context of the biphasic paradigm of ROP pathophysiology. As in this study, drugs with a vasoconstrictive effect on the retinal vasculature may potentially exacerbate ROP when given during the initial hyperoxic phase of the process, although they may have an opposite effect if given later. Thus, the trend toward increased ROP may reflect the timing of the ibuprofen exposure together with its retinal vasoconstrictive effect. There is no known effect of paracetamol on the retinal vasculature.

In summary, the prospective randomized trial by Oncel et al is an important first step in showing paracetamol and ibuprofen to be of similar overall efficacy in mediating ductal closure. We believe that the existing data support the use of paracetamol as a first-line therapeutic option in the pharmacologic approach to the hemodynamically significant patent ductus arteriosus in the premature neonate. Furthermore, judging from the rapidly growing number of publications reporting on the use of paracetamol for ductal closure, the scientific community at large seems to agree. We attribute the burgeoning popularity of paracetamol to several factors. As one of most commonly used over-the-counter drugs worldwide, it offers familiarity, availability, and financial feasibility. Furthermore, it presents certain practical as well as theoretical advantages over both ibuprofen and indomethacin, including the potential to treat those with contraindications to the use of COX inhibitors and the absence of any known peripheral vasoconstrictive effects.

Nevertheless, many issues remain unresolved. Further studies are clearly needed to look at optimal paracetamol dosing levels for PDA closure, to prove noninferiority versus COX inhibitors, and to look at possible long-term safety effects of early paracetamol exposure. However, these basic questions notwithstanding, we believe that the concerns must be evaluated in relation to the fact that COX inhibitors are associated with safety concerns of their own, which are no less troubling than the hypothetical concerns raised regarding paracetamol administration.

A. Bin-Nun, MD

C. Hammerman, MD

References

1. Hammerman C, Bin-Nun A, Markovitch E, Schimmel MS. Ductal Closure With Paracetamol: A Surprising New Approach to Patent Ductus Arteriosus Treatment. *Pediatrics*. 2011;128:e1-e4.
2. Oncel MY, Yurttutan S, Erdeve O, et al. Oral Paracetamol versus Oral Ibuprofen in the Management of Patent Ductus Arteriosus in Preterm Infants: A Randomized Controlled Trial. *J Pediatr*. 2014.
3. Ogilvie J, Rieder MJ, Lim R. Acetaminophen Overdose in Children. *CMAJ*. 2012; 184:1492-1496.

Effect of Fluconazole Prophylaxis on Candidiasis and Mortality in Premature Infants: A Randomized Clinical Trial
Benjamin DK Jr, for the Fluconazole Prophylaxis Study Team (Duke Clinical Res Inst, Durham, NC; et al)
JAMA 311:1742-1749, 2014

Importance.—Invasive candidiasis in premature infants causes death and neurodevelopmental impairment. Fluconazole prophylaxis reduces candidiasis, but its effect on mortality and the safety of fluconazole are unknown.

Objective.—To evaluate the efficacy and safety of fluconazole in preventing death or invasive candidiasis in extremely low-birth-weight infants.

Design, Setting, and Patients.—This study was a randomized, blinded, placebo-controlled trial of fluconazole in premature infants. Infants weighing less than 750 g at birth (N = 361) from 32 neonatal intensive care units (NICUs) in the United States were randomly assigned to receive either fluconazole or placebo twice weekly for 42 days. Surviving infants were evaluated at 18 to 22 months corrected age for neurodevelopmental outcomes. The study was conducted between November 2008 and February 2013.

Interventions.—Fluconazole (6 mg/kg of body weight) or placebo.

Main Outcomes and Measures.—The primary end point was a composite of death or definite or probable invasive candidiasis prior to study day 49 (1 week after completion of study drug). Secondary and safety outcomes included invasive candidiasis, liver function, bacterial infection, length of stay, intracranial hemorrhage, periventricular leukomalacia, chronic lung disease, patent ductus arteriosus requiring surgery, retinopathy of prematurity requiring surgery, necrotizing enterocolitis, spontaneous intestinal perforation, and neurodevelopmental outcomes—defined as a Bayley-III cognition composite score of less than 70, blindness, deafness, or cerebral palsy at 18 to 22 months corrected age.

Results.—Among infants receiving fluconazole, the composite primary end point of death or invasive candidiasis was 16% (95% CI, 11%-22%) vs 21% in the placebo group (95% CI, 15%-28%; odds ratio, 0.73 [95% CI, 0.43-1.23]; *P* =.24; treatment difference, −5% [95% CI, −13% to 3%]). Invasive candidiasis occurred less frequently in the fluconazole group (3% [95% CI, 1%-6%]) vs the placebo group (9% [95% CI, 5%-14%]; *P* =.02; treatment difference, −6% [95% CI, −11% to −1%]). The cumulative incidences of other secondary outcomes were not statistically different between groups. Neurodevelopmental impairment did not differ between the groups (fluconazole, 31% [95% CI, 21%-41%] vs placebo, 27% [95% CI, 18%-37%]; *P* =.60; treatment difference, 4% [95% CI, −10% to 17%]).

Conclusions and Relevance.—Among infants with a birth weight of less than 750 g, 42 days of fluconazole prophylaxis compared with placebo did not result in a lower incidence of the composite of death or invasive candidiasis. These findings do not support the universal use of prophylactic fluconazole in extremely low-birth-weight infants.

Trial Registration.—clinicaltrials.gov Identifier: NCT00734539.

▶ The history of neonatology prominently features disastrous consequences of prophylactic antibiotic therapy. These consequences most notably include kernicterus and death with the use of prophylactic sulfonamides, and gray baby syndrome and death with the use of chloramphenicol.[1,2] Fortunately, such is not the case with prophylactic fluconazole to prevent invasive fungal infections.

Fungi represent the third-leading cause of late-onset sepsis in very low-birth-weight infants (VLBWI) and have a high rate of infection-associated mortality. Randomized, single and multiple-center, placebo-controlled trials found intravenous fluconazole prophylaxis to be effective in decreasing fungal colonization and sepsis for at-risk preterm infants <1500 g birth weight. In these trials, fluconazole prophylaxis demonstrated efficacy without side effects or emergence of resistance.[3,4]

Benjamin et al, in the trial abstracted here, wished to determine whether prophylactic fluconazole for 42 days in infants with a birth weight < 750 grams would not only reduce invasive fungal disease but also reduce the combined outcome of infection and death. In a well-designed and executed trial, despite no evidence of harm, they documented reduced rates of invasive *Candida* infection, but no reduction in the composite of death or invasive candidiasis. They were therefore forced to reluctantly conclude that the findings do not support the universal use of prophylactic fluconazole in extremely low-birth-weight infants. In analyzing the study, they found some unanticipated differences between the treatment and control groups. More babies in the control group were the beneficiaries of antenatal corticosteroids and were delivered by Caesarean section. Both these events would increase survival and influence one of the primary outcome variables. Indeed, mortality overall was lower than anticipated, a good outcome. Infection rates were also lower, a reflection of increased attention to hand hygiene and improved efforts to prevent central line blood stream infections.

Of interest is the report from Aliaga et al,[5] who examined data from 709 325 infants at 322 neonatal intensive care units (NICUs) managed by the Pediatrix Medical Group from 1997 to 2010. Over the study period, the annual incidence of invasive candidiasis decreased from 3.6 episodes per 1000 patients to 1.4 episodes per 1000 patients among all infants, from 24.2 to 11.6 episodes per 1000 patients among infants with a birth weight of 750 to 999 g, and from 82.7 to 23.8 episodes per 1000 patients among infants with a birth weight < 750 g. Fluconazole prophylaxis use increased, and the use of broad-spectrum antibacterial antibiotics decreased among all infants during this time period, which may have contributed to these findings.

A report from Adams-Chapman[6] on the follow-up of the Eunice Kennedy Shriver National Institute of Child Health and Development Neonatal Network *Candida* study confirmed that infants with invasive *Candida* infection and/or meningitis had higher rates of neurodevelopmental impairment than infants with non-*Candida* sepsis and infants without infection.

Candida remains a significant contributor to mortality and morbidity in extremely low-birth-weight infants. Unfortunately, despite some early promise, fluconazole prophylaxis is not the answer to preventing these outcomes.

A. A. Fanaroff, MD

References

1. Andersen DH, Blanc WA, Crozier DN, Silverman WA. A difference in mortality rate and incidence of kernicterus among premature infants allotted to two prophylactic antibacterial regimens. *Pediatrics*. 1956;18:614-625.
2. Sutherland JM. Fatal cardiovascular collapse of infants receiving large amounts of chloramphenicol. *AMA J Dis Child*. 1959;97:761-767.
3. Manzoni P, Mostert M, Latino MA, et al. Italian Task Force for the Study and Prevention of Neonatal Fungal Infections, Italian Society of Neonatology. Clinical characteristics and response to prophylactic fluconazole of preterm VLBW neonates with baseline and acquired fungal colonisation in NICU: data from a multi-centre RCT. *Early Hum Dev*. 2012;88:S60-S64.

4. Kaufman DA, Morris A, Gurka MJ, Kapik B, Hetherington S. Fluconazole prophylaxis in preterm infants: a multicenter case-controlled analysis of efficacy and safety. *Early Hum Dev.* 2014;90:S87-S90.
5. Aliaga S, Clark RH, Laughon M, et al. Changes in the incidence of candidiasis in neonatal intensive care units. *Pediatrics.* 2014;133:236-242.
6. Adams-Chapman I, Bann CM, Das A, et al. Neurodevelopmental outcome of extremely low-birth-weight infants with Candida infection. *J Pediatr.* 2013;163: 961-967.e3.

2010 Perinatal GBS Prevention Guideline and Resource Utilization

Mukhopadhyay S, Dukhovny D, Mao W, et al (Boston Children's Hosp, MA; Beth Israel Deaconess Med Ctr, Boston, MA; et al)
Pediatrics 133:196-203, 2014

Objectives.—To quantify differences in early-onset sepsis (EOS) evaluations, evaluation-associated resource utilization, and EOS cases detected, when comparing time periods before and after the implementation of an EOS algorithm based on the Centers for Disease Control and Prevention (CDC) 2010 guidelines for prevention of perinatal Group B *Streptococcus* (GBS) disease.

Methods.—Retrospective cohort study of infants born at ≥ 36 weeks' gestation from 2009 to 2012 in a single tertiary care center. One 12-month period during which EOS evaluations were based on the CDC 2002 guideline was compared with a second 12-month period during which EOS evaluations were based on the CDC 2010 guideline. A cost minimization analysis was performed to determine the EOS evaluation-associated costs and resources during each time period.

Results.—During the study periods, among well-appearing infants ≥ 36 weeks' gestation, EOS evaluations for inadequate GBS prophylaxis decreased from 32/1000 to <1/1000 live births; EOS evaluation-associated costs decreased by $6994 per 1000 live births; and EOS evaluation-associated work hours decreased by 29 per 1000 live births. We found no increase in EOS evaluations for other indications, total NICU admissions, frequency of infants evaluated for symptoms before hospital discharge, or incidence of EOS during the 2 study periods.

Conclusions.—Implementation of an EOS algorithm based on CDC 2010 GBS guidelines resulted in a 25% decrease in EOS evaluations performed among well-appearing infants ≥ 36 weeks' gestation, attributable to decreased evaluation of infants born in the setting of inadequate indicated GBS prophylaxis. This resulted in significant changes in EOS evaluation-associated resource expenditures.

▶ The Centers for Disease Control and Prevention (CDC) guidelines for the use of intrapartum antibiotic prophylaxis to prevent perinatal Group B streptococcus (GBS) infection were revised in 2010. The revision contained 1 significant change: the evaluation of infants born to GBS-positive mothers who were inadequately treated with intrapartum antibiotic prophylaxis is now recommended

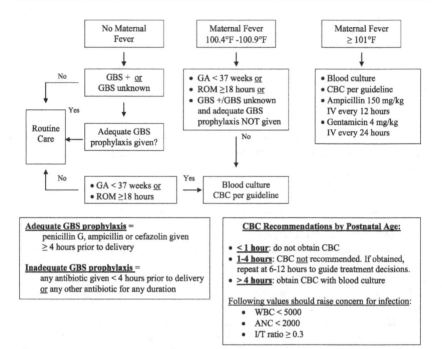

Adequate GBS prophylaxis =
penicillin G, ampicillin or cefazolin given
≥ 4 hours prior to delivery

Inadequate GBS prophylaxis =
any antibiotic given < 4 hours prior to delivery
or any other antibiotic for any duration

CBC Recommendations by Postnatal Age:

- **< 1 hour**: do not obtain CBC
- **1-4 hours**: CBC not recommended. If obtained,
  repeat at 6-12 hours to guide treatment decisions.
- **> 4 hours**: obtain CBC with blood culture

Following values should raise concern for infection:
- WBC < 5000
- ANC < 2000
- I/T ratio ≥ 0.3

Additional Notes:

1. Chorioamnionitis is an obstetrical clinical diagnosis made on the basis of clinical findings, laboratory data and fever. If obstetrical staff diagnose chorioamnionitis, the infant should be evaluated for sepsis and receive empiric antibiotic treatment.
2. Maternal fever that occurs within 1 hour of delivery should be treated like intrapartum fever, and the infant should be evaluated as outlined above.
3. Women with a previous infant with GBS disease should receive intrapartum GBS prophylaxis.
4. Blood cultures should consist of aerobic and anaerobic bottles with minimum 1 mL blood in each bottle.
5. To facilitate family bonding and initiation of breastfeeding, the sepsis evaluation can be delayed for up to 1 hour after birth, at the discretion of the obstetrical and neonatal caregivers.

FIGURE 1.—Guidelines for the management of asymptomatic infants born at ≥36 weeks' gestation at risk for EOS. Local algorithm used at BWH since March 2011, based on the CDC 2010 perinatal GBS prevention guidelines.[3] ANC, absolute neutrophil count; I/T, immature neutrophil to total neutrophil. *Editor's Note*: Please refer to original journal article for full references. (Reprinted from Mukhopadhyay S, Dukhovny D, Mao W, et al. 2010 perinatal GBS prevention guideline and resource utilization. *Pediatrics*. 2014;133:196-203, with permission from the American Academy of Pediatrics.)

only if there are additional risk factors. These risk factors include gestational age < 37 weeks, rupture of membranes > 18 hours, and chorioamnionitis (Fig 1).

Mukhopadhyay et al studied the impact of this guideline change among well-appearing infants ≥36 weeks' gestation. They found that early-onset sepsis (EOS) evaluation frequency decreased from 12.6% to 6.8% and empiric antibiotic administration decreased from 7.2% to 5.2% after implementation of the revised guidelines. They reported that this change was not associated with an increase in infants who became symptomatic later, but the authors did not provide an estimate of the risk difference or its 95% confidence interval. This information would have allowed readers to estimate how large a difference may have been missed.

The observed decrease in the rate of evaluated and tested infants is favorable given the current low incidence of EOS and reflects an improvement in the revised guideline over its predecessor. Nonetheless, the current Centers for Disease Control and Prevention (CDC) guideline still falls short of an evidence-based approach to identifying infants most in need of further evaluation or empiric treatment.

The decision to evaluate an infant for EOS should be based on the pretest probability of infection. Similarly, the decision to treat with empiric antibiotics should be based on the posttest probability of EOS (after adjusting the pretest probability based on the evolving clinical picture and laboratory results) and the relative costs of unnecessary versus delayed treatment.

The CDC guidelines do not attempt to quantify any of these factors. The dichotomization of risk factors makes for a simple flow cart but leads to loss of information and increases the risk of misclassification. For example, the CDC guidelines mandate diagnostic workup for all infants born to mothers with "chorioamnionitis." However, there is no validated approach for diagnosing chorioamnionitis. That diagnosis is presumably made by the obstetrician when the estimated benefits of treating the mother exceed the risks and costs. However, the risk-benefit ratio for treating the infant is most likely different and needs to be assessed separately.

There are now clinical tools available that can take into account objective maternal risk factors as continuous variables and explicitly estimate the probability of infection based on maternal risk factors, neonatal clinical presentation,[1,2] and complete blood count results.[3] These prediction models are more accurate than the CDC guidelines in estimating EOS probabilities.

The next steps for an evidence-based approach to newborns at risk of EOS will require further changes in treatment guidelines to reflect a more sophisticated approach to pretest and posttest probability estimation. Additional steps include refining treatment thresholds so that these improved probability estimates can be translated to recommended courses of action.[4] This study by Mukhopadhyay et al suggests that this work is well worth doing, because clinicians seem to be willing to follow EOS guidelines that lead to fewer evaluations and less treatment.

M. Steurer, MD, MAS

T. B. Newman, MD, MPH

References

1. Puopolo KM, Draper D, Wi S, et al. Estimating the probability of neonatal early-onset infection on the basis of maternal risk factors. *Pediatrics.* 2011;128(5): e1155-1163.
2. Escobar GJ, Puopolo KM, Wi S, et al. Stratification of risk of early-onset sepsis in newborns >=34 weeks' gestation. *Pediatrics.* 2014;133(1):30-36.
3. Newman TB, Draper D, Puopolo KM, Wi S, Escobar GJ. Combining immature and total neutrophil counts to predict early onset sepsis in term and late preterm newborns: use of the I/T². *Pediatr Infect Dis J.* 2014 Feb 5 [Epub ahead of print].
4. Newman TB, Kohn MA. *Evidence-based Diagnosis.* New York: Cambridge University Press; 2009:52-60.

Effects of Caffeine on Intermittent Hypoxia in Infants Born Prematurely: A Randomized Clinical Trial

Rhein LM, The Caffeine Pilot Study Group (Boston Children's Hosp, MA; et al)

JAMA Pediatr 168:250-257, 2014

Importance.—Preterm infants have immature respiratory control and resulting intermittent hypoxia (IH). The extent of IH after stopping routine caffeine treatment and the potential for reducing IH with extended caffeine treatment are unknown.

Objectives.—To determine (1) the frequency of IH in premature infants after discontinuation of routine caffeine treatment and (2) whether extending caffeine treatment to 40 weeks' postmenstrual age (PMA) reduces IH.

Design, Setting, and Participants.—A prospective randomized clinical study was conducted at 16 neonatal intensive care units in the United States, with an 18-month enrollment period. Preterm infants (<32 weeks' gestation) previously treated with caffeine were randomized to extended caffeine treatment or usual care (controls) at a PMA of at least 34 weeks but less than 37 weeks. Continuous pulse oximeter recordings were obtained through 40 weeks' PMA. Oximeter data were analyzed by persons masked to patient group.

Intervention.—Continued treatment with caffeine.

Main Outcomes and Measures.—Number of IH events and seconds with less than 90% hemoglobin oxygen saturation (SaO_2) per hour of recording.

Results.—Our analysis included 95 preterm infants. In control infants, the mean (SD) time at less than 90% SaO_2 at 35 and 36 weeks' PMA was 106.3 (89.0) and 100.1 (114.6) s/h, respectively. The number of IH events decreased significantly from 35 to 39 weeks' PMA ($P = .01$). Extended caffeine treatment reduced the mean time at less than 90% SaO_2 by 47% (95% CI, −65% to −20%) to 50.9 (48.1) s/h at 35 weeks and by 45% (95% CI, −74% to −17%) to 49.5 (52.1) s/h at 36 weeks.

Conclusions and Relevance.—Substantial IH persists after discontinuation of routine caffeine treatment and progressively decreases with increasing PMA. Extended caffeine treatment decreases IH in premature infants.

Trial Registration.—clinicaltrials.gov Identifier: NCT01875159.

▶ Adults with obstructive sleep apnea associated with frequent episodes of intermittent hypoxia (IH) show loss of gray matter in multiple brain regions on brain imaging studies and have early cognitive impairment. We know that episodes of IH in newborn and adult models without associated upper airway obstruction or apnea, increases reactive oxidative species (ROS),[7] and ROS unbalanced by antioxidant defenses is associated with significant tissue damage, especially in developing tissues (for review, see[1]).

It is undisputed that chronic IH occurs in premature infants,[2] and reducing the frequency of IH theoretically may decrease short- and long-term morbidities that are known to occur in premature infants. For example, infants with the greater frequency of IH are more likely to have retinopathy of prematurity that was treated with laser therapy.[2] Whether IH is an independent cause of poor neurodevelopmental outcome in premature infants is less clear. Nevertheless, if extending caffeine therapy beyond the usual duration of the treatment of apnea of prematurity (approximately 34 weeks' postmenstrual age [PMA]), reduces the frequency of IH and morbidities, then it is reasonable to treat premature infants beyond 34 weeks' PMA.

Rhein and colleagues present a well-designed, multicenter prospective randomized trial showing that IH events are frequent past 34 weeks' PMA in premature infants born between 25 0/7 and 32 0/7 weeks of gestation, and the frequency of IH decreases with increasing PMA.[8] Moreover, they show that in those premature infants between 34 and 37 weeks' PMA who were clinically assessed to no longer need caffeine or oxygen therapy and who did not have chronic lung disease or severe intracranial hemorrhage had IH that significantly improved in the group that had caffeine restarted. Restarting caffeine was associated with a reduction in the frequency of IH with a threshold of < 80% SaO_2 by 64% at 35 weeks' PMA ($P = .002$) and by 45% at 36 weeks' PMA ($P = .05$) as shown in Fig 2 of the original article.

Although these results show that continued caffeine therapy reduces the incidence of IH in premature infants, the way the study was designed does not easily translate into how to implement therapy into clinical practice for the following reasons: (1) The correlation between the Masimo pulse oximeter data and the pulse oximeters used as standard of care was not reported. (2) Acceptable SaO_2 limits in premature infants not requiring oxygen therapy for each of the participating centers was not reported, bringing into question what is considered a clinically acceptable level of SaO_2 at each PMA that leads to discontinuation of supplemental oxygen. (3) The duration of therapy postdischarge is not presented, and neither are suggested guidelines for when and how to discontinue caffeine therapy. (4) Finally, caffeine therapy was discontinued for 5 days before restarting therapy, which does not equate with extending therapy through 36 weeks' PMA or longer. Thus, if standard measurement devices do not detect the IH episodes that are short and self-resolving or the clinical team did not consider IH episodes of less than 90% or 85% SaO_2 as problematic warranting therapy, determining which infants need to be to treated and for how long is unclear.

It is particularly important to understand that the efficacy of reducing the frequency of IH with continued caffeine therapy may not be the same as having a "drug holiday" and restarting therapy, as was done in by these investigators. Caffeine therapy in premature infants increases central respiratory drive, thereby decreasing periodic breathing and apnea frequency via adenosine receptor blocked in the central respiratory network and peripheral arterial chemoreceptors. Caffeine binds to G-protein coupled receptors (GPCRs). Specifically, it blocks both adenosine A1 receptors, which are negatively coupled to adenylyl cyclase and A2a-receptor, which are positively coupled to adenylyl cyclase. Adenosine binding to A1 receptors on respiratory-related neurons or binding to A2a receptors on inhibitory gamma-aminobutyric acid interneurons leads to respiratory depression. When caffeine blocks 1 or both of these receptors, respiratory drive increases.

Persistent blockade of GPRCs causes an upregulation of the receptor, often leading to drug tolerance. Removal of the drug allows for resetting of the receptors with improved efficacy after restarting of the drug. Multiple acute physiologic responses to caffeine are attenuated over time with continued use. Respiratory system tolerance to caffeine has been well demonstrated in rhesus monkeys in which the initial respiratory stimulant effects of caffeine were no longer observed after 1 week of chronic therapy and with sensitivity to caffeine returning after 9 days of discontinuation.[6] Because chronic caffeine therapy did not affect pharmacokinetics of caffeine in these animals, the effect is likely related to pharmacodynamics potentially occurring at level of the adenosine receptor or intracellular signaling. In newborn rats treated with chronic caffeine from postnatal day 2 to 6, adenosine A1 and A2a receptor gene and protein expression was upregulated in pontine-medullary brainstem regions that are involved in control of breathing.[5] Thus, collectively these animal studies suggest extending the therapy with caffeine may not be as effective as the stop and restart design outlined in this clinical trial in premature infants. It is also important to note that although short pauses in breathing are common in term and preterm infants, the associated hypoxemia can only occur if there is simultaneous ventilation/perfusion mismatch or an intrapulmonary or intracardiac shunt leading to right to left shunting. Premature infants are prone to both of these conditions. Thus, there are multiple mechanisms through which caffeine might be improving the frequency of IH events that are not directly related to changes in ventilatory drive.

Caffeine therapy is relatively safe in premature infants. Symptomatic apnea and bradycardia occur more frequently and persist longer in premature infants born at the lower gestational ages,[4] and these events are often associated with hemoglobin (Hgb) saturations of ≤90%. The study reviewed here shows that IH still persists in premature infants at 35 and 36 weeks' gestation who otherwise appear well and who had previously had caffeine therapy discontinued. The novel observation is that restarting caffeine reduces the frequency of IH events in this population. It is unclear whether the definition of the threshold for Hgb saturation for "asymptomatic" events in the study population was the same between the participating centers, and thus the threshold Hgb-saturation for discontinuing oxygen therapy is unknown. The lower the baseline Hgb saturation, the more frequent and more rapid the desaturation episodes will be with short apneic pauses.[3,9]

The findings from this study suggest that restarting caffeine in a subpopulation of infants stabilizes oxygen saturation, which the authors speculate might lead to improved neurodevelopmental outcomes in premature infants. Although the pharmacokinetics and pharmacodynamics of caffeine in infants aged over 34 weeks should be established to better guide therapy, the findings from this study also suggest that an alternative dosing strategy for caffeine may be beneficial for in premature infants who have intractable cardiorespiratory events on prolonged caffeine therapy. Specifically, these infants might benefit from a drug holiday and then restarting caffeine, which could theoretically reduce the frequency of symptomatic and asymptomatic cardiorespiratory events. As noted by the authors, follow-up studies are essential to determine whether reducing the frequency and severity of IH is associated with improved neurodevelopmental outcomes.

E. B. Gauda, MD

References

1. Davis JM, Auten RL. Maturation of the antioxidant system and the effects on preterm birth. *Semin Fetal Neonatal Med.* 2010;15:191-195.
2. Di Fiore JM, Bloom JN, Orge F, et al. A higher incidence of intermittent hypoxemic episodes is associated with severe retinopathy of prematurity. *J Pediatr.* 2010; 157:69-73.
3. Di Fiore JM, Walsh M, Wrage L, et al. Low oxygen saturation target range is associated with increased incidence of intermittent hypoxemia. *J Pediatr.* 2012;161: 1047-1052.
4. Eichenwald EC, Aina A, Stark AR. Apnea frequently persists beyond term gestation in infants delivered at 24 to 28 weeks. *Pediatrics.* 1997;100:354-359.
5. Gaytan SP, Pasaro R. Neonatal caffeine treatment up-regulates adenosine receptors in brainstem and hypothalamic cardio-respiratory related nuclei of rat pups. *Exp Neurol.* 2012;237:247-259.
6. Howell LL, Landrum AM. Effects of chronic caffeine administration on respiration and schedule-controlled behavior in rhesus monkeys. *J Pharmacol Exp Ther.* 1997;283:190-199.
7. Prabhakar NR. Oxygen sensing during intermittent hypoxia: cellular and molecular mechanisms. *J Appl Physiol.* 2001;90:1986-1994.
8. Rhein LM, Dobson NR, Darnall RA, et al. Effects of caffeine on intermittent hypoxia in infants born prematurely: a randomized clinical trial. *JAMA Pediatr.* 2014;168:250-257.
9. Weintraub Z, Alvaro R, Kwiatkowski K, Cates D, Rigatto H. Effects of inhaled oxygen (up to 40%) on periodic breathing and apnea in preterm infants. *J Appl Physiol.* 1992;72:116-120.

Dextrose gel for neonatal hypoglycaemia (the Sugar Babies Study): a randomised, double-blind, placebo-controlled trial

Harris DL, Weston PJ, Signal M, et al (Waikato District Health Board, Hamilton, New Zealand; Univ of Canterbury, Christchurch, New Zealand; et al)
Lancet 382:2077-2083, 2013

Background.—Neonatal hypoglycaemia is common, and a preventable cause of brain damage. Dextrose gel is used to reverse hypoglycaemia in individuals with diabetes; however, little evidence exists for its use in babies. We aimed to assess whether treatment with dextrose gel was more effective than feeding alone for reversal of neonatal hypoglycaemia in at-risk babies.

Methods.—We undertook a randomised, double-blind, placebo-controlled trial at a tertiary centre in New Zealand between Dec 1, 2008, and Nov 31, 2010. Babies aged 35—42 weeks' gestation, younger than 48-h-old, and at risk of hypoglycaemia were randomly assigned (1:1), via computer-generated blocked randomisation, to 40% dextrose gel 200 mg/kg or placebo gel. Randomisation was stratified by maternal diabetes and birthweight. Group allocation was concealed from clinicians, families, and all study investigators. The primary outcome was treatment failure, defined as a blood glucose concentration of less than 2·6 mmol/L after two treatment attempts. Analysis was by intention to treat. The trial is registered with Australian New Zealand Clinical Trials Registry, number ACTRN12608000623392.

Findings.—Of 514 enrolled babies, 242 (47%) became hypoglycaemic and were randomised. Five babies were randomised in error, leaving 237 for analysis: 118 (50%) in the dextrose group and 119 (50%) in the placebo group. Dextrose gel reduced the frequency of treatment failure compared with placebo (16 [14%] *vs* 29 [24%]; relative risk 0·57, 95% CI 0·33—0·98; $p = 0·04$). We noted no serious adverse events. Three (3%) babies in the placebo group each had one blood glucose concentration of 0·9 mmol/L. No other adverse events took place.

Interpretation.—Treatment with dextrose gel is inexpensive and simple to administer. Dextrose gel should be considered for first-line treatment to manage hypoglycaemia in late preterm and term babies in the first 48 h after birth.

▶ In a novel study from Auckland, New Zealand, Harris et al showed in a mixed group of infants at risk for neonatal hypoglycemia that the number of episodes of "hypoglycemia" could be reduced, as well as recurrence and need for admission to the neonatal intensive care unit (NICU) to treat hypoglycemia, with a simple treatment of dextrose gel massaged into the buccal mucosa. This is important because hypoglycemia is one of the most frequently encountered problems in the newborn period and has the potential, if untreated and worsens, to lead to irreparable neurological injury.

Current guidelines suggest screening preterm (early and late), large for gestational age (LGA), small for gestational age (SGA) and/or intrauterine growth restricted (IUGR) infants, and infants of a diabetic mother (IDMs) for low glucose concentrations.[1] The incidence of low glucose concentrations in these infants who are at risk for hypoglycemia will depend on the age and frequency at which measurements are made, as well as the concentrations used to define normal and abnormal glucose concentrations, but the incidence of hypoglycemia in such infants is high enough that many require more aggressive treatment than simply providing oral feedings.

Most low glucose concentrations will be found in asymptomatic newborns, the significance of which for long-term outcomes is unknown.[1] Novel treatments for mild asymptomatic hypoglycemia have been lacking. Frequent milk feeding with repeated glucose measurements is the current standard treatment because this allows mothers and babies to remain together and provides nutrient substrates to support gluconeogenesis as it develops. If low glucose concentrations persist or the newborn becomes symptomatic, a continuous intravenous dextrose infusion, often preceded by an intravenous dextrose bolus, is indicated. This approach always involves discomfort from the placement of an intravenous catheter and almost always necessitates admission to a neonatal intensive care unit. Preventing the separation of mother and child while safely managing asymptomatic low glucose concentrations has many benefits. However, until now there have been no large studies to inform this type of management.

Harris et al have addressed this limitation and present the results of a large, randomized, placebo-controlled, double-blinded study of buccal dextrose gel.

Dextrose gel massaged into the buccal mucosa may be rapidly absorbed and thereby raise blood sugar concentrations. Furthermore, stimulation of insulin release and rebound hypoglycemia from buccal mucosal dextrose gel may be reduced, because there would be less gastric and intestinal glucose absorption with less incretin release by these organs. These theoretical benefits in the newborn population have remained largely untested until now.

In the study by Harris et al, at-risk newborns were randomized to receive buccal dextrose gel or placebo gel, followed by oral milk feeding in both groups to treat hypoglycemia, defined as < 2.6 mmol/L (< 47 mg/dL). Treatment failure was defined as a persistently low blood glucose concentration despite 2 doses of dextrose gel or placebo gel. Treatment failure was less common in the dextrose gel group compared with the placebo gel group, thus establishing efficacy. There were no adverse events reported with the dextrose gel and recurrent hypoglycemia was less common in this group, establishing safety.

Although safety and efficacy were established in this study, admission rates to the NICU for all causes were not significantly different between groups, 38% in the dextrose gel group versus 46% with placebo gel (relative risk: 0.83; 95% confidence interval 0.61–1.11; P value = .24). The reason for this is unclear because admissions to the NICU for hypoglycemia and the use of supplemental dextrose from sources other than the study gel were lower in the dextrose gel group. It is possible that the sample size was too small to show a difference in a secondary outcome as common as NICU admission rates in this population that is at risk for many disorders that not only require NICU admission but often are accompanied by hypoglycemia. Despite the similar NICU admission rates, other secondary outcomes did show benefit of the dextrose gel. Perhaps the most important of these is that at 2 weeks of age, those babies in the dextrose gel group were significantly less likely to be formula feeding (5 [4%] vs 15 [13%]; Relative risk 0.34; 95% confidence interval: 0.13–0.90; P = .03). Given the many benefits of breastfeeding, this is an important improvement compared with standard practice of NICU admission or switching to formula feeding when lactation is delayed.

Another interesting feature of this study is the use of continuous interstitial glucose monitoring (CGMS). CGMS for neonatal glucose management remains largely a research tool,[2,3] and the caregivers for patients in this study were blinded to the CGMS measurements. This study, like several others, continues to show the accuracy and promise of this method. CGMS data demonstrated that correction of hypoglycemia with dextrose gel was essentially as rapid as has been reported for correction with intravenous dextrose, about 20 minutes. It also showed that rebound hypoglycemia was rare in both groups and recurrent hypoglycemia was lower in the dextrose gel group, thus supporting the safety and efficacy established by intermittent glucose sampling. Perhaps even more intriguing is that many episodes of low glucose concentrations, documented by both blood and CGMS measurement, resolved spontaneously. This demonstrates the potential that CGMS has to reduce treatment for hypoglycemia by indicating which episodes have resolved before intervention.

However, not reported in the Harris et al article is the number of episodes of low glucose concentrations documented by CGMS that went undocumented by routine clinical blood sampling. In other publications, the number of these episodes is high. The significance of these episodes for long-term outcomes is unclear. It is possible, therefore, that finding many more episodes of hypoglycemia with CGMS could increase the risk of overtreatment, which might outweigh the benefits of documenting all or most low glucose concentrations with standard clinical use of CGMS in this population, at least until further studies with long-term outcomes can be performed.[4]

When considering the adoption of dextrose gel into clinical practice based on this study, it must be remembered that the study was conducted at a single center in New Zealand. Mitigating this concern are the relatively large number of infants in the study and the broad representation of the major at-risk groups. Other features to note when considering using dextrose gel is that the treatment cutoff (2.6 mmol/L or 47 mg/dL, irrespective of age) is higher than what is recommended by the American Academy of Pediatrics for the types of infants studied.[1] Also, this study only included asymptomatic or mildly symptomatic (poor-feeding) newborns. Dextrose gel was not studied in moderately or severely symptomatic patients, and intravenous dextrose should remain the treatment of choice for these infants. It also is not clear that patients in these at-risk groups will benefit long term from this treatment. Furthermore, although increased rates of breastfeeding at 2 weeks may be enough of a benefit to adopt this treatment, it should be remembered that the rates of intent to breastfeed and actual breastfeeding rates at 2 weeks were extremely high in the population studied in New Zealand. It is not certain that this benefit would be found in a population where formula feeding is more prevalent.

Despite these concerns, it may be reasonable to include buccal dextrose gel in the management plan of asymptomatic neonatal hypoglycemia. There currently is no consensus or evidence to determine when a glucose concentration is too low and what duration of such low glucose concentrations is necessary to cause permanent neurological injury. Nor is there consensus regarding when treatment would make any difference. In light of such uncertainties and lack of evidence, making current guidelines safe, simple, and easy to follow, while at the same time promoting increased maternal-infant interactions that lead to increased breastfeeding, may be worthwhile to pursue. Buccal dextrose gel, which is relatively inexpensive (approximately $2 per dose) compared with a NICU admission for hypoglycemia, appears to have a promising role in achieving these goals.

P. J. Rozance, MD

W. W. Hay, Jr, MD

References

1. Adamkin DH. Postnatal glucose homeostasis in late-preterm and term infants. *Pediatrics.* 2011;127:575-579.
2. Beardsall K, Vanhaesebrouck S, Ogilvy-Stuart AL, et al. Validation of the continuous glucose monitoring sensor in preterm infants. *Arch Dis Child Fetal Neonatal Ed.* 2013;98:F136-F140.
3. Harris DL, Battin MR, Weston PJ, Harding JE. Continuous glucose monitoring in newborn babies at risk of hypoglycemia. *J Pediatr.* 2010;157:198-202.
4. Hay WW Jr, Rozance PJ. Continuous glucose monitoring for diagnosis and treatment of neonatal hypoglycemia. *J Pediatr.* 2010;157:180-182.

Probiotic Effects on Late-onset Sepsis in Very Preterm Infants: A Randomized Controlled Trial

Jacobs SE, for the ProPrems Study Group (The Royal Women's Hosp, Melbourne, Australia; et al)

Pediatrics 132:1055-1062, 2013

Background and Objective.—Late-onset sepsis frequently complicates prematurity, contributing to morbidity and mortality. Probiotics may reduce mortality and necrotizing enterocolitis (NEC) in preterm infants, with unclear effect on late-onset sepsis. This study aimed to determine the effect of administering a specific combination of probiotics to very preterm infants on culture-proven late-onset sepsis.

Methods.—A prospective multicenter, double-blinded, placebo-controlled, randomized trial compared daily administration of a probiotic combination (*Bifidobacterium infantis*, *Streptococcus thermophilus*, and *Bifidobacterium lactis*, containing 1×10^9 total organisms) with placebo (maltodextrin) in infants born before 32 completed weeks' gestation weighing <1500 g. The primary outcome was at least 1 episode of definite late-onset sepsis.

Results.—Between October 2007 and November 2011, 1099 very preterm infants from Australia and New Zealand were randomized. Rates of definite late-onset sepsis (16.2%), NEC of Bell stage 2 or more (4.4%), and mortality (5.1%) were low in controls, with high breast milk feeding rates (96.9%). No significant difference in definite late-onset sepsis or all-cause mortality was found, but this probiotic combination reduced NEC of Bell stage 2 or more (2.0% versus 4.4%; relative risk 0.46, 95% confidence interval 0.23 to 0.93, $P = .03$; number needed to treat 43, 95% confidence interval 23 to 333).

Conclusions.—The probiotics *B infantis*, *S thermophilus*, and *B lactis* significantly reduced NEC of Bell stage 2 or more in very preterm infants, but not definite late-onset sepsis or mortality. Treatment with this combination of probiotics appears to be safe (Tables 2 and 3).

▶ Despite recent advances in neonatal medicine, including ventilation and surfactant therapy, necrotizing enterocolitis (NEC) and late-onset sepsis (LOS) continue to be important causes of mortality and morbidity in premature neonates.[1,2] The mortality related to definite NEC (Bell's criteria Stage II and greater) is ~25% in very low birth weight (VLBW: birth weight <1500 grams) and ~45% in extremely low birth weight (ELBW: birth weight <1000 grams) neonates, increasing to ~100% in those with full-thickness widespread gut necrosis.[1] The morbidity of definite NEC is significant and includes prolonged hospitalization, complications associated with short bowel syndrome and long-term neurodevelopmental impairment (NDI), especially in ELBW neonates needing surgery for the illness. The economic burden of NEC is also significant, considering its complications that often prolong the hospital stay. In the United States, it is estimated to be as high as 1 billion dollars per year.[3] Neonatal infection and the associated inflammatory response contribute to various long-term

TABLE 2.—Late-onset Sepsis Outcomes

	Probiotic Group, $n = 548$	Control Group, $n = 551$	RR (95% CI)	P Value
Primary outcome				
Infants with at least 1 episode of definite late-onset sepsis, n (%)	72 (13.1)	89 (16.2)	0.81 (0.61 to 1.08)	.16
Subgroup analyses:				
Gestational age				.03[a]
<28 wk, n (%)	54 (24.7)	55 (23.4)	1.05 (0.76 to 1.46)	.75
≥28 wk, n (%)	18 (5.5)	34 (10.8)	0.51 (0.29 to 0.88)	.01
Birth weight				.24[a]
<1000 g, n (%)	53 (22.6)	58 (24.3)	0.93	
≥1000 g, n (%)	19 (6.1)	31 (9.9)	0.61	
Secondary outcomes				
Infants with at least 1 episode of definite late-onset sepsis with pathogens, n (%)	38 (6.9)	48 (8.7)	0.80 (0.53 to 1.20)	.27
Infants with at least 1 episode of definite late-onset sepsis with CoNS, n (%)	40 (7.3)	43 (7.8)	0.94 (0.62 to 1.42)	.75
Infants with at least 1 episode of definite late-onset sepsis with probiotic species, n (%)	0	0		
Infants with clinical late-onset sepsis, n (%)	75 (13.7)	83 (15.1)	0.91 (0.68 to 1.21)	.52
Infants with late-onset sepsis (definite or clinical), n (%)	129 (23.5)	146 (26.5)	0.89 (0.72 to 1.09)	.26
Courses of antibiotics, median (IQR)	1 (0–1)	1 (0–1)		.78
Days of antibiotic treatment, median (IQR)	2 (0–7)	2 (0–8)		.64

Late-onset sepsis >48 h after birth and before discharge home or term postmenstrual age.
Pathogens isolated included the following:
Pathogens: Staphylococcus aureus (n = 21), Escherichia coli (n = 20), Group B Streptococcus (n = 11), Enterococcus faecalis (n = 10), Klebsiella spp (n = 7), Enterobacter spp (n = 6), Candida spp (n = 5), Pseudomonas aeruginosa (n = 4), Pseudomonas spp (n = 2), Stenotrophomonas maltophilia (n = 2), Serratia spp (n = 2), Enterococcus spp (n = 1), Bacillus cereus (n = 1), Clostridium perfringens (n = 1), group A Streptococcus (n = 1), Streptococcus viridans (n = 1). Coagulasenegative Staphylococcus spp (CoNS spp) (n = 87; not speciated CoNS [n = 57]), Staphylococcus epidermidis (n = 24), Staphylococcus capitis (n = 5), Staphylococcus warneri (n = 1). IQR, interquartile range (25–75).
[a]Interaction P value.
Reprinted from Jacobs SE, for the ProPrems Study Group. Probiotic Effects on Late-onset Sepsis in Very Preterm Infants: A Randomized Controlled Trial. Pediatrics. 2013;132:1055-1062. Copyright © 2013, by the American Academy of Pediatrics.

complications, including bronchopulmonary dysplasia, central nervous system injury, and adverse neurodevelopmental outcome.[2]

Recent systematic reviews (30 randomized controlled trials [RCTs], $N = 6000$) have shown that probiotics reduce NEC and all-cause mortality; however, there was no difference in LOS.[4,5] Based on the current evidence, a change in practice has been recommended;[4,5] however, others have argued about limitations of the meta-analyses, including heterogeneity of the probiotic strain(s) and supplementation protocols and paucity of data from large, randomized, controlled trials and on breast-milk-fed very preterm neonates.[6]

This RCT was unique in several areas. To date, this is the largest trial in this field ($N = 1099$). Nearly 42% of neonates had birth weight < 1000 g. More than 90% of neonates have received at least 1 dose of antenatal glucocorticoid. The

TABLE 3.—Other Secondary Outcomes

	Probiotic Group, $n = 548$	Control Group, $n = 551$	RR (95% CI)	P Value
NEC				
NEC (Bell stage 2 or more), n (%)	11 (2.0)	24 (4.4)	0.46 (0.23 to 0.93)	.03
Subgroup analyses:				
Gestational age				[a]
<28 wk, n (%)	11 (5.0)	17 (7.2)	0.69	
≥28 wk, n (%)	0	7 (2.2)		
Birth weight				.08[b]
<1000 g, n (%)	10 (4.3)	14 (5.9)	0.73	
≥1000 g, n (%)	1 (0.3)	10 (3.2)	0.10	
Age at NEC (Bell stage 2 or more), d, median (IQR)	20.5 (15.5–34.5)	21 (17.0–30.5)		.99
Mortality				
Death, n (%)	27 (4.9)	28 (5.1)	0.97 (0.58 to 1.62)	.91
Age at death, d, mean (SD)	21.7 (18.5)	23.3 (16.7)		.75
Death during primary hospitalization, n (%)	30 (5.5)	31 (5.6)	0.97 (0.60 to 1.58)	.91
Age at death during primary hospitalization, d, median (IQR)	21 (7–40)	24.5 (10–42·5)		.49
Causes of death, n (%)				
Late-onset sepsis	6 (1.1)	4 (0.7)	1.55 (0.43 to 5.32)	.52
NEC	4 (0.7)	11 (2.0)	0.37 (0.12 to 1.14)	.07
Composite of death or NEC (Bell stage 2 or more), n (%)	33 (6.0)	41 (7.4)	0.81 (0.52 to 1.26)	.35
Other secondary outcomes				
Length of primary hospital admission, d, median (IQR)	71 (54–92)	74 (58–93)		.09
Duration on parenteral nutrition, d, median (IQR)	12 (8–17)	12 (8–18)		.29
Days to full enteral feeds, median (IQR)	12 (9–16)	12 (10–17)		.31
Days to regain birth weight, mean (SD)	11.1 (4.5)	11.7 (4.8)	−0.5 (−1.1 to 0)	.06
Weight at 28 d, g, mean (SD)	1495.0 (401.2)	1446.0 (379.2)	48.9 (2.0 to 95.9)	.04
Weight at discharge, g, mean (SD)	2870.5 (748.8)	2864.0 (738.9)	6.5 (−84.2 to 97.2)	.89
Any breast milk, n (%)	520 (95.6)	532 (96.9)	0.99 (0.96 to 1.01)	.25
Exclusive breast milk at discharge home, n (%)	266 (51.6)	292 (56.5)	0.91 (0.82 to 1.02)	.11
Any breast milk at discharge home, n (%)	370 (71.7)	379 (73.3)	0.98 (0.91 to 1.05)	.56

Secondary outcomes during study period (before discharge or term postmenstrual age, whichever occurs sooner), unless specified otherwise. IQR, interquartile range (25–75).
[a]Interaction P value unable to be calculated.
[b]Interaction P value.

Reprinted from Jacobs SE, for the ProPrems Study Group. Probiotic Effects on Late-onset Sepsis in Very Preterm Infants: A Randomized Controlled Trial. Pediatrics. 2013;132:1055-1062. Copyright © 2013, by the American Academy of Pediatrics.

taxonomy of the probiotic strains (*Bifidobacterium infantis Streptococcus thermophiles and Bifidobacterium lactis*) were confirmed independently. Rates of definite LOS (16.2%), definite ($\geq$ Stage II) NEC (4.4%), and mortality (5.1%) were low in controls, and the breast milk feeding rates were high (96.9%). The study methods, including randomization and blinding, were sound. The primary and secondary outcomes were well defined. The results showed no significant differences in definite LOS or mortality between both groups (Table 2); however, probiotics reduced definite NEC (2.0% vs 4.4%; Table 3). This combination of probiotic strains was safe and well tolerated in the study population. Surviving children are undergoing allergy and neurodevelopmental assessments after 2 years of age, and their outcomes will be of interest.

There are some limitations of this trial. The expected incidence of LOS turned out to be lower than its actual incidence during the trial period (23% vs 16%). The trial is thus underpowered to detect a significant difference in the primary outcome. LOS was predominantly (n = 87) related to coagulase negative staphylococci (CONS); however, it is unclear whether there was any difference in non-CONS related LOS between the two arms of the trial. Overall, the results of this study confirm that probiotics do not reduce CONS related LOS. The inability of probiotics alone to overcome the burden of LOS may relate to the presence of not only a single (gut) but multiple (endotracheal tubes, central venous catheters, TPN solutions, lipid infusions, breakdown of skin integrity etc.) sources of various pathogens (eg, CONS, gram negative organisms, fungi) in presence of frequent prolonged exposure to broad spectrum antibiotics, suboptimal enteral nutrition, and an immature innate immune system in this high-risk population.[7]

The possibility of cross contamination resulting in acquisition of probiotic strains by neonates in the placebo arm should also not be forgotten. Kitajima et al have reported colonization rates of 73% and 91% in the probiotic vs 12% and 44% in the no probiotic group neonates at 2 and 6 weeks, respectively.[8] So a third of neonates in the placebo group could potentially be exposed to probiotics, resulting in possible underestimation of real benefits. The Proprems study team plans to analyze the colonization in a small subgroup. Although NEC was the secondary outcome for which this trial did not have an adequate power, the results were consistent with earlier systematic reviews in that probiotics reduced the incidence of definite NEC by 50%. The trial results confirm that probiotics can reduce NEC even when the background incidence of the illness is low in presence of high rates of breast-milk feeding. Overall, the results of this trial provide important additional evidence supporting routine probiotic supplementation for preterm neonates.

G. Deshpande, FRACP, MSc

L. Downe, FRACP

S. Patole, DrPh, FRACP

References

1. Lin PW, Stoll BJ. Necrotising enterocolitis. *Lancet*. 2006;368:1271-1283.
2. Adams-Chapman I. Long-term impact of infection on the preterm neonate. *Semin Perinatol*. 2012;36:462-470.

3. Bisquera JA, Cooper TR, Berseth CL. Impact of necrotizing enterocolitis on length of stay and hospital charges in very low birth weight infants. *Pediatrics.* 2002;109: 423-428.
4. Deshpande G, Rao S, Patole S, Bulsara M. Updated meta-analysis of probiotics for preventing necrotizing enterocolitis in preterm neonates. *Pediatrics.* 2010;125: 921-930.
5. Alfaleh K, Anabrees J. Probiotics for prevention of necrotizing enterocolitis in preterm infants. *Cochrane Database Syst Rev.* 2014:CD005496.
6. Millar M, Wilks M, Fleming P, Costeloe K. Should the use of probiotics in the preterm be routine? *Arch Dis Child Fetal Neonatal Ed.* 2012;97:F70-F74.
7. Strunk T, Richmond P, Simmer K, Currie A, Levy O, Burgner D. Neonatal immune responses to coagulase-negative staphylococci. *Curr Opin Infect Dis.* 2007;20: 370-375.
8. Kitajima H, Sumida Y, Tanaka R, Yuki N, Takayama H, Fujimura M. Early administration of Bifidobacterium breve to preterm neonates: randomised control trial. *Arch Dis Child Fetal Neonatal Ed.* 1997;76:F101-F107.

Safety and Efficacy of Filtered Sunlight in Treatment of Jaundice in African Neonates

Slusher TM, Vreman HJ, Olusanya BO, et al (Univ of Minnesota, Minneapolis; Stanford Univ, CA; Ctr for Healthy Start Initiative, Ikoyi, Lagos, Nigeria; et al)
Pediatrics 133:e1568-e1574, 2014

Objectives.—Evaluate safety and efficacy of filtered-sunlight phototherapy (FS-PT).

Methods.—Term/late preterm infants ≤14 days old with clinically significant jaundice, assessed by total bilirubin (TB) levels, were recruited from a maternity hospital in Lagos, Nigeria. Sunlight was filtered with commercial window-tinting films that remove most UV and significant levels of infrared light and transmit effective levels of therapeutic blue light. After placing infants under an FS-PT canopy, hourly measurements of axillary temperatures, monitoring for sunburn, dehydration, and irradiances of filtered sunlight were performed. Treatment was deemed safe and efficacious if infants were able to stay in FS-PT for ≥5 hours and rate of rise of TB was ≤0.2 mg/dL/h for infants ≤72 hours of age or TB decreased for infants >72 hours of age.

Results.—A total of 227 infants received 258 days of FS-PT. No infant developed sunburn or dehydration. On 85 (33%) of 258 treatment days, infants were removed briefly from FS-PT due to minor temperature-related adverse events. No infant met study exit criteria. FS-PT was efficacious in 92% (181/197) of evaluable treatment days. Mean ± SD TB change was -0.06 ± 0.19 mg/dL/h. The mean ± SD (range) irradiance of FS-PT was 38 ± 22 (2−115) $\mu W/cm^2/nm$, measured by the BiliBlanket Meter II.

Conclusions.—With appropriate monitoring, filtered sunlight is a novel, practical, and inexpensive method of PT that potentially offers safe and efficacious treatment strategy for management of neonatal jaundice in tropical countries where conventional PT treatment is not available.

▶ In the United States and the rest of the world's higher income countries, turning on the "bilirubin lights" to deliver phototherapy is a daily occurrence, But in low- and middle-income countries, where lack of appropriate equipment and an unpredictable supply of electricity often preclude the use of phototherapy, calling on nature in the form of sunshine is the only available alternative for treating the severely jaundiced newborn. To this end, doctors Vreman and Slusher have been working for some time to develop a system that uses sunshine in a practical, inexpensive, safe, and effective way to deliver phototherapy to jaundiced newborns, and this study shows that they have succeeded.

In their original description of phototherapy, Cremer et al,[1] in addition to designing their own phototherapy unit, exposed 13 infants to sunlight for an average of 2.5 hours. This produced a decrease in the total serum bilirubin (TSB) level from 17.4 mg/dL to 13.5 mg/dL, a response that is as good or better than can be achieved with current intensive phototherapy systems. Salih[2] exposed bilirubin solutions to sunlight and demonstrated an 80% reduction in bilirubin levels within 30 minutes.

Commercially available window tinting films filter out virtually all of the ultraviolet (UV)-B and UV-A radiation and therefore avoid sunburn, yet they allow sufficient penetration of the wavelengths responsible for isomerizing bilirubin to provide effective phototherapy. Exposing infants to this filtered sunlight (Fig 1 in the original article), Slusher et al were able to prevent the TSB rising by ≥ 0.2 mg/dL per hour in infants less than 72 hours old and could achieve a decline in the TSB in infants > 72 hours old.

If sunlight works in this manner, why does the American Academy of Pediatrics[3] (AAP) discourage pediatricians from recommending this treatment for our newborns? The AAP does this for 2 reasons: the first is that this advice has often been given to parents of a jaundiced neonate, without appropriate monitoring of TSB levels, in the belief that this exposure will take care of the problem. In some cases, the TSB has continued to rise while the parents are falsely reassured that everything is under control. The second and more important reason is that, in northern climes, it is almost impossible to operationalize this advice. The Nigerian infants were placed naked in the filtered sun but, during most of the year, this cannot be done in most parts of North America and Europe, and the advice to "expose the infant to sun" leads to a fully clothed and blanketed infant being placed near a window, an intervention that will not affect the bilirubin level.

Of course no system is perfect, and the vicissitudes of the weather, even in Nigeria, will determine just how often and how effectively this treatment can be used. Nevertheless, over a period of 243 days, the average irradiance ranged from 8 to 65 μW/cm^2/nm, sufficient to provide adequate, if not always intensive, phototherapy. The investigators also note that they have not yet tested this in a group of infants with higher bilirubin levels.

I congratulate Drs Slusher, Vreman, and colleagues for this important study. There is no reason why similar phototherapy systems cannot be developed and used in many other parts of the equatorial world, where the ready availability of sunshine can be used to treat jaundiced newborns. A randomized Nigerian trial is ongoing, and we look forward to the results of that study.

M. J. Maisels, MB, BCh, DSc

References

1. Cremer RJ, Perryman PW, Richards DH. Influence of light on the hyperbilirubinemia of infants. *Lancet.* 1958;1:1094-1097.
2. Salih FM. Can sunlight replace phototherapy units in the treatment of neonatal jaundice? An *in vitro* study. *Photodermatol Photoimmunol Photomed.* 2001;17: 272-277.
3. Maisels MJ, Baltz RD, Bhutani V, et al. Management of hyperbilirubinemia in the newborn infant 35 or more weeks of gestation. *Pediatrics.* 2004;114:297-316.

Bilirubin Uridine Diphosphate-Glucuronosyltransferase Variation Is a Genetic Basis of Breast Milk Jaundice

Maruo Y, Morioka Y, Fujito H, et al (Shiga Univ of Med Science, Otsu, Japan; Hanwasumiyoshin General Hosp, Osaka, Japan; Hino Memorial Hosp, Kozukeda, Japan; et al)
J Pediatr 165:36-41, 2014

Objective.—To evaluate the role of bilirubin *UDP-glucuronosyltransferase family 1, polypeptide A1 (UGT1A1)* gene variations on prolonged unconjugated hyperbilirubinemia associated with breast milk feeding (breast milk jaundice [BMJ]).

Study Design.—*UGT1A1* gene allelic variation was analyzed in 170 Japanese infants with BMJ with polymerase chain reaction-direct sequencing, and their genotypes compared with serum bilirubin concentrations. In 62 of 170 infants, serum bilirubin concentration was followed after 4 months of life. Genotypes were examined in 55 infants without BMJ.

Results.—Of 170 infants with BMJ, 88 (51.8%) were homozygous *UGT1A1*6.* Serum bilirubin concentrations (21.8 ± 3.65 mg/dL) were significantly greater than in infants with other genotypes ($P < .0001$). The Gilbert *UGT1A1*28* allele was not detected in infants with BMJ, except in an infant who was compound heterozygous with *UGT1A1*6.* At 4 months of age, serum bilirubin concentration improved to >1 mg/ dL, except in 2 infants who were homozygous *UGT1A1*7.* Homozygous *UGT1A1*6* was not detected in the control group.

Conclusion.—One-half of the infants with BMJ were homozygous *UGT1A1*6* and exhibited a serum bilirubin concentration significantly greater than other genotypes. This finding indicates that *UGT1A1*6* is a major cause of BMJ in infants in East Asia. Previous finding have demonstrated that 5β-pregnane-3α,20β-diol present in breast milk inhibits p.G71R-UGT1A1 bilirubin glucuronidation activity. Thus, prolonged unconjugated hyperbilirubinemia may develop in infants with *UGT1A1*6* who are fed breast milk.

▶ Breast milk jaundice was introduced as a clinical diagnosis in 1963 by Newman and Gross[1] based on a report of 5 exclusively breastfed newborns who were compared with those who were also supplemented with cow's milk. In the subsequent landmark study that linked the diagnosis to decreased UDP-glucuronosyltransferase (UGT) activity, Arias et al[2] described a syndrome of severe and a prolonged unconjugated hyperbilirubinemia associated with breastfeeding in 7 full-term, unrelated newborn infants. Curiously, the study cohort included "3 Jewish, 2 Italian, 1 Negro, and 1 Chinese mothers."[2] A case report in the *New England Journal of Medicine*[3] coined the phrase "breast milk jaundice."

Over the years, this term was clinically overused to include any jaundice in breastfed infants such that Newman et al[4] reported an odds ratio of 6 for severe hyperbilirubinemia as clinical risk factor for any exclusively breastfed infant. Winfield and Macfaul[5] challenged the prevailing impression that prolonged unconjugated jaundice (PUJ) and breast milk jaundice were more common. In their study of 893 births, the incidence of PUJ was 2.4% in all breastfed infants compared with 0% in bottle-fed infants. In most of their cohort, the jaundice faded while the infants were still being breastfed. Gourley et al[6] demonstrated that the key factor in cow's milk was not just the effect of casein but that both L-aspartic acid and enzymatically hydrolyzed casein act as competitive beta-glucuronidase inhibitors and promote bilirubin elimination through prevention of enterohepatic circulation of bilirubin.

Jaundice persisting beyond age 14 days, often in combination with late prematurity, may be a sign of "breast milk jaundice," sustained bruising, unrecognized hemolysis (eg, glucose-6-phosphate dehydrogenase [G6PD] deficiency, ABO incompatibility, Rh disease), hypothyroidism, urosepsis, and inborn errors of metabolism including galactosemia and Crigler Najjar syndromes. Recently, Gundur et al[7] attempted to define the natural history of PUJ in 66 infants who were cared for in northern India. Of these, 42% were preterm, and 40% were small for gestational age (SGA); 82% were exclusively breastfed, and 72% were male or had a history of a sibling with PUJ. Concurrent inciting factors included G6PD deficiency (27%) and blood group incompatibilities (16.5%). As a follow-up, 1 infant died, but in most, the outcome was benign and associated with a disappearance of jaundice between 5 and 8 weeks of age. The mean peak total bilirubin (TB) levels were 15.8 ± 4.3 mg/dL. In a more recent study, Bhutani et al[8] have reported that by age 14 days, the 95th and 99th percentile for TB is 14.4 and 17.2 mg/dL, respectively. It is to be noted that PUJ was not fully characterized for a substantial number of the infants.

Genetic considerations regarding the delayed resolution and higher than expected peak TB levels is a fertile area of inquiry. It is in the context of this background that the report by Maruo et al serves as a seminal contribution. Their study demonstrated a causal relationship between infants with PUJ (who were exclusively breastfed) and homozygosity for UGT1A1*6. Using

TABLE 1.—Differences in UGT1A1 Genotypes Between Infants with and Without BMJ

| Genotype | | Infants with BMJ, | | Infants without BMJ, | |
Allele 1	Allele 2	n = 170	%	n = 55	%
UGT1A1*6	*UGT1A1*6*	88	51.7	0	0
UGT1A1*6	*UGT1A1*60*	23	13.5	2	3.6
UGT1A1*6	*UGT1A1*1*	26	15.2	15	27.2
UGT1A1*6	*UGT1A1*28*	1	0.58	3	5.4
UGT1A1*28	*UGT1A1*28*	0	0	1	1.8
UGT1A1*28	*UGT1A1*60*	0	0	2	3.6
UGT1A1*28	*UGT1A1*1*	0	0	7	12.7
UGT1A1*60	*UGT1A1*60*	4	2.3	1	1.8
UGT1A1*60	*UGT1A1*1*	5	2.9	7	12.7
UGT1A1*1	*UGT1A1*1*	8	4.7	17	30.9
Other	Other*	15	9.4	0	0

UGT1A1*1, wild-type allele; UGT1A1*6, pG71R; UGT1A1*28, c.-3279T>G+A(TA)7TAA; UGT1A1*60, c.-3279T>G.
*Other/other genotype in the BMJ group includes homozygous for p.Y486D (UGT1A1*7) (3 cases), compound heterozygous for UGT1A1*6 and UGT1A1*7 (4 cases), compound heterozygous for UGT1A1*60 and c.-3279T>G+p.P364L (UGT1A1*63) (2 cases), compound heterozygous for UGT1A1*6 and UGT1A1*63 (1 case), heterozygous for p.A471V (c.1412C>T) (1 case), homozygous UGT1A1*63 (1 case), UGT1A1*6/p.[G71R;Y486D] (2 cases), and UGT1A1*7/ p.[G71R;Y486D] (1 case).

Reprinted from Journal Pediatrics. Maruo Y, Morioka Y, Fujito H, et al. Bilirubin Uridine Diphosphate-Glucuronosyltransferase Variation Is a Genetic Basis of Breast Milk Jaundice. J Pediatr. 2014;165:36-41, Copyright 2014, with permission from Elsevier.

polymerase chain reaction—directed sequencing, they analyzed the allelic variations of the UGT1A1 gene in 170 Japanese infants. They designated a control group of 55 infants UGT1A1 genotypes that did not have the phenotypic manifestations of PUJ. Homozygous UGT1A1*6 infants were not detected in this control group. Fifty-two percent of infants with UGT1A1 genotypes with phenotypic manifestations of PUJ were homozygous for UGT1A1*6 (Table 1). This subset of infants had significant hyperbilirubinemia (TB = 21.8 ± 3.65 mg/dL). These values were greater than in infants with other genotypes (Table 2 in the original article).

The authors' conclusion that UGT1A1*6 is a major cause of breast milk jaundice in infants in East Asia is consistent with observations in reports from other investigators. In infants of other ethnic backgrounds, Gilbert syndrome (OMIM#143500) has been recognized as a heterogeneous group of disorders that exhibit < 50% of hepatic UGT activity.

Our understanding of the UGT1A1 gene (which encodes bilirubin, phenol, uridine diphosphate glucuronosyltransferase isoenzymes) led to the recognition of mutations or polymorphisms of UGT1A1 being associated with this group of disorders. In Caucasians, the homozygous finding of an additional TA repeat in the promoter region was linked to Gilbert syndrome. Here, in the TATA box, the (TA)7TAA rather than (TA)6TAA of the UGT1A1 gene was necessary for the Gilbert designation. Individuals who are heterozygous for 7 TA repeats had higher TB levels than infants with the homozygous wild-type 6 TA repeats. In Asian populations, (TA)7TAA mutations are rare; however, mutations involving the exon 1 of the UGT1A1 gene most commonly present as Gly71Arg mutation (known as UGT1A1*6). In a nested study of North Indian babies, Agrawal et al[9] observed that the incidence of the variant (TA)n polymorphism was higher in hyperbilirubinemic infants (TB $\geq$ 18 mg/dL) with an allele frequency of 49.7%; none were identified as having UGT1A1*6 mutations. These authors also identified a novel polymorphism (Ala72Pro) at codon position 72 of exon 1 of the UGT1A1 gene, but it was unrelated to hyperbilirubinemia. Kaplan et al[10] have reported a significant superimposition of (TA)n promoter variants in infants with G6PD deficiency and shown an allele dose-dependent response for severe hyperbilirubinemia. In combination with clinical risk factors, these superimposed genotypes may result in an unpredictable phenotype of fulminant and rapidly rising TB levels.

The Maruo et al study provides the evidentiary basis to expand the inquiry for a spectrum of genetic disorders that lead to PUJ as well as to commence the retirement of "breast milk jaundice" as a clinical diagnosis. Whether breast milk intake leads to an unmasking of an underlying genetic disorder or the use of beta-glucuronidase inhibitors in casein, the optimization of UGT activities remains a clinical conundrum in the management of PUJ. Nevertheless, it is time to refrain from using the term "breast milk jaundice" as a clinical disorder.

V. K. Bhutani, MD, FAAP

R. J. Wong

References

1. Newman AJ, Gross S. Hyperbilirubinemia in breast-fed infants. *Pediatrics*. 1963; 32:995-1001.
2. Arias IM, Gartner LM, Seifter S. Neonatal unconjugated hyperbilirubinemia associated with breast-feeding and a factor in milk that inhibits glucuronide formation *in vitro*. *J Clin Invest*. 1963;42:913.
3. Katz HP, Robinson TA. Breast-milk hyperbilirubinemia: report of a case. *N Engl J Med*. 1965;273:546-547.
4. Newman TB, Xiong B, Gonzales VM, Escobar GJ. Prediction and prevention of extreme neonatal hyperbilirubinemia in a mature health maintenance organization. *Arch Pediatr Adolesc Med*. 2000;154:1140-1147.
5. Winfield CR, MacFaul R. Clinical study of prolonged jaundice in breast- and bottle-fed babies. *Arch Dis Child*. 1978;53:506-507.
6. Gourley GR, Li Z, Kreamer BL, Kosorok MR. A controlled, randomized, double-blind trial of prophylaxis against jaundice among breastfed newborns. *Pediatrics*. 2005;116:385-391.
7. Gundur NM, Kumar P, Sundaram V, Thapa BR, Narang A. Natural history and predictive risk factors of prolonged unconjugated jaundice in the newborn. *Pediatr Int*. 2010;52:769-772.
8. Bhutani VK, Wong RJ. Bilirubin neurotoxicity in preterm infants: risk and prevention. *J Clin Neonatol*. 2013;2:61-69.
9. Agrawal SK, Kumar P, Rathi R, et al. UGT1A1 gene polymorphisms in North Indian neonates presenting with unconjugated hyperbilirubinemia. *Pediatr Res*. 2009;65:675-680.
10. Kaplan M, Renbaum P, Levy-Lahad E, Hammerman C, Lahad A, Beutler E. Gilbert syndrome and glucose-6-phosphate dehydrogenase deficiency: a dose-dependent genetic interaction crucial to neonatal hyperbilirubinemia. *Proc Natl Acad Sci U S A*. 1997;94:12128-12132.

In-Hospital Formula Use Increases Early Breastfeeding Cessation Among First-Time Mothers Intending to Exclusively Breastfeed

Chantry CJ, Dewey KG, Peerson JM, et al (Univ of California Davis Med Ctr, Sacramento; Univ of California Davis; et al)

J Pediatr 164:1339-1345.e5, 2014

Objective.—To evaluate in-hospital formula supplementation among first-time mothers who intended to exclusively breastfeed and determined if in-hospital formula supplementation shortens breastfeeding duration after adjusting for breastfeeding intention.

Study Design.—We assessed strength of breastfeeding intentions prenatally in a diverse cohort of expectant primiparae and followed infant feeding practices through day 60. Among mothers planning to exclusively breastfeed their healthy term infants for ≥ 1 week, we determined predictors, reasons, and characteristics of in-hospital formula supplementation, and calculated the intention-adjusted relative risk (ARR) of not fully breastfeeding days 30-60 and breastfeeding cessation by day 60 with in-hospital formula supplementation (n = 393).

Results.—Two hundred ten (53%) infants were exclusively breastfed during the maternity stay and 183 (47%) received in-hospital formula supplementation. The most prevalent reasons mothers cited for in-hospital formula supplementation were: perceived insufficient milk supply (18%), signs of inadequate intake (16%), and poor latch or breastfeeding (14%). Prevalence of not fully breastfeeding days 30-60 was 67.8% vs 36.7%, ARR 1.8 (95% CI, 1.4-2.3), in-hospital formula supplementation vs exclusively breastfed groups, respectively, and breastfeeding cessation by day 60 was 32.8% vs 10.5%, ARR 2.7 (95% CI, 1.7-4.5). Odds of both adverse outcomes increased with more in-hospital formula supplementation feeds (not fully breastfeeding days 30-60, $P = .003$ and breastfeeding cessation, $P = .011$).

Conclusions.—Among women intending to exclusively breastfeed, in-hospital formula supplementation was associated with a nearly 2-fold greater risk of not fully breastfeeding days 30-60 and a nearly 3-fold risk of breastfeeding cessation by day 60, even after adjusting for strength of breastfeeding intentions. Strategies should be sought to avoid unnecessary in-hospital formula supplementation and to support breastfeeding when in-hospital formula supplementation is unavoidable.

▶ Formula use during the birth hospitalization is a compelling area of research because formula use can be both a cause and a result of early breastfeeding problems. On the one hand, feeding formula can satiate newborns so that they have reduced interest in breastfeeding. Additionally, using a bottle to feed formula may cause nipple confusion so that newborns can no longer latch well at the breast.[1] On the other hand, mothers who have problems with breastfeeding such as pain or difficulty latching their infants may be more likely to have excess weight loss and use formula.[2] Thus formula use can both cause and be caused by breastfeeding problems, leading to a lack of definitive evidence about the risks associated with early formula.[3]

In this article, Chantry et al begin to disentangle these causal relationships. In confirmation of previous observational research, the authors report that using formula during the birth hospitalization is associated with 3 times the risk of breastfeeding cessation before 2 months of age. In this cohort, adjusting for the strength of maternal breastfeeding intention did not substantially affect the risk of cessation. However, the authors also report that the 2 most common reasons for formula supplementation were maternal perception of inadequate milk supply and signs of inadequate infant intake (Table 3).

Of note, whether the formula was used because of maternal preference or because of clinician recommendation had no predictive value for breastfeeding cessation. Higher volumes of formula feedings more strongly predicted breastfeeding cessation and that the use of a bottle interfered with breastfeeding much more than an alternate method such as a syringe or cup for feeding.

This study provides confirmatory evidence that in-hospital formula use is a strong predictor of breastfeeding problems and provides important new information on the risks of higher volume feeding and the use of a bottle. However, the available data did not allow the authors to assess the effect of breastfeeding difficulties on the decision to use formula and the duration of breastfeeding. Mothers whose babies breastfeed easily without causing pain may be less likely to use formula and more likely to continue breastfeeding, whereas mothers who have pain or have difficulty in latching or difficulty with newborn weight loss may be less likely to continue breastfeeding.

In addition, because this study analyzed only predictors available during the birth hospitalization, the authors were unable to report whether discouraging

TABLE 3.—Main Categories and Prevalence of Maternally Reported Reasons for in-Hospital Formula Supplementation*

Main Category	Prevalence (%) of Main Category[†,‡]			
	0-24 h	24-48 h	48-72 h	Overall 0-72 h
Low maternal supply	7.4	13.7	16.4	18.1
Signs of inadequate infant intake (eg, excess weight loss, hypoglycemia)	6.3	10.1	21.7	16.3
Poor infant breastfeeding behavior	6.6	8.8	14.6	13.7
Separation of dyad	6.6	2.3	4.0	9.4
Psychosocial reasons	2.8	3.6	3.5	5.3
Breastfeeding pain	0.5	3.1	4.4	4.1
Maternal incapacitation	2.8	1.0	1.3	3.6
Maternal medication	0.8	0.8	1.3	1.5

*Mothers (n = 393) were asked at the day 3 interview to provide reasons for formula supplementation (if any) for each 24-hour interval since birth. Reasons for formula supplementation were missing for 4 mothers whose babies received in-hospital formula supplementation, resulting in n = 389 mothers with complete in-hospital formula supplementation reason data.

†Number of mothers reporting a reason under specified category at each time interval/number of mothers in the hospital at each time interval: n = 112/393, 0-24 h; N = 142/388, 24-48 h; n = 117/226, 48-72 h; n = 179/393, overall 0-72 h.

‡Mothers could give multiple reasons in their open-ended response, and some reasons were coded under more than 1 main category.

Reprinted from Journal Pediatrics. Chantry CJ, Dewey KG, Peerson JM, et al. In-Hospital Formula Use Increases Early Breastfeeding Cessation Among First-Time Mothers Intending to Exclusively Breastfeed. J Pediatr. 2014;164:1339-1345.e5, Copyright 2014, with permission from Elsevier.

formula use during the birth hospitalization may have sometimes resulted in delayed formula use after discharge from the birth hospitalization or on whether delayed formula use was an effective method preventing breastfeeding cessation. It is possible that formula use delayed until after discharge from the birth hospitalization might have interfered with the successful establishment of breastfeeding even more than formula use during the birth hospitalization.

A main challenge of research in this area is that although some mothers may worry about milk supply even though their baby is feeding well and their milk supply is adequate, others may be noting subtle cues from their infant and their own bodies that breast milk production is inadequate. In some cases, maternal formula use may represent a correct maternal impression that the baby is not receiving enough intake.[4] Currently, physicians and researchers alike are often unable to tell the difference. Pre- and postfeeding weights on a research-quality scale can be helpful in describing milk transfer, but these are time-consuming to obtain and are often not available. Measuring breast milk sodium has the potential to further characterize the copiousness of maternal milk supply, but further research is needed to validate this as a predictor of adequate milk supply. In addition, future studies should consider comparing the effect of in-hospital formula supplementation with that of formula supplementation delayed until shortly after hospital discharge. If formula is eventually necessary to prevent dehydration, it may be better to begin formula use early and discontinue it once mature milk is available than to wait until signs of dehydration develop and the infant needs to be rescued from dehydration by formula.[5]

V. Flaherman, MD, MPH

References

1. Neifert M, Lawrence R, Seacat J. Nipple confusion: toward a formal definition. *J Pediatr.* 1995;126(6):S125-129.
2. Dewey KG, Nommsen-Rivers LA, Heinig MJ, Cohen RJ. Risk factors for suboptimal infant breastfeeding behavior, delayed onset of lactation, and excess neonatal weight loss. *Pediatrics.* 2003;112(3 Pt 1):607-619.
3. Becker GE, Remmington S, Remmington T. Early additional food and fluids for healthy breastfed full-term infants. *Cochrane Database Syst Rev.*12:CD006462.
4. Hill PD. The enigma of insufficient milk supply. *MCN Am J Matern Child Nurs.* 1991;16(6):312-316.
5. Flaherman VJ, Aby J, Burgos AE, Lee KA, Cabana MD, Newman TB. Effect of early limited formula on duration and exclusivity of breastfeeding in at-risk infants: an RCT. *Pediatrics.* 2013;131(6):1059-1065.

Microbial Contamination of Human Milk Purchased Via the Internet
Keim SA, Hogan JS, McNamara KA, et al (The Res Inst at Nationwide Children's Hosp, Columbus, OH; The Ohio State Univ, Columbus, OH; et al)
Pediatrics 132:e1227-e1235, 2013

Objective.—To quantify microbial contamination of human milk purchased via the Internet as an indicator of disease risk to recipient infants.

Methods.—Cross-sectional sample of human milk purchased via a popular US milk-sharing Web site (2012). Individuals advertising milk were contacted to arrange purchase, and milk was shipped to a rented mailbox in Ohio. The Internet milk samples ($n = 101$) were compared with unpasteurized samples of milk donated to a milk bank ($n = 20$).

Results.—Most (74%) Internet milk samples were colonized with Gramnegative bacteria or had $>10^4$ colony-forming units/mL total aerobic count. They exhibited higher mean total aerobic, total Gram-negative, coliform, and *Staphylococcus* sp counts than milk bank samples. Growth of most species was positively associated with days in transit (total aerobic count [$\log_{10}$ colony-forming units/mL] $\beta = 0.71$ [95% confidence interval: 0.38−1.05]), and negatively associated with number of months since the milk was expressed ($\beta = -0.36$ [95% confidence interval: -0.55 to -0.16]), per simple linear regression. No samples were HIV type 1 RNA-positive; 21% of Internet samples were cytomegalovirus DNA-positive.

Conclusions.—Human milk purchased via the Internet exhibited high overall bacterial growth and frequent contamination with pathogenic bacteria, reflecting poor collection, storage, or shipping practices. Infants consuming this milk are at risk for negative outcomes, particularly if born preterm or are medically compromised. Increased use of lactation support services may begin to address the milk supply gap for women who want to feed their child human milk but cannot meet his or her needs.

▶ Human milk sharing via the Internet is increasingly popular but may be dangerous for infants and children. Milk-sharing websites abound (for example, "Eats on Feets" and "Human milk for human babies—or HM4HB)"[1,2] connecting mothers with an abundant supply of nonpasteurized donor milk to those seeking milk for their child. Some individuals even advertise their milk using terms such as "safest" or "best quality." Both the US Food and Drug Administration and the American Academy of Pediatrics strongly recommend against this practice.[3,4]

Pediatricians must be aware that this recent phenomenon of casual milk sharing exists and that there are remarkable infectious risks associated with this practice. In contradistinction, human milk donated to and dispensed by human milk banks in the United States is pasteurized. The pasteurization process used by US milk banks eradicates all the harmful bacteria and viruses in the donated milk, including cytomegalovirus (CMV), hepatitis B virus (HBV), and human immunodeficiency virus (HIV). In addition, US human milk banks screen all of their milk donors with serological testing for HBV and HIV.[5]

In this article, investigators from several academic institutions in Ohio provide data describing high rates of pathogenic bacterial contamination found in human milk purchased via the Internet. Compared with milk donated to a local human milk bank, the Internet-acquired samples had much higher colony counts of Gram-negative coliforms and *Staphylococcus* species (Table 1 in the original article).

In addition, 21% of purchased samples were CMV DNA-positive compared with only 5% of the milk bank samples (Fisher's exact test $P = .12$). All milk samples were expressed outside of the clinical setting and handled and stored in the home environment. However, samples from milk bank donors differed in that these mothers were instructed on hygienic milk collection and storage techniques and optimal shipping procedures, such as overnight shipping on dry ice. Purchased Internet-acquired milk samples often arrived completely thawed or warm.

The majority of the Internet-acquired milk samples showed high overall bacterial growth and frequent contamination, reflecting poor collection, storage and, or shipping practices. The rates of bacterial isolation of *Salmonella* species, coliforms (lactose-fermenting Gram-negative bacteria), other Gram-negative bacteria, and *Streptococcus* and *Staphylococcus* species ranged widely, from 3% to 72% of Internet-acquired milk samples. Rates of similar bacterial isolation from milk bank samples (before pasteurization) were much lower, ranging from 0% to 35%. The Internet samples had contamination rates predicted by time-in-transit and the age of the milk. Information that Internet milk sellers conveyed in their advertisements about their health and behaviors were poor indicators of milk quality.

When advocating for breastfeeding and feeding human milk to babies, pediatricians need to explain to new mothers the hazards of acquiring donor milk via the Internet. They should advise strongly against this practice and instruct interested mothers to seek donor milk, or to donate their excess milk, only in conjunction with established US human milk banks. For example, on its website (https://www.hmbana.org) the Human Milk Banking Association of North America lists contact information for member milk banks and describes procedures and practices used to screen donors and collect, store, pasteurize, and transport donor milk, all at no cost to donor mothers.

S. Landers, MD

References

1. Eats on Feets Community Breastmilk Sharing. http://www.eatsonfeets.org/. Accessed July 27, 2014.
2. Human Milk 4 Human Babies. Informed Milksharing Network. http://hm4hb.net/. Accessed July 27, 2014.
3. United States Food and Drug Administration. Use of Donor Human Milk. http://www.fda.gov/ScienceResearch/SpecialTopics/PediatricTherapeuticsResearch/ucm235203.htm. Accessed July 28, 2014.
4. American Academy of Pediatrics, Section on Breastfeeding. Breastfeeding and the use of human milk. *Pediatrics.* 2012;129:e827-e841.
5. Landers S, Hartman BT. Donor human milk banking and the emergence of milk sharing. *Pediatr Clin North Am.* 2013;60:247-260.

Effects of Home Visits by Paraprofessionals and by Nurses on Children: Follow-up of a Randomized Trial at Ages 6 and 9 Years
Olds DL, Holmberg JR, Donelan-McCall N, et al (Univ of Colorado Denver, Aurora; et al)
JAMA Pediatr 168:114-121, 2014

Importance.—The Nurse-Family Partnership delivered by nurses has been found to produce long-term effects on maternal and child health in replicated randomized trials. A persistent question is whether paraprofessional home visitors might produce comparable effects.

Objective.—To examine the impact of prenatal and infancy/toddler home visits by paraprofessionals and by nurses on child development at child ages 6 and 9 years.

Design, Setting, and Participants.—Randomized trial in public and private care settings in Denver, Colorado, of 735 low-income women and their first-born children (85% of the mothers were unmarried; 47% were Hispanic, 35% were non-Hispanic white, 15% were African American, and 3% were American Indian/Asian).

Interventions.—Home visits provided from pregnancy through child age 2 years delivered in one group by paraprofessionals and in the other by nurses.

Main Outcomes and Measures.—Reports of children's internalizing, externalizing, and total emotional/behavioral problems, and tests of children's language, intelligence, attention, attention dysfunction, visual attention/task switching, working memory, and academic achievement. We hypothesized that program effects on cognitive-related outcomes would be more pronounced among children born to mothers with low psychological resources. We report paraprofessional-control and nurse-control differences with $P < .10$ given similar effects in a previous trial, earlier effects in this trial, and limited statistical power.

Results.—There were no significant paraprofessional effects on emotional/behavioral problems, but paraprofessional-visited children born to mothers with low psychological resources compared with control group counterparts exhibited fewer errors in visual attention/task switching at age 9 years (effect size $= -0.30$, $P = .08$). There were no statistically significant paraprofessional effects on other primary outcomes. Nurse-visited children were less likely to be classified as having total emotional/behavioral problems at age 6 years (relative risk [RR] $= 0.45$, $P = .08$), internalizing problems at age 9 years (RR $= 0.44$, $P = .08$), and dysfunctional attention at age 9 years (RR $= 0.34$, $P = .07$). Nurse-visited children born to low-resource mothers compared with control-group counterparts had better receptive language averaged over ages 2, 4, and 6 years (effect size $= 0.30$, $P = .01$) and sustained attention averaged over ages 4, 6, and 9 years (effect size $= 0.36$, $P = .006$). There were no significant nurse effects on externalizing problems, intellectual functioning, and academic achievement.

Conclusions and Relevance.—Children born to low-resource mothers visited by paraprofessionals exhibited improvement in visual attention/task switching. Nurse-visited children showed improved behavioral functioning, and those born to low-resource mothers benefited in language and attention but did not improve in intellectual functioning and academic achievement.

Trial Registration.—clinicaltrials.gov Identifier: NCT00438282 and NCT00438594.

▶ This new paper by Olds and colleagues adds to 3 decades of scientific evidence he has led on the benefits of early-life home visitation for maternal–child outcomes. Indeed, the innovative Nurse Family Partnership (NFP) program, which visits low-income women during pregnancy and follows mother–infant pairs through age 2 years, has served as much of the justification for the Maternal Infant and Early Childhood Home Visiting Program (MIECHVP) funded under the Patient Protection and Affordable Care Act.

The current article describes outcomes at child ages 6 and 9 years of a 3-arm trial in which primiparous women were randomized to receive either postnatal child developmental screening through age 2 years, such screening plus regular home visitation from paraprofessional visitors who shared social characteristics of the families, or such screening plus home visitation from registered nurses. Although modest benefits were shown for paraprofessional-visited children of mothers with low psychological resources compared with controls, the results were more impressive for those visited by nurses, a finding seen in previous trials. Nurse-visited children had fewer emotional/behavioral problems, internalizing problems, and dysfunctional attention, although with no long-term improvement in intellectual functioning or academic achievement.

Perinatal home visitation programs have been used domestically and abroad since as early as the 1800s. In England, for example, a program was initiated in the 1850s to promote cleanliness for newborns as a means to control epidemics.[1] Since that time, many models of perinatal visitation programs have been proposed with the majority of the efforts focused on a multivisit model that encompasses both prenatal and postnatal visitation. The NFP program is the most well-known model, having demonstrated for mothers improved knowledge about contraception, fewer subsequent pregnancies, and more time between subsequent pregnancies.[2–5] Their infants also have fewer emergency department visits, unintentional injuries, ingestions, and poisonings.[4,6,7] Similarly, there is a reduced incidence of child abuse and neglect in those infants participating in such programs.[3,6,8] Importantly, this model of home visitation, although initially expensive, has been proven to be highly cost-effective over time, with actual significant savings because participants are less likely over time to require government-based financial assistance programs.[9]

Although these collective results are impressive, a provocative editorial accompanied the new article.[10] Shonkoff highlighted that most early-life intervention programs do not match the intensity of the NFP and are not evidence-based. Furthermore, the evidence base for most early-life programs to improve long-term behavioral and educational outcomes is thin, yet cries for investment in early childhood programs are common. Minkovitz et al. responded to this editorial with a letter describing how the MIECHVP is addressing the evidence gap through state evaluations conducted as part of the MIECHVP, national evaluation of the MIECHVP, and a Home Visiting Research Network.[11] This approach hopefully will build on the findings of Olds and colleagues to advance knowledge, but, most important, to improve the lives of underprivileged mothers and their children.

I. M. Paul, MD, MSc

References

1. Kamerman SB, Kahn AJ. Home health visiting in Europe. *Future Child*. 1993;3: 39-52.
2. Olds DL. Home visitation for pregnant women and parents of young children. *Am J Dis Child*. 1992;146:704-708.
3. Olds DL, Eckenrode J, Henderson CR Jr, et al. Long-term effects of home visitation on maternal life course and child abuse and neglect. Fifteen-year follow-up of a randomized trial. *JAMA*. 1997;278:637-643.
4. Kitzman H, Olds DL, Henderson CR Jr, et al. Effect of prenatal and infancy home visitation by nurses on pregnancy outcomes, childhood injuries, and repeated childbearing. A randomized controlled trial. *JAMA*. 1997;278:644-652.
5. Olds DL, Robinson J, O'Brien R, et al. Home visiting by paraprofessionals and by nurses: a randomized, controlled trial. *Pediatrics*. 2002;110:486-496.
6. Olds DL, Henderson CR Jr, Chamberlin R, Tatelbaum R. Preventing child abuse and neglect: a randomized trial of nurse home visitation. *Pediatrics*. 1986;78: 65-78.
7. Olds DL, Henderson CR Jr, Kitzman H. Does prenatal and infancy nurse home visitation have enduring effects on qualities of parental caregiving and child health at 25 to 50 months of life? *Pediatrics*. 1994;93:89-98.
8. Eckenrode J, Ganzel B, Henderson CR Jr, et al. Preventing child abuse and neglect with a program of nurse home visitation: the limiting effects of domestic violence. *JAMA*. 2000;284:1385-1391.
9. Olds DL, Henderson CR Jr, Phelps C, Kitzman H, Hanks C. Effect of prenatal and infancy nurse home visitation on government spending. *Med Care*. 1993; 31:155-174.
10. Shonkoff JP. Changing the narrative for early childhood investment. *JAMA Pediatr*. 2014;168:105-106.
11. Minkovitz CS, O'Neill KM, Duggan AK. Home visiting narrative: rewrite is in progress. *JAMA Pediatr*. 2014;168:584-585.

15 Nutrition and Metabolism

Day-patient treatment after short inpatient care versus continued inpatient treatment in adolescents with anorexia nervosa (ANDI): a multicentre, randomised, open-label, non-inferiority trial

Herpertz-Dahlmann B, Schwarte R, Krei M, et al (Univ Hosp of the RWTH Aachen, Germany; et al)

Lancet 383:1222-1229, 2014

Background.—In-patient treatment (IP) is the treatment setting of choice for moderately-to-severely ill adolescents with anorexia nervosa, but it is costly, and the risks of relapse and readmissions are high. Day patient treatment (DP) is less expensive and might avoid problems of relapse and readmission by easing the transition from hospital to home. We investigated the safety and efficacy of DP after short inpatient care compared with continued IP.

Methods.—For this multicentre, randomised, open-label, non-inferiority trial, we enrolled female patients (aged 11–18 years) with anorexia nervosa from six centres in Germany. Patients were eligible if they had a body-mass index (BMI) below the tenth percentile and it was their first admission to hospital for anorexia nervosa. We used a computer generated randomisation sequence to randomly assign patients to continued IP or DP after 3 weeks of inpatient care (1:1; stratified for age and BMI at admission). The treatment programme and treatment intensity in both study groups were identical. The primary outcome was the increase in BMI between the time of admission and a 12-month follow-up adjusted for age and duration of illness (non-inferiority margin of $0 \cdot 75$ kg/m^2). Analysis was done by modified intention to treat. This trial is registered with the International Standard Randomised Controlled Trial Number Register, number ISRCTN67783402, and the Deutsches Register Klinischer Studien, number DRKS00000101.

Findings.—Between Feb 2, 2007, to April 27, 2010, we screened 660 patients for eligibility, 172 of whom we randomly allocated to treatment: 85 to IP and 87 to DP. DP was non-inferior to IP with respect to the primary outcome, BMI at the 12-month follow-up (mean difference $0 \cdot 46$ kg/m^2 in favour of DP (95% CI, $-0 \cdot 11$ to $1 \cdot 02$; $p_{\text{non-inferiority}} < 0 \cdot 0001$). The number of treatment-related serious adverse events was similar in both study groups (eight in the IP group, seven in the DP group). Three serious adverse

events in the IP group and two in the DP group were related to suicidal idea-
tion; one patient in the DP attempted suicide 3 months after she was
discharged.

Interpretation.—DP after short inpatient care in adolescent patients
with non-chronic anorexia nervosa seems no less effective than IP for
weight restoration and maintenance during the first year after admission.
Thus, DP might be a safe and less costly alternative to IP. Our results justify the broad implementation of this approach.

▶ Anorexia nervosa (AN) is a serious psychiatric disorder with high rates of
psychiatric and medical morbidity and has one of the highest mortality rates
among psychiatric disorders. Identifying efficacious treatments for AN should
therefore be a top priority. To date, fewer than 10 randomized clinical trials
(RCT) for adolescents with AN have been published. This dire state of affairs
is exacerbated in that several of these published RCTs are underpowered and
therefore provide less than definitive findings.

Consequently, it remains somewhat of a challenge to make conclusive statements about the relative efficacy of one particular treatment compared to
another for this patient population. Without clear guidance from RCTs, treatment decisions are often based on clinical wisdom and experience rather than
firm research evidence. Moreover, different treatment options are often pursued
based on a specific country, its health care system, or untested but trusted
modus operandi. For instance, adolescents with AN in Europe may typically
be admitted to a psychiatric facility for 20 weeks or longer, whereas the same
adolescent in the United States will spend only about 2 weeks in hospital.

Until recently, most such treatment decisions were not based on findings
generated by RCTs. In 2007, Simon Gowers and his colleagues published the
first RCT that compared the relative efficacy of refeeding in an inpatient psychiatric facility to outpatient psychosocial treatments for this patient population.
Results from their relatively large RCT allowed these authors to conclude that
first-line inpatient psychiatric treatment does not provide advantages over outpatient management. Moreover, outpatient treatment failures did poorly on
transfer to inpatient facilities.

Against this backdrop, the study by Herpertz-Dahlman and her colleagues is 1
of only 2 additional published RCTs for this patient population comparing inpatient treatment to another treatment modality (See Madden et al[1] for a comparison of inpatient pediatric admission and outpatient family-based treatment).
The Herpertz-Dahlman study is the largest RCT to date. It is adequately powered
and well designed, and the authors were therefore well placed to evaluate their
primary research aim—to investigate the safety and efficacy of day-patient treatment after short inpatient treatment compared with continued inpatient
treatment.

All treatments were provided in psychiatric facilities. A psychiatric admission
for refeeding is the first-line treatment for adolescent AN in many parts of the
world. Therefore, day-patient treatment, a relatively less intensive alternative
intervention, is an appropriate comparison and a helpful step toward treatments
that do not remove adolescents from their families for prolonged periods of time.

Of note, this RCT is a multicenter noninferiority design, which enrolled 172 female patients between the ages of 11 and 18, all of whom met *Diagnostic and Statistical Manual of Mental Disorders* (4th edition; DSM-IV) criteria for AN. Qualifying patients were randomized to continued inpatient treatment or day-patient treatment after 3 weeks of inpatient care.

Once patients were discharged from either arm of the study, they received what the authors referred to as an identical multimodal multidisciplinary treatment program based on weight restoration. This program included nutritional counseling, cognitive-behavior therapy, and family therapy. All patients were followed up at 12 months postadmission with increase in body mass index (BMI) as the primary outcome.

The authors found that day-patient treatment was not inferior to inpatient treatment (Fig 2) and that there were few, if any, meaningful differences between these 2 groups in terms of their secondary outcome measures (Table 2). These findings led the authors to conclude that day-patient treatment after a short inpatient admission is no less effective than inpatient treatment in terms of weight gain and maintenance of these gains during the 12-month follow-up period. Day-patient treatment for adolescents with nonchronic AN may be safe and less costly than inpatient treatment. Therefore, the authors recommend a broader implementation of day-patient treatment for this patient population.

This impressive study is not without its limitations. The authors highlight a few of these shortcomings such as short follow-up period, and restrictions to the generalizability of their findings. However, a few additional limitations should be considered before embarking on a broader implementation of their findings. Patients were included in this study when they met DSM-IV criteria for AN and were below the 10th BMI percentile. However, the authors do not mention medical instability per se as a reason for being included in the study or whether medical instability is the primary reason for inpatient care. Instead, it would appear, and this is where intercontinental treatment philosophy might come into play, that patients were unwell but not necessarily medically unstable to justify a prolonged period of psychiatric hospital stay. It is not clear from this study whether all participating treatment centers provided psychiatric rather than pediatric medical care. Also unclear is how the authors defined "moderately-to-

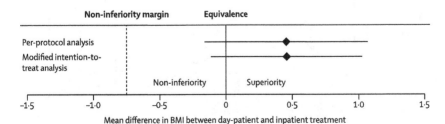

FIGURE 2.—Primary endpoint analysis. Error bars are 95% CIs. The dashed line is the predefined non-inferiority margin (-0.75 kg/m^2). BMI = body-mass index. (Reprinted from Soll RF, Edwards EM, Badger GJ, et al. Obstetric and neonatal care practices for infants 501 to 1500 g from 2000 to 2009. *Pediatrics.* 2013;132:222-228.)

TABLE 2.—Outcomes at 12-Month Follow-Up

	Inpatient Treatment Value	n*	Day-Patient Treatment Value	n*	Difference (95% CI)*	p Value[†]
Primary outcome						
BMI (kg/m²)	17·8 (1·7)	75	18·1 (2·0)	86	0·46 (−0·11 to 1·02)	<0·0001[‡]
Secondary outcomes						
General Morgan and Russell Score		75		82		0·92[§]
Good	19 (25%)		25 (31%)			
Intermediate	14 (19%)		8 (10%)			
Poor	42 (56%)		49 (60%)			
MRAOS	7·3 (2·6)	69	8·4 (1·9)	71	0·64 (−0·05 to 1·34)	0·07
MRAOS subscales		69		71		
Scale A (food intake)	6·6 (3·2)		7·7 (3·1)		1·02 (−0·03 to 2·08)	0·06
Scale B (menstruation)	4·2 (4·9)		4·1 (5·0)		−0·52 (−2·19 to 1·16)	0·54
Scale C (mental state)	8·0 (3·1)		10·1 (2·6)		1·05 (0·09 to 2·02)	0·03
Scale D (psychosexual adjustment)	7·5 (3·5)		9·1 (2·7)		1·29 (0·34 to 2·24)	0·008
Scale E (socioeconomic status)	9·8 (2·1)		10·5 (1·5)		0·46 (−0·12 to 1·04)	0·12
Number of readmissions for eating disorders	19 (25·3%)	75	13 (15·1%)	86	−10·2% (−22·7 to 2·2)	0·12[|]
EDI-2 global score	256·2 (78·2)	69	248·2 (71·1)	74	6·3 (−15·5 to 28·2)	0·57
BSI (global severity index)	0·6 (0·5)	68	0·5 (0·5)	73	0·01 (−0·15 to 0·17)	0·91
Costs (€)	39 481[¶] (16 174)	85	31 114[¶] (16 246)	87	−8367 (−13 247 to −3487)	0·002
Loss to follow-up	10 (11·8%)	85	1 (1·1%)	87	−10·6% (−19·2 to −3·3)	0·0046[|]

Data are mean (SD) or n (%). BMI = body-mass index. BSI = Brief Symptom Inventory. EDI-2 = Eating Disorder Inventory-2. MRAOS = Morgan and Russell average outcome score.
*Number of patients for whom data were available for analysis (in particular, some patients refused weight assessment or questionnaires).
[†]Linear model adjusted for age, duration of illness, and baseline value.
[‡]For the non-inferiority hypothesis.
[§]Cochran-Armitage test for trend.
[¶]Mean costs correspond to US$51 629 or 33 687 pounds (inpatient treatment) and $40 687 or 26 548 (day-patient treatment; exchange rates as of April 10, 2013).
[|]Fisher's exact test. 12-month follow-up data are either at 52 (±6) weeks from the time of admission or to relapse (readmission for eating disorder).
Reprinted from Soll RF, Edwards EM, Badger GJ, et al. Obstetric and neonatal care practices for infants 501 to 1500 g from 2000 to 2009. Pediatrics. 2013;132:222-228.

severely" ill adolescents with AN, and why 3 weeks of inpatient care came to be the defined marker for randomization to either ongoing inpatient care or the day-patient treatment arm. Was this perhaps the time point when a medically unstable adolescent with AN typically reaches vital sign stability? (See Garber et al[2] and Le Grange[3] for a discussion on length of stay in a pediatric setting). The authors do not mention much about what sounds like a rather complex multimodal multi-disciplinary treatment program that consisted of several components other than to say that this program was "identical."

Multisite RCTs are challenging especially in the domain of providing identical treatment across more than 1 site. In this remarkable study, 5 sites participated, which no doubt compounds this challenge by quite a few margins. Yet there is no description of this standard treatment program and how the authors went about making sure that it was indeed identical from 1 site to the next (or as identical as one could hope for across 5 sites). For instance, what was the rate of refeeding across sites, how was adherence to cognitive-behavior therapy or to family therapy verified, who supervised the clinical teams, and how was treatment fidelity across sites established?

Finally, an impressive 660 patients across the 5 sites were assessed for eligibility, and the authors ought to be commended for embarking and successfully completing such an endeavor. However, 114 patients were excluded because this was not their first admission; what was the rationale for excluding these patients, especially given that this was a study of "moderately-to-severely-ill" adolescents with AN. Also, a rather large number of patients ($n = 95$) refused to participate; what were some of the reasons for not participating?

Notwithstanding these limitations, this is an extraordinary study and a must-read for all those involved in the care of adolescents with eating disorders. Interpreting findings from this study should be done with the appropriate caution required when looking at a first comparison of these 2 treatments. That said, it still allows us to deduce that inpatient weight restoration for adolescent AN, especially in a psychiatric setting, is not warranted quite as often as the accepted status quo would dictate. This study adds to the growing evidence that inpatient psychiatric refeeding for adolescent AN has its limitations.[4] Finally, this study serves as a pathway for more vigorous exploration of outpatient treatments for a patient population still ensconced within resourceful families.

D. Le Grange, PhD

References

1. Madden S, Miskovic-Wheatley J, Wallis A, et al. A Randomized Controlled Trial of Inpatient Treatment for Anorexia Nervosa in Medically Unstable Adolescents. *Psychol Med.* Jul 2014; http://dx.doi.org/10.1017/S0033291714001573.
2. Garber AK, Mauldin K, Michihata N, Buckelew SM, Shafer MA, Moscicki AB. Higher calorie diets increase rate of weight gain and shorten hospital stay in hospitalized adolescents with anorexia nervosa. *J Adolesc Health.* 2013;53:579-584.
3. Le Grange D. Examining refeeding protocols for adolescents with anorexia nervosa (Again). Challenging clinical practice (Editorial). *J Adolesc Health.* 2013;53: 555-556.
4. Gowers SG, Clark A, Roberts C, et al. Clinical effectiveness of treatments for anorexia nervosa in adolescents: randomized controlled trial. *Br J Psychiatry.* 2007; 191:427-435.

Higher Calorie Diets Increase Rate of Weight Gain and Shorten Hospital Stay in Hospitalized Adolescents With Anorexia Nervosa

Garber AK, Mauldin K, Michihata N, et al (Univ of California, San Francisco; San José State Univ, CA; Natl Ctr for Child & Health Development, Tokyo, Japan)
J Adolesc Health 53:579-584, 2013

Purpose.—Current recommendations for refeeding in anorexia nervosa (AN) are conservative, beginning around 1,200 calories to avoid refeeding syndrome. We previously showed poor weight gain and long hospital stay using this approach and hypothesized that a higher calorie approach would improve outcomes.

Methods.—Adolescents hospitalized for malnutrition due to AN were included in this quasi-experimental study comparing lower and higher calories during refeeding. Participants enrolled between 2002 and 2012; higher calories were prescribed starting around 2008. Daily prospective measures included weight, heart rate, temperature, hydration markers and serum phosphorus. Participants received formula only to replace refused food. Percent Median Body Mass Index (% MBMI) was calculated using 50th percentile body mass index for age and sex. Unpaired t-tests compared two groups split at 1,200 calories.

Results.—Fifty-six adolescents with mean ($\pm$SEM) age 16.2 ($\pm$.3) years and admit %MBMI 79.2% ($\pm$1.5%) were hospitalized for 14.9 ($\pm$.9) days. The only significant difference between groups (N = 28 each) at baseline was starting calories (1,764 [$\pm$60] vs. 1,093 [$\pm$28], $p < .001$). Participants on higher calories had faster weight gain (.46 [$\pm$.04] vs. .26 [$\pm$.03] %MBMI/day, $p < .001$), greater daily calorie advances (122 [$\pm$8] vs. 98 [$\pm$6], $p = .024$), shorter hospital stay (11.9 [$\pm$1.0] vs. 17.6 [$\pm$1.2] days, $p < .001$), and a greater tendency to receive phosphate supplementation (12 vs. 8 participants, $p = .273$).

Conclusions.—Higher calorie diets produced faster weight gain in hospitalized adolescents with AN as compared with the currently recommended lower calorie diets. No cases of the refeeding syndrome were seen using phosphate supplementation. These findings lend further support to the move toward more aggressive refeeding in AN.

▶ Recently, there has been great interest in exploring the most efficient, effective, and safe way of refeeding hospitalized adolescents with anorexia nervosa (AN). Garber et al was among one of the first groups to explore this important question in adolescents with AN and, more important, the first group to do a prospective, observational study comparing high and low baseline calorie intake protocols. Not surprisingly, the adolescents in the higher calorie group gained weight faster than the comparison group, leading to hospital discharge nearly 6 days earlier. The authors concluded that this study lends support to more aggressive meal-based protocols for moderately malnourished adolescents with AN.

Although there is growing support for this important finding,[1] it is critical to underscore a cautionary fact that must be considered when implementing nutritional rehabilitation in this population. Approximately 45% of the adolescents in Garber's study developed "low serum phosphorus level in hospital" or refeeding hypophosphatemia (RH)—an important and medically concerning metabolic finding of the refeeding syndrome. RH is the most well-known and significant element of the refeeding syndrome and can potentially have a harmful impact on all metabolic processes in the body. RH can result in sudden death, rhabdomyolysis, delirium, red cell and leukocyte dysfunction, arrhythmias, heart failure, and respiratory insufficiency.[2] Symptoms of RH are often nonspecific. Therefore, recognizing RH can be challenging. In a recent systematic review of hospitalized adolescents with AN, the average incidence of RH in adolescents was 14% (range 0% to 38%)—not an insignificant complication.[3]

Although not all hospitalized adolescents with AN who are refed develop RH, it is important to be aware that it can occur. Garber and others[4-7] have endeavored to understand who is at most risk for the development of RH in this population. Based on the literature to date, studies[4,6,7] have shown that the degree of RH at presentation is correlated with degree of malnutrition (<70% median body mass index) on admission to hospital, as opposed to the quantity of calories consumed.[2]

Although most clinicians would agree that careful monitoring and treatment of electrolyte imbalances is of particular importance in an adolescent with AN, there are currently no evidence-based guidelines to guide this process. How frequently and when should one monitor serum electrolytes? What are the standard phosphate replacement regimens for adolescents with AN who develop RH? Should we consider prophylactic oral phosphate supplementation in this group? What are the risks and benefits of prescribing prophylactic oral phosphate supplementation during nutritional rehabilitation in this population? In addition to the degree of malnutrition, does the method of nutritional rehabilitation (oral, enteral, parenteral) have an impact on the development of RH? Does the composition of the diet (ie, macronutrient and micronutrient content) have an impact on the safety and efficacy of nutritional rehabilitation? The answers to these questions remain unknown, and further study is necessary to help us understand the implications of these issues on RH.

One thing is certain: nutritional rehabilitation will remain a fundamental first-line treatment for hospitalized adolescents with AN, and it is not without its complications. RH is a potentially life-threatening complication of nutritional rehabilitation in malnourished adolescents with AN. Being aware that RH can result from refeeding severely malnourished inpatients with AN will allow the clinician to look for this complications.

Garber's study has opened the door to further considerations about how we think about nutritional rehabilitation and RH in adolescents with AN, and highlights the need to exercise caution as we move forward. Most important, it has prompted us to ask more questions as we strive to provide the most efficient, effective, and safe treatment for young people with these disorders.

D. K. Katzman, MD

References

1. Katzman DK. Refeeding hospitalized adolescents with anorexia nervosa: is "start low, advance slow" urban legend or evidence based? *J Adolesc Health*. 2012;50: 1-2.
2. Katzman DK, Garber A, Kohn M, Golden NH, Society for Adolescent Medicine Position Statement. Refeeding hypophosphatemia in hospitalized adolescents with anorexia nervosa: a position statement of the society for adolescent health and medicine. *J Adolesc Health*. 2014;55:455-457.
3. O'Connor G, Nicholls D. Refeeding hypophosphatemia in adolescents with anorexia nervosa: a systematic review. *Nutr Clin Pract*. 2013;28:358-364.
4. Whitelaw M, Gilbertson H, Lam PY, Sawyer SM. Does aggressive refeeding in hospitalized adolescents with anorexia nervosa result in increased hypophosphatemia? *J Adolesc Health*. 2010;46:577-582.
5. Leclerc A, Turrini T, Sherwood K, Katzman DK. Evaluation of a nutrition rehabilitation protocol in hospitalized adolescents with restrictive eating disorders. *J Adolesc Health*. 2013;53:585-589.
6. Garber AK, Michihata N, Hetnal K, Shafer MA, Moscicki AB. A prospective examination of weight gain in hospitalized adolescents with anorexia nervosa on a recommended refeeding protocol. *J Adolesc Health*. 2012;50:24-29.
7. Golden NH, Keane-Miller C, Sainani KL, Kapphahn CJ. Higher caloric intake in hospitalized adolescents with anorexia nervosa is associated with reduced length of stay and no increased rate of refeeding syndrome. *J Adolesc Health*. 2013;53: 573-578.

Breastfeeding and Obesity Among Schoolchildren: A Nationwide Longitudinal Survey in Japan

Yamakawa M, Yorifuji T, Inoue S, et al (Okayama Univ Graduate School of Medicine, Japan; Okayama Univ Graduate School of Environmental and Life Science, Japan)
JAMA Pediatr 167:919-925, 2013

Importance.—Although it is suggested that breastfeeding is protective against obesity in children, the evidence remains inconclusive because of possible residual confounding by socioeconomic status or children's lifestyle factors. Most of the participants in the previous studies were children in Western developed countries, so studies in a different context are awaited.

Objective.—To examine the associations of breastfeeding with overweight and obesity among schoolchildren in Japan, with adjustment for the potential confounders.

Design.—Secondary data analyses of a nationwide longitudinal survey ongoing since 2001, with results collected from 2001 to 2009.

Setting.—All over Japan.

Participants.—A total of 43 367 singleton children who were born after 37 gestational weeks and had information on their feeding during infancy.

Exposures.—Five mutually exclusive infant feeding practice categories.

Main Outcomes and Measures.—Underweight, normal weight (referent group), overweight, and obesity at 7 and 8 years of age defined by using international cutoff points of body mass index by sex and age.

Results.—In multinomial logistic regression models with adjustment for children's factors (sex, television viewing time, and computer game playing time) and maternal factors (educational attainment, smoking status, and working status), exclusive breastfeeding at 6 to 7 months of age was associated with decreased risk of overweight and obesity compared with formula feeding. The adjusted odds ratios were 0.85 (95% CI, 0.69-1.05) and 0.55 (95% CI, 0.39-0.78) for overweight and obesity, respectively, at 7 years of age. Similar results were observed at 8 years of age.

Conclusions and Relevance.—Breastfeeding is associated with decreased risk of overweight and obesity among schoolchildren in Japan. Therefore, it would be better to encourage breastfeeding even in developed countries.

▶ In this article, Yamakawa and colleagues demonstrate that exclusive breastfeeding is associated with decreased risk for obesity and overweight.[1] Their study is based on the 21st Century Longitudinal Survey of Newborns, an ongoing national cohort study administered by the Ministry of Health, Labor and Welfare of Japan in which surveys are mailed annually to parents of children born during two 1-week periods in 2001. Breastfeeding duration was categorized on the basis of maternal report on the first survey mailed when infants were aged 6 to 7 months. Obesity was defined according to body mass index (BMI) cutoff points proposed by the International Obesity Task Force, using BMI calculated from height and weight reported at the seventh and eighth surveys when the children were 7 and 8 years old. As reported by the authors, any breastfeeding, with and without adjustment for other factors, was associated with decreased risk for obesity. For 8-year-olds, the odds ratio ranged from 0.55 to 0.56 for children breastfed for 1 to 2 months and 0.36 to 0.44 for children breastfed for 6 to 7 months.

Japan, like other industrialized nations, suffers from an evolving epidemic of obesity. The proportions of adults who are obese (BMI ≥30) are 3.8% in men and 3.2% in women, and the proportion of adults who are overweight (BMI ≥25) are 30.4% in men and 21.1% in women.[2] Inclusion of overweight is critical because of recent research demonstrating relationships between overweight and lifestyle-related diseases such as diabetes, hypertension, and hyperlipidemia.[3] Among children aged 6 to 14 years, the proportions who are overweight and obese are 16.2% and 4.1% in boys and 14.2% and 2.5% in girls, respectively.[4] To effectively address obesity, it is helpful to understand factors that both protect against and contribute to obesity. This study is significant in that nearly 4% of parents of newborns in Japan were systematically sampled and that cohort continues to be relatively intact after 7 to 8 years. In addition, of the 53 575 parents receiving the initial survey, 88% responded. Among the 43 367 parents of eligible children in year 1, 77% responded in year 8. The results are significant in that the protective effects of breastfeeding on obesity remained unchanged after adjustment for potential proxies of social factors commonly cited as predictors of obesity, such as socioeconomic status; current analyses also included adjustments for maternal education, maternal smoking, maternal work status, sex of child, and child screen time.

The purpose of the 21st Century Longitudinal Survey of Newborns was to collect information about the environment and lifestyles of children between birth and age 20 years; because the specific objective was not to study obesity, critical information was not collected in the surveys including maternal weight, child nutrition, and physical activities. Factors associated with continuation of breastfeeding, such as maternal age, length of maternity leave, and postpartum depression were also not considered.[5] Furthermore, key measures, such as weight and height were based on parent report. While there is no reason to suspect that parents of breastfed children would report results differently from parents of formula-fed children, the accuracy of parent report remains unknown.

Finally, although the response rate was high and loss of sample relatively small, there may be critical differences between participants and nonparticipants. As discussed by the authors, children included in the analyses at age 7 and 8 years were more likely to have been breastfed and less likely to have mothers who smoked, compared with all eligible children in the first survey. If smokers are less likely to breastfeed and more likely to have children who are obese,[6] their exclusion from this analysis may have magnified the protective effect of breastfeeding.

Our knowledge about obesity, however, is rapidly changing. BMI may not be as accurate a measure of body fat in people of differing ethnicity.[7] Recent reports indicate that waist size may be an additional measurement to consider that is more likely to be associated with complications of obesity such as diabetes.[8]

Although this study does not technically meet the current international standards of a cohort study to determine antecedent factors associated with the development of obesity in children, the unlikely scenario of a systematic bias in parent report and the large sample size make the results of this study credible. Using the 21st Century Longitudinal Survey of Newborns, which includes 1 in 25 newborn infants in Japan, the authors have demonstrated that breastfeeding, ranging from 1 to 2 months to 6 to 7 months of life, confers protection against subsequent development of obesity at age 7 and 8 years.

J. I. Takayama, MD, MPH

N. Matsuo, MD

References

1. Yamakawa M, Yorifuji T, Inoue S, Kato T, Doi H. Breastfeeding and obesity among schoolchildren: a nationwide longitudinal survey in Japan. *JAMA Pediatr.* 2013;167:919-925.
2. Yoshiike N, Miyoshi M. [Epidemiologic aspects of overweight and obesity in Japan - international comparisons]. *Nihon Rinsho.* 2013;71:207-216.
3. Kanazawa M, Yoshiike N, Osaka T, Numba Y, Zimmet P, Inoue S. Criteria and classification of obesity in Japan and Asia-Oceania. *Word Rev Nutr Diet.* 2005; 94:1-12.
4. Inokuchi M, Matsuo N, Takayama JI, Hasegawa T. Official Japanese reports significantly underestimate prevalence of overweight in Japanese children: inappropriate definition of standard weight and calculation of excess weight. *Ann Hum Bio.* 2009;36:139-145.
5. Haku M. Breastfeeding: factors associated with the continuation of breastfeeding, the current situation in Japan, and recommendations for further research. *J Med Invest.* 2007;54:224-234.

6. Yang S, Decker A, Kramer MS. Exposure to parent smoking and child growth and development: a cohort study. *BMC Pediatr.* 2013;13:104.
7. Carpenter CL, Yan E, Chen S, et al. Body fat and body-mass index among a multiethnic sample of college-age men and women. *J Obes.* 2013.
8. Anzo M, Inokuchi M, Matsuo N, Takayama JI, Hasegawa T. Waist circumference centiles by age and sex for Japanese children based on the 1978-1981 cross-sectional national survey data. *Ann Hum Biol.* 2014:1-6 [Epub ahead of print].

Bottle-Weaning Intervention and Toddler Overweight

Bonuck K, Avraham SB, Lo Y, et al (Albert Einstein College of Medicine, Bronx, NY)

J Pediatr 164:306-312.e2, 2013

Objective.—To evaluate 3 research questions: (1) Does a Women, Infants, and Children (WIC)-based counseling intervention reduce (milk) bottle use?; (2) Does this intervention reduce energy intake from bottles?; and (3) Does this intervention reduce the risk of a child being >85th percentile weight-for-length?

Study Design.—Parents of n = 300 12-month-olds consuming >2 bottles/d were randomized to a bottle-weaning intervention or control group. Nutritionists at WIC Supplemental Feeding Program sites delivered the intervention. Researchers assessed dietary intake and beverage container use via computer-guided 24-hour recalls, and anthropometrics at 15, 18, 21, and 24 months old. Intent-to-treat analyses controlled for baseline measures of outcomes and months post-baseline.

Results.—At 1 year follow-up, the intervention group had reduced use of any bottles (OR = 0.23, 95% CI = 0.08-0.61), calories from milk bottles (OR = 0.36, 95% CI = 0.18-0.74), and total calories ($\beta = -1.15$, $P = .043$), but did not differ from controls in risk of overweight status (ie, >85th percentile weight-for-length (OR = 1.02, 95% CI = 0.5-2.0). The intervention group's decreased bottle usage at 15 and 18 months was paralleled by increased "sippy cup" usage.

Conclusion.—A brief intervention, during WIC routine care, reduced early childhood risk factors for overweight—bottle use and energy intake—but not risk of overweight. The intervention group's increased use of sippy cups may have attenuated an intervention effect upon risk of overweight. Toddlers consume a high proportion of their calories as liquid. Parents should be counseled about excess intake from bottles and sippy cups. WIC is an ideal setting for such interventions.

▶ Prolonged bottle use by a toddler is a risk factor for negative health outcomes, including dental caries,[1] iron insufficiency due to excessive milk intake,[2] and obesity.[3] As a result, the American Academy of Pediatrics recommends that families wean toddlers off of bottles by 15 months of age.[1] Yet it is not uncommon to see preschool-age children still using a bottle. Data from the 2001 birth cohort of the Early Childhood Longitudinal Study noted that 22% of toddlers at 2 years of age still use a bottle at least once a day, including 11% of toddlers who were described as "regular" bottle users.[3]

This study by Bonuck et al evaluates an intervention delivered through the Women Infants and Children's Program (WIC; a program that provides nutrition counseling and assistance to low-income women and children in the United States) to decrease bottle use as a strategy to address pediatric obesity. The primary outcome was bottle use frequency, and a secondary outcome was the proportion of children >85% weight for length. The study enrolled children 11 to 13 months of age seen at WIC who were consuming more than 2 bottles of milk or juice per day. There was a single, standardized educational intervention delivered by a nutritionist. In addition, intervention families received a handout and a lidded, 6-ounce sippy cup. Although the intervention was successful in decreasing the primary outcome of interest—infant bottle use—there was no difference in the secondary outcome of overweight status between the intervention and control groups.

This study and results are similar to the TARGet Kids bottle-weaning study for 9-month-old infants.[4] One major difference was setting of the different studies. The TARGet Kids study was delivered in a primary care practice setting, whereas the intervention described by Bonuck et al was delivered at WIC Supplemental Feeding Program sites. Similarly, although there was a decrease in bottle use in the TARGet study, there was no change in the main health outcome—iron deficiency status.

Prolonged use of bottles has been associated with overweight in both cross-sectional and cohort studies. Bottles are thought to be associated with obesity because they facilitate easy consumption of excess liquid calories. Although influencing the route of beverage intake is important, it is also critical to focus on the type of beverage that is being placed into a bottle or sippy cup. One limitation of the current study is that the type of beverage consumed was not described. In addition to whole milk or formula, some parents may fill bottles and sippy cups with fruit juice or sugar-sweetened beverages (soda, fruit drinks, and other drinks with added sugar), which are associated with obesity and obesity-related comorbidities.

If the bottle is going to be used, why not also remove calories and cariogenic properties from the beverage? Health providers, including pediatricians and WIC nutritionists, may want to encourage parents to offer only water in bottles or lidded sippy cups after 12 months of age. Water provides a noncaloric source of hydration that is low cost and that can prevent obesity and dental caries among children. Although it is important to decrease bottle use, the results of this study suggest a need to also combine bottle-weaning interventions with messages to change type of beverage provided to the young children. As children develop their dietary preferences and drinking habits at an early age, there may also be benefits in influencing long-term beverage consumption patterns.

Finally, it is important to ensure that these messages are culturally appropriate and do not exacerbate health disparities. For example, from 2003 to 2009, the percentage of children aged 2 to 5 years in California consuming sugar-sweetened beverages declined from 40% to 16% (2003 to 2009; $P < .001$). In the same age group, although consumption of 100% fruit juice per day decreased among white children, consumption increased among Latinos.[5] It is concerning that the increase in fruit juice consumption among minority children may be an unintended consequence of efforts to reduce sugar-sweetened beverage consumption because public health messages may have different interpretations in different communities.

This study by Bonuck et al is important and demonstrates that it is possible to influence parental use of bottles in the short-term. The intervention is feasible and can potentially be implemented in WIC centers throughout the country. Further work is needed to understand how behavior changes achieved by this intervention can be reinforced and sustained, and possibly adapted for other settings, such as child care or clinics, that young children frequent.

A. Patel, MD, MSPH

M. D. Cabana, MD, MPH

References

1. Section on Pediatric Dentistry and Oral Health. Preventive oral health intervention for pediatricians. *Pediatrics.* 2008;122:1387-1394.
2. Bonuck KA, Kahn R. Prolonged bottle use and its association with iron deficiency anemia and overweight: a preliminary study. *Clin Pediatr.* 2002;41:603-607.
3. Gooze RA, Anderson SE, Whitaker RC. Prolonged bottle use and obesity at 5.5 years of age in US children. *J Pediatr.* 2011;159:431-436.
4. Maguire JL, Birken CS, Jacobson S, et al. Office-based intervention to reduce bottle use among toddlers: TARGet Kids! Pragmatic, randomized trial. *Pediatrics.* 2010;126:e343-e350.
5. Beck AL, Patel A, Madsen K. Trends in sugar-sweetened beverage and 100% fruit juice consumption among California children. *Acad Pediatr.* 2013;13:364-370.

Prevalence of Childhood and Adult Obesity in the United States, 2011-2012
Ogden CL, Carroll MD, Kit BK, et al (Ctrs for Disease Control and Prevention, Hyattsville, MD)
JAMA 311:806-814, 2014

Importance.—More than one-third of adults and 17% of youth in the United States are obese, although the prevalence remained stable between 2003-2004 and 2009-2010.

Objective.—To provide the most recent national estimates of childhood obesity, analyze trends in childhood obesity between 2003 and 2012, and provide detailed obesity trend analyses among adults.

Design, Setting, and Participants.—Weight and height or recumbent length were measured in 9120 participants in the 2011-2012 nationally representative National Health and Nutrition Examination Survey.

Main Outcomes and Measures.—In infants and toddlers from birth to 2 years, high weight for recumbent length was defined as weight for length at or above the 95th percentile of the sex-specific Centers for Disease Control and Prevention (CDC) growth charts. In children and adolescents aged 2 to 19 years, obesity was defined as a body mass index (BMI) at or above the 95th percentile of the sex-specific CDC BMI-for-age growth charts. In adults, obesity was defined as a BMI greater than or equal to 30. Analyses

TABLE 6.—Unadjusted Tests of Linear Trends of High Weight for Length[a] and Obesity[b,c] by Age. United States, 2003-2012[d]

	2003-2004	2005-2006	% (95% CI) 2007-2008	2009-2010	2011-2012	Change 2003-2004 to 2011-2012, Point (95% CI)[e]	P Value[f]
High weight for length (birth-< 2y)							
All	9.5 (7.1 to 12.7)	8.2 (6.1 to 10.9)	9.5 (7.5 to 12)	9.7 (7.6 to 12.3)	8.1 (5.8 to 11.1)	-1.4 (-4.9 to 2.1)	.72
Childhood obesity, 2-19y							
2-19	17.1 (14.6 to 20)	15.4 (12.8 to 18.5)	16.8 (14.3 to 19.7)	16.9 (15.4 to 18.4)	16.9 (14.9 to 19.2)	-0.2 (-3.4 to 3)	.78
2-5	13.9 (10.8 to 17.6)	10.7 (8.5 to 13.3)	10.1 (7.8 to 12.9)	12.1 (9.9 to 14.8)	8.4 (5.9 to 11.6)	-5.5 (-9.6 to -1.4)	.03
6-11	18.8 (16.2 to 21.7)	15.1 (11.3 to 20.1)	19.6 (17.2 to 22.4)	18.0 (16.3 to 19.8)	17.7 (14.5 to 21.4)	-1.1 (-5.2 to 3.0)	.88
12-19	17.4 (14 to 21.3)	17.8 (14.2 to 22)	18.1 (14.7 to 22)	18.4 (15.8 to 21.3)	20.5 (17.1 to 24.4)	3.1 (-1.7 to 7.9)	.20
Adult obesity, ≥20y							
≥20	32.2 (29.7 to 34.8)	34.3 (31.5 to 37.3)	33.7 (31.5 to 36.1)	35.7 (33.8 to 37.7)	34.9 (32 to 37.9)	2.8 (-0.8 to 6.4)	.09
20-39	28.5 (25.3 to 31.9)	29.1 (25 to 33.7)	30.7 (26.6 to 35.1)	32.6 (29 to 36.4)	30.3 (26.6 to 34.4)	1.9 (-2.8 to 6.6)	.20
40-59	36.8 (33 to 40.8)	40.4 (36.1 to 44.7)	36.2 (32.8 to 39.8)	36.6 (34.5 to 38.7)	39.5 (36.1 to 43)	2.7 (-2.1 to 7.5)	.78
≥60	31.0 (28.2 to 33.9)	33.4 (31.1 to 35.9)	35.1 (32.9 to 37.3)	39.7 (36.6 to 42.9)	35.4 (31.3 to 39.6)	4.4 (-0.3 to 9.1)	.004

[a]High weight for length defined as at or above the 95th percentile on the sex-specific Centers for Disease Control and Prevention (CDC) 2000 growth charts.
[b]Obesity for youth aged 2 to 19 years defined as body mass index (BMI) at or above the 95th percentile on the CDC sex-specific BMI for age growth charts.
[c]Obesity in adults defined as BMI ≥ 30.
[d]Data from the National Health and Nutrition Examination Survey.
[e]Percentage points.
[f]From the t test.
Reprinted from Ogden CL, Carroll MD, Kit BK, et al. Prevalence of Childhood and Adult Obesity in the United States, 2011-2012. JAMA. 2014;311:806-814. Copyright 2014, American Medical Association. All rights reserved.

of trends in high weight for recumbent length or obesity prevalence were conducted overall and separately by age across 5 periods (2003-2004, 2005-2006, 2007-2008, 2009-2010, and 2011-2012).

Results.—In 2011-2012, 8.1% (95% CI, 5.8%-11.1%) of infants and toddlers had high weight for recumbent length, and 16.9% (95% CI, 14.9%-19.2%) of 2- to 19-year-olds and 34.9% (95% CI, 32.0%-37.9%) of adults (age-adjusted) aged 20 years or older were obese. Overall, there was no significant change from 2003-2004 through 2011-2012 in high weight for recumbent length among infants and toddlers, obesity in 2- to 19-year-olds, or obesity in adults. Tests for an interaction between survey period and age found an interaction in children ($P = .03$) and women ($P = .02$). There was a significant decrease in obesity among 2- to 5-year-old children (from 13.9% to 8.4%; $P = .03$) and a significant increase in obesity among women aged 60 years and older (from 31.5% to 38.1%; $P = .006$).

Conclusions and Relevance.—Overall, there have been no significant changes in obesity prevalence in youth or adults between 2003-2004 and 2011-2012. Obesity prevalence remains high and thus it is important to continue surveillance (Table 6).

▶ Identifying a change in trend can be difficult and hazardous. This article by Ogden et al generated attention when the authors reported that "there was a significant decrease in obesity among 2-to 5-year-old children (from 13.9% to 8.4%; $P = .03$)." After years of steadily increasing rates of pediatric obesity, is it possible that we have turned a corner? Are health care providers and public health practitioners now starting to see the results of pediatric interventions and public health campaigns to address obesity by improving childhood activity and nutrition?

The study included children aged 2 to 19 years, and separate subanalyses were conducted for children 2 to 5 years, 6 to 11 years, and 12 to 19 years. In the 2- to 5-year age group, when the frequencies for obesity were compared from the 2003—2004 period through the 2011—2012 period, a downward trend was detected (13.9% to 8.4%; $P = .03$; Table 6). In the article, the authors provide a thoughtful discussion of this issue and point out several potential limitations.

One reason for noting a decline may be the selection of the specific year for the initial comparison point. The obesity rate of 13.9% in 2003 may have been unusually elevated and, as a result, may create the impression of a relative short-term decline. This point is further illustrated by another study, also published in 2014.[1] This study used the same data set and a similar analysis was completed, but the time frame was expanded to 1999. In 1999—2000, the prevalence of obesity was 11.1% for girls and 10.0% for boys. In a comparison of 1999—2000 with 2011—2012, the results suggested that no change or downward trend in obesity prevalence had occurred for the 2- to 5-year-old age group during this broader time frame.[1]

Another potential issue is the use of multiple tests or comparisons being conducted within the same study. When a P value of .05 is used, a significant difference can occur simply by chance in 1 of 20 tests.[2] In this study, multiple comparisons using different age groups and different demographic characteristics were conducted using the same data set. Is it possible that this difference simply occurred by chance? When multiple comparisons are being conducted, it is important to consider the broader context of the analyses and to assess whether the results are clinically plausible or simply serendipitous.

If one were to expect a change in obesity trends, one might imagine that the children 2 to 5 years of age might be the first group to demonstrate a decline in obesity rates. As greater attention has been placed on pediatric obesity in recent years, this group would be more likely to benefit from the recent increase in rates of breastfeeding, efforts to decrease sugar-sweetened beverage consumption or efforts to emphasize fruits and vegetables in subsidized food programs such as the Women Infants and Children Program.[3]

In the end, only time will tell if the results reported by Ogden et al. were merely a 'blip' or the start of a true trend. In two years, the next set of data from the 2013—14 NHANES will be released, and I am sure that many follow-up studies will reassess for the presence of any trends. In the meantime, one thing that is certain from this study is that obesity continues to be a problem. Approximately 1 in 6 children (17%) are obese. Trend or no trend, there is still much more work to do.

M. D. Cabana, MD, MPH

References

1. Skinner AC, Skelton JA. Prevalence and trends in obesity and severe obesity among children in the United States, 1999–2012. *JAMA Pediatr.* 2014;168:561-566.
2. Mills JL. Data torturing. *N Engl J Med.* 1993;329:1196-1199.
3. US Department of Agriculture. Fresh fruit and vegetable program. http://www.fns.usda.gov/ffvp/program-history. Accessed August 19, 2014

Incidence of Childhood Obesity in the United States

Cunningham SA, Kramer MR, Narayan KM (Emory Univ, Atlanta, GA)
N Engl J Med 370:403-411, 2014

Background.—Although the increased prevalence of childhood obesity in the United States has been documented, little is known about its incidence. We report here on the national incidence of obesity among elementary-school children.

Methods.—We evaluated data from the Early Childhood Longitudinal Study, Kindergarten Class of 1998–1999, a representative prospective cohort of 7738 participants who were in kindergarten in 1998 in the United States. Weight and height were measured seven times between 1998 and 2007. Of the 7738 participants, 6807 were not obese at baseline; these participants were followed for 50,396 person-years. We used standard thresholds from the Centers for Disease Control and Prevention to define "overweight" and "obese" categories. We estimated the annual incidence of obesity, the cumulative incidence over 9 years, and the incidence

density (cases per person-years) overall and according to sex, socioeconomic status, race or ethnic group, birth weight, and kindergarten weight.
Results.—When the children entered kindergarten (mean age, 5.6 years), 12.4% were obese and another 14.9% were overweight; in eighth grade (mean age, 14.1 years), 20.8% were obese and 17.0% were overweight. The annual incidence of obesity decreased from 5.4% during kindergarten to 1.7% between fifth and eighth grade. Overweight 5-year-olds were four times as likely as normal-weight children to become obese (9-year cumulative incidence, 31.8% vs. 7.9%), with rates of 91.5 versus 17.2 per 1000 person-years. Among children who became obese between the ages of 5 and 14 years, nearly half had been overweight and 75% had been above the 70th percentile for body-mass index at baseline.
Conclusions.—Incident obesity between the ages of 5 and 14 years was more likely to have occurred at younger ages, primarily among children who had entered kindergarten overweight. (Funded by the Eunice Kennedy Shriver National Institute of Child Health and Human Development.)

▶ Although the problem of pediatric obesity is well identified and well known to health care providers,[1] the typical patterns related to the "timing" of obesity during childhood are less well documented. At what age do children typically transition from being normal weight to being obese? In this study, Cunningham et al analyze data from the Early Childhood Longitudinal Study (from kindergarten to eighth grade) to describe the incidence of obesity.

Being overweight in kindergarten seems to be a harbinger of future obesity, as overweight 5-year-olds were 4 times more likely to become obese compared with normal-weight 5-year-olds. During the 9-year observation period, of those children who became obese, 75% had been above the 70th percentile for body mass index at 5 years of age. Although the incidence of obesity was highest at 5 to 9 years of age, the incidence subsequently declines with increasing age (Fig 1 in the original article).

Is the development of future obesity inevitable? To paraphrase Robert Fulghum, who wrote *All I Really Need to Know I Learned in Kindergarten*,[2] is all you really need to know about future obesity what you learn from a kindergarten BMI? What can a clinician do to prevent obesity among children before kindergarten?

There are few clinical interventions, if any, that are regularly effective in preventing obesity.

Perhaps the kindergarten well-child visit is too late for obesity prevention efforts. As suggested by the study authors and organizations such as the American Academy of Pediatrics and the Institute of Medicine,[3,4] obesity prevention should start as early as possible. Although there are few randomized controlled trials focused on infants and toddlers, increasingly interventions are targeting a variety of settings (eg, home; child care; Women, Infants, and Children) that young children frequent. To date, the most successful interventions include a parental component and also target multiple behaviors (eg, increasing physical activity, decreasing sedentary behaviors, increasing intake of healthy foods and beverages).[5,6] However, to most effectively prevent early childhood obesity will require population-based approaches that target multiple levels (eg, home, clinics, parks, child care), include both environment and policy change, and involve multiple disciplines and sectors (eg, public health, medicine, private industry, transportation).

It really does take a village to raise a healthy child.

M. D. Cabana, MD, MPH

A. I. Patel, MD, MSPH

References

1. Singh GK, Kogan MD, van Dyck PC. Changes in state-specific childhood obesity and overweight prevalence in the United States from 2003 to 2007. *Arch Pediatr Adolesc Med.* 2010;164:598-607.
2. Fulghum R, All I. *Really Need To Know I Learned in Kindergarten.* New York: Villard Books; 1988.
3. Institute of Medicine (IOM). *Early Childhood Obesity Prevention Policies.* Washington, DC: The National Academies Press; 2011.
4. American Academy of Pediatrics. http://www.aap.org/en-us/advocacy-and-policy/aap-health-initiatives/HALF-Implementation-Guide/Pages/The-Case-for-Early-Obesity-Prevention.aspx. Accessed August 10, 2014.
5. Hesketh KD, Campbell KJ. Interventions to prevent obesity in 0–5 year olds: an updated systematic review of the literature. *Obesity (Silver Spring).* 2010;18: S27-S35.
6. Robert Wood Johnson Foundation. *Preventing Obesity Among Preschool Children: How Can Child-care Settings Promote Healthy Eating and Physical Activity?.* Princeton, NJ: Robert Wood Johnson Foundation; 2011.

Consuming calories and creating cavities: beverages NZ children associate with sport

Smith M, Jenkin G, Signal L, et al (Univ of Otago, Wellington, New Zealand; et al)
Appetite 81:209-217, 2014

Sugar-sweetened beverages (SSBs) are widely available, discounted and promoted, and despite recommendations to the contrary, frequently consumed by children. They provide few nutritional benefits, and their consumption is implicated in a number of poor health outcomes. This study examined the nature of the beverages that sport-playing New Zealand (NZ) children associate with sport. It assessed how well the beverages aligned with nutrition guidelines and relevant regulations, and their likely impacts on health. Eighty-two children (38 girls and 44 boys) aged 10–12 years were purposively selected from netball, rugby and football clubs in low and high socioeconomic neighbourhoods, in Wellington, New Zealand (NZ). Children photographed beverages they associated with sport. The beverages were then purchased and analysed in accordance with NZ nutrition guidelines, and relevant content and labelling regulations, by: package and serving size; energy, sugar, sodium and caffeine content; pH; and advisory statements. The beverages the children associated with sport overwhelmingly had characteristics which do not support children in adhering to NZ nutrition guidelines. Implementing public health mechanisms, such as healthy food and beverage policies, widely promoting water as the beverage of choice in sport, and implementing healthy eating and drinking campaigns in sports clubs, would assist children who play organised sport to select beverages that are in keeping with children's nutrition guidelines. As part of a comprehensive public health approach they would also reduce the substantial, unnecessary and potentially harmful contribution sugar-sweetened beverages make to their diet.

▶ Nearly a decade of research demonstrates an association between intake of sugar-sweetened beverages (SSBs) and obesity.[1] According to a 2012 Institute of Medicine report, 20% of pounds gained by the American public over the past 30 years are attributable to intake of SSBs.[2] Children are particularly vulnerable because consumption of 1 additional serving of SSB per day may increase a child's obesity risk by 60%.[3]

Sports drinks (flavored beverages with added carbohydrates, minerals, electrolytes, and often vitamins) are a particular subset of SSBs that is increasingly consumed by children.[4] Although sports drinks contain added sugar, these beverages are often perceived as healthier than other SSBs because they contain nutrients (eg, potassium, sodium, calcium, and magnesium) and are marketed as choice drinks for active living.[5] With the growing market share of these beverages, professional organizations, including the American Academy of Pediatrics, have concerns about excessive intake among children and adolescents.[4]

Smith et al attempt to shed light on the types of beverages marketed to children participating in sports.[6] This study uses an innovative approach of data from both child originated photos of beverages in their environment and focus groups to highlight beverage availability and marketing and child perceptions of beverages. Specifically, a convenience sample of 82 children aged 10 to 12 were recruited for the study from netball, rugby, and football clubs in Wellington, New Zealand. These youth who played sports were asked to photograph beverages they saw in both the physical environment and the marketing environment and also to comment on their perceptions of the beverages they photographed.

Although this study included a small convenience sample (only 82 children who photographed 148 beverages in their sports environment) and did not document actual beverage consumption, study findings are revealing. Based on New Zealand Beverage Standards for Youth, 83% of the beverages photographed were classified as "for limited consumption" by youth. Further, 52% of beverages photographed exceeded New Zealand serving size recommendations of 250 mL per serving. One-third of the beverages had advisory statements on nutrition labels; however, the majority of "statements were in small font on the back of the container." Youth reported that their main reasons for consuming beverages identified by photograph were because they quench thirst, provide energy, were available at sports venues or were endorsed by athletes.

The most dramatic finding from this study was the high proportion of beverages photographed that were either not recommended for youth (caffeinated) or recommended to be limited (defined as sugary drinks with added sugars).

In concordance with New Zealand beverage standards, the American Academy of Pediatrics recommends that water should be the beverage of choice for children and adolescents who are participating in sports. Sports drink consumption is appropriate only for youth who are participating in vigorous physical activity for more than 90 minutes.[4] Further, energy drinks, which often contain sugar and stimulants such as caffeine or guarana, are not ever recommended for children.[4]

To address these concerns, the authors propose a variety of public health solutions including beverage policies for sports venues, uncoupling of sport and beverage marketing, regulation of portion size, taxation of sugary beverages, and improved labeling.[6] Although the policy solutions are necessary, they are not sufficient. The authors indicated that New Zealand had labeling and marketing regulations that were not implemented with fidelity (eg, proper labeling on containers). Education regarding beverage policies along with enforcement could help improve compliance with beverage standards. Education of parents can also be key to replacing sports drinks, energy drinks and other sugary beverages offerings with water in physical activity and sports settings.

While the authors recommendations were excellent, they failed to point out an excellent resource in the promotion of healthy lifestyle behaviors - pediatric providers.[6] According to the AAP recommendations, pediatricians should inform families that water is the best source of hydration for most children.[4] Pediatric providers can equip families with concrete steps for increasing child water intake (eg, have a reusable water bottle with water for easy access by children, role model water intake). Additionally, providers should discuss the limited indications for sports drink use (ie, extended periods of vigorous physical activity) and highlight the risks of energy drink consumption.[4] Only a third of pediatric providers in a 2014 US study reported regularly counseling patients on sports and energy drink consumption.[7] There is a need to elevate the importance of this counseling in light of the current obesity crisis.

Involvement of pediatricians is important because they also play an important role through advocacy in their local communities. Advocacy opportunities include efforts to increase the availability of healthy beverages in sports venues and practices; limit marketing of SSBs, including endorsement of unhealthy beverages by athletes and celebrities; reduce portion sizes for SSBs; and institute standards to ensure clear information about health impacts and ideal portion sizes on beverage labels.

Although public health efforts have been successful in reducing soda intake over the past decade, consumption of sports drinks and energy drinks are on the rise.[8] Moving forward, it is important that we apply lessons from successes in reducing soda intake to help curb consumption of sports drinks and energy drinks as well. Pediatric providers can play a critical role in this effort by counseling families as early as possible that water is the beverage of choice for children.

A. I. Patel, MD, MSHS
P. B. Crawford, DrPH, RD

References

1. Woodward-Lopez G, Ritchie LD, Gerstein D, Crawford PB. *Obesity: Dietary and Developmental Influences.* Boca Raton, LA: CRC Press; 2006.
2. Institute of Medicine. Accelerating Progress in Obesity Prevention. Solving the Weight of the Nation. http://forthealthcare.com/LetsDoThis/wp-content/uploads/2012/12/Institute_of_Medicine-Obesity_Prevention.pdf. Accessed July 24, 2014.
3. Ludwig DS, Peterson KE, Gortmaker SL. Relation between consumption of sugar-sweetened drinks and childhood obesity: a prospective, observational analysis. *Lancet.* 2001;357(9255):505-508.
4. Committee on Nutrition and the Council on Sports Medicine and Fitness. Sports drinks and energy drinks for children and adolescents: are they appropriate? *Pediatrics.* 2011;127:1182-1189.
5. Sugary Drink Facts. Yale Rudd Center for Food Policy & Obesity Website. http://www.sugarydrinkfacts.org/resources/SugaryDrinkFACTS_Report_Conclusions.pdf. Accessed July 24, 2014.
6. Smith M, Jenkin G, Signal L, McLean R. Consuming calories and creating cavities: beverages NZ children associate with sport. *Appetite.* 2014;81:209-217.
7. Xiang N, Wethington H, Onufrak S, Belay B. Characteristics of US health care providers who counsel adolescents on sports and energy drink consumption. *Int J Pediatr.* 2014;2014:987082.
8. Larson N, Dewolfe J, Story M, Neumark-Sztainer D. Adolescent consumption of sports and energy drinks: linkages to higher physical activity, unhealthy beverage patterns, cigarette smoking, and screen media use. *J Nutr Educ Behav.* 2014;46:181-187.

Perioperative outcomes of adolescents undergoing bariatric surgery: the Teen-Longitudinal Assessment of Bariatric Surgery (Teen-LABS) study

Inge TH, Teen-LABS Consortium (Cincinnati Children's Hosp Med Ctr, OH; et al)
JAMA Pediatr 168:47-53, 2014

Importance.—Severe obesity in childhood is a major health problem with few effective treatments. Weight-loss surgery (WLS) is being used to treat severely obese adolescents, although with very limited data regarding surgical safety for currently used, minimally invasive procedures.

Objective.—To assess the preoperative clinical characteristics and perioperative safety outcomes of severely obese adolescents undergoing WLS.

Design, Setting, and Participants.—This prospective, multisite observational study enrolled patients from February 28, 2007, through December 30, 2011. Consecutive patients aged 19 years or younger who were approved to undergo WLS (n = 277) were offered enrollment into the study at 5 academic referral centers in the United States; 13 declined participation and 22 did not undergo surgery after enrollment, thus the final analysis cohort consisted of 242 individuals. There were no withdrawals.

Main Outcomes and Measures.—This analysis examined preoperative anthropometrics, comorbid conditions, and major and minor complications occurring within 30 days of operation. All data were collected in a standardized fashion. Reoperations and hospital readmissions were adjudicated by independent reviewers to assess relatedness to the WLS procedure.

Results.—The mean (SD) age of participants was 17.1 (1.6) years and the median body mass index (calculated as weight in kilograms divided by height in meters squared) was 50.5. Fifty-one percent demonstrated 4 or more major comorbid conditions. Laparoscopic Roux-en-Y gastric bypass, vertical sleeve gastrectomy, and adjustable gastric banding were performed in 66%, 28%, and 6% of patients, respectively. There were no deaths during the initial hospitalization or within 30 days of operation; major complications (eg, reoperation) were seen in 19 patients (8%). Minor complications (eg, readmission for dehydration) were noted in 36 patients (15%). All reoperations and 85% of readmissions were related to WLS.

Conclusions and Relevance.—In this series, adolescents with severe obesity presented with abundant comorbid conditions. We observed a favorable short-term complication profile, supporting the early postoperative safety of WLS in select adolescents. Further longitudinal study of this cohort will permit accurate assessment of long-term outcomes for adolescents undergoing bariatric surgery.

▶ The prevalence of severe obesity among adolescents remains high, putting millions of youth at risk for a host of comorbid conditions and a shortened life expectancy.[1-3] Current behavioral approaches to treatment have only achieved modest effects.[4] Bariatric surgery has the potential to be the most effective means of achieving significant weight loss for numerous patients who have been unable to achieve success with other interventions, but many clinicians question the appropriateness and safety of performing bariatric surgery among adolescents. Indeed, our survey of primary care physicians (pediatricians and family physicians) showed that approximately half would not refer their severely obese adolescent patients for bariatric surgery until age 18.[5] Although this perspective likely reflects concern regarding the possible risks of bariatric surgery among youth, it may lead to decreased access to a potentially effective means of treatment. Data about the risks and benefits of these procedures for young patients are crucial to provide the best care for affected youth.

Numerous studies among adults demonstrate the benefits of bariatric surgery in both weight reduction and improvement in the comorbidities of obesity.[6,7] However, to date there has been a lack of rigorous prospective studies regarding the safety and effectiveness of bariatric surgery for adolescents. Thus, the Teen-LABS study is valuable and these results fill a gap in the literature and will help to inform decision making for adolescents, their parents, and their physicians. The findings are particularly useful because procedure-specific findings are provided. Among the literature available on adolescent bariatric surgery, the majority of studies address the Roux-en-Y (Tables 3 and 4 in the original article). Thus, additional information regarding the vertical sleeve gastrectomy and the adjustable gastric band offers valuable comparative data. Furthermore, the evidence from this study of the high number of comorbidities (including conditions not used as selection criteria) experienced by the patient population provides support regarding the critical need for interventions to improve the health of severely obese adolescents. This finding highlights the fact that severe obesity does not merely lead to long-term health risks, but it affects patients' health even during the adolescent years.

While the study addresses a significant question, it has some pertinent limitations. As African American and Hispanic populations have a disproportionately high prevalence of obesity, the fact that the sample was not representative of the national population of severely obese adolescents is unfortunate. Indeed, the study raises questions regarding referral patterns and access to bariatric surgery for minorities that warrant exploration. Furthermore, the mean age of the patients in Teen-LABS was 17.7 years old. However, severe obesity affects younger adolescents as well, and it is in the younger age group that most clinical hesitation and concern exists. Although 27% of the patients in Teen-LABS were 13 to 15 years old, findings were not reported by age group, which would be helpful for those treating younger teens.

This report from the Teen-LABS study is an important step in providing information about the risks of bariatric surgery. The relatively low complication rate may help to alleviate concerns about adolescent bariatric surgery and lead to a larger number of patients and providers considering this option. Furthermore, it serves as a benchmark for hospitals that might offer this option to teens. Because there was not a standard protocol across sites, additional details regarding the treatment protocols from the sites with the best outcomes (or from all sites if outcomes were similar) would be of great benefit to emerging programs. However, these results are just a piece of the puzzle.

As additional data (particularly about long-term medical and psychosocial outcomes) are gleaned from the Teen-LABS study, it will be possible to gain a more complete picture regarding the ramifications of adolescent bariatric surgery and ways to optimize care. Patients, clinicians, and researchers will benefit most if future results from Teen-LABS are reported with age stratification. Furthermore, follow-up investigations in this clinical arena should prioritize recruitment of subjects in ways that generate study samples who more closely resemble the population of severely obese adolescents in the United States.

S. J. Woolford, MD, MPH

References

1. Skinner AC, Skelton JA. Prevalence and trends in obesity and severe obesity among children in the United States, 1999-2012. *JAMA Pediatr.* 2014;168:561-566.
2. Dietz WH. Health consequences of obesity in youth: childhood predictors of adult disease. *Pediatrics.* 1998;101:518-525.
3. Olshansky SJ, Passaro DJ, Hershow RC, et al. "A potential decline in life expectancy in the United States in the 21st century". *New England Journal of Medicine.* 2005;352:1138-1145.
4. Savoye M, Shaw M, Dziura J, et al. Effects of a weight management program on body composition and metabolic parameters in overweight children: a randomized controlled trial. *JAMA.* 2007;297:2697-2704.
5. Woolford SJ, Clark SJ, Freed G. To Cut or Not to Cut: Physicians' Perspectives on Referring Adolescents for Bariatric Surgery. *Obesity Surg.* 2010;20:937-942.
6. Sjöström L, Narbro K, Sjöström CD, et al. Effects of bariatric surgery on mortality in Swedish obese subjects. *N Engl J Med.* 2007;357:741-752.
7. Sjöström L, Lindroos A-K, Peltonen M, et al. Lifestyle, diabetes, and cardiovascular risk factors 10 years after bariatric surgery. *N Engl J Med.* 2004;351:2683-2693.

16 Oncology

Cancer Risk among Children Born after Assisted Conception
Williams CL, Bunch KJ, Stiller CA, et al (Univ College London, UK; Univ of Oxford, UK; et al)
N Engl J Med 369:1819-1827, 2013

Background.—Accurate population-based data are needed on the incidence of cancer in children born after assisted conception.

Methods.—We linked data on all children born in Britain between 1992 and 2008 after assisted conception without donor involvement with data from the United Kingdom National Registry of Childhood Tumours to determine the number of children in whom cancer developed before 15 years of age. Cohort cancer rates were compared with population-based rates in Britain over the same period, with stratification for potential mediating and moderating factors, including sex, age at diagnosis, birth weight, singleton versus multiple birth, parity, parental age, type of assisted conception, and cause of parental infertility.

Results.—The cohort consisted of 106,013 children born after assisted conception (700,705 person-years of observation). The average duration of follow-up was 6.6 years. Overall, 108 cancers were identified, as compared with 109.7 expected cancers (standardized incidence ratio, 0.98; 95% confidence interval [CI], 0.81 to 1.19; $P = 0.87$). Assisted conception was not associated with an increased risk of leukemia, neuroblastoma, retinoblastoma, central nervous system tumors, or renal or germ-cell tumors. It was associated with an increased risk of hepatoblastoma (standardized incidence ratio, 3.64; 95% CI, 1.34 to 7.93; $P = 0.02$; absolute excess risk, 6.21 cases per 1 million person-years) and rhabdomyosarcoma (standardized incidence ratio, 2.62; 95% CI, 1.26 to 4.82; $P = 0.02$; absolute excess risk, 8.82 cases per 1 million person-years), with hepatoblastoma developing in 6 children and rhabdomyosarcoma in 10 children. The excess risk of hepatoblastoma was associated with low birth weight.

Conclusions.—There was no increase in the overall risk of cancer among British children born after assisted conception during the 17-year study period. Increased risks of hepatoblastoma and rhabdomyosarcoma were detected, but the absolute risks were small. (Funded by Cancer Research UK and others.)

▶ This article brings up the risk of cancer as a possible long-term consequence of in vitro fertilization (IVF) including intracytoplasmic sperm injection (ICSI). Such studies are important but difficult to perform. Why would one expect such an effect? Infants born after IVF have an increased risk for various neonatal morbidity including preterm birth and low birth weight, low Apgar score, respiratory complications, neonatal sepsis, cerebral hemorrhage, and neonatal convulsions.[1-3] These negative outcomes are, to some extent, due to multiple births, but even among singletons an increased morbidity exists. There is some evidence that parental subfertility is a major cause of the latter effects. Such neonatal conditions may affect later morbidity in life, including cancer risk. To this list one can add the much discussed possibility that IVF may increase the risk for disturbances of epigenetic mechanisms. Such effects have been seen after IVF in the form of rare congenital malformations (eg, Beckwith-Wiedemann syndrome) and may play a role also for cancer development.

To study cancer risk after fertility treatments, large numbers of patients are needed.[4] Until recently only 2 studies were large enough to identify about 50 cancer cases, and 1 of them[5] did not study IVF but instead the use of ovulation-stimulating drugs. The second study[6] concerned children born after IVF in Sweden. Table 1 compares some characteristics and results of the latter study with that of Williams et al. The Swedish study found a significant risk increase; however, the larger British study found no risk increase. How come?

In the British study, the linkage of cancer cases with birth registration and information on IVF was performed by rather complicated methods, involving probability linkage. A number of characteristics such as birth weight, date of birth, and maternal and paternal date of birth were used to identify potential matches, and further linkage was made with father's surname and mother's forename and recorded surnames. Mislinkage will cause a risk estimate bias toward null. The authors have rejected this possibility.[7] In the Swedish study, linkage was easily made, because every child born has a unique identification number, which is used in all health care, and mislinkage is nearly impossible.

In the British study, the expected number of cancer cases was calculated from the incidence rates in the general population (probably including immigrants), in the Swedish study from observed number of cancer cases in children born in Sweden. In both studies, analysis was made according to year of birth.

The British study found 6 cases of hepatoblastomas against an expected number of 1.8 and ten cases of rhabdomyomas against the expected number of 3.8. In the Swedish material, there was 1 case for each of these diagnoses.

TABLE 1.—Comparison of Two Large Studies on Cancer Risks in Infants Born After IVF

Characteristics	Källén et al., 2011 [6]	Williams et al., 2013
Number of infants after IVF	26,692	106,013
Number of infants with cancer	47*	108
Average follow-up time	7.3 years	6.6 years
Risk estimate	1.34 (1.02-1.76)	0.98 (0.81-1.19)
Specific cancer types increased	None except histiocytosis*	Rhabdomyosarcoma, Hepatoblastoma

Editor's Note: Please refer to original journal article for full references.
*In this Table data on histiocytosis are excluded as they may not qualify as malignant and usually are not counted.
Reprinted from Williams CL, Bunch KJ, Stiller CA, et al. Cancer Risk among Children Born after Assisted Conception. N Engl J Med. 2013;369:1819-1827, © 2013, Massachusetts Medical Society.

The simplest explanation to the divergent results between the 2 studies is that the 2 estimates are random variations of a common estimate, which would be based on 155 observed and 145 expected cases, a nonsignificant risk of 1.07, 95% confidence interval 0.91–1.25. This risk estimate is included in both confidence intervals. Nothing speaks against this interpretation, and it would illustrate a classical rule in epidemiology: never to trust the results of a single study. Perhaps even 2 studies are too few to permit a definite conclusion. Anyway, it seems evident that the cancer risk after IVF, however interesting it is from a theoretical point of view, is hardly high enough to play any practical role, a conclusion drawn also in our previous review.[4]

B. Källén, MD, PhD

References

1. Helmerhorst FM, Perquin DAM, Donker D, Keirse MJNC. Perinatal outcome of singletons and twins after assisted conception: a systematic review of controlled studies. *BMJ.* 2004;328:261.
2. Källén B, Finnström O, Nygren K-G, Olausson PO. In vitro fertilization (IVF) in Sweden: infant outcome after different fertilization methods. *Fertil Steril.* 2005; 84:611-617.
3. Pinborg A, Wennerholm UB, Romundstad LB, et al. Why do singletons conceived after assisted reproduction technology have adverse perinatal outcome? Systematic review and meta-analysis. *Hum Reprod Update.* 2013;19:87-104.
4. Källén B, Finnström O, Nygren K-G, Olausson PO. The link between IVF children and cancer: what do we know so far? *Reprod Sys Sexual Disorders.* 2012;(S5):1-8.
5. Brinton LA, Krüger Kjaer S, Thomsen BL, et al. Childhood tumor risk after treatment with ovulation-stimulatinig drugs. *Fertil Steril.* 2004;81:1083-1091.
6. Källén B, Finnström O, Lindam A, Nilsson E, Nygren K-G, Otterblad Olausson P. Cancer risk in children and young adults conceived by in vitro fertilizartion. *Pediatrics.* 2010;126:270-276.
7. Williams CL, Bunch KJ, Sutcliffe AG. Cancer risk among children born after assisted conception. *N Engl J Med.* 2014;370:975-976.

Early-Onset Basal Cell Carcinoma and Indoor Tanning: A Population-Based Study
Karagas MR, Zens MS, Li Z, et al (Children's Environmental Health and Disease Prevention Res Ctr at Dartmouth, Hanover, NH; et al)
Pediatrics 134:e4-e12, 2014

Objective.—Indoor tanning with UV radiation—emitting lamps is common among adolescents and young adults. Rising incidence rates of basal cell carcinoma (BCC) have been reported for the United States and elsewhere, particularly among those diagnosed at younger ages. Recent epidemiologic studies have raised concerns that indoor tanning may be contributing to early occurrence of BCC, and younger people may be especially vulnerable to cancer risk associated with this exposure. Therefore, we sought to address these issues in a population-based case—control study from New Hampshire.

Methods.—Data on indoor tanning were obtained on 657 cases of BCC and 452 controls ≤50 years of age.

Results.—Early-onset BCC was related to indoor tanning, with an adjusted odds ratio (OR) of 1.6 (95% confidence interval, 1.3–2.1). The strongest association was observed for first exposure as an adolescent or young adult, with a 10% increase in the OR with each age younger at first exposure (OR per year of age ≤23 = 1.1; 95% confidence interval, 1.0–1.2). Associations were present for each type of device examined (ie, sunlamps, tanning beds, and tanning booths).

Conclusions.—Our findings suggest early exposure to indoor tanning increases the risk of early development of BCC. They also underscore the importance of counseling adolescents and young adults about the risks of indoor tanning and for discouraging parents from consenting minors to this practice.

▶ Karagas and colleagues describe the association of tanning indoors with the early-onset (defined in this article as occurring before 50 years of age) of basal cell carcinoma (BCC). The researchers controlled for key confounding factors such as outdoor exposures and skin type. This large study, with results strikingly similar to an earlier study in Connecticut,[1] examined exposures from different types of tanning devices. Early-onset BCC was related to exposures for each type of device; the strongest association was seen when the first exposure occurred in adolescence or young adulthood. The adverse effects of these early life exposures underscore the relevance of indoor tanning to pediatricians and others who provide health care to young people.

BCC is the most common cancer in humans, arising from basal cells in the epidermis. Basal cells and squamous cells together comprise keratinocytes. BCC and squamous cell carcinoma (SCC) comprise "keratinocyte carcinoma" or "nonmelanoma skin cancer (NMSC)." There are about 3.5 million keratinocyte cancers in 2.2 million Americans each year; about 80% are BCC.[2] Not long ago, BCC was found almost entirely in middle-aged and older adults. Recently, BCC has occurred with increasing frequency in younger people.[3] Although BCC is entirely treatable in most people and rarely results in fatality, its treatment results in morbidity and cost.

Tanning in salons is surprisingly common, especially among adolescent girls and women. In a 2011 national survey of 5600 high school students, 13.3% reported using indoor tanning devices at least once in the previous year; girls' use was 20.9%. Use increased with age with more than one-quarter of 17-year-old girls reporting exposure.[4] Among 17-year-old white girls who reported indoor tanning, 62% said they did so 10 or more times in 2011,[5] dispelling the notion that this practice is merely a "pre-prom" or "prevacation" phenomenon. Salon tanning is low-cost, and salons that offer tanning are easy to find, often located near high schools and colleges. There are more tanning salons in an average US city than Starbucks or McDonalds.[6]

Many studies of tanning devices and their relationship to cancer have focused on cutaneous melanoma. Although melanoma comprises just 4% to 5% of skin cancers, it accounts for 80% of skin cancer fatalities. Melanoma incidence has risen dramatically in young women, more so than in young men,[7] and is considered to be an epidemic by some experts. There will be an expected

78 100 new cases of melanoma in the United States in 2014.[8] Although melanoma is treatable when found early, approximately 9710 melanoma fatalities are expected in the United States in 2014[8]; some of these deaths will occur in young people. Melanoma is now the second most common cancer in women aged 20 to 29.[9] Many authorities believe this rise is related, at least in part, to the far higher prevalence of indoor tanning in adolescent girls and young women compared with adolescent boys and young men.

In 2009, the International Agency for Research on Cancer (IARC, part of the World Health Organization) classified ultraviolet-emitting tanning devices as "carcinogenic to humans."[10] This was based on IARC's analyses of epidemiologic studies showing that exposure to ultraviolet (UV) radiation emitted from tanning devices increased the risk of developing cutaneous melanoma; risk increased by 75% when use started before 35 years of age. Subsequent studies confirmed this association.[11,12] Tanning device use also raises the risk of developing SCC.[13]

Because of increased skin cancer risks, the World Health Organization, the American Academy of Pediatrics, American Medical Association, American Academy of Dermatology, American Cancer Society and others recommend banning access to tanning salons for consumers under age 18. Many nations ban minors' access. Because indoor tanning raises cancer risks for all people, a population-wide ban of tanning beds takes effect throughout Australia on January 1, 2015. Australia will become the second country, after Brazil, to completely ban use of these devices.

In May 2014, the US Food and Drug Administration (FDA) issued an order requiring that sunlamp products used in tanning salons carry a visible blackbox warning stating: "Attention: This sunlamp product should not be used on persons under the age of 18 years."[14] The new order came with the FDA's reclassification of UV sunlamp products. Although a warning label is now required, the FDA did not require an outright ban on minors' access. It therefore still falls to states to enact such bans. Of all available legislative approaches, age restrictions are most effective in preventing adolescents from tanning.[15] Increasingly, US states are passing legislation banning minors under age 18 from indoor tanning. As of July 2014, one-fifth of states had passed these under-18 bans, and most others had some kind of legislation concerning adolescents and tanning salons.[16]

The Karagas study gives clinicians more reason to include discussions about skin cancer and its prevention in well-child and well-adolescent visits, and during "teachable moments" such as when adolescents present with sunburns. The US Preventive Services Task Force recommends that clinicians counsel fair-skinned persons between the ages of 10 and 24 years about UV protection. Evidence indicates that this advice will result in behavior change in some patients.[17] Because young adolescents often visit salons with their mothers, discussions should also include parents. Clinicians can stress the point of the Karagas article: early exposure—at the ages adolescents are seen in the pediatric office—increases the risk of developing skin cancer. There is no reason for any adolescent to visit a tanning salon.

The study also suggests that pediatricians and colleagues—including dermatologists and surgical and medical oncologists—should continue to wage legislative campaigns in states that currently do not have strong laws to protect children and adolescents.[18] All states should pass under-18 tanning bans. Because indoor tanning also raises cancer risk in the adult population, it is hoped that in the future, advocates will urge policy makers to pass a population-wide ban in the United States, as has been done in Brazil and Australia.

S. J. Balk, MD

References

1. Ferrucci LM, Cartmel B, Molinaro AM, Leffell DJ, Bale AE, Mayne ST. Indoor tanning and risk of early-onset basal cell carcinoma. *J Am Acad Dermatol.* 2012;67:552-562.
2. American Cancer Society. What are the key statistics about basal and squamous cell skin cancers? http://www.cancer.org/cancer/skincancer-basalandsquamouscell/detailedguide/skin-cancer-basal-and-squamous-cell-key-statistics. Accessed July 23, 2014.
3. Christenson LJ, Borrowman TA, Vachon CM, et al. Incidence of basal cell and squamous cell carcinomas in a population younger than 40 years. *JAMA.* 2005;294:681-690.
4. Guy GP Jr, Berkowitz Z, Tai E, Holman DM, Everett Jones S, Richardson LC. Indoor tanning among high school students in the United States, 2009 and 2011. *JAMA Dermatol.* 2014;150:501-511.
5. Guy GP, Berkowitz Z, Watson M, Holman DM, Richardson LC. Indoor tanning among young non-Hispanic white females. *JAMA Intern Med.* 2013;173:1920-1922.
6. Hoerster KD, Garrow RL, Mayer JA, et al. Density of indoor tanning facilities in 116 large U.S. cities. *Am J Prev Med.* 2009;36:243-246.
7. Purdue MP, Freeman LE, Anderson WF, Tucker MA. Recent trends in incidence of cutaneous melanoma among US Caucasian young adults. *J Invest Dermatol.* 2008;128:2905-2908.
8. American Cancer Society. What are the key statistics about melanoma skin cancer? http://www.cancer.org/cancer/skincancer-melanoma/detailedguide/melanoma-skin-cancer-key-statistics. Accessed July 27, 2014.
9. CDC Wonder. United States Cancer Statistics, 1999-2010 Incidence Results. http://wonder.cdc.gov/cancer-v2010.HTML. Accessed July 27, 2014.
10. International Agency for Research on Cancer. Sunbeds and UV Radiation. http://www.iarc.fr/en/media-centre/iarcnews/2009/sunbeds_uvradiation.php. Accessed July 23, 2014.
11. Lazovich D, Vogel RI, Berwick M, Weinstock MA, Anderson KE, Warshaw EM. Indoor tanning and risk of melanoma: a case-control study in a highly exposed population. *Cancer Epidemiol Biomarkers Prev.* 2010;19:1557-1568.
12. Cust AE, Armstrong BK, Goumas C, et al. Sunbed use during adolescence and early adulthood is associated with increased risk of early-onset melanoma. *Int J Cancer.* 2011;128:2425-2435.
13. The International Agency for Research on Cancer Working Group on Artificial Ultraviolet (UV) Light and Skin Cancer. The association of use of sunbeds with cutaneous malignant melanoma and other skin cancers: a systematic review. *Int J Cancer.* 2006;120:1116-1122.
14. Department of Health and Human Services. Food and Drug Administration. 21 CFR Part 878. [Docket No. FDA-2013-N-0461]. General and Plastic Surgery Devices: Reclassification of Ultraviolet Lamps for Tanning, Henceforth to Be Known as Sunlamp Products and Ultraviolet Lamps Intended for Use in Sunlamp Products. http://www.gpo.gov/fdsys/pkg/FR-2014-06-02/pdf/2014-12546.pdf. Accessed July 13, 2014.

15. Guy GP, Berkowitz A, Jones SE, et al. State indoor tanning laws and adolescent indoor tanning. *Am J Public Health*. 2014;104:e69-e74.
16. National Conference of State Legislatures. Indoor Tanning Restrictions for Minors - A State-by-State Comparison. http://www.ncsl.org/research/health/indoor-tanning-restrictions.aspx. Accessed July 27, 2014.
17. Moyer VA, United States Preventive Services Task Force. Behavioral counseling to prevent skin cancer: U.S. Preventive Services Task Force recommendation statement. *Ann Intern Med*. 2012;157:59-65.
18. Balk SJ, Fisher DE, Geller AC. Stronger laws are needed to protect teens from indoor tanning. *Pediatrics*. 2013;131:586-588.

A Longitudinal, Randomized, Controlled Trial of Advance Care Planning for Teens With Cancer: Anxiety, Depression, Quality of Life, Advance Directives, Spirituality

Lyon ME, Jacobs S, Briggs L, et al (George Washington Univ School of Medicine and Health Sciences, DC; Gundersen Med Foundation, Inc, La Crosse, WI)

J Adolesc Health 54:710-717, 2014

Purpose.—To test the feasibility, acceptability and safety of a pediatric advance care planning intervention, Family-Centered Advance Care Planning for Teens With Cancer (FACE-TC).

Methods.—Adolescent (age 14—20 years)/family dyads (N = 30) with a cancer diagnosis participated in a two-armed, randomized, controlled trial. Exclusion criteria included severe depression and impaired mental status. Acceptability was measured by the Satisfaction Questionnaire. General Estimating Equations models assessed the impact of FACE-TC on 3-month post-intervention outcomes as measured by the Pediatric Quality of Life Inventory 4.0 Generic Core Scale, the Pediatric Quality of Life Inventory 4.0 Cancer-Specific Module, the Beck Depression and Anxiety Inventories, the Spiritual Well-Being Scale of the Functional Assessment of Chronic Illness Therapy—IV, and advance directive completion.

Results.—Acceptability was demonstrated with enrollment of 72% of eligible families, 100% attendance at all three sessions, 93% retention at 3-month post-intervention, and 100% data completion. Intervention families rated FACE-TC worthwhile (100%), whereas adolescents' ratings increased over time (65%—82%). Adolescents' anxiety decreased significantly from baseline to 3-months post-intervention in both groups ($\beta = -5.6$; $p = .0212$). Low depressive symptom scores and high quality of life scores were maintained by adolescents in both groups. Advance directives were located easily in medical records (100% of FACE-TC adolescents vs. no controls). Oncologists received electronic copies. Total Spirituality scores ($\beta = 8.1$; $p = .0296$) were significantly higher among FACE-TC adolescents versus controls. The FACE-TC adolescents endorsed the best time to bring up end-of-life decisions: 19% before being sick, 19% at diagnosis, none when first ill or hospitalized, 25% when dying, and 38% for all of the above.

Conclusions.—Family-Centered Advance Care Planning for Teens With Cancer demonstrated feasibility and acceptability. Courageous adolescents willingly participated in highly structured, indepth pediatric advance care planning conversations safely.

▶ Although the American Academy of Pediatrics and the Institute of Medicine encourage palliative care consultation for all patients at diagnosis with a potentially life-limiting illness, it rarely occurs in pediatric oncology before the immediate end-of-life period. This lack of referral is consistent with oncologists' reluctance to have goals-of-care conversations with families, or do advanced care planning. There are a variety of explanations for this reluctance, including lack of training in how to conduct these conversations, the emotional challenge for providers of having a difficult conversation and managing families' intense emotions, and the worry that these conversations indicate to families that oncologists have given up on finding a cure for patients.

There is much fear that advanced care planning will be perceived by families as giving up on the patients and, as a result, will destroy families' hopes for recovery. However, families consistently indicate that they want more open, honest communication with their medical providers and that they learn that their child has incurable cancer up to weeks after providers are aware of this. Importantly, families are more likely to have a clearer sense of what their adolescent or young adult child would want done if they were to worsen and be unable to participate in conversations about their care if they have had advanced care planning discussions with their parents and providers earlier in their treatment course.[1]

Lyon et al have conducted the first randomized controlled trials to determine the impact of an early advanced care planning intervention and whether adolescent cancer patients and their surrogate parents would vote with their feet. Would they agree to participate and continue to show up? The answer seems to be a resounding yes. Although oncologists have long feared patients and families would refuse to have these conversations and that they would make patients and families more upset and anxious, Lyon found the opposite, which in the end isn't that surprising. People often want to prepare for the worst and hope for the best. Much anxiety arises when people feel like they are not allowed to talk about something that they are thinking a lot about. It is also common to worry that one's wishes won't be honored, but there are taboos that prevent open discussions of topics like death.

There are several reasons why the intervention described in the article by Lyon et al was largely successful at keeping people enrolled. First, by standardizing the timing of the intervention near diagnosis, it allowed families and providers to believe the intervention was not a result of treatment failure. This routine protocol likely reduced the anxiety around the discussion and kept it largely hypothetical. This may also explain the similar lowering of rates of anxiety for patients in both the intervention and control arms. Although the surrogates' anxiety did rise for the intervention group, the authors claim that it was not a clinically significant increase. It is reasonable that having these conversations did make the reality of their child's potential mortality more real, but overall this did not have a significantly negative impact on parents in the intervention arm. Second, the intervention was done with trained facilitators, which ensured there was less of a concern about self-efficacy or inadequate skills in conducting the conversations, as is often described by oncology providers who have little formal training in communication skills. Third, the intervention was adapted from another previously tested intervention for a similarly aged population of chronically ill patients and was iteratively improved based on early feedback.

In addition to showing up for the session, the majority of participants rated the 3 sessions as worthwhile, and, more important, 100% of patients in the interventions and their surrogates filled out the advanced care planning document and had it readily available to the medical team in the medical record. Any provider who has cared for patients near the end of life in the intensive care unit or even on the cancer unit floor understands how incredibly stressful it is to initiate these conversations with families when they are in the midst of a crisis. Having these documents readily available can be an incredibly powerful tool for how to best support patients and families in these stressful times. It also reduces uncertainty so the family is more confident about what the child would have wanted in these circumstances.

Some limitations of the study include the fact that the sample size was small and that it recruited patients who were willing to engage in advanced care planning discussions at entry to the study, limiting the study's generalizability to all adolescent cancer patients. Also, the authors do not explain why they hypothesize the intervention will positively affect a patient's spirituality, which leaves one to assume that increased spirituality is perceived to be a positive attribute for cancer patients.

Despite these minor limitations, the study takes a large step forward in developing and refining an advanced care planning intervention for adolescents with cancer. It was successful in enrolling and sustaining enrollment across multiple sessions. There was completion of advanced directives without seriously compromising patient or family anxiety, patient quality of life, or increasing the likelihood of depression. As a result, this is a safe and important study to expand on.

J. K. Walter, MD, PhD, MS

C. Feudtner, MD, PhD, MPH

Reference

1. Lyon ME, Jacobs S, Briggs L, Cheng YI, Wang J. Family centered advanced care planning for teens with cancer. *JAMA Pediatr.* 2013:943. http://dx.doi.org/10.1001/jamapediatrics.

17 Ophthalmology

Choroidal Thickness in Patients With a History of Retinopathy of Prematurity

Wu W-C, Shih C-P, Wang N-K, et al (Chang Gung Memorial Hosp, Taoyuan, Taiwan; Chang Gung Univ, Taoyuan, Taiwan; et al)
JAMA Ophthalmol 131:1451-1458, 2013

Importance.—The cause of reduced vision in patients with a history of retinopathy of prematurity (ROP) is not yet fully understood. The role of the choroid in ROP remains unknown and existing studies of choroidal thickness in patients with a history of ROP are limited. It might be helpful to understand the association of the choroid with ROP by measuring the choroidal thickness in patients with a history of ROP and correlating these findings with the visual outcome of these patients.

Objective.—To examine choroidal thickness by spectral-domain optical coherence tomography in children with a history of ROP and assess the impact of choroidal thickness on visual acuity.

Design.—A prospective cross-sectional analysis from August 2011 to September 2012.

Setting.—Institutional referral centers.

Participants.—Children aged 6 to 14 years with a history of ROP were classified into the following 2 groups: patients with a history of threshold ROP and treatment with laser or cryotherapy (treated group) and those with regressed ROP who had not received any treatment (nontreated group). All of the patients had a normal-appearing posterior pole.

Intervention.—Examinations of visual acuity, refractive errors, and optical components and measurement of choroidal thickness.

Main Outcomes and Measures.—Best-corrected visual acuity, optical components, and optical coherence tomography findings.

Results.—In total, 49 patients were enrolled in the study. Patients in the treated group had a significantly thinner choroidal thickness than the patients in the nontreated group after adjusting for age, axial length, and spherical power. Choroidal thickness was found to be positively associated with spherical power and spherical equivalent and negatively associated with axial length and vitreous depth. In addition, a thin choroidal thickness was associated with a worse best-corrected visual acuity.

Conclusions and Relevance.—Choroidal thickness is thinner in patients with threshold ROP compared with the patients with spontaneously regressed ROP. A thinner choroid is associated with worse vision in these patients. This study might imply the association of choroid circulation with ROP.

▶ Retinopathy of prematurity (ROP) remains one of the most common causes of permanent visual impairment among children in the developed world. In this condition abnormal development of the retinal blood vessels develop after pre-term delivery, which, if sufficiently severe, can lead to retinal distortion and detachment. With the advent of ablative retinal treatments (specifically, cryother-apy and retinal photocoagulation) in the 1980s and 1990s, the number of chil-dren with catastrophic visual loss has been greatly reduced.[1,2] However, some children with spontaneously regressed ROP or postablation treated have nor-mal-appearing retinas on direct and indirect ophthalmoscopy, yet the child's vision is reduced.[3] Even after excluding developmental and cognitive issues this unfavorable outcome persists.

The most visually sensitive portion of the retina is the fovea, less than 1 mm in diameter, which is located at the center of the macula. Characteristically there is a light reflection from the fovea when viewed with the direct ophthalmoscope. Beneath the retina is the choroid, which is a highly vascular layer of the eye, sup-plying oxygen and nutrition to the outer retina.

Recently, investigators have begun exploring microscopic changes to the retinal capillaries in children with ROP. The hypothesis is that there may be vas-cular changes in smaller retinal vessels not seen with the ophthalmoscope. For instance the development of the normal pattern of fine capillaries around the fovea and the necessary thinning of the fovea are altered in some premature chil-dren.[4] Such changes could produce clinically significant changes in best-corrected visual acuity.

Beneath the fovea, other investigators have been studying the choroid to determine if prematurity can alter development of the choroidal vasculature. Damage or loss of choroid leads to loss of photoreceptors and presumably loss of visual acuity. Wu and colleagues explored the impact of prematurity and ROP on the choroid of human infants. The authors imaged the retina and choroid of 49 children with a history of ROP in the area of the fovea using optical coher-ence tomography. This noninvasive imaging technique provides a cross-sectional view of the eye showing highly detailed renderings of the retinal layers as well as the choroid (Fig 1 in the original article), in many ways comparable to histology.

The study included children aged 6 to 14 years; all had ROP as infants. Some had been treated for ROP as infants, and others experienced spontaneous regres-sion. The investigators found that the children, who were treated and therefore are presumed to have had more serious retinal disease, had on average signifi-cantly thinner choroids (Fig 2 in the original article). This finding persisted under the fovea and for the entire macula.

They developed a multivariate analytical model and found a negative correla-tion of choroidal thickness and visual acuity. As the choroid thinned, visual acuity declined. They concluded that ROP was associated with a significant adverse impact on choroidal development. They felt it biologically plausible that an abnormally thin choroid could reduce visual acuity potential, at least in children with severe ROP requiring surgery.

There are important limitations of the research. First, the study cannot demonstrate causation. Furthermore, we do not know if the choroidal thinning was related to the severity of ROP, the greater degree of prematurity in the treatment group, or the ablative treatment itself. This study did not include children without any ROP, which would have helped establish normal values of subfoveal choroidal thickness for previously premature infants. Such data could help determine if prematurity, ROP, or ablative therapy was associated with the changes in the choroid. Lastly, we do not know if the fovea was actually damaged by the thinned choroid.

These data encourage ophthalmologists to pursue a better understanding of the impact of prematurity and ROP on choroidal development and ultimately visual acuity. Better noninvasive imaging could be used to detect variations in the normal development of the choroid and the fovea, which could lead to improvement in management. In addition, with the increasing interest and use of bevacizumab, a vascular endothelial growth factor inhibitor, for the treatment of ROP,[5,6] there may be additional unanticipated adverse effects on retinal and choroidal development and consequent impairment of vision. Such an adverse effect of bevacizumab on development of the retinal microvasculature has recently been reported.[7] The ability to study the choroid with noninvasive imaging allows future research concerning ROP therapy to explore the potential positive and negative impacts of bevacizumab theory before wholesale adoption.

M. X. Repka, MD, MBA

References

1. Palmer EA, Hardy RJ, Dobson V, et al. 15-year outcomes following threshold retinopathy of prematurity: final results from the multicenter trial of cryotherapy for retinopathy of prematurity. *Arch Ophthalmol.* 2005;123:311-318.
2. Hunter DG, Repka MX. Diode laser photocoagulation for retinopathy of prematurity: a randomized study. *Ophthalmology.* 1993;100:238-244.
3. Siatkowski RM, Good WV, Summers CG, Quinn GE, Tung B. Clinical characteristics of children with severe visual impairment but favorable retinal structural outcomes from the Early Treatment for Retinopathy of Prematurity (ETROP) study. *J AAPOS.* 2013;17:129-134.
4. Yanni SE, Wang J, Chan M, et al. Foveal avascular zone and foveal pit formation after preterm birth. *Br J Ophthalmol.* 2012;96:961-966.
5. Mintz-Hittner HA, Kennedy KA, Chuang AC, BEAT-ROP Cooperative Group. Efficacy of intravitreal bevacizumab for stage 3+ retinopathy of prematurity. *N Engl J Med.* 2011;364:603-615.
6. Micieli JA, Surkont M, Smith AF. A systematic analysis of the off-label use of bevacizumab for severe retinopathy of prematurity. *Am J Ophthalmol.* 2009;148:536-543.
7. Lepore D, Quinn GE, Molle F, et al. Intravitreal bevacizumab versus laser treatment in type 1 retinopathy of prematurity: report on fluorescein angiographic findings. *Ophthalmology.* 2014 [Epub ahead of print].

18 Respiratory Tract

Infant Deaths and Injuries Associated with Wearable Blankets, Swaddle Wraps, and Swaddling

McDonnell E, Moon RY (Children's Natl Med Ctr, Washington, DC; George Washington Univ School of Medicine and Health Sciences, DC)
J Pediatr 164:1152-1156, 2014

Objective.—To assess risks involved in using wearable blankets, swaddle wraps, and swaddling.

Study Design.—This was a retrospective review of incidents reported to the Consumer Product Safety Commission between 2004 and 2012.

Results.—A total of 36 incidents involving wearable blankets and swaddle wraps were reviewed, including 10 deaths, 2 injuries, and 12 incidents without injury. The median age at death was 3.5 months; 80% of the deaths were attributed to positional asphyxia related to prone sleeping, and 70% involved additional risk factors, usually soft bedding. Two injuries involved tooth extraction from the zipper. The 12 incidents without injury reported concern for strangulation/suffocation when the swaddle wrap became wrapped around the face/neck, and a potential choking hazard when the zipper detached. All 12 incidents involving swaddling in ordinary blankets resulted in death. The median age at death was 2 months; 58% of deaths were attributed to positional asphyxia related to prone sleeping, and 92% involved additional risk factors, most commonly soft bedding.

Conclusion.—Reports of sudden unexpected death in swaddled infants are rare. Risks can be reduced by placing infants supine and discontinuing swaddling as soon as an infant's earliest attempts to roll are observed. Risks can be further reduced by removing soft bedding and bumper pads from the sleep environment. When using commercial swaddle wraps, fasteners must be securely attached.

▶ In the 1990s, the national Back-to-Sleep Campaign, aimed at getting all infants in the supine position for sleep, led to an impressive decrease in infant mortality in the United States. But sudden infant death syndrome (SIDS) and other sleep-related deaths remain the leading cause of postneonatal infant mortality (death of infants more than 1 month of age). These deaths likely result, at least in part, from the fact that those who take care of infants continue to place them in a position other than the supine for sleep; to share a bed, sofa, or other unsafe sleep surface; and to place soft bedding around the infants.

TABLE 1.—Deaths Associated with Wearable Blankets and Swaddle Wraps (Total: 10 Infants)

Age	Sex	Race/Ethnicity	Wrap Type	Location	Position	Hazards	Cause of Death
3 d	F	Hispanic	Swaddle wrap	Bassinet	Supine	None	Undetermined
2 mo	M	White	Wearable blanket	Infant glider seat (unrestrained)	Side	Found with face partially covered by side of glider seat	Undetermined
3 mo	F	White	Wearable blanket	Crib	Prone	Thick blankets and pillows under baby	Positional asphyxia
3 mo	M	White	Swaddle wrap	Car seat on floor	Sitting in seat; rolled out of seat to prone	Floor covered with piles of clothes, blankets, pillows	Positional asphyxia
3 mo	M	White	Unknown	Crib	Side; rolled to prone	Placed in sleep positioner between foam wedges, blanket by head, crib bumper pads	Positional asphyxia
4 mo	M	White	Swaddle wrap	Portable crib	Supine; rolled to prone	Soft homemade foam pad instead of mattress	Positional asphyxia
5 mo	M	White	Swaddle wrap	Crib	Supine; rolled to prone	Wrap was removed from product; extra blanket wrapped around baby, crib bumper pads, toys in crib	Positional asphyxia
5 mo	F	White	Swaddle wrap	Crib	Supine; rolled to prone	Crib bumper pads	Positional asphyxia
5.5 mo	F	White	Swaddle wrap	Portable crib	Supine; rolled to prone	Unknown	Positional asphyxia
6.5 mo	M	White	Swaddle wrap	Portable crib	Supine; rolled to prone	Unknown	Positional asphyxia

F, female; M, male.

Reprinted from Journal Pediatrics. McDonnell E, Moon RY. Infant Deaths and Injuries Associated with Wearable Blankets, Swaddle Wraps, and Swaddling. J Pediatr. 2014;164:1152-1156, Copyright 2014, with permission from Elsevier.

TABLE 2.—Deaths Associated with Swaddling in Ordinary Blankets (Total, 12 Infants)

Age	Sex	Race/Ethnicity	Sleep Location	Position	Hazards	Cause of Death
13 d	F	Unknown	Car seat	Sitting in car seat	Sleeping in car seat, covered with quilt, room temperature in 90s	Hyperthermia
2 wk	F	Biracial	Crib	Supine, with head on standard adult pillow	Crib bumper pads, multiple blankets, pillows, stuffed animals; smoke exposure	Suffocation
3 wk	M	White	Adult bed	Supine, with head on nursing pillow	Pillow, comforter; bed-sharing	Suffocation
5 wk	F	White	Bassinet	Supine; rolled to prone	Fleece blanket	Positional asphyxia
1.5 mo	F	Black	Bassinet	Prone	Blankets and stuffed animals	Suffocation
2 mo	F	White	Unknown	Unknown - found with swaddling blanket covering nose and mouth	Unknown	Mechanical asphyxia
2 mo	F	Black	Bassinet	Supine; rolled to prone	Multiple blankets, crib bumper pads, clothes	Positional asphyxia
2.5 mo	F	White	Car seat	Sitting face-up in car seat, but flipped to prone and head-down	Sleeping unstrapped in car seat	Positional asphyxia
3 mo	M	Black	Bassinet	Prone	Multiple blankets, smoke exposure	Positional asphyxia
4 mo	M	Unknown	Portable crib	Supine; rolled to prone	Soft comforter folded underneath baby	Positional asphyxia
4.5 mo	F	Asian	Crib	Supine; rolled to prone	Additional blanket, pillow	Positional asphyxia
8 mo	M	Unknown	Crib	Supine; rolled to prone	Large blanket for swaddling, comforter, crib bumper pads	Positional asphyxia

Most health care providers recommend safe sleep practices to families of infants. But what about swaddling? What should health care providers recommend? Many families like to swaddle their infants because the infants sleep better. Health care providers often model this behavior by swaddling infants during the postpartum hospital stay. Special swaddle blankets, even those with Velcro straps, are popular among consumers of infant products. But is this practice safe? In this article, McDonnell and colleagues take on this question by examining closely deaths related to swaddling.

This study is unique because to date no other study has examined in depth deaths related to swaddling over this many years. In addition, the authors of the study include some details of the incidents, making it somewhat easier to develop recommendations that health care providers can use to keep the swaddled infant safe (Tables 1 and 2).

There are some limitations to the study that should be noted. The authors used data from the Consumer Product Safety Commission from volunteer sources. As a result, the number of injuries and deaths may be underreported. Additionally, the authors acknowledge the absence of data regarding specific product designs that may be associated with varying risk. There was also no way for them to determine the relative risk of death associated with these products because it is impossible to know the overall number of infants using wearable blankets, swaddle wraps, or ordinary blankets.

There are several take-home messages from this study. First, the current public health and provider-level education regarding the safe-sleep environment for infants that includes placing the infant in the supine position, discouraging soft bedding and bumper pads, and maintaining a clutter-free crib or bassinet needs to continually be reinforced. Prone sleeping and soft bedding appear to increase the risk of swaddling. Second, health care providers, and others who serve as important sources of advice, should discuss ways to make swaddling safe. In addition to being told to follow safe sleep recommendations when swaddling, families should know that infants who can roll should not be swaddled because rolling while in a swaddle appears to be dangerous. That means that families should stop swaddling the infants when they turn 3 months of age or start to roll, whichever comes first. Finally, the consistent message for safe swaddling should be both modeled and delivered during the postpartum hospital stay, a critical time for establishing behaviors that will continue at home. Until studies are done to further elucidate the dangers of swaddling, it appears to be prudent to approach this practice with some caution.

E. R. Colson, MD

J. Loyal, MD, MS

Influence of Bedsharing Activity on Breastfeeding Duration Among US Mothers

Huang Y, Hauck FR, Signore C, et al (Univ of Maryland, Baltimore; Univ of Virginia School of Medicine, Charlottesville; Eunice Kennedy Shriver Natl Inst of Child Health and Human Development, Bethesda, MD; et al)
JAMA Pediatr 167:1038-1044, 2013

Importance.—Some professional associations advocate bedsharing to facilitate breastfeeding, while others recommend against it to reduce the risk of sudden infant death syndrome and suffocation deaths. A better understanding of the quantitative influence of bedsharing on breastfeeding duration is needed to guide policy.

Objective.—To quantify the influence of bedsharing on breastfeeding duration.

Design, Setting, and Participants.—Longitudinal data were from the Infant Feeding Practices Study II, which enrolled mothers while pregnant and followed them through the first year of infant life. Questionnaires were sent at infant ages 1 to 7, 9, 10, and 12 months, and 1846 mothers answered at least 1 question regarding bedsharing and were breastfeeding at infant age 2 weeks.

Exposures.—Bedsharing, defined as the mother lying down and sleeping with her infant on the same bed or other sleeping surfaces for nighttime sleep or during the major sleep period.

Main Outcomes and Measures.—Survival analysis to investigate the effect of bedsharing on duration of any and exclusive breastfeeding.

Results.—Longer duration of bedsharing, indicated by a larger cumulative bedsharing score, was associated with a longer duration of any breastfeeding but not exclusive breastfeeding, after adjusting for covariates. Breastfeeding duration was longer among women who were better educated, were white, had previously breastfed, had planned to breastfeed, and had not returned to work in the first year postpartum.

Conclusions and Relevance.—Multiple factors were associated with breastfeeding, including bedsharing. Given the risk of sudden infant death syndrome related to bedsharing, multipronged strategies to promote breastfeeding should be developed and tested.

▶ The benefits of breastfeeding for both mother and baby are well known. Babies are protected from infections, including gastroenteritis, otitis media, and pneumonia; they are less likely to become obese or die of sudden infant death syndrome (SIDS). Mothers who breastfeed have a decreased risk of breast and ovarian cancers.

Despite this, US breastfeeding rates remain low. Although 75% of US mothers initiate breastfeeding, < 15% of babies are exclusively breastfed at the end of 6 months. Additionally, rates are significantly lower for African American infants. According to the Centers for Disease Control and Prevention 2012 Breastfeeding Report Card, these rates are slowly rising. Breastfeeding initiation increased from 74.6% in 2008 to 76.9% in 2009. This improvement in initiation represents the

A

B

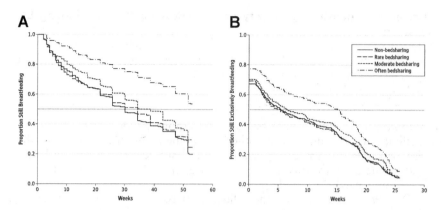

FIGURE.—Kaplan-Meier Curves on the Duration of Any Breastfeeding Within the First Year (A) and Exclusive Breastfeeding Within the First 6 Months (B). Categories are as follows: non-bedsharing (score = 0), rare bedsharing (score = 1 or 2), moderate bedsharing (score = 3 or 4), and often bedsharing (score = 5, 6, or 7). (Reprinted from Huang Y, Hauck FR, Signore C, et al. Influence of bedsharing activity on breastfeeding duration among US mothers. *JAMA Pediatr.* 2013;167:1038-1044.)

largest annual increase over the previous decade. Breastfeeding at 6 months increased from 44.3% to 47.2%; breastfeeding at 12 months increased from 23.8% to 25.5%.

There is still much work to be done to reach the Healthy People 2020 goals for US breastfeeding rates. Compared with 2006 levels, the goals include increasing any breastfeeding from 74% to 81.9%, exclusive 3-month rates from 33.6% to 46.2%, exclusive 6-month rates from 14.1% to 25.5%, and 1-year rates from 22.7% to 34.1%.

If further increases in sustained breastfeeding are to be achieved, it is critical to determine factors that promote breastfeeding success. One way to acquire understanding is through study of the underlying characteristics that are associated with longer versus shorter duration of breastfeeding. The study by Huang explores factors that affect breastfeeding duration and focuses on the controversial variable of bed sharing.

The study confirms the relationship between bed sharing and prolonged partial breastfeeding (ie, "any breastfeeding") but does not show a longer duration of exclusive breastfeeding if one bed shares. Both these relationship are illustrated in the Kaplan-Meier curves (Figure). Importantly, the study also confirms that many other factors are critical to the success of long-term breastfeeding. Mothers were more likely to sustain breastfeeding if they had some college education, were non-Hispanic white, were married, did not return to work in the first year of infancy, had breastfed another child, did not smoke postpartum, had prenatally planned to exclusively breastfeed, and had no neonatal breastfeeding problems (Table 3 in the original article). These findings are consistent with results found in previous studies.

Because it is difficult to accurately measure the true duration of bed sharing, the authors used a rigorous cumulative bed sharing score as a proxy for duration of bed sharing. Additionally, the authors controlled for numerous covariates to better identify the association between bed sharing and duration of breastfeeding. They found that for each 1-level increase in the cumulative bed-sharing score, the likelihood of stopping any breastfeeding within the first year was reduced by 15.5% (Table 3 in the original article).

The study is limited by an overrepresentation of Caucasian women of higher socioeconomic status and inclusion of only healthy singleton infants, which may limit extrapolating the results to families of other races and ethnicities and infants with health issues. In addition, the duration of breastfeeding was not defined by a continuous duration but by how often the question was asked during the study.

This study does not prove a causal link between breastfeeding and bed sharing. Other factors common to both, such as parenting style, may also be important. Furthermore, some mothers may not wish to or are not able (for work or other reasons) to breastfeed for prolonged duration, and this issue was not explored. Additionally, this study does not evaluate whether room sharing without bed sharing can achieve the same breastfeeding benefit without putting the baby at risk for sleep-related death.

Numerous studies have documented that bed sharing increases the risk of SIDS. The growing body of evidence led the American Academy of Pediatrics in 2005 to recommend that parents should sleep in the same room, but not sleep on the same bed or surface with their infants. Additional evidence continues to accumulate, with studies showing the combined odds ratio of approximately 2.8 for SIDS when bed sharing. The risk of bed sharing is highest for infants <12 weeks of age (odds ratios 5.1—10.3).

The study by Huang can help health care providers identify mothers who are at higher risk for not breastfeeding—for example, those who are younger, of lower education and socioeconomic status, returning to work soon after giving birth, non-white race, and first-time mothers. Targeted, culturally sensitive interventions promoting the benefits of breastfeeding and providing assistance to achieve longer breastfeeding duration may be helpful.

At the end of the day, parents want to be the best they can be and provide the best for their babies. As providers and child advocates, we want to assist parents by providing the best information to allow infants to not just be healthy but to thrive and reach their full potential. This study places public health officials and providers (and perhaps parents) in a difficult situation; on the one hand, we want to promote breastfeeding, and bed sharing appears to be a way to increase its duration. On the other hand, epidemiologic studies show a clear association of bed sharing and increased risk of SIDS.

The challenge will be in finding the equipoise between the conflicting ideals of maximizing breastfeeding and minimizing the risk of sleep-related death as we provide education for families. If promoting the benefits of breastfeeding rather than the benefits of bed sharing can achieve the same outcome, it would be worthwhile to avoid the increased risk of a sleep-related death for the infant. Perhaps after these interventions have been exhausted, there could be further discussion of balancing the risks and benefits to bed sharing, but until we reach that point, safety would dictate the promotion of safe sleep over the benefit of prolonged breastfeeding through bed sharing. Additional research is needed to explore the impact of the safer alternative of room sharing on breastfeeding duration. Further efforts are needed to determine the most effective messages providers can give parents to achieve optimal outcomes for infants: breastfeeding and a safe sleep environment.

M. H. Goodstein, MD

R. Y. Moon, MD

Readmissions Among Children Previously Hospitalized With Pneumonia
Neuman MI, Hall M, Gay JC, et al (Boston Children's Hosp, MA; The Children's Hosp Association, Overland Park, KS; Monroe Carell Jr. Children's Hosp at Vanderbilt, Nashville, TN; et al)
Pediatrics 134:100-109, 2014

Background and Objectives.—Pneumonia is a leading cause of hospitalization and readmission in children. Understanding the patient characteristics associated with pneumonia readmissions is necessary to inform interventions to reduce avoidable hospitalizations and related costs. The objective of this study was to characterize readmission rates, and identify factors and costs associated with readmission among children previously hospitalized with pneumonia.

Methods.—Retrospective cohort study of children hospitalized with pneumonia at the 43 hospitals included in the Pediatric Health Information System between January 1, 2008, and December 31, 2011. The primary outcome was all-cause readmission within 30 days after hospital discharge, and the secondary outcome was pneumonia-specific readmission. We used multivariable regression models to identify patient and hospital characteristics and costs associated with readmission.

Results.—A total of 82 566 children were hospitalized with pneumonia (median age, 3 years; interquartile range 1—7). Thirty-day all-cause and pneumonia-specific readmission rates were 7.7% and 3.1%, respectively. Readmission rates were higher among children <1 year of age, as well as in patients with previous hospitalizations, longer index hospitalizations, and complicated pneumonia. Children with chronic medical conditions were more likely to experience all-cause (odds ratio 3.0; 95% confidence interval 2.8—3.2) and pneumonia-specific readmission (odds ratio 1.8; 95% confidence interval 1.7—2.0) compared with children without chronic medical conditions. The median cost of a readmission ($11 344) was higher than that of an index admission ($4495; $P = .01$). Readmissions occurred in 8% of pneumonia hospitalizations but accounted for 16.3% of total costs for all pneumonia hospitalizations.

Conclusions.—Readmissions are common after hospitalization for pneumonia, especially among young children and those with chronic medical conditions, and are associated with substantial costs.

▶ Hospitals are currently at financial risk for excess adult readmissions for heart failure, heart attack, or pneumonia. This Center for Medicaid and Medicare

Services (CMS) program started in October 2012 and has been associated with a decrease in these readmissions nationally. However, the CMS program only started after extensive work had been done studying adult readmissions, understanding who was at risk and how hospitals or outpatient programs might prevent them, and after hospital-level readmission rates had been publicly reported for some time. In light of the success of the adult program, and with some evidence for variation in pediatric readmission rates,[1] there is interest in pediatric readmissions as a potential quality measure. This article by Neuman et al contributes to our understanding of whether pneumonia readmission rates may be important measures of hospital quality.

The study takes the first steps toward quality measurement development—describing overall rates of readmissions and variation across hospitals and assessing whether there are patient or hospital characteristics that are associated with higher readmission rates, to find potentially modifiable factors to help reduce readmissions. The strength of the article is that it captures data from a large group of hospitals, caring for approximately 15% of pediatric hospitalizations nationally. The study found variation in hospital readmission rates (range: 5%–13%), and found that hospitals with higher volumes for pneumonia admissions had lower readmission rates (Fig 1 in the original article). The study concludes that pneumonia readmissions at 30 days are common and costly and that they are a valid focus for CMS readmission reduction efforts in pediatrics (Fig 2 in the original article).

Although the work is foundational, there are few important caveats to the conclusions the authors draw. The study used data from only 43 high-volume children's hospitals, which means that the other 600-plus hospitals in the United States that admit children for pneumonia are not represented,[2] and patterns may be quite different. Because a CMS program would focus on all hospitals, we need some information on non—children's hospitals before spending resources on developing a pneumonia-specific readmissions program, especially given that children with pneumonia at children's hospitals may be different from the otherwise healthy pediatric pneumonia patient admitted to a community hospital.[3]

In addition, more work needs to be done to better understand which readmissions are preventable. From our experience, having reviewed each readmission to our institution over the previous 2 years, approximately 20% to 25% of unplanned, related readmissions were preventable. However, this study does not exclude planned readmissions, which would have decreased the readmission rates. If, similar to our institution, only 25% of study readmissions were preventable, the numbers of unplanned, preventable readmissions, which should be the focus of quality improvement programs, could be as low as <1% of related readmissions and <2% of unrelated readmissions (based on the study rates of 3.1% and 7.7%, respectively). These numbers would make it difficult to detect meaningful variation in preventable readmissions across hospitals,[2,4] defeating the purpose of measurement to drive improved care. This illustrates the need for additional data from other institutions on preventability and planned versus unplanned readmissions to achieve a more complete picture.

Another important step toward a useful quality measure, particularly when there is talk of linking performance and financial incentives, is demonstrating that interventions can change readmission risk. The article has 2 findings that suggest areas for potential intervention. One compelling finding is that children with complicated pneumonia who underwent drainage were less likely to be readmitted than children not drained. That argues for preventability. In addition, the finding that higher volumes of pneumonia cases was associated with lower readmission rates implies that hospitals with greater experience with pneumonia may have clinical practices that are more successful in preventing readmissions. However, much more work needs to be done in this area. For adult heart failure, there are known interventions to prevent readmissions, including care coordination and close follow-up.[5] Without known interventions to prevent them, it would be premature to consider pediatric pneumonia readmissions a potential area for financial penalties.

An alternative to a financial penalty program would be to start by making hospital performance rates publicly available. This would allow hospitals to benchmark themselves against peer institutions. This may allow for collaboration and shared learnings as we continue to assess whether pediatric readmissions are potentially preventable and develop and test interventions to try to reduce them.

N. S. Bardach, MD, MAS
A. Bekmezian, MD

References

1. Berry JG, Toomey SL, Zaslavsky AM, et al. Pediatric readmission prevalence and variability across hospitals. *JAMA*. 2013;309:372-380.
2. Bardach NS, Vittinghoff E, Asteria-Penaloza R, et al. Measuring hospital quality using pediatric readmission and revisit rates. *Pediatrics*. 2013;132:429-436.
3. Wise PH. The transformation of child health in the United States. *Health Aff (Millwood)*. 2004;23:9-25.
4. Lee HC, Chien AT, Bardach NS, Clay T, Gould JB, Dudley RA. The impact of statistical choices on neonatal intensive care unit quality ratings based on nosocomial infection rates. *Arch Pediatr Adolesc Med*. 2011;165:429-434.
5. Coleman EA, Parry C, Chalmers S, Min SJ. The care transitions intervention: results of a randomized controlled trial. *Arch Intern Med*. 2006;166:1822-1828.

Traffic-Related Air Pollution and Asthma Hospital Readmission in Children: A Longitudinal Cohort Study
Newman NC, Ryan PH, Huang B, et al (Cincinnati Children's Hosp Med Ctr, OH)
J Pediatr 164:1396-1402, 2014

Objective.—To examine the association between exposure to traffic-related air pollution (TRAP) and hospital readmission for asthma or bronchodilator-responsive wheezing.

Study Design.—A population-based cohort of 758 children aged 1-16 years admitted for asthma or bronchodilatorresponsive wheezing was assessed for asthma readmission within 12 months. TRAP exposure was estimated with a land use regression model using the home address at index admission, with TRAP dichotomized at the sample median $(0.37\ \mu g/m^3)$. Covariates included allergen-specific IgE, tobacco smoke exposure, and social factors obtained at enrollment. Associations between

TRAP exposure and readmission were assessed using logistic regression and Cox proportional hazards models.

Results.—The study cohort was 58% African American and 32% white; 19% of the patients were readmitted within 12 months of the original admission. Higher TRAP exposure was associated with a higher readmission rate (21% vs 16%; $P = .05$); this association was not significant after adjusting for covariates (aOR, 1.4; 95% CI, 0.9-2.2). Race modified the observed association; white children with high TRAP exposure had 3-fold higher odds of asthma readmission (OR, 3.0; 95% CI, 1.1-8.1), compared with white children with low TRAP exposure. In African American children, TRAP exposure was not associated with increased readmission (OR, 1.1; 95% CI, 0.6-1.8). In children with high TRAP exposure, TRAP exposure was associated with decreased time to readmission in white children (hazard ratio, 3.2; 95% CI, 1.5-6.7) compared with African American children (hazard ratio, 1.0; 95% CI, 0.7-1.4). African American children had a higher readmission rate overall.

Conclusion.—TRAP exposure is associated with increased odds of hospital readmission in white children, but not in African American children.

▶ Although inclusion of race as a covariate in epidemiologic analyses is considered to be reflexive, the significance of race as a construct, particularly for pediatric asthma, merits further deliberation.

Recently, race has been advanced as a biological risk factor for asthma. Genetic analysis and sequencing have demonstrated that alleles that are racially patterned may confer vulnerability to environmental insults or increase responsiveness to certain medication. More commonly, and often erroneously, race is considered as a proxy for socioeconomic status (SES), particularly for studies conducted in the United States. However, because poverty rates for black children are significantly higher compared with those of white children,[1] the social patterning of race and poverty in the United States has important implications for understanding asthma-related morbidity.

Although race and poverty frequently appear as risk factors for acute care encounters, these covariates may serve as surrogates of true etiologic risk factors: lack of access to adequate health care, adverse physical environmental exposures, fractured social support systems, and contextual barriers to engaging in healthful behaviors. A wealth of research had shown that these are all risk factors for pediatric-asthma exacerbations and that they coincide frequently in urban communities. The challenge is to understand the relative contribution of these factors and develop strategies to reduce unnecessary morbidity.

Through their careful work, Newman et al have demonstrated that high levels of residential diesel exhaust exposure resulted in significant increased odds of a repeated readmission to the hospital for an asthma exacerbation. Adjustment for covariates did not result in a significant association between diesel exhaust exposure and readmission in a multivariable model. However, stratification by race demonstrated a significant relation between high diesel exhaust exposure (or traffic-related air pollution exposure) and readmission, although this association was limited to white children (Table 2).

TABLE 2.—Association Between TRAP and Asthma Readmission

Model	OR (95% CI)	P Value
Unadjusted	1.5 (1.0-2.1)	.05
Adjusted*	1.4 (0.9-2.2)	.08
Model Including race × TRAP interaction†		.07‡
White	3.0 (1.1-8.1)	.03
African American	1.1 (0.6-1.8)	.70

*n = 621, adjusted for age, race, gender, household income, maternal education, controller medication use, and allergic sensitization.

†n = 556, includes white and African American only, adjusted for age, sex, household income, maternal education, controller medication use, and allergic sensitization.

‡P value for interaction term.

Reprinted from Journal Pediatrics. Newman NC, Ryan PH, Huang B, et al. Traffic-Related Air Pollution and Asthma Hospital Readmission in Children: A Longitudinal Cohort Study. J Pediatr. 2014;164:1396-1402, Copyright 2014, with permission from Elsevier.

Given that black children had higher readmission prevalence and higher than average diesel exhaust exposure compared with white children, it seems counterintuitive that the race-exposure would be not only elevated and significant for white children but close the null value for black children. However, the authors found that black children, on average, were exposed to other competing risk factors that were likely to contribute to hospital readmission for asthma. Irrespective of category of diesel exhaust exposure (high or low), black children were more likely to have additional exposure to environmental risk factors (ie, presence of cockroaches in the homes, cracks or holes in walls, carpeting in the child's bedroom) and sociodemographic risk factors (ie, caregivers with high burden of psychological stress, residence in census tracts with high poverty concentration) compared with white children. Given that all of these exposures are meaningful contributors to asthma-related morbidity, they may potentially obscure the effect of exposure to diesel exhaust for black children.

The authors did not provide main effect estimates for the association between these other environmental and sociodemographic covariates and odds of readmission, so this hypothesis cannot be tested directly. However, a cautious interpretation of these results suggest that white children may not be more vulnerable to the effects of diesel exhaust exposure but have a limited set of other potential risk factors that may be more closely associated with hospital readmission compared to black children.

This article offers the opportunity to consider several important aspects in how we study the roles of environmental exposures and social status in pediatric asthma morbidity.

Potential measurement error in the determining exposure: Many epidemiologic studies that investigate the role of ambient air pollution exposure on acute health events have used a time-series or a case-crossover approach. These strategies leverage the natural temporal variation of air pollution concentrations to better understand temporal changes in health care utilization. The land use regression model used in this study offers a comprehensive understanding of the spatial variation of diesel exhaust exposure across the study area. However, the exposure estimate represents an averaged pollution estimate over multiple years; temporal variation in the air pollution levels cannot be ascertained. Evidence of increased diesel exhaust exposure levels immediately before an admission or readmission event may help to clarify the etiologic role of diesel exhaust exposure on asthma-related morbidity.

The role of health insurance and primary care: the National Asthma Education and Prevention Program Guidelines stress the importance of the primary care provider in household asthma management strategies. Given appropriate pharmaceutical and behavioral modifications, the majority of acute care encounters for pediatric asthma are considered to be avoidable. Because the study site was an urban tertiary care hospital, it is likely that primary care records for subjects enrolled in the study were not available. However, given that controller use was a strong protective factor in readmission (odds ratio: 0.5, 95% confidence interval: 0.3—0.83), it is likely that children who had established a continuum of care were less likely to experience readmission.

The role of income: Although the race-exposure term was marginally significant in this model, the household income main effect term was associated significantly with the odds of readmission (odds ratio: 3.1, 95% confidence interval: 1.1—8.2). More than one-third of the families enrolled in this study would be considered to be below the 2010 poverty threshold for a single-parent family.[2] It would have been informative to understand how diesel exhaust exposure varied over household income levels and if that pattern was similar to the association found for race.

This article is illustrative of the ongoing challenges for urban families of children with asthma. Although the authors focused on the role of ambient air pollution, an important modifiable risk factor, it is clear that subjects enrolled in this study—particularly black children—are exposed to multiple risk factors linked to asthma-related morbidity. The study highlights 2 important issues: developing the best methodologic approaches for understanding the role of cumulative risk factors and identifying potential interventions to reduce avoidable health care utilization for vulnerable populations.

S. Magzamen, PhD

References

1. Poverty in the United States: Frequently Asked Questions. National Poverty Center, University of Michigan.
2. US Census Bureau, 2010.

Seasonality of Asthma: A Retrospective Population Study
Cohen HA, Blau H, Hoshen M, et al (Pediatric Ambulatory Community Clinic, Petach Tikva, Israel; Tel Aviv Univ, Israel; Clalit Res Inst, Tel Aviv, Israel; et al)
Pediatrics 133:e923-e932, 2014

Objectives.—Seasonal variations in asthma are widely recognized, with the highest incidence during September. This retrospective population study aimed to investigate whether this holds true in a large group of asthmatic children in primary care and to assess the impact of age, gender, urban/rural living, and population sector.

Methods.—The key study outcomes were the diagnosis of asthma exacerbations and asthma medication prescriptions, recorded by family physicians during 2005 to 2009. These were analyzed by "week of diagnosis" in Clalit Health Services' electronic medical record database. Regression models were built to assess relative strength of secular trends, seasonality, and age-group in explaining the incidence of asthma exacerbations.

Results.—A total of 919 873 children aged 2 to 15 years were identified. Of these, 82 234 (8.9%) were asthmatic, 61.6% boys and 38.4% girls; 49.1% aged 2 to 5 years, 24.1% 6 to 9 years, and 26.8% 10 to 15 years. We observed a 2.01-fold increase in pediatric asthma exacerbations and 2.28-fold increase in prescriptions of asthma bronchodilator medications during September (weeks 37—39 vs weeks 34—36) compared with August. The association between the opening of school and the incidence of asthma-related visits to the primary care physician was greatest in children aged 2 to 5 years (odds ratio, 2.15) and 6 to 11 years (1.90-fold). Adolescents (age 12—15 years) had a lesser peak (1.81-fold). In late fall there was a second rise, lasting with fluctuations throughout winter, with a trough in summer.

Conclusions.—Returning to school after summer is strongly associated with an increased risk for asthma exacerbations and unscheduled visits to the primary care physician.

▶ This article extends previous studies of the "September epidemic" by examining a large database including close to 1 million children in Israel. The study not only confirms the large increase in asthma exacerbations that occur annually among children after returning to school from summer vacations (Fig 1 in the original article) but shows that this is seen equally strongly in primary care practice as was previously documented in hospital admissions or emergency department visits in studies undertaken in Canada.[1] Furthermore, this study clearly shows the effect is greatest in younger children in that 49% of asthma visits occurred in 2- to 5-year-olds who comprised only 29% of the asthmatic children. Interestingly, no differences were found between children living in urban and rural settings.

The study illustrates well the advantages of a uniform system of electronic medical records allowing many aspects of disease epidemiology and management to be evaluated. As expected from other epidemiologic studies, boys were overrepresented in both the asthmatic children and the asthma visits (both 61% of the total), although they comprised just 51% of all children in the database. However, the Arab population seemed less affected, providing only 28% of asthmatics and asthmatic exacerbations despite comprising 38% of the overall pediatric database.

The availability of a drug-dispensing database greatly enhances the study. This clearly demonstrates the decline in asthma medication dispensing during the summer and the sharp upturn at the onset of the epidemic. Indeed, the prescription data show a progressive decline in all asthma-related prescriptions from the winter peak in early January to the lowest level just immediately before the September epidemic strikes. This decline was more than a 60% reduction in bronchodilator use (which may be appropriate because symptoms are less in warmer weather) but also a major reduction (60%) in use of inhaled corticosteroid and more than 40% reduction in leukotriene receptor antagonist therapy. These reductions in regular treatments may allow asthma to become less well controlled and the child to be unprotected against the multiple triggers that are encountered on school return. Prescription data from one insurer in the Canadian study did indicate the same phenomenon of children having "drug holidays" during the summer.

As noted in this and other publications, the triggers of September exacerbations of asthma are likely dominated by viral infections but may also include allergen exposures both in the school and the general environment and the stress of school return. The authors demonstrate a greater likelihood of primary care visits related to upper respiratory infections in younger compared with older children and again suggest young children may be the vectors transmitting increased risk of such infections and resulting asthma to older children a few days later. There is a more attenuated epidemic in older children, who may be siblings, although presumably the anonymized database did not allow investigators to examine the detail of family relationships.

What messages does this article bring? First, the September peak of asthma exacerbations noted in many countries in hospital and emergency department visits is also evident in primary care where most asthma management occurs. Second, younger children are at highest risk during this period. Third, there is progressive reduction of controller medications during the months before the epidemic. Hence, there is opportunity to reduce the epidemic by ensuring asthma controller medication is taken especially at the time of school return. We demonstrated in a randomized double-blind placebo-controlled 6-week study among community asthmatics in Canada that the simple strategy of providing montelukast once daily reduced the prevalence of days with worse asthma symptoms by 53%, with an even more dramatic reduction in unscheduled doctor visits of 78%.[2] This occurred despite the fact that many of these children were already prescribed inhaled corticosteroid therapy, which, in the event, was often not being taken. Losing time from school at the beginning of a school year due to an exacerbation of asthma should be largely avoidable by awareness of the predictability of the phenomenon and ensuring appropriate asthma controller therapy is not only prescribed but taken.

M. Sears, MB, ChB

References

1. Sears MR, Johnson NW. Understanding the September asthma epidemic. *J Allergy Clin Immunol.* 2007;120:526-529.
2. Johnson NW, Mandhane PJ, Dai J, et al. Attenuation of the September epidemic of asthma exacerbations in children: a randomized, controlled trial of montelukast added to usual therapy. *Pediatrics.* 2007;120:e702-e712.

Demonstrating and Assessing Metered-Dose Inhaler-Spacer Technique: Pediatric Care Providers' Self-Reported Practices and Perceived Barriers
Reznik M, Jaramillo Y, Wylie-Rosett J (Children's Hosp at Montefiore, Bronx, NY) *Clin Pediatr* 53:270-276, 2014

The National Asthma Education and Prevention Program recommends that providers demonstrate and assess metered-dose inhaler-spacer (MDI-S) technique at each medical visit. To examine practice behaviors and perceived barriers to demonstrating and assessing MDI-S technique, we surveyed pediatric providers (n = 114) at an inner-city academic medical center. While 82% of providers demonstrated MDI-S technique, only 5% of providers demonstrate the technique at every visit. Although 67% of providers assessed MDI-S technique, only 13% assess the technique at every visit. None of the providers used MDI-S checklist for assessment. Attendings were more likely than residents to demonstrate with illustrations (24% vs 6%, $P =.01$) and when patient's asthma was not well controlled (68% vs 47%, $P =.05$). Provider-identified barriers included limited access to MDI-S device, lack of time, and inadequate knowledge. Suggestions to address barriers include in-service training, device access, and nurse/health educators to alleviate the time constraints. Clinic modifications and education are needed.

▶ When used correctly, there are medications that can keep asthma under control or quiet symptoms during an exacerbation. The majority of these asthma medications are designed to be delivered directly to the lung, the site of concern. However, the delivery mechanism for these medications (ie, respiratory inhaler devices) can be difficult to use correctly.[1-3] Therefore, guideline recommendations exist that encourage providers to assess and teach respiratory inhaler technique at all health care encounters.[4] Although previous work has shown that providers have often not been formally taught and do not know correct inhaler technique,[5-10] there are few data that outline how often providers attempt to adhere to guideline recommendations to assess and demonstrate inhaler technique. This study adds to the literature on the topic of inhaler technique by asking the providers directly whether they follow these guidelines and, if so, how often. The results are not surprising; providers fail to adhere to guidelines the majority of the time. However, it is imperative to document the current state of practice, as this study did, to outline the scope of the problem. Further, to begin to improve guideline adherence, it is important to understand the providers' barriers to assessing and demonstrating correct inhaler technique. By outlining these barriers, Reznik et al provide a blueprint to address and overcome these barriers so that providers are enabled to adhere to the guidelines and provide critical education to patients and their families on correct inhaler technique.

Among the most common barriers were lack of access to teaching devices and/or knowledge to provide education and time limitations to provide the teaching even if these other barriers were not present. This study helped to outline solutions to these barriers, including providing access to demonstration devices and provider education on inhaler technique. Time limitations, though, may seem more insurmountable. However, providing patient education has been proven beneficial[11,12] and may not be as time-consuming as expcted.[13] Furthermore, providers may not understand how to document and bill for their counseling time, which may limit their inclination or belief that they have time to provide this education.[13] Therefore, to truly provide guideline-recommended, self-management counseling, providers need improved education not only for inhaler instruction but also on how to efficiently use an office visit to provide this critical education and then document and bill appropriately for these services.

Although this study helps to outline the scope of the problem, there are a few limitations. First, the self-reported nature of the study may overinflate the reports of assessing and/or demonstrating inhaler technique. Therefore, adherence to guidelines may be even worse than stated. Furthermore, as noted in the article, providers may lack the correct knowledge themselves of how to demonstrate technique. Thus, self-report of technique demonstration may not, in and of itself, be enough. Verification that the self-reported demonstration is correct would be necessary to truly understand the scope of how many patients and their families have access to correct inhaler technique.

Despite these limitations, it is clear that a critical component of asthma care—assessing and demonstrating to patients and their families how to use respiratory inhaler devices—is underaddressed in the clinical setting. Therefore, this study helps to shape the direction that future research should take to truly begin to address this critical aspect of asthma disease management. In addition, larger studies should evaluate pediatric providers' ability to assess and demonstrate inhaler technique, develop and test educational programs designed to teach providers, and study programs that incorporate interdisciplinary programs, including asthma educators, are just a few of the areas of investigation that this article inspire. Together, this field of inquiry can help us attain our ultimate goal: truly informed patients and families, ensuring delivery of life-saving medications from inhaler devices into the lungs.

V. G. Press, MD, MPH

References

1. van der Palen J, Klein JJ, van Herwaarden CLA, Zielhuis GA, Seydel ER. Multiple inhalers confuse asthma patients. *Eur Respir J.* 1999;14:1034-1037.
2. Melani AS, Bonavia M, Cilenti V, et al. Inhaler mishandling remains common in real life and is associated with reduced disease control. *Respir Med.* 2011;105: 930-938.
3. Press VG, Arora VM, Shah LM, et al. Misuse of respiratory inhalers in hospitalized patients with asthma or COPD. *J Gen Intern Med.* 2011;26:635-642.
4. Guidelines for the diagnosis and management of asthma (EPR-3). http://www.nhlbi.nih.gov/guidelines/asthma/. Accessed June 25, 2014.
5. Press VG, Pincavage AT, Pappalardo AA, et al. The Chicago Breathe Project: a regional approach to improving education on asthma inhalers for resident physicians and minority patients. *J Natl Med Assoc.* 2010;102:548-555.
6. Interiano B, Guntupalli KK. Metered-dose inhalers. Do health care providers know what to teach? *Arch Intern Med.* 1993;153:81-85.

7. Jones JS, Holstege CP, Riekse R, White L, Bergquist T. Metered-dose inhalers: do emergency health care providers know what to teach? *Ann Emerg Med.* 1995;26: 308-311.
8. Fink JB, Rubin BK. Problems with inhaler use: a call for improved clinician and patient education. *Respir Care.* 2005;50:1360-1374.
9. Guidry GG, Brown WD, Stogner SW, George RB. Incorrect use of metered dose inhalers by medical personnel. *Chest.* 1992;101:31-33.
10. Amirav I, Goren A, Pawlowski NA. What do pediatricians in training know about the correct use of inhalers and spacer devices? *J Allergy Clin Immunol.* 1994;94:669-675.
11. Partridge MR, Hill SR. Enhancing care for people with asthma: the role of communication, education, training and self-management. 1998 World Asthma Meeting Education and Delivery of Care Working Group. *Eur Respir J.* 2000; 16:333-348.
12. Clark NM, Gong M, Schork MA, et al. Impact of education for physicians on patient outcomes. *Pediatrics.* 1998;101:831-836.
13. Cabana MD, Bradley J, Meurer JR, Holle D, Santiago C, Clark NM. Coding for asthma patient education in the primary care setting. *J Med Pract Manage.* 2005; 21:115-119.

Financial Barriers to Care Among Low-Income Children With Asthma: Health Care Reform Implications

Fung V, Graetz I, Galbraith A, et al (Massachusetts General Hosp, Boston; Kaiser Permanente Northern California, Oakland; Harvard Med School and Harvard Pilgrim Health Care Inst, Boston, MA; et al)
JAMA Pediatr 168:649-656, 2014

Importance.—The Patient Protection and Affordable Care Act (ACA) includes subsidies that reduce patient cost sharing for low-income families. Limited information on the effects of cost sharing amongchildren is available to guide these efforts.

Objective.—To examine the associations between cost sharing, income, and care seeking and financial stress among children with asthma.

Design, Setting, and Participants.—A telephone survey in 2012 about experiences during the prior year within an integrated health care delivery system. Respondents included 769 parents of childrenaged 4 to 11 years with asthma. Of these, 25.9% of children received public subsidies; 21.7% were commercially insured with household incomes at or below 250% of the federal poverty level (FPL) and 18.2% had higher cost-sharing levels for all services (eg, ≥$75 for emergency department visits). We classified children with asthma based on (1) current receipt of a subsidy (ie, Medicaid or Children'sHealth Insurance Program) or potential eligibility for ACA low-income cost sharing or premium subsidies in 2014 (ie, income ≤250%, 251%-400%, or >400% of the FPL) and (2) cost-sharing levels for prescription drugs, office visits, and emergency department visits. We examined the frequency of changes in care seeking and financial stress due to asthma care costs across these groups using logistic regression, adjusted for patient/family characteristics.

Main Outcomes and Measures.—Switching to cheaper asthma drugs, using less medication than prescribed, delaying/avoiding any office or emergency department visits, and financial stress (eg, cutting back on necessities) because of the costs of asthma care.

Results.—After adjustment, parents at or below 250% of the FPL with lower vs higher cost-sharing levels were less likely to delay or avoid taking their children to a physician's office visit (3.8% vs 31.6%; odds ratio, 0.07 [95% CI, 0.01-0.39]) and the emergency department (1.2% vs 19.4%; 0.05 [0.01-0.25]) because of cost; higher-income parents and those whose children were receiving public subsidies (eg, Medicaid) were also less likely to forego their children's care than parents at or below 250% of the FPL with higher cost-sharing levels. Overall, 15.6% of parents borrowed money or cut back on necessities to pay for their children's asthma care.

Conclusions and Relevance.—Cost-related barriers to care among children with asthma were concentrated among low-income families with higher cost-sharing levels. The ACA's low-income subsidies could reduce these barriers for many families, but millions of dependents for whom employer-sponsored family coverage is unaffordable could remain at risk for cost-related problems because of ACA subsidy eligibility rules.

▶ As the Patient Protection and Affordable Care Act (ACA) is being rolled out, the immense complexity of the implementation of the ACA for children is becoming more evident.[1] Yet the outcome of the ACA on the care of children with a chronic condition, such as asthma, is largely unknown. Because the cost of care related to a child with a chronic condition is high, expansion of coverage and subsidies for these children is imperative, especially for low-income children. Medical costs for children covered by Medicaid and the Children's Health Insurance program (CHIP) are subsidized without cost sharing for children in the lowest income levels. Commercially insured families with low to moderate income are also at risk for higher health care costs due to potential increased cost sharing (copays) for drugs, office visits, and emergency department (ED) visits under the ACA. Further complicating the cost of care for children with chronic conditions is that cost sharing will vary by state exchange and the uncertainty of CHIP reauthorization.

Fung et al examined the relationship between adherence to controller medication and delay or avoiding office and ED visits and financial stress among families of children with asthma enrolled in an integrated health care delivery system (Kaiser Permanente of Northern California). Families were stratified by cost sharing levels based on type of subsidy received from Medicaid, CHIP or the ACA. They concluded that families at or below 250% of the poverty limit and those who had higher cost sharing were more likely to delay or avoid an office or ED visit than families with higher income levels or low-income families with lower levels of cost sharing through Medicaid and CHIP subsidies.

Why is this important? As the ACA is implemented, advocacy for policy addressing the scope and depth of pediatric coverage is critical for children with chronic conditions because they were prone to discriminatory insurer coverage standards in the past.[2] Furthermore, the US Department of Health and Human Services may require coverage linked to commercial insurance market standards and not the unique coverage provided by Medicaid resulting in precarious care-seeking and medication adherence behaviors.[2]

Asthma is particularly elucidative of the effects of cost sharing in a chronic disease model. For example, prescribing generic medications is limited in children with asthma. Because of the switch to hydrofluoroalkane inhalers in 2009, all inhalers (controller and rescue) are widely available as branded products.[3] There are few generic controller medications available. Without significant cost-sharing copays covered by insurance, families of children with asthma may incur a significant high cost burden for asthma medications.

Will high cost sharing for medication and office visits costs for families of children with asthma result in behavior that may lead to unhealthy outcomes for children? The evidence is unclear. Fung et al report that medication adherence, defined as switching to a cheaper asthma controller medication or using less medication than prescribed, was not significantly different by income or level of cost sharing. Few families switched their child's asthma medication to a cheaper asthma medication, which may be a result of the low availability of generic controller medications rather than low rate of parental decision to switch to cheaper medication. What is more disturbing is that almost 1 out of 10 families reported using less medication than prescribed, which is likely to result in worse asthma control. Furthermore, 7.6% reported delaying or avoiding taking their child to any physician's office visit due to cost of care (Figure in the original article). These results indicate that increased cost sharing for pediatric asthma care may result in worse asthma outcomes and higher long-term costs related to poor asthma control.

The study's strength is the use of a large insurance data set for cost-sharing levels for medications, office visits, and ED visits. However, the data are limited to children enrolled in an integrated health care delivery system from 1 state and who were primary commercially insured. Furthermore, parent report of using less medication than prescribed or not refilling a prescription is biased by not asking about other factors associated with medication nonadherence such as parent beliefs in medication side effects and sharing medication among family members.

Identifying and understanding family health-seeking decisions is imperative for clinicians. This can only occur when an open discussion of cost is encouraged during office visits. Pediatric clinicians often do not have the knowledge of the financial burdens of health care costs on families and are not trained in how to discuss health care costs during visits. Moreover, there is little evidence how to prepare clinicians to conduct these discussions. Research is needed regarding effective methods to teach clinicians to have a cost discussion with families.

The results of Fung el al have important implications for ACA implementation and child health. First, pediatric clinicians need to be informed about their individual state ACA coverage, subsidies, and cost sharing, especially for children with chronic conditions. Second, clinicians may need to advocate for families with incomes 200% to 250% of the federal poverty limit (FPL) who are eligible for cost-sharing subsidies but whose subsidies may be modest. This advocacy will need to include a discussion of cost of care decisions with families and the financial burden of health care costs. As the ACA is implemented and cost sharing becomes a more widely accepted practice, clinicians must be educated on how to discuss cost of care with families and consider costs when recommending medication regimens and plan of asthma care.

M. M. Tschudy, MD, MPH

A. M. Butz, ScD, MSN, CRNP

References

1. Health Reform and the AAP: What the New Law Means for Children and Pediatricians Fact Sheet. http://www.aap.org/en-us/advocacy-and-policy/federal-advocacy/Documents/ACAImplementationFactSheets.pdf. Accessed July 28, 2014.
2. Goldstein MM, Rosenbaum S. From EPSDT to EHBs: The future of pediatric coverage design under government financed health insurance. *Pediatrics*. 2013;131: S142-S148.
3. Peters S. Hydrofluoroalkane mandate in effect January 1, 2009: Switch from Chlorofluorocarbon- to hydrofluoroalkane-propelled inhalers requires active transition. *Clin Cornerstone*. 2009;9:50-53.

Outpatient Course and Complications Associated With Home Oxygen Therapy for Mild Bronchiolitis

Flett KB, Breslin K, Braun PA, et al (Boston Children's Hosp, MA; Denver Health, CO)

Pediatrics 133:769-775, 2014

Background.—Home oxygen has been incorporated into the emergency department management of bronchiolitis in high-altitude settings. However, the outpatient course on oxygen therapy and factors associated with subsequent admission have not been fully defined.

Methods.—We conducted a retrospective cohort study in consecutive patients discharged on home oxygen from the pediatric emergency department at Denver Health Medical Center from 2003 to 2009. The integration of inpatient and outpatient care at our study institution allowed comprehensive assessment of follow-up rates, outpatient visits, time on oxygen, and subsequent admission. Admitted and nonadmitted patients were compared by using a χ^2 test and multivariable logistic regression.

Results.—We identified 234 unique visits with adequate follow-up for inclusion. The median age was 10 months (interquartile range [IQR]: 7—14 months). Eighty-three percent of patients were followed up within 24 hours and 94% within 48 hours. The median length of oxygen use was 6 days (IQR: 4—9 days), and the median number of associated encounters was 3 (range: 0—9; IQR: 2—3). Ninety-three percent of patients were on room air at 14 days. Twenty-two patients (9.4%) required subsequent admission. Fever at the initial visit (>38.0°C) was associated with admission ($P < .02$) but had a positive predictive value of 15.4%. Age, prematurity, respiratory rate, oxygen saturation, and history of previous bronchiolitis or wheeze were not associated with admission.

Conclusions.—There is a significant outpatient burden associated with home oxygen use. Although fever was associated with admission, we

TABLE 1.—Criteria for Discharge on Home Oxygen for Mild Bronchiolitis

1. Meets all inclusion criteria
   - Upper airway infection associated with wheezing ± crackles
   - Age 2 months to 2 years (at least 44 weeks' gestational age)
   - First time wheezing
   - ED visit between December and April
   - Secretions manageable with bulb suctioning by caregivers
   - Smoke-free home environment
   - Reliable family with access to emergency medical care
   - Lives at an altitude ≤6000 feet
2. No identified exclusion criteria
   - Toxic appearance or evidence of bacterial disease
   - Apparent life-threatening event occurring with illness
   - Cardiac, chronic lung, or neuromuscular disease
   - Oxygen requirement at baseline
   - Immunodeficiency
3. Clinical evidence of mild illness after suctioning, oxygen, and observation for >4 hours
   - Alert, active, and feeding well
   - None to minimal retractions
   - Respiratory rate <50 breaths/minute
   - Adequate oxygenation (~90%) on ≤0.5 L/minute of oxygen

(Reprinted from Flett KB, Breslin K, Braun PA, et al. Outpatient Course and Complications Associated With Home Oxygen Therapy for Mild Bronchiolitis. Pediatrics. 2014;133:769-775. Copyright © 2014, by the American Academy of Pediatrics.)

were unable to identify predictors that could modify current protocols (Tables 1 and 2).

▶ "Your baby has bronchiolitis and low oxygen levels. Would you like your supplemental oxygen for here or to go?" This is not a question parents hear often, but maybe it should be. After the introduction of widespread pulse oximetry use several decades ago, hospitalization rates for young infants with respiratory syncytial virus bronchiolitis tripled.[1] Evidence suggests that pediatric emergency department physicians rely heavily on the oxygen saturation to drive admission decisions,[2] and once infants are hospitalized, the use of continuous pulse oximetry drives length of stay.[3,4] The fact that the hospitalization burden has increased without any change in mortality rates[1] suggests that in many cases, the hypoxemia that is detected in bronchiolitis is overdiagnosed.

Home oxygen therapy has emerged as a promising alternative to hospitalization in some cases. Published research on this intervention, however, generally has been limited to centers at high altitude, where hypoxemia is more common.[5-7] Nonetheless, initial reports have suggested that hospitalization can be avoided in a substantial proportion of infants—generally infants who are somewhat hypoxemic (< 88%–90% oxygen saturation) but lack any other indications for hospitalization such as intravenous hydration, frequent suctioning, or increased respiratory support (Table 1). For this practice to catch on, better information was needed on outpatient outcomes.[8]

By reviewing records of 234 patients with bronchiolitis treated with home oxygen therapy in an integrated health system (Denver Health Medical Center), Flett et al provide some valuable information regarding the outpatient course

TABLE 2.—Characteristics of Children Discharged on Home Oxygen

Characteristic	Total ($n = 234$), n (%)	Not Admitted ($n = 212$), n (%)	Subsequently Admitted ($n = 22$), n (%)	P
Age				.88
<6 months	30 (12.8)	27 (12.7)	3 (13.6)	
6−18 months	175 (74.8)	158 (74.5)	17 (77.3)	
>18 months	29 (12.4)	27 (12.7)	2 (9.1)	
Gender				.79
Female	102 (43.6)	93 (43.9)	9 (40.9)	
Male	132 (56.4)	119 (56.1)	13 (59.1)	
Language				.21
Non-English	98 (41.9)	86 (40.6)	12 (54.5)	
English	136 (58.1)	126 (59.4)	10 (45.5)	
Race/ethnicity				.19
Hispanic	132 (56.4)	116 (54.7)	16 (72.7)	
White	65 (27.7)	60 (28.3)	5 (22.7)	
Other	37 (15.8)	36 (17.0)	1 (4.5)	
Gestational age				.996
30−36 weeks	32 (13.7)	29 (13.7)	3 (13.6)	
≥37 weeks	202 (86.3)	183 (86.3)	19 (86.4)	
Highest respiratory rate				.46
≥60 breaths/minute	79 (33.8)	70 (33.0)	9 (40.9)	
<60 breaths/minute	155 (66.2)	142 (67.0)	13 (59.1)	
Highest respiratory rate				.07
≥70 breaths/minute	26 (11.1)	21 (9.9)	5 (22.7)	
<70 breaths/minute	208 (88.9)	191 (90.1)	17 (77.3)	
Lowest O_2 saturation				.39
<85%	57 (24.4)	50 (23.6)	7 (31.8)	
≥85%	177 (75.6)	162 (69.2)	15 (68.1)	
Lowest O_2 saturation				.31
<80%	11 (4.7)	9 (4.2)	2 (9.1)	
≥80%	223 (95.3)	203 (95.8)	20 (90.9)	
Amount of O_2				.06
0.5 or 1 L/minute	148 (63.2)	130 (61.3)	18 (81.8)	
0.125 or 0.25 L/minute	86 (36.8)	82 (38.7)	4 (18.2)	
Previous wheeze or bronchiolitis	43 (18.4)	39 (18.4)	4 (18.2)	.98
Fever (≥38.0°C)	117 (50.0)	99 (46.7)	18 (81.8)	.002

Reprinted from Flett KB, Breslin K, Braun PA, et al. Outpatient Course and Complications Associated With Home Oxygen Therapy for Mild Bronchiolitis. Pediatrics. 2014;133:769-775. Copyright © 2014, by the American Academy of Pediatrics.

(Table 2). The integrated nature of this health system allowed for reliable measurements of outpatient outcomes. The median number of outpatient encounters was 3, and the median length of supplemental oxygen use was 6 days. The readmission rate was 9.4%, which is somewhat higher than previous reports. Although this readmission rate might be alarming to some, the optimist will note that >90% of patients were spared hospitalization.

Although the definitive need for supplemental oxygen in these infants and young children remains undetermined, home oxygen therapy certainly represents a better option than hospitalization from the perspective of the family, the patient, and the health care system. With increasing economic pressures to limit hospitalizations in the era of accountable care, the intensification of outpatient services is inevitable. Home oxygen therapy might pose some additional burden on outpatient providers, but the system must adapt.

Before the advent of pulse oximetry, many of these infants would have been discharged home from the emergency department without oxygen, and the data suggest that they ultimately would have fared no differently. Although intermittent oxygen desaturation may have some association with adverse cognitive outcomes in children with chronic diseases, it is highly unlikely that the transient episodes of hypoxemia that are so common in acute bronchiolitis have any long-term implications. Therefore, although home oxygen therapy is certainly a better alternative to hospitalization, perhaps the broader question is this: Why have we become so beholden to the pulse oximeter? Why do we have such precise thresholds for oxygenation but not for other vitals signs such as heart rate, respiratory rate, and temperature? Is it because oxygenation is one of the few things we can actually fix in this otherwise frustrating disease? Other than fixing an abnormal number, are we providing any true benefit to the patient? These are the difficult questions, and we still don't have good answers. In the meantime, the "to go" variety of supplemental oxygen is a promising solution.

A. R. Schroeder, MD

References

1. Shay DK, Holman RC, Newman RD, Liu LL, Stout JW, Anderson LJ. Bronchiolitis-associated hospitalizations among US children, 1980–1996. *JAMA.* 1999; 282:1440-1446.
2. Mallory MD, Shay DK, Garrett J, Bordley WC. Bronchiolitis management preferences and the influence of pulse oximetry and respiratory rate on the decision to admit. *Pediatrics.* 2003;111:e45-e51.
3. Schroeder AR, Marmor AK, Pantell RH, Newman TB. Impact of pulse oximetry and oxygen therapy on length of stay in bronchiolitis hospitalizations. *Arch Pediatr Adolesc Med.* 2004;158:527-530.
4. Unger S, Cunningham S. Effect of oxygen supplementation on length of stay for infants hospitalized with acute viral bronchiolitis. *Pediatrics.* 2008;121:470-475.
5. Bajaj L, Turner CG, Bothner J. A randomized trial of home oxygen therapy from the emergency department for acute bronchiolitis. *Pediatrics.* 2006;117:633-640.
6. Halstead S, Roosevelt G, Deakyne S, Bajaj L. Discharged on supplemental oxygen from an emergency department in patients with bronchiolitis. *Pediatrics.* 2012; 129:e605-e610.
7. Sandweiss DR, Mundorff MB, Hill T, et al. Decreasing hospital length of stay for bronchiolitis by using an observation unit and home oxygen therapy. *JAMA Pediatr.* 2013;167:422-428.
8. Sandweiss DR, Kadish HA, Campbell KA. Outpatient management of patients with bronchiolitis discharged home on oxygen: a survey of general pediatricians. *Clin Pediatr (Phila).* 2012;51:442-446.

Comparison of high-frequency oscillatory ventilation and conventional mechanical ventilation in pediatric respiratory failure

Gupta P, Green JW, Tang X, et al (Univ of Arkansas Med Ctr, Little Rock)
JAMA Pediatr 168:243-249, 2014

Importance.—Outcomes associated with use of high-frequency oscillatory ventilation (HFOV) in children with acute respiratory failure have not been established.

Objective.—To compare the outcomes of HFOV with those of conventional mechanical ventilation (CMV) in children with acute respiratory failure.

Design, Setting, and Participants.—We performed a retrospective, observational study using deidentified data obtained from all consecutive patients receiving mechanical ventilation aged 1 month to 18 years in the Virtual PICU System database from January 1, 2009, through December 31, 2011. The study population was divided into 2 groups: HFOV and CMV. The HFOV group was further divided into early and late HFOV. Propensity score matching was performed as a 1-to-1 match of HFOV and CMV patients. A similar matching process was performed for early HFOV and CMV patients.

Exposure.—High-frequency oscillatory ventilation.

Main Outcomes and Measures.—Length of mechanical ventilation, intensive care unit (ICU) length of stay, ICU mortality, and standardized mortality ratio (SMR).

Results.—A total of 9177 patients from 98 hospitals qualified for inclusion. Of these, 902 (9.8%) received HFOV, whereas 8275 (90.2%) received CMV. A total of 1764 patients were matched to compare HFOV and CMV, whereas 942 patients were matched to compare early HFOV and CMV. Length of mechanical ventilation (CMV vs HFOV: 14.6 vs 20.3 days, $P < .001$; CMV vs early HFOV: 14.6 vs 15.9 days, $P < .001$), ICU length of stay (19.1 vs 24.9 days, $P < .001$; 19.3 vs 19.5 days, $P = .03$), and mortality (8.4% vs 17.3%, $P < .001$; 8.3% vs 18.1%, $P < .001$) were significantly higher in HFOV and early HFOV patients compared with CMV patients. The SMR in the HFOV group was 2.00 (95% CI, 1.71-2.35) compared with an SMR in the CMV group of 0.85 (95% CI, 0.68-1.07). The SMR in the early HFOV group was 1.62 (95% CI, 1.31-2.01) compared with an SMR in the CMV group of 0.76 (95% CI, 0.62-1.16).

Conclusions and Relevance.—Application of HFOV and early HFOV compared with CMV in children with acute respiratory failure is associated with worse outcomes. The results of our study are similar to recently published studies in adults comparing these 2 modalities of ventilation for acute respiratory distress syndrome.

▶ Acute respiratory distress syndrome (ARDS) is an uncommon pediatric illness that occurs primarily in medically complicated patients who continue to suffer high morbidity and mortality.[1] Mechanical ventilation with supplemental oxygen are the mainstay of support, but these very factors can lead to irreversible ventilator induced lung injury (VILI) depending on the ventilation strategy used and patient-related comorbid conditions. Randomized clinical trials consistently demonstrate that conventional mechanical ventilation (CMV) using low tidal volumes (TV; < 6 mL/kg) decreases mortality and long-term morbidity compared with use of high TV[2]; this "lung-protective" ventilation strategy is widely accepted as standard care for ARDS.

High-frequency oscillatory ventilation (HFOV) is, theoretically, a way to minimize secondary lung injury by delivering very small TV (approximately 1–2 mL/kg) at high rates (measured in cycles per second, aka, hertz) and constant mean airway pressure, thus potentially minimizing both volutrauma and alveolar damage due to repetitive opening and closing during conventional ventilation. However, TV is not measured during HFOV, and the use of lower hertz, which increases effective ventilation and CO_2 elimination, may also contribute to VILI. HFOV presents additional challenges for patient care because of increased need of sedation and neuromuscular blocking agent use and decreased clearance of respiratory secretions. HFOV remains a rescue strategy, and thus provider experience is lower compared with adjusting CMV.

Clinical trials comparing HFOV and CMV in children and adults have yielded inconsistent results. One recent systematic review in adults and children and 2 recent meta-analyses, one in adults and children, and the other in adults only, reached inconclusive summaries but differed between positive and negative benefit. HFOV possibly improves survival or HFOV is unlikely to inflict harm.[3-5] Clinical studies in pediatric patients are hampered by small sample size[6] and wide practice variability in HFOV use among pediatric critical care physicians.[7] Two very recent randomized adult clinical trials of ARDS were published in 2013. One failed to show either benefit or harm from HFOV use compared with CMV,[8] and the other was stopped early because of increased mortality among patients randomized to HFOV.[9] A recently published follow-up study of extreme premature infants, now 11 to 14 years of age, found that among surviving children, those treated with HFOV had better lung function.[10]

Gupta et al. chose a different approach to answer this complex question: how does survival of HFOV compare with CMV in children, many of whom had comorbid conditions that increased their risk of death from acute respiratory failure? They devised a retrospective analysis as an observational cohort and adjusted for risk factors associated with death by propensity matching. By using the Virtual PICU Systems, LLC database (VPS) the authors were able to include 9177 pediatric patients from 98 pediatric intensive care units in the United States—clearly the largest cohort of children or adults included in a study on this topic. The authors used extensive and rigorous statistical methods to account for missing data and control for center differences to analyze a matched cohort of children who received HFOV versus CMV. Based on their analyses, they concluded that HFOV was associated with worse outcomes, including increased mortality, compared with CMV.

For rescue therapies to be successful in ARDS, they must be instituted before development of severe VILI. Because VILI occurs over time exposed to high ventilator setting, most trials exclude patients who have received mechanical ventilation for more than a week before the study intervention. The present study has a fundamental and critical study limitation related to timing and dose of HFOV and CMV. Children were included in the HFOV group if they received HFOV for more than 24 hours, whereas the CMV group required receipt of CMV for more than 96 hours. In other words, if a child received HFOV for 30 hours after receiving CMV for 10 days, they were assigned to the HFOV group. In fact, the authors state that the "median time of HFOV initiation after intubation was 20.5 hours; [and] the median duration of HFOV use was 4.7 days," whereas the mean total duration of mechanical ventilation in the HFOV group was 20.3 days, indicating a substantial exposure to CMV within this group of children who were analyzed in the HFOV group. The authors divided HFOV initiation to starting in the first day of ventilation or later but did not further quantitate timing or proportion of HFOV ventilation.

The recent multicenter trial of adults with ARDS comparing HFOV management (guided by general recommendations rather than a detailed algorithm) to CMV found that providers used relatively high mean airway pressures, causing greater rates of hemodynamic compromise, need for vasoactive medications, and higher mortality compared to CMV.[10] Gupta et al clearly demonstrate wide variability of HFOV use in children with respiratory failure compared with CMV by center but did not report any information on settings used, oxygenation, or complications. Is the complexity of HFOV management causing harm in children with respiratory failure? The authors do not report other information to further evaluate this concern. They did not report use of vasoactive medications, and the propensity matching included invasive monitoring, so this clinical risk factor cannot be assessed.

Nevertheless, Gupta et al used a novel strategy to examine a complex topic. By using a pediatric critical care network database, the authors were able to evaluate a large sample of children treated at multiple centers. The results call into question use of HFOV as a rescue therapy in pediatric acute respiratory failure.

R. R. Dixon, MD

S. L. Bratton, MD, MPH

References

1. Lopez-Fernandez Y, Azagra AM, de la Oliva P, et al. Pediatric acute lung injury epidemiology and natural history study: incidence and outcome of the acute respiratory distress syndrome in children. *Crit Care Med.* 2012;40:3238-3245.
2. Ventilation with lower tidal volumes as compared with traditional tidal volumes for acute lung injury and the acute respiratory distress syndrome. The Acute Respiratory Distress Syndrome Network. *N Engl J Med.* 2000;342:1301-1308.
3. Sud S, Sud M, Friedrich JO, et al. High-frequency ventilation versus conventional ventilation for treatment of acute lung injury and acute respiratory distress syndrome. *Cochrane Database Syst Rev.* 2013;28:CD004085.
4. Sud S, Sud M, Friedrich JO, et al. High frequency oscillation in patients with acute lung injury and acute respiratory distress syndrome (ARDS): systematic review and meta-analysis. *BMJ.* 2010;340:c2327.
5. Maitra S, Bhattacharjee S, Khanna P, Baidya DK. High-frequency ventilation does not provide mortality benefit in comparison with conventional lung-protective ventilation in acute respiratory distress syndrome: a meta-analysis of the randomized controlled trials. *Anesthesiology.* 2014 [Epub ahead of print].
6. Arnold JH, Hanson JH, Toro-Figuero LO, Gutiérrez J, Berens RJ, Anglin DL. Prospective, randomized comparison of high-frequency oscillatory ventilation and conventional mechanical ventilation in pediatric respiratory failure. *Crit Care Med.* 1994;22:1530-1539.
7. Arnold JH, Anas NG, Luckett P, et al. High-frequency oscillatory ventilation in pediatric respiratory failure: a multicenter experience. *Crit Care Med.* 2000;28:3913-3919.
8. Young D, Lamb SE, Shah S, et al. High-frequency oscillation for acute respiratory distress syndrome. *N Engl J Med.* 2013;368:806-813, http://www.ncbi.nlm.nih.gov/pubmed/23339638.
9. Ferguson ND, Cook DJ, Guyatt GH, et al. High-frequency oscillation in early acute respiratory distress syndrome. *N Engl J Med.* 2013;368:795-805.
10. Zivanovic S, Peacock J, Alcazar-Paris M, et al. Late outcomes of a randomized trial of high-frequency oscillation in neonates. *N Engl J Med.* 2014;370:1121-1130.

19 Therapeutics and Toxicology

Communicating Doses of Pediatric Liquid Medicines to Parents/Caregivers: A Comparison of Written Dosing Directions on Prescriptions with Labels Applied by Dispensed Pharmacy

Shah R, Blustein L, Kuffner E, et al (Univ of the Sciences in Philadelphia, PA; McNeil Consumer Healthcare, Fort Washington, PA)

J Pediatr 164:596-601, 2014

Objective.—To identify and compare volumetric measures used by healthcare providers in communicating dosing instructions for pediatric liquid prescriptions to parents/caregivers.

Study Design.—Dosing instructions were retrospectively reviewed for the 10 most frequently prescribed liquid medications dispensed from 4 community pharmacies for patients aged ≤12 years during a 3-month period. Volumetric measures on original prescriptions (ie, milliliters, teaspoons) were compared with those utilized by the pharmacist on the pharmacy label dispensed to the parent/caregiver.

Results.—Of 649 prescriptions and corresponding pharmacy labels evaluated, 68% of prescriptions and 62% of pharmacy labels communicated dosing in milliliters, 24% of prescriptions and 29% of pharmacy labels communicated dosing in teaspoonfuls, 7% of prescriptions and 0% of pharmacy labels communicated dosing in other measures (ie, milligrams, cubic centimeters, "dose"), and 25% of dispensed pharmacy labels did not reflect units as written in the prescription.

Conclusion.—Volumetric measures utilized by healthcare professionals in dosing instructions for prescription pediatric oral liquid medications are not consistent. Healthcare professionals and parents/caregivers should be educated on safe dosing practices for liquid pediatric medications. Generalizability to the larger pediatric population may vary depending on pharmacy chain, location, and medications evaluated.

▶ Parent errors in dosing medications for their children occur frequently.[1] Inconsistent and confusing medication instructions have been cited as a contributor to this problem. For a single prescribed medication, different units of measurement, including milliliters, teaspoons, and tablespoons, may be used as part of counseling by the prescribing health care provider and the pharmacist dispensing the medication, and these units may also appear differently on the prescription or

TABLE 1.—Volumetric Measures on HCP-Prescribed Prescriptions and Pharmacy-Dispensed Labels

| HCP-Prescribed Prescriptions | Pharmacy-Dispensed Labels* | | | |
	Milliliters Only (n)	Teaspoons Only (n)	Milliliters and Teaspoons (n)	Total n (%)
Milliliters only (n)	364	40	36	440 (67.8)
Teaspoons only (n)	12	124	20	156 (23.7)
Milliliters and teaspoons (n)	2	4	1	7 (1.1)
Other (n)	24	17	5	46 (7.1)
Total n (%)	402 (61.9)	185 (28.5)	62 (9.6)	649 (100.0)

*No units other than milliliters or teaspoons appear on pharmacy-dispensed labels.
Reprinted from Journal Pediatrics. Shah R, Blustein L, Kuffner E, et al. Communicating Doses of Pediatric Liquid Medicines to Parents/Caregivers: A Comparison of Written Dosing Directions on Prescriptions with Labels Applied by Dispensed Pharmacy. J Pediatr. 2014;164:596-601, Copyright 2014, with permission from Elsevier.

medication bottle label. Written instructions may also include a range of abbreviations for these volumetric measures (eg, ml, mL, ML, tsp, TSP, tbsp, TBSP).

Confusion between units increases the likelihood of multifold errors. Teaspoon and tablespoon terms may be especially confusing for parents. The terms sound alike, and their abbreviations appear to be similar; teaspoon and tablespoon terms also inadvertently endorse the use of kitchen spoons, which are known to be inaccurate for dosing.[2] Although it is recognized that health care providers' use of different units of measurement may lead to parent misunderstanding of medication instructions, there has been limited study of which units are typically used by providers, and the extent to which the units of measurement used on providers' written prescriptions differ from the medication bottle labels printed by the dispensing pharmacy.

In this study's sample of more than 600 prescriptions from 4 community pharmacies in Philadelphia, about 1 in 4 prescriptions and nearly 1 in 3 bottle labels used teaspoons (Table 1). Overall, 1 in 4 medication labels contained units that were not the same as those on the prescriptions written by providers. There was variability across pharmacies in the percentage of prescriptions that had their volumetric measures changed, with nearly half of prescriptions changed in 1 pharmacy, and in another pharmacy, less than 10% of prescriptions were changed. The pharmacy in which the most changes occurred served a lower income population than the other pharmacies. These study findings suggest that terms such as teaspoon are commonly used, and that changes in units from the prescription to the medication label may occur frequently in some pharmacies.

As this study took place in just 4 community pharmacies in 1 state, examined a specific subset of medications, and focused on English-language prescriptions and labels only, the results may not be generalizable. Further study is needed to examine why pharmacists may change the units used on a provider's prescription, explore health care provider perceptions of patient understanding of the term "milliliter," and evaluate parent/patient understanding of units of measurement. This study focused only on prescriptions and labels and did not examine units of measurement used as part of counseling by physicians or pharmacists. The study also did not specifically examine the extent to which different abbreviations were used for each term.

Importantly, the study helps document the problem of inconsistent use of units of measurement by health care providers, illustrating the benefit of a potential move to a standard unit of measurement system. The study is timely in that there is currently growing support to move toward greater consistency in units of measurement for medication instructions, with milliliter as the preferred unit of measurement for liquid medicines. Under the leadership of the Centers for Disease Control and Prevention PROTECT (Prevention of Overdoses and Therapeutic Errors in Children Taskforce) initiative, a number of groups, including the American Academy of Pediatrics, American Association of Poison Control Centers, the Consumer Healthcare Products Association, and the Institute for Safe Medication Practices have come out in support of a milliliter-preferred system.[3]

Improving consistency in dosing instructions by moving to a standard unit of measurement system could be especially beneficial for those with low health literacy as well as non-English speakers, who are at particular risk for medication dosing errors. A move to a milliliter-preferred system would also likely benefit health care providers; a number of cases have been reported in which health care provider confusion with units of measurement have resulted in harm to children. Buy-in from physicians, nurses, pharmacists, and other health care providers related to the issue of standardization of dosing units will be critical if a move to a milliliter-preferred system is to be successful.

H. S. Yin, MD, MS

References

1. Yin HS, Dreyer BP, Ugboaja D, et al. Units of measurement used and parent medication dosing errors. *Pediatrics.* 2014;134:1-8.
2. Rothman RL, Yin HS, Mulvaney S, et al. Health Literacy and Quality: Focus on Chronic Illness Care and Patient Safety. *Pediatrics.* 2009;124:S315-S326.
3. NCPDP Recommendations and Guidance for Standardizing the Dosing Designations on Prescription Container Labels of Oral Liquid Medications. National Council for Prescription Drug Programs. http://www.ncpdp.org/NCPDP/media/pdf/wp/DosingDesignations-OralLiquid-MedicationLabels.pdf. Accessed April 1, 2014.

Environmental Phthalate Exposure and Preterm Birth
Ferguson KK, McElrath TF, Meeker JD (Univ of Michigan School of Public Health, Ann Arbor; Brigham and Women's Hosp, Boston, MA)
JAMA Pediatr 168:61-67, 2014

Importance.—Preterm birth is a leading cause of neonatal mortality, with a variety of contributing causes and risk factors. Environmental exposures represent a group of understudied, but potentially important, factors. Phthalate diesters are used extensively in a variety of consumer products worldwide. Consequently, exposure in pregnant women is highly prevalent.

Objective.—To assess the relationship between phthalate exposure during pregnancy and preterm birth.

Design, Setting, and Participants.—This nested case-control study was conducted at Brigham and Women's Hospital, Boston, Massachusetts. Women were recruited for a prospective observational cohort study from 2006-2008. Each provided demographic data, biological samples, and information about birth outcomes. From within this group, we selected 130 cases of preterm birth and 352 randomly assigned control participants, and we analyzed urine samples from up to 3 time points during pregnancy for levels of phthalate metabolites.

Exposure.—Phthalate exposure during pregnancy.

Main Outcomes and Measures.—We examined associations between average levels of phthalate exposure during pregnancy and preterm birth, defined as fewer than 37 weeks of completed gestation, as well as spontaneous preterm birth, defined as preterm preceded by spontaneous preterm labor or preterm premature rupture of the membranes (n = 57).

Results.—Geometric means of the di-2-ethylhexyl phthalate (DEHP) metabolites mono-(2-ethyl)-hexyl phthalate (MEHP) and mono-(2-ethyl-5-carboxypentyl) phthalate (MECPP), as well as mono-n-butyl phthalate (MBP), were significantly higher in cases compared with control participants. In adjusted models, MEHP, MECPP, and Σ DEHP metabolites were associated with significantly increased odds of preterm birth. When spontaneous preterm births were examined alone, MEHP, mono-(2-ethyl-5-oxohexyl) phthalate, MECPP, Σ DEHP, MBP, and mono-(3-carboxypropyl) phthalate metabolite levels were all associated with significantly elevated odds of prematurity.

Conclusions and Relevance.—Women exposed to phthalates during pregnancy have significantly increased odds of delivering preterm. Steps should be taken to decrease maternal exposure to phthalates during pregnancy.

► Fetal growth and length of gestation, especially low birth weight and preterm birth (PTB), are highly important predictors of health in later life. Consequences of PTB can include infant and childhood mortality; cardiovascular dysfunction, hypertension, and diabetes in adulthood; and other adverse cognitive, psychological, behavioral, and educational outcomes in later life. Although substantial progress in reducing PTB has been made since 2006, rates (11.5% in 2010) remain higher than the Healthy People 2010 goal of < 7.6%.

Although PTB is multifactorial (with risk factors including maternal age, prenatal care, race, socioeconomic status, and preeclampsia), most of these risk factors are not amenable to modification or avoidance. If environmental chemicals can be more convincingly identified and quantified as important predictors of birth outcomes, then clinical and public health efforts to avoid or reduce exposures to these pollutants could result in positive and lifelong benefits for future birth cohorts in the United States.

Phthalates are esters of phthalic acid that are used in a broad array of consumer products and foods. Laboratory studies have found that phthalates increase release of pro-inflammatory cytokines, and biomarkers of phthalate exposure have also been associated with increases in C-reactive protein and the oxidative stress markers malondialdehyde and 8-hydroxydeoxyguanosine. Because oxidative stress can contribute to intrauterine inflammation and PTB, phthalates represent biologically plausible risk factors.

Ferguson et al examined phthalate exposure at up to 3 time points in pregnancy in a nested case-control study and found strong associations of metabolites of di-2-ethylhexylphthalate (DEHP) with PTB, and especially spontaneous PTB (PTB preceded by premature labor or rupture of membranes. These associations are of particular interest because industrial processes to produce food frequently use plastic products containing DEHP. This is a carefully conducted study that correctly measured these short half-life chemicals at multiple time points. Absent those frequent measurements, exposure imprecision could have biased the results to the null. Unmeasured confounders include dietary factors that could have contributed both to DEHP exposure and PTB.

Although regulatory action can reduce DEHP exposure, behavioral change can also produce reductions in DEHP metabolites as measured in urine. An intervention substituting packaged/canned foods with fresh foods reduced DEHP metabolites by 53% to 56%.[1] Increasing concern about phthalates and links to obesity, insulin resistance, and neurodevelopmental and cardiovascular risks have prompted increasing replacement of DEHP with diisodecylphthalate (DIDP) and diisononylphthalate (DINP), phthalates that have not been designated as hazardous by regulatory agencies.

Indeed, DEHP biomarkers decreased by 17% to 37% between 2001 and 2010 based on national survey samples; however, the 1976 Toxic Substances Control Act does not require toxicity testing before approval and widespread use of chemicals. Effects of DIDP and DINP may be identical to DEHP, which shares substantial structural similarity. The Food, Drug and Cosmetic Act permits food manufacturers to attest safety for additives such as DEHP, DINP, and DIDP without similar data.

There are simple steps pediatricians can suggest to reduce exposure to phthalates. Plastic containers should not be placed in the microwave and should be washed with soap and water rather than in the dishwasher with harsher detergents. Containers should be disposed when there is obvious etching or cracking. The recycling number is a good guide as well for beverage containers; the number 3 represents polyvinyl chloride plastics, which use phthalates as part of the manufacturing process. Avoiding the use of food and beverage containers made of PVC can reduce phthalate exposure.

Clearly, more research examining environmental risks for PTB, such as air pollution and other environmental oxidant stressors, are needed as well. As advocated by the American Academy of Pediatrics, reform of chemical regulation is urgently needed. Otherwise, epidemiologic studies will take decades to document effects of chemical exposures that could have been identified through a more rigorous premarket testing approach. Food additives oversight should also be strengthened. Failure to do so could produce further increases in significant morbidities such as PTB.

L. Trasande, MD, MPP

Reference

1. Rudel RA, Gray JM, Engel CL, et al. Food packaging and bisphenol a and bis(2-ethylhexyl) phthalate exposure: findings from a dietary intervention. *Environ Health Perspect.* 2011;119:914-920.

Bisphenol A Exposure Is Associated with Decreased Lung Function

Spanier AJ, Fiorino EK, Trasande L, et al (Penn State Univ, Hershey, PA; Cohen Children's Med Ctr, NY; New York Univ School of Medicine)
J Pediatr 164:1403-1408, 2014

Objective.—To examine the associations of bisphenol A (BPA) exposure with lung function measures and exhaled nitric oxide (FeNO) in children.

Study Design.—We performed a cross-sectional analysis of a subsample of US children age 6-19 years who participated in the 2007-2010 National Health and Nutrition Examination Survey. We assessed univariate and multivariable associations of urinary BPA concentration with the predicted pulmonary function measures for age, sex, race/ethnicity and height (forced expiratory volume in 1 second [FEV1], forced vital capacity [FVC], forced expiratory flow 25%-75%, and FEV1 divided by FVC) and with FeNO.

Results.—Exposure and outcome data were available for 661 children. Median BPA was 2.4 ng/mL (IQR: 1.3, 4.1). In multivariable analysis, a larger urinary BPA concentration was associated with significantly decreased percent predicted forced expiratory flow 25%-75% (% FEF2575) (3.7%, 95% CI 1.0, 6.5) and percent predicted FEV1 divided by FVC (%FEV1/FVC) (0.8%, 95% CI 0.1, 1.7) but not percent predicted FEV1, percent predicted FVC, or FeNO. A child in the top quartile of BPA compared with the bottom quartile had a 10% decrease in %FEF2575 (95% CI −1, −19) and 3% decrease in %FEV1/FVC (95% CI −1, −5).

Conclusions.—BPA exposure was associated with a modest decrease in %FEF2575 (small airway function) and %FEV1/FVC (pulmonary obstruction) but not FEV1, FVC, or FeNO. Explanations of the association cannot rule out the possibility of reverse causality.

▶ The rise in use of chemicals in modern-day life coupled with the rise in asthma prevalence in recent decades leads to a justifiable concern that the 2 trends may be linked. Epidemiologic studies may shed light on the relationships between environmental chemical exposure and the development of asthma. Thus, the question of whether exposure to the chemical bisphenol A (BPA) is associated with asthma and related outcomes as posed by the authors of this study is both provocative and relevant. In using the 2007—2010 National Health and Nutrition Examination Survey (NHANES) data set, the authors had the unique opportunity to assess a nationally represented cohort of children to attempt to answer this question.

The findings of this study are of particular interest because there were significant associations between BPA exposure and lung function measured by spirometry, but other findings seem to conflict with previously published work. To put in context, most environmental asthma studies fail to find links between changes in exposures with changes in lung function. Therefore, the positive finding is a unique feature and strength of this particular study. Interestingly, findings were significant between some (such as forced expiratory volume in 1 second/force vital capacity ratio [%FEV1/FVC] and forced expiratory flow 25—75% [%FEF25—75]), but not all spirometry measurements, possibly highlighting a small airway obstructive effect of BPA exposure. However, it is intriguing that this study failed to replicate the association between urinary BPA measures and diagnosis of asthma as previously published by Vaidya et al,[1] who used earlier 2005—2006 NHANES data. The conflicting results may be explained by the fact that Vaidya's outcome measurement was allergic asthma, defined by history of asthma, high eosinophil count, and high total immunoglobulin E or atopy, whereas Spanier did not specify a particular asthma phenotype. Similarly, the association between urinary BPA concentrations and fractional exhaled nitric oxide (FeNO) that was reported by our birth cohort group at the Columbia Center for Children's Environmental Health[2] also was not replicated in this study. Although dissimilarities between study designs, including assessment of varied asthma phenotypes, may play a role, the inconsistencies across studies offer more confusion rather than clarity.

Clarity is also needed in understanding the relationship between timing of BPA exposure and the development of wheeze, asthma, and related outcomes. As the authors highlight in their introduction, there is conflicting evidence regarding prenatal versus postnatal BPA exposure and the development of wheeze. However, a major limitation of this study was the cross-sectional design that did not allow for assessing this important question regarding the role of timing of BPA exposure. Similarly, using a single measurement of urinary BPA may not accurately reflect long-term exposure, and single measurements of lung function and FeNO do not account for natural variability with these measurements over time and with acute illness.

We found this study noteworthy and informative because it established a link between BPA exposure and decreased lung function (%FEV1/FVC and %FEF25—75), a relationship that strengthens the argument for reducing BPA exposure in our daily lives. The stated association should be investigated further in clinical studies to address the hypothesis posed by the authors that BPA is associated with small airway obstruction. For example, impulse oscillometry may offer better lung function assessment of the small airways. In addition, the measurement of FeNO at different flow rates can dissect fractions from alveolar and bronchial segments of the lung that may produce meaningful differences. Further mechanistic studies are also necessary and may be more informative if multiple pollutants are studied in combination to address the complexity of multiple environmental exposures and the risk of asthma. Overall, this study definitely offers firm footing to launch future studies and advance the field of environmental asthma research.

S. Lovinsky-Desir, MD

R. L. Miller, MD

References

1. Vaidya SV, Kulkarni H. Association of urinary bisphenol A concentration with allergic asthma: results from the National Health and Nutrition Examination Survey 2005–2006. *J Asthma.* 2012;49:800-806.
2. Donohue KM, Miller RL, Perzanowski MS, et al. Prenatal and postnatal bisphenol A exposure and asthma development among inner-city children. *J Allergy Clin Immunol.* 2013;131:736-742.

Predictors and Patterns of Cigarette and Smokeless Tobacco Use Among Adolescents in 32 Countries, 2007–2011
Agaku IT, Ayo-Yusuf OA, Vardavas CI, et al (Harvard School of Public Health, Boston, MA)
J Adolesc Health 54:47-53, 2014

Purpose.—This study compared data from 32 countries to assess predictors and patterns of cigarette and smokeless tobacco (SLT) use among students aged 13–15 years old.

Methods.—Data from the 2007–2008 Global Youth Tobacco Surveys were analyzed for students aged 13–15 years in 31 countries located in all six World Health Organization regions. In addition, the 2011 National Youth Tobacco Survey was analyzed for U.S. students aged 13–15 years. Country specific prevalence of current smoking, current SLT use, and concurrent use patterns were assessed.

Results.—The national prevalence of current cigarette smoking among students aged 13–15 years ranged from 1.8% (Rwanda) to 32.9% (Latvia), whereas current SLT use ranged from 1.1% (Montenegro) to 14.4% (Lesotho). In the U.S. and most European countries surveyed, current smoking prevalence was significantly higher than SLT prevalence, in contrast to patterns observed in low- and middle-income countries. Also, in most of the surveyed countries outside of Europe and the United States, SLT use among girls was as common as their use of cigarettes, and not significantly different from use by boys. When compared with U.S. adolescents, the odds of SLT use were highest among African adolescents (adjusted odds ratio = 3.98; 95% CI: 2.19–7.24) followed by those in the Southeast Asian region (adjusted odds ratio = 2.76; 95% CI: 1.38–5.53).

Conclusions.—Region-specific patterns of tobacco use were noticed. Furthermore, it is alarming that in several low- and middle-income countries, the prevalence of SLT use among females did not differ from that

TABLE 1.—Characteristics of the National Tobacco Surveys Among Adolescents (GYTS-NYTS) in 32 Countries During 2007—2011

Region/Country	Income Category[a]	Survey Year	Total Sample of All Students	Overall Response Rate, %	% of all Students Aged 13—15 Years	% Composition of Girls[b]
African region						
Botswana	Upper-middle income	2008	2,207	96.0	72.8	58.4
Lesotho	Lower- middle income	2008	3,426	83.2	49.8	62.5
Madagascar	Low-income	2008	1,991	83.3	62.0	54.8
Rwanda	Low-income	2008	2,284	91.8	30.2	52.8
Seychelles	Upper-middle income	2007	1,508	86.0	57.0	50.6
South Africa	Upper-middle income	2008	8,602	77.9	46.0	57.7
Togo	Low-income	2007	4,262	89.9	46.9	40.4
Eastern Mediterranean region						
Islamic Republic of Iran	Upper-middle income	2007	1,996	85.9	66.6	47.9
Qatar	High-income	2007	1,434	87.3	68.8	67.0
Tunisia	Upper-middle income	2007	2,155	92.4	70.3	49.9
Yemen	Lower-middle income	2008	1,219	83.5	52.7	37.5
European region						
Croatia	High-income	2007	4,108	90.9	88.0	49.7
Estonia	High-income	2007	3,145	68.2	73.2	50.7
Hungary	Upper-middle income	2008	3,861	81.6	82.9	50.4
Kyrgyzstan	Low-income	2008	4,038	93.2	74.4	52.6
Latvia	High-income	2007	3,362	81.4	73.1	56.6
FYR Macedonia	Upper-middle income	2008	5,824	90.1	73.5	49.1
Republic of Moldova	Lower-middle income	2008	4,703	84.3	75.1	55.6
Montenegro	Upper-middle income	2008	5,723	92.9	58.5	51.9
Serbia	Upper-middle income	2008	4,727	89.4	67.4	54.6
Slovenia	High-income	2007	3,532	80.8	73.3	50.9
Region of the Americas (exclusive of the United States)						
Barbados	High-income	2007	1,499	79.4	74.7	52.8
Belize	Upper-middle income	2008	1,751	93.9	61.1	53.0
Panama	Upper-middle income	2008	3,543	80.0	80.3	52.9
Trinidad and Tobago	High-income	2007	2,841	74.0	69.4	51.0
Southeast Asia						
Myanmar	Low-income	2007	3,118	95.2	69.5	51.2
Sri Lanka	Lower-middle income	2007	1,764	85.0	79.8	49.8
Western Pacific						
Cook Islands	Upper-middle-income	2008	734	91.1	82.6	53.7
Republic of South Korea	High-income	2008	6,046	93.5	87.7	47.2
Mongolia	Lower-middle income	2007	1,831	51.9	77.8	53.4
Philippines	Lower-middle income	2007	5,919	80.9	56.4	55.8
United States of America	High-income	2011	18,866	72.7	45.5	49.4

GYTS = Global Youth Tobacco Survey; NYTS = National Youth Tobacco Survey.
[a]Based on the World Bank's economic groups using countries' 2011 gross national incomes.
[b]Among students aged 13—15 years.

among males, suggesting the possibility of a future shared burden of disease between both males and females.

▶ Worldwide, there has been some overall progress in cigarette smoking rates. An analysis of data from 1980 to 2012 suggests that "large reductions in the estimated prevalence of daily smoking were observed at the global level for both men and women".[1] However, within this overall worldwide trend, there are pediatric-specific patterns that merit concern. This study by Agaku and colleagues, describes trends regarding adolescents in 32 countries in more recent years (2007—2011). They also include trends in smokeless tobacco use as well as cigarette use.

One issue is the difference in tobacco use in low- and middle-income countries (LMIC) compared with developed countries. Country income classification of LMIC was based on the World Bank data on 2011 gross national incomes and groups included high-income (eg, United States, South Korea, Barbados), upper-middle income (eg, Botswana, Panama), lower-middle income (eg, Sri Lanka, Philippines) and low-income countries (eg, Myanmar, Rwanda). The survey included a large sample of adolescent participants and an impressive range of countries (Table 1).

Adolescent tobacco use may differ across countries due to factors such as cost, availability, and cultural norms. Previously, with only a few exceptions, such as northern Thailand, certain areas of India, and Papua New Guinea, cultural norms in the developing world made smoking socially unacceptable for women. Urbanization, as well as aggressive marketing that fuels the perception that smoking is associated with affluence and sophistication, has been associated with increased tobacco use by women.[2]

This study documents that for adolescents who use tobacco products, the use of smokeless tobacco (SLT) is becoming much more common in Africa, Southeast Asia, and the Western Pacific. In Europe and the United States, cigarette smoking is the more commonly used tobacco product. In addition, in several LMIC, Agaku et al note that the frequency of SLT use by adolescent females is similar to the frequency of use by males. The "gender gap" in SLT use by adolescents in the United States is not present in many of these LMIC countries.

These findings have several implications. For clinicians, with the increased use of SLT use in adolescent females, there will be a corresponding increased risk of low-birth-weight infants,[3] heart disease,[4] and caries, as well as oral cancer.[5] The patterns of tobacco use are different worldwide. As a result, in terms of developing policies and strategies to curb pediatric tobacco use, this study suggests that "one size does not fit all." Different policies and strategies to address adolescent tobacco use will need to be tailored to specific countries, cultures, and environments.

In 1968, the Phillip Morris Company launched Virginia Slims, a cigarette brand designed for and marketed to young women. To emphasize the association with modern sophistication and economic progress, the company used the slogan, "You've come a long way, baby."[6] Almost half a century later, this study by Agaku and colleagues documents a new and growing trend in tobacco use by women: the use of SLT, particularly in LMIC. As a result, many of the associated diseases of SLT will be shared equally by young men and women in those countries.

You've come a long way, baby, indeed.

M. D. Cabana, MD, MPH

References

1. Ng M, Freeman MK, Fleming TD, et al. Smoking Prevalence and Cigarette Consumption in 187 Countries, 1980-2012. *JAMA.* 2014;311(2):183-192.
2. Chollat-Traquet C. *Women and Tobacco.* Geneva, Switzerland: World Health Organization; 1992.
3. Ratsch A, Bogossian F. Smokeless tobacco use in pregnancy: an integrative review of the literature. *Int J Public Health.* 2014;59:599-608.
4. Gupta R, Gurm H, Bartholomew JR. Smokeless tobacco and cardiovascular risk. *Arch Intern Med.* 2004;164:1845-1849.
5. Greer RO. Oral manifestations of smokeless tobacco use. *Otolaryngol Clin North Am.* 2011;44:31-56.
6. Weinstein H. *How an Agency Builds a Brand: the Virginia Slims Story.* http://legacy.library.ucsf.edu/tid/efc64e00/pdf. Accessed July 20, 2014.

Exposure to Electronic Cigarette Television Advertisements Among Youth and Young Adults

Duke JC, Lee YO, Kim AE, et al (RTI International, Research Triangle Park, NC; et al)
Pediatrics 134:e29-e36, 2014

Background and Objective.—Currently, the US Food and Drug Administration does not regulate electronic cigarette (e-cigarette) marketing unless it is advertised as a smoking cessation aid. To date, the extent to which youth and young adults are exposed to e-cigarette television advertisements is unknown. The objective of this study was to analyze trends in youth and young adult exposure to e-cigarette television advertisements in the United States.

Methods.—Nielsen data on television household audiences' exposure to e-cigarette advertising across US markets were examined by calendar quarter, year, and sponsor.

Results.—Youth exposure to television e-cigarette advertisements, measured by target rating points, increased 256% from 2011 to 2013. Young adult exposure increased 321% over the same period. More than 76% of all youth e-cigarette advertising exposure occurred on cable networks and was driven primarily by an advertising campaign for 1 e-cigarette brand.

Conclusions.—E-cigarette companies currently advertise their products to a broad audience that includes 24 million youth. The dramatic increase in youth and young adult television exposure between 2011 and 2013 was driven primarily by a large advertising campaign on national cable networks. In the absence of evidence-based public health messaging, the current e-cigarette television advertising may be promoting beliefs and behaviors that pose harm to the public health. If current trends in e-cigarette television advertising continue, awareness and use of e-cigarettes are likely to increase among youth and young adults.

▶ Cigarette advertising on television has been banned since 1971 because of a broad social and political consensus that it was inappropriate to use mass media to push products that caused cancer, heart, and other diseases. After a 40-year hiatus, however, in 2012, aggressive promotion of recreational inhaled nicotine—in the form of e-cigarettes—returned to television.[1] E-cigarette ads contain the same messages and themes cigarette ads used in the heyday of cigarette television advertising: rebellion, sex, stylishness, freedom, and, for kids, looking adult.[1-4] For the 168 million Americans (61% of the entire population) born between 1971 and 2012,[5] e-cigarette ads were their first exposure to what appears to be smoking in television advertising.

Duke et al[1] reported rapidly increasing exposure to e-cigarette advertising on television among US adolescents (ages 12–17 years old) and young adults (ages 18–24 years old) between 2011 and 2013: a 256% increase for adolescents and a 321% increase for young adults. Between October 2012 and September 2013, the total population-level exposure (measured as "total rating points") was intense enough to expose half of all adolescents to 21 e-cigarette advertisements, 10% of all adolescents to 105 advertisements, or 80% of all US adolescents to 13 ads. Young adult exposure was even higher: the advertising was intense enough to expose half of all young adults to 35 e-cigarette television advertisements during the same 11-month period.

These estimates likely underestimate exposure to adolescents and young adults because e-cigarette ads appeared during several programs that were among the top 100 youth-rated programs on television for 2012–2013 (eg, *Big Brother, The Bachelor,* and *Survivor*). The vast majority of television e-cigarette advertising directed at adolescents (81.7%) and young adults (80.4%) in 2013 was for Blu e-cigarettes, which is owned by the Lorillard tobacco company. The majority of e-cigarette advertising is produced by tobacco companies for the e-cigarette brands they own.[1,6]

Rapid increases in e-cigarette use by adolescents and young adults[7,8] have tracked rapid increases in e-cigarette advertising, which is not surprising given that the Surgeon General concluded in 2012 that tobacco advertising and sponsorship causes youth smoking.[9] E-cigarette use doubled among middle and high school students between 2011 and 2012.[7] E-cigarettes are introducing a substantial number of adolescents to nicotine addiction: in 2011, 48% of adolescent e-cigarettes users were nonsmokers. In 2012, this figure had risen to 63%. The 2013 Utah Prevention Needs Assessment (PNA), Utah's largest survey of students in grades 6, 8, 10, and 12, found that nearly one-third of the students who had used e-cigarettes in the past 30 days had never tried a cigarette.[10] The Utah PNA also found that current e-cigarette use among 6th-, 8th-, 10th-, and 12th-graders was 3 times that of adults, suggesting faster market penetration among adolescents than adults.[10]

Dual use of cigarettes and e-cigarettes is high among both adolescents and adults.[8,11-16] Adolescents who use e-cigarettes are less likely to have recently stopped smoking cigarettes.[11,12] Although 1 cross-sectional population study of English adults who had actively tried to quit smoking in the past 12 months found that e-cigarette users were more likely to report not smoking at the time of data collection than participants who purchased nicotine replacement therapy or had not used any smoking cessation aid,[17] a meta-analysis of 5 studies (4 of which were longitudinal) of adult smokers (not exclusively those making an active quit attempt) revealed that e-cigarette users were about one-third less likely to have stopped smoking cigarettes than non-e-cigarette users.[18]

E-cigarette advertising is likely not only contributing to e-cigarette use among adolescents and young adults but, because of the similarities in advertising for e-cigarettes and cigarettes, may be promoting cigarette smoking initiation, relapse, and maintenance.[19,20] E-cigarette advertising often makes unsubstantiated claims about the benefits of e-cigarette use and promotes dual use and e-cigarettes as a way to circumvent smoke-free laws.[4,20]

As of July 2014 there are no restrictions on e-cigarette advertising on television (or anywhere else). In particular, neither the federal Food and Drug Administration (FDA), nor the Federal Trade Commission or Federal Communications Commission, have taken any actions in dealing with the rapidly growing threat to public health that e-cigarette advertising represents. Despite pressure from Democrats in Congress,[2,21] the White House has been dragging its feet on regulating e-cigarettes. In addition, as of June 2014, the Department of Transportation's proposal to prohibit e-cigarettes on airlines, which was issued as a draft in September 2011,[22] still had not been finalized.[23]

The FDA-proposed "deeming" rule in which the agency asserts jurisdiction over e-cigarettes contains no mention of regulating e-cigarette advertising.[24] The proposed deeming rule represents a watered-down version of the FDA's original modest attempt due to the White House Office of Management and Budget's heavy editing, which protects e-cigarette and other tobacco interests.[25] As time continues to pass without an effective federal response to growing and aggressive e-cigarette marketing, more adolescents and young adults are becoming addicted to nicotine. The industry is moving rapidly to create a sustained e-cigarette use pattern reminiscent of cigarette use resulting from intense cigarette marketing on television in the 1950s and 1960s.

L. M. Dutra, ScD

S. A. Glantz, PhD

References

1. Duke JC, Lee YO, Kim AE, et al. Exposure to electronic cigarette television advertisements among youth and young adults. *Pediatrics*. 2014;134:e29-e36.
2. Durbin RJ, Waxman HA, Harkin T, Rockefeller JD IV, et al. Gateway to addiction? A survey of popular electronic cigarette manufacturers and targeted marketing to youth. 2014.
3. Bauld L, Angus K, de Andrade M. *E-Cigarette Uptake and Marketing A Report Commissioned by Public Health England*. London: Public Health England; 2014.
4. Grana R, Ling P. Smoking Revolution? A content analysis of electronic cigarette retail websites. *Am J Prev Med*. 2014;46:395-403.
5. United States Census Bureau. Annual Estimates of the Resident Population for Selected Age Groups by Sex for the United States, States, Counties, and Puerto Rico Commonwealth and Municipios: April 1, 2010 to July 1, 2013 *American FactFinder*

2014. http://factfinder2.census.gov/faces/tableservices/jsf/pages/productview.xhtml? pid=PEP_2013_PEPAGESEX&prodType=table. Accessed July 24, 2014.

6. Kim AE, Arnold KY, Makarenko O. E-cigarette advertising expenditures in the U.S., 2011–2012. *Am J Prev Med.* 2014;46:409-412.

7. Corey C, Wang B, Johnson SE, et al. Electronic cigarette use among middle and high school students- United States, 2011-2012. *MMWR Morb Mortal Wkly Rep.* 2013;62:729-730.

8. King BA, Alam S, Promoff G, Arrazola R, Dube SR. Awareness and ever use of electronic cigarettes among U.S. adults, 2010–2011. *Nicotine Tob Res.* 2013;15: 1623-1627.

9. U.S. Department of Health and Human Services. *The Health Consequences of Smoking—50 Years of Progress: A Report of the Surgeon General.* Atlanta, GA: U.S. Department of Health and Human Services, Centers for Disease Control and Prevention, National Center for Chronic Disease Prevention and Health Promotion, Office on Smoking and Health; 2014.

10. Utah Department of Health. *Utah Health Status Update: Electronic Cigarette Use Among Utah Students (Grades, 8, 10 and 12) and Adults.* Salt Lake City, UT: Utah Department of Public Health; 2013.

11. Dutra LM, Glantz SA. Electronic cigarettes and conventional cigarette use among US adolescents a cross-sectional study. *JAMA Pediatr.* 2014;168:610-617.

12. Lee S, Grana R, Glantz S. Electronic-cigarette use among Korean adolescents: a cross-sectional study of market penetration, dual use, and relationship to quit attempts and former smoking. *J Adolesc Health.* 2014;54:684-690.

13. Pearson JL, Richardson A, Niaura RS, Vallone DM, Abrams DB. e-cigarette awareness, Use, and harm perceptions in US adults. *Am J Public Health.* 2012; 102:1758-1766.

14. McMillen R, Maduka J. Use of emerging tobacco products in the United States. *J Environ Public Health.* 2012;2012:989474.

15. Sutfin EL, McCoy TP, Morrell HE, Hoeppner BB, Wolfson M. Electronic cigarette use by college students. *Drug Alcohol Depend.* 2013;131:214-221.

16. Regan AK, Promoff G, Dube SR, Arrazola R. Electronic nicotine delivery systems: adult use and awareness of the 'e-cigarette' in the USA. *Tob Control.* 2013;22:19-23.

17. Brown J, Beard E, Kotz D, Michie S, West R. Real-world effectiveness of e-cigarettes when used to aid smoking cessation: a cross-sectional population study. *Addiction.* 2014;109:1531-1540.

18. Grana RA, Popova L, Ling PM. A longitudinal analysis of electronic cigarette use and smoking cessation. *JAMA Intern Med.* 2014;174:812-813.

19. Ritchel M. A bolder effort by big tobacco on e-cigarettes. http://www.cnbc.com/ id/101766575. Accessed July 23, 2014.

20. de Andrade M, Hastings G, Angus K. Promotion of electronic cigarettes: tobacco marketing reinvented? *BMJ.* 2013;347:f7473.

21. DeLauro R. Letter to Hamburg II on tobacco regulation. In: MA Hamburg, ed. Washington, DC: 2014; 2.

22. United States Department of Transportation. *DOT Policy on e-Cigarettes.* Washington, DC: Aviation Consumer Protection Division; 2010.

23. Reuters. Senators urge ban on e-cigarettes on airplanes. *Huffington Post.* http:// www.huffingtonpost.com/2014/06/10/senators-e-cigarettes-airplanes_n_5481548. html. Accessed July 29, 2014.

24. Department of Health and Human Services. Deeming tobacco products to be subject to the Federal Food, Drug, and Cosmetic Act, as amended by the Family Smoking Prevention and Tobacco Control Act; regulations on the sale and distribution of tobacco products and required warning statements for tobacco products; proposed rule. In: Administration USFaD, ed. April 25, 2014. Vol 79. No 802014.

25. Clarke T, Begley S. White House weakened draft of FDA's proposed tobacco regulations. *Reuters.* http://www.reuters.com/article/2014/06/25/us-usa-ecigarettes-whitehouse-idUSKBN0F006O20140625. Accessed July 29, 2014.

The impact of electronic cigarettes on the paediatric population
Durmowicz EL (US Food and Drug Administration, Rockville, MD)
Tob Control 23:ii41-ii46, 2014

Objective.—To review the impact of electronic cigarettes (e-cigarettes) on children.

Methods.—Five electronic databases were searched through 31 December 2013. Studies in English that included data for children younger than 18 years of age were included. In addition, relevant data from articles identified during searches of the e-cigarette literature, relevant state survey data and paediatric voluntary adverse event reports submitted to the US Food and Drug Administration (FDA) were reviewed and included.

Results.—Use of e-cigarettes by youth is increasing and is not limited to traditional cigarette smokers. Data regarding the reasons for youth e-cigarette initiation and ongoing use are limited. The effects of e-cigarette marketing and the availability of flavoured e-liquids on youth use are unknown. The abuse liability of e-cigarettes in youth is also not known. Unintentional exposures to e-cigarettes and e-liquids have been reported in children. The number of e-cigarette-related reports received by poison centres is increasing. No data are available on secondhand and thirdhand e-cigarette aerosol exposures in children.

Conclusions.—Data on the impact of e-cigarettes on children are extremely limited. The available data indicate that youth awareness is high and use is increasing rapidly. The extent to which e-cigarette use in youth will result in nicotine dependence and subsequent use of other tobacco products is unknown. e-cigarettes present risks of unintentional nicotine exposure and are potential choking hazards. A greater understanding of the impact of e-cigarettes on children is needed and will be important in the evaluation of the effects of these products on the public health.

▶ The prevalence of electronic cigarette (e-cigarette) use among adolescents is increasing exponentially. In fact, current reports may drastically underestimate actual use because adolescents often use different terms to describe these devices than the researchers conducting the surveys (eg, "hookah pens," "or "vape pipes"). Although the actual number of adolescent e-cigarette users is still well below that of traditional cigarettes, the rapid rise in popularity among teens coupled with the lack of information on their safety is cause for concern.

Using aerosolized nicotine rather than combustion, e-cigarettes likely produce fewer toxins than traditional cigarettes and are even marketed as a safer alternative to traditional cigarettes. Consequently, many researchers and public health officials believe that e-cigarettes may help reduce the risk from tobacco smoking in adult smokers. However, although e-cigarettes may be part of the solution to adult smoking by promoting cessation and/or acting as an agent of harm reduction, there are concerns about use in children.

First, because some e-cigarettes look strikingly similar to traditional cigarettes, there is concern about the "renormalization" of traditional smoking as teens view adults using these products. E-cigarettes that mimic traditional cigarettes may also provide social and behavioral triggers to reinforce use among teen tobacco smokers who are still in the process of developing nicotine dependence. Finally, some e-cigarettes include flavor additives that are believed to promote smoking in children and are consequently banned from traditional cigarettes.

Owing to the availability of youth-friendly flavors (eg, chocolate, grape, and cotton candy) and the widespread marketing of e-cigarettes on the Web and on social media sites, there is growing concern that the manufacturers of these products may actually be encouraging use among youth. Some have also worried that e-cigarettes may be a gateway to traditional cigarette smoking for nonsmoking youth. In fact, use of e-cigarettes among adolescents who have never smoked traditional cigarettes is on the rise.

Despite all of the unknowns, to date there is surprisingly little government oversight or regulation of these products. The US Food and Drug Administration (FDA) has made some proposals to limit the sales of e-cigarettes to those over 18 years of age but has yet to ban the sale of youth-friendly flavorings or marketing as they have done with traditional cigarettes. Consequently, the e-cigarette industry is somewhat of a "Wild West" atmosphere with hundreds of brands, of which many are sold online to anyone claiming to be over 18 years of age. On their website, the FDA acknowledges that "e-cigarettes have not been fully studied," and so the actual quantity of nicotine or other potential toxins inhaled from these products is unknown.[1]

This review is the first article to comprehensively examine the existing data on adolescent e-cigarette use. The researchers included both national and international data (from France, Hungary, Lithuania, Poland, and Korea). This distinction is important given the differences in access to and regulation of e-cigarettes in other countries. This review does an excellent job of summarizing the scant data that is available, providing a well-rounded report of myriad issues related to these largely unregulated products.

One of the strengths of this article is that it illustrates some of the important areas for which there are no available data, helping to define future areas of investigation. The author raises important points that seem to be unique to these products, including the limitations of quantifying use given the lack of standardized dosing of e-cigarettes. For example, should dosing be measured by puffs per day, e-cigarette cartridges consumed per week, or some other methodology? She also raises some issues that may not be on everyone's radar, such as the ability to use these products with marijuana and the risks of nicotine overdose (both for users and small children) given the large amount of nicotine contained in some of the refill cartridges. Because the search was limited to English-language articles only, it is likely that the international data on e-cigarette use was underrepresented.

E-cigarettes are becoming more popular among youth. There are many unanswered questions regarding their safety for both the user and those around them, potential addictiveness, and the possibility that they may be a gateway to traditional cigarettes for adolescent nonsmokers. More research needs to be conducted to answer many of these questions, and this review article provides a jumping-off point for these important efforts.

M. L. Rubinstein, MD

Adolescent dosing and labeling since the Food and Drug Administration Amendments Act of 2007
Momper JD, Mulugeta Y, Green DJ, et al (US Food and Drug Administration, Silver Spring, MD; et al)
JAMA Pediatr 167:926-932, 2013

Importance.—During pediatric drug development, dedicated pharmacokinetic studies are generally performed in all relevant age groups to support dose selection for subsequent efficacy trials. To our knowledge, no previous assessments regarding the need for an intensive pharmacokinetic study in adolescents have been performed.

Objectives.—To compare U.S. Food and Drug Administration (FDA)-approved adult and adolescent drug dosing and to assess the utility of allometric scaling for the prediction of drug clearance in the adolescent population.

Design.—Adult and adolescent dosing and drug clearance data were obtained from FDA-approved drug labels and publicly available databases containing reviews of pediatric trials submitted to the FDA. Dosing information was compared for products with concordant indications for adolescent and adult patients. Adolescent drug clearance was predicted from adult pharmacokinetic data by using allometric scaling and compared with observed values.

Main Outcomes and Measures.—Adolescent and adult dosing information and drug clearance.

Results.—There were 126 unique products with pediatric studies submitted to the FDA since the FDA Amendments Act of 2007, of which 92 had at least 1 adolescent indication concordant with an adult indication. Of these 92 products, 87 (94.5%) have equivalent dosing for adults and adolescent patients. For 18 of these 92 products, a minimum weight or body surface area threshold is recommended for adolescents to receive adult dosing. Allometric scaling predicted adolescent drug clearance with an overall mean absolute percentage error of 17.0%.

Conclusions and Relevance.—Approved adult and adolescent drug dosing is equivalent for 94.5% of products with an adolescent indication studied since the FDA Amendments Act of 2007. Allometric scaling may be a useful tool to avoid unnecessary dedicated pharmacokinetic studies in the adolescent population during pediatric drug development, although each development program in adolescents requires a full discussion of drug dosing with the FDA.

▶ Historically, children have represented an understudied, "orphan" population in the field of pharmacotherapy. To help guide drug prescribing, the US Food and

Drug Administration (FDA) drug "label" (or "package insert") provides information on what a drug is used for, who should take it, known side effects, instructions for use (including dosing), and safety information. However, for the majority of drugs used in children, pediatric-specific information in the drug "label" is lacking. Therefore, health care providers for children have been left to routinely use drugs "off-label."[1] The evidence to support the safe and efficacious use of a drug in children is lacking compared with that available for adults.

Recognizing this gap in pediatric pharmacotherapy, a series of policies over the past 2 decades have been enacted by the federal government and implemented by the FDA under the current umbrella of laws known as the Best Pharmaceuticals for Children Act (BPCA) and the Pediatric Research Equity Act (PREA). BPCA and PREA provide incentives and requirements to the pharmaceutical industry for conducting pediatric drug trials. Together, they have led to more than 500 drug "label" revisions adding pediatric specific information,[2] and this new pediatric information to the drug "label" should be considered a significant development in the care of children. The information and data provided by the studies conducted under BPCA and PREA can also provide additional opportunities to advance our general understanding of pediatric pharmacotherapy and help improve the design and conduct of future drug studies.

Fundamental to the safe and efficacious use of a drug is an understanding of its pharmacokinetics. This understanding is critical in the selection of an appropriate dose to achieve the desired exposure across patient populations. Accordingly, during drug development, substantial time, effort, and money are invested in conducting pharmacokinetics studies in children. Minimizing the number of children needed to adequately define the pharmacokinetics of a drug is an ethical imperative.

As health care providers for children, we all follow the tenet, "Children are not little adults," but from a pharmacokinetic perspective, adolescents and adults may be similar enough. Most major drug clearance pathways have matured by adolescence. Therefore, adult pharmacokinetic data may provide significant a priori information for adolescents. The report by Momper et al used data from 92 products approved in both adults and adolescents under BPCA and PREA to examine whether drug dose needs are similar in adults and adolescents. In addition, they explored whether drug clearance in an adult can be used to predict the clearance in adolescents using allometric scaling (ie, adjusting clearance only based on the size of the patient). Interestingly, they found that 95% of products had the same "labeled" dose in adults and adolescents. Allometric scaling predicted adolescent clearance within 25% of the observed value for 21 of 27 (78%) drugs. This study demonstrates that for many drugs, the impact of adolescence on drug pharmacokinetics is minimal and is likely not clinically relevant after scaling for size, and drug dose selection during drug development can be guided from adult data. Such understanding could be applied to reduce the number of adolescent patients necessary for enrollment in pharmacokinetic trials, allowing for more efficient progression to Phase II/III trials and establishment of efficacy.

Of course, caution is warranted and a drug's specific clearance pathway must be considered when assessing the appropriateness of scaling from adults. For example, have previous drugs that used the same elimination pathway been successfully predicted from adult data? Is there anything that makes this drug different or unique? In addition, our understanding on the impact of a child's growth and development on the action and response to drugs (including side effects) is grossly inadequate, and simply matching exposure of a drug to adults may be a framework for therapeutic misadventure. A deeper understanding on the pharmacodynamics of drugs including long-term safety and effectiveness is critically needed in children.[3] Hopefully, further advancements will continue with the passing of the FDA Safety and Innovation Act in 2012, which makes permanent BPCA and PREA and solidifies the importance of pediatric pharmacotherapy in the future of drug development.

A. Frymoyer, MD

References

1. Bazzano ATF, Mangione-Smith R, Schonlau M, Suttorp MJ, Brook RH. Off-label prescribing to children in the United States outpatient setting. *Acad Pediatr.* 2009; 9(2):81-88.
2. New Pediatric Labeling Information Database. http://www.accessdata.fda.gov/scripts/sda/sdNavigation.cfm?sd=labelingdatabase. Accessed July 15, 2014.
3. IOM (Institute of Medicine). *Safe and Effective Medicines for Children: Pediatric Studies Conducted Under the Best Pharmaceuticals for Children Act and the Pediatric Research Equity Act.* Washington, DC: The National Academies Press; 2012.

Article Index

Chapter 1: Adolescent Medicine

Chapter 2: Allergy and Dermatology

Chapter 3: Blood

Chapter 8: Genitourinary Tract

Chapter 9: Heart and Blood Vessels

Chapter 10: Infectious Diseases and Immunology

Chapter 11: Miscellaneous

Chapter 12: Musculoskeletal

Chapter 13: Neurology Psychiatry

Chapter 14: Newborn

Chapter 15: Nutrition and Metabolism

Chapter 16: Oncology

Chapter 17: Ophthalmology

Chapter 18: Respiratory Tract

Chapter 19: Therapeutics and Toxicology

Author Index